ANNUAL PROGRESS IN
CHILD PSYCHIATRY AND
CHILD DEVELOPMENT
1997

ANNUAL PROGRESS IN CHILD PSYCHIATRY AND CHILD DEVELOPMENT 1997

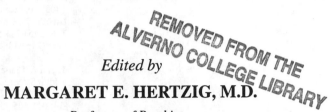

Edited by

MARGARET E. HERTZIG, M.D.

Professor of Psychiatry
Cornell University Medical College

and

ELLEN A. FARBER, Ph.D.

Assistant Professor of Psychology in Psychiatry
Cornell University Medical College

BRUNNER/MAZEL
Taylor & Francis Group

USA	Publishing Office:	BRUNNER/MAZEL *A Member of the Taylor & Francis Group* 325 Chestnut Street Suite 800 Philadelphia, PA 19106 Tel: (215) 625-8900 Fax: (215) 625-2940
	Distribution Center:	BRUNNER/MAZEL *A Member of the Taylor & Francis Group* 1900 Frost Road, Suite 101 Bristol, PA 19007-1598 Tel: (215) 785-5800 Fax: (215) 785-5515
UK		Taylor & Francis Ltd. 4 John Street London WC1N 2ET Tel: 071 405 2237 Fax: 071 831 2035

ANNUAL PROGRESS IN CHILD PSYCHIATRY AND CHILD DEVELOPMENT 1997

1 2 3 4 5 6 7 8 9 0

Printed by Braun-Brumfield, Ann Arbor, MI.

A CIP catalog record for this book is available from the British Library.
⊗ The paper in this publication meets the requirements of the ANSI Standard Z39.48-1984 (Permanence of Paper)

ISBN 0-87630-870-1

CONTENTS

Part I

DEVELOPMENTAL ISSUES

In the first of the five papers in this section, Dahl presents an extensive review of the literature on sleep. Dahl's goal is to present a model linking sleep and arousal regulation to developmental psychopathology. The review includes a description of the restorative function of sleep, the ways in which sleep is a part of the arousal system, normative sleep–wake cycles, the association of sleep and affect, and the effects of sleep deprivation. He uses clinical vignettes to illustrate the links between sleep, depression, and behavior problems. Dahl raises an important issue: the need to differentiate between depression, which results in sleep problems, and erratic sleep habits, which can lead to behavior and mood problems, and he presents studies of EEG sleep measures in depressed children.

In the second half of the paper, Dahl proposes a model in which the prefrontal cortex is the primary regulatory system responsible for the interface of sleep, affect, and attention. He acknowledges that his model is not able to fully address a question that he finds of primary interest: "Why is sleep so important during early brain development?" Overall, this paper presents much information and intriguing ideas about an important but often overlooked topic.

In the second paper in this section, Belsky et al. describe a study of temperament. Temperament is one of the major constructs in development. Although controversy remains about the dimensions of temperament, such as whether to include activity level and sociability, the measurement of emotional tone tends to be central to all proposed definitions. In fact, much of the interest in temperament has focused on negative emotionality and its effects on parenting. As Belsky and his colleagues point out, the failure to account for the child's degree of positive emotionality is a limitation of many studies and may explain inconsistent findings across studies.

In this paper, Belsky et al. examine the notion that positive and negative emotionality are two dimensions, not a single bipolar construct. A sample of 122 boys between ages 12 months and 20 months was studied. Parental reports and laboratory observations of temperament were obtained. In a series of sophisticated analyses, the authors demonstrate that a two-dimensional model fit the data better than a single construct model. Children who were high in negative emotionality were not necessarily low in positive emotionality, and vice versa. Consistent with other studies, parental reports of temperament were considered unreliable. This is a carefully conducted study with an interesting discussion of the two-dimensional model of emotionality.

The next three papers complement one another. The first two are reviews and the last is an empirical study, all of social development. Judy Dunn has conducted numerous studies of peer, parent, and sibling relationships. In her paper, an invited lecture, she pulls together much of the recent literature to demonstrate the interplay between cognitive and social development. She contends that new cognitive research, such as theory of mind studies, is important for researchers trying to understand social development and, vice versa, that cognitive researchers need to understand children's social interactions and relationships. In one example of the cognitive–social interplay, Dunn highlights how naturalistic studies have been critical to understanding children's early cognitive capacities for mind reading. She notes that laboratory theory-of-mind studies using hypothetical situations reveal understanding of family and peer relationships at later ages than occurs in the natural environment. Some of the social interaction research that can unearth mind-reading (cognitive) abilities has included studies of teasing, jokes, sharing a pretend world in play, comforting, and deception. All of these "skills" involve understanding another's point of view. Dunn goes on to describe the social processes—such as joint pretend play, arguments, and conversations about the social world and inner states—that enhance emotional understanding. She also discusses the role of various social partners. Of note, children do not demonstrate the same level of understanding across partners (parents, siblings, and friends).

The next paper by Hartup is an excellent, highly readable summary of the developmental significance of friendship. As Hartup points out, more is known about the importance of acceptance–rejection by peers than about friendships. The sociometric literature is much larger than the literature on friendships. He contends that researchers need to distinguish between (a) having friends, (b) the identity (personality) of the child's friends, and (c) friendship quality. He describes how "having friends" is measured, including dichotomous (friend v. nonfriend) and continuous (best friend, good friend, etc.) variables. He describes some interesting studies of the significance of friends, including the higher quality of collaborative school work completed by friends compared with nonfriends. He concludes that there is no clear picture of the developmental significance of having friends.

In studying the second topic, the identity of children's friends, investigators have found that children are similar to their friends in attributes with "reputational salience" such as prosocial behavior, antisocial behavior, and shyness. The third topic discussed is friendship quality. Friendship quality has been assessed in two main ways. Dimensional analysis looks at features of the relationship, such as intimacy, companionship, and conflict. The typological analysis examines patterns of social interactions among friends.

In the next paper, Crick and Grotpeter present some of their research on victimization. There have been many reports describing the characteristics of bullies, but little is known about the victims of peer aggression. The authors attempt to remedy this by differentiating the types of aggression that occur among peers and the characteristics of the victims.

The study presents a large sample of third- through sixth-grade children drawn from four schools. The measures include the Social Experiences Questionnaire, a 15-item self-report measure designed for this study. It has three subscales: Relational Victimization, Overt Victimization, and Receipt of Prosocial Acts. Overt victimization includes hitting, name calling, and verbal threats. Relational aggression is defined as harming others through manipulation of or damage to their peer relationships, such as spreading rumors. Other measures include self-reports of loneliness, depression, and social anxiety. Peer sociometric nominations were used to assign children to status groups: popular, average, neglected, rejected, and controversial.

Victims were defined as falling 1 standard deviation above the sample mean on the victimization scales. Sixty-three percent of the students experienced either relational victimization or overt victimization, but not both. Boys were more likely to be the victims of overt aggression, but both boys and girls experienced relational aggression.

Rejected children were more likely to be the recipients of both types of victimization than were children in the other status groups. Popular children received more prosocial acts than rejected children. This is an interesting line of research that contributes to the understanding of peer socialization.

1

The Regulation of Sleep and Arousal: Development and Psychopathology

Ronald E. Dahl

Western Psychiatric Institute & Clinic, University of Pittsburgh School of Medicine, Department of Psychiatry

Throughout early development, a child spends more time asleep than in any waking activity. Yet, the specific role of sleep in brain maturation is a complete mystery. In this article, the developmental psychobiology of sleep regulation is conceptualized within the context of close links to the control of arousal, affect, and attention. The interactions among these systems are considered from an ontogenetic and evolutionary biological perspective. A model is proposed for the development of sleep and arousal regulation with the following major tenets:

1. *Sleep and vigilance represent opponent processes in a larger system of arousal regulation.*

2. *The regulation of sleep, arousal, affect, and attention overlap in physiological, neuroanatomical, clinical, and developmental domains.*

3. *Complex interactions among these regulatory systems are modulated and integrated in regions of the prefrontal cortex (PFC).*

4. *Changes at the level of PFC underlie maturational shifts in the relative balance across these regulatory systems (such as decreases in the depth/length of sleep and increased capacity for vigilance and attention), which occur with normal development.*

5. *The effects of sleep deprivation (including alterations in attention, emotions, and goal-directed behaviors) also involve changes at the level of PFC integration across regulatory systems.*

This model is then discussed in the context of developmental pathology in the control of affect and attention, with an emphasis on sleep changes in depression.

Reprinted with permission from *Development and Psychopathology*, 1996, Vol. 8, 3–27. Copyright © 1996 by the Cambridge University Press.

The author gratefully acknowledges support from NIH# 41712 and NIH# 46510. The author also thanks Dan Buysee and Dante Cicchetti for many helpful suggestions in the writing and editing of this paper.

At first glance, sleep regulation may not appear to be a very promising conceptual framework for investigating development and psychopathology. There is a tendency from common experience to regard sleep as a period when the most interesting processes of brain and behavior are, in effect, shut down. The lack of overt behaviors during sleep often leads to an impression that sleep regulation has little connection to the control of attention, arousal, emotions, and behavior—the domains of focus for much research in development and psychopathology. However, when one looks more deeply at the regulation of sleep, particularly from a developmental perspective, it becomes readily apparent that sleep occupies a relatively central role in early maturational processes.

In fact, it can be argued that sleep is the *primary* activity of the brain during the early years of development. By age 2 years, the average child has spent almost 10,000 hr (nearly 14 months) asleep and approximately 7,500 hr (about 10 months) in waking activities (Anders, Sadeh, & Appareddy, 1995). In these 2 years, the brain has reached 90% of adult size (Chugani, Phelps, & Mazziota, 1987), and the child has attained remarkable complexity in areas such as cognitive skills, language, concept of self, socio-emotional development, and physical skills (Cicchetti & Beeghly, 1990; Kagan, 1987). Yet, for the majority of the interval during which these maturational advances have occurred, the brain has been in a state of sleep. During the next 3 years (ages 2–5), there will be approximately an even balance between sleep and wakefulness. Thus, by early school age a child has spent more time asleep than in social interactions, exploring the environment, eating, or any other single waking activity. Why has evolution favored the predominance of sleep in development? Why would it not have been more advantageous to permit more waking time to acquire knowledge, language, and experiences, to practice motor skills, and to refine social and cognitive abilities—*unless sleep itself directly serves some fundamental role in brain development?* To address these questions requires that one move beyond the concept that sleep is simply a period of rest or inactivity. Merely relaxing the mind and body is insufficient to create the restorative state of sleep. For example, if one is permitted to lie quietly, physically relaxed, with eyes closed and no tasks or activities for the entire night, but not permitted to fall asleep, the replenished feeling of having slept will not occur. On a behavioral level, *the essence of sleep (in contrast to rest) is a categorical diminution of awareness and responsiveness to the external environment.* During the deepest non-rapid eye movement (non-REM) sleep (stages 3 and 4), there is nearly complete loss of awareness, and virtual inability to respond rapidly to stimuli in the external environment (Busby & Pivik, 1983). Why does the brain—particularly the developing brain—require long intervals of relative unresponsiveness? This is even more puzzling when one considers the evolutionary perspective including the adaptational pressures in the human ancestral environment. For example, early hominids living in an open savanna region were surrounded by large nocturnal-hunting carnivores and minimal access to safe sleeping sites (Brain, 1981). Why then would the human brain have evolved a regulatory system that shuts down awareness and responsiveness for most of the night? A strong argument can be made that sleep must serve some essential aspect of brain function or it would not have been conserved across such conditions.

SLEEP AND AROUSAL

In many ways, it is useful to conceptualize sleep as the nadir in a larger cycle of arousal regulation. That is, sleep and arousal[1] represent closely linked, opponent processes. Sleep is incompatible with a state of high responsiveness (vigilance), while a high arousal state precludes the ability to sleep. On a

---

[1] Arousal is not a consistently defined construct in cognitive neuroscience or physiological psychology. Some elements of arousal overlap with broad constructs such as emotional state and attentional processes. The term is used here to denote the state of awareness and responsiveness to the external environment.

daily basis, the brain regularly cycles through patterns of higher and lower arousal states influenced by both the circadian system and the sleep/wake system. On a moment-to-moment basis, however, arousal state is strongly influenced by emotional state, vigilance, and attentional processes (Lang, 1995; LeDoux, 1989; Posner & Petersen, 1990). Short-term surges of arousal occur in response to threat, demand, effort, of emotionally salient experiences. These short-term changes in arousal that are closely linked with affect and attention are of great interest to most investigators studying development and psychopathology.

In some ways, however, to investigate the regulation of arousal, affect, and attention without addressing sleep, is a bit like a respiratory physiologist examining changes in inhalation without considering exhalation. To extend this analogy another step, an asthma attack appears clinically as distress from an inability to take in sufficient air; however, the primary pathophysiology is actually trouble getting air *out* of the lungs. The point is that the mechanisms underlying pathology in the control of arousal, affect, and attention may be most evident when one considers the full cycle of sleep and arousal regulation.

Sleep and Vigilance

An important conceptual framework for these opponent processes of sleep and arousal comes from further considering the perspective of evolutionary biology and the relation of arousal to vigilance. Because sleep represents a period of turning off awareness and responsiveness, it is adaptive for sleep to be restricted to times and places relatively safe from predators or other dangers. Within species, sleep often occurs in the context of nests, burrows, or other safe sites, and sleep onset is linked to behaviors that favor the selection of safe locations. For an individual, at any one moment, the brain must choose a state of relative vigilance versus sleep, as the two states are mutually exclusive. The pendulum of arousal moving between sleep and vigilance is largely influenced by a relative sense of safety versus threat. Any perception of threat in the environment will raise arousal and inhibit sleep. Most threatening or negative affective experiences are also associated with increased arousal (Lang, 1995). Thus, short-term demands for vigilance, or attention, and acute surges of arousal secondary to emotions, involve increased arousal, which pulls the system in the opposite direction from sleep. Over a longer temporal frame, however, the brain has fundamental requirements for periods of sleep (low-arousal and unresponsive states). Although sleep needs can be transiently put off to meet the needs for vigilance or attention, research has demonstrated that the drive for sleep becomes extremely powerful over extended periods of wakefulness (Anders & Roffwarg, 1973; Bonnet, 1994) and longterm sleep loss is incompatible with life (Rechtshaffen, Bergman, Everson, Kushida, & Gilliland, 1989). Thus, sleep, arousal, affect, and attention are closely intertwined in a dynamic regulatory system. Aspects of the system that increase arousal dominate in short time frames permitting the individual to accommodate acute threats, affective responses, and demands for attention. Over longer intervals, however, the sleep and circadian systems must predominate to achieve a balance regarding alternative physiologic requirements.

Early in development, the balance in this system is heavily skewed toward sleep. In infancy, demands for vigilance and attention are relatively low, because safety and other needs are largely conferred by caretakers. As maturation occurs, however, periods of wakefulness become longer, and the needs for attention and vigilance become more sustained and complex. These increasing requirements for arousal repeatedly "stretch" the sleep/arousal loops further in the dimension toward higher and more sustained arousal. The dynamics within sleep reflect, to some degree, the "release" of the preceding "stretch" during wakefulness. For example, power in delta electroen-cephalogram (EEG) frequency during non-REM sleep is largely determined by the length of wakefulness preceding sleep (Dijk, Brunner, & Borbely, 1991; Borbely & Wirz-Justice, 1982).

The premise of this article is that considering the full cycle (the upward extension of arousal to meet increased demands for vigilance and attention and the subsequent release into low-arousal, sleep states) may provide a more complete picture of the development of these regulatory systems. In a similar manner, developmental investigations of *dysregulation* of affect and attention may benefit from a conceptual framework that includes this broad view of sleep and arousal regulation. For example, one critical question relevant to affective dysregulation concerns the issue of sensitive periods of development. What is the influence of repetitively stressful or threatening experiences that distort this sleep/arousal loop in the direction of chronic high arousal during early development—during maturational periods when the relationships among these regulatory systems are being established? Could such experiences during sensitive periods of development alter sleep and affective regulation over long intervals of time?

NORMATIVE SLEEP

Prior to considering the interactions between sleep regulation and the control of affect and attention, it may be helpful to briefly review the physiology, stages, and normal development of sleep. Sleep stages are defined by three electrophysiologic measures; the EEG, the electromyogram (EMG), and the electroocculogram (EOG). The patterning of these measures (EEG, muscle tone, and eye movements) divides state into three broad categories: awake, REM sleep, and non-REM sleep. A brief overview of REM and non-REM physiology reveals a number of contrasts.

REM sleep is also called paradoxical sleep because it has aspects of both deep sleep and light sleep. The body and brain-stem show dramatic sleep-related changes during REM with a huge drop in muscle tone and altered subcortical and autonomic functions, such as increased variability in the control of heart rate, blood pressure, respiration, and temperature (Parmeggiani, 1994). Cortical areas during REM show activity levels similar to waking states; however, this cortical activity is not connected to the same inputs and outputs. For example, motor cortex activity does not create body movements during REM (Chase & Morales, 1990), and cognitive activity (dreaming) is not largely influenced by sensory input regarding the external environment. When a person is awakened from REM sleep, alertness returns relatively briskly. REM periods occur in cycles of approximately 60–90 min throughout the night, with the longest and most intense REM periods occurring just after the body temperature reaches a minimum (around 5 a.m. in an individual on a normal sleep/wake schedule).

Non-REM sleep is further subdivided into stages 1, 2, 3, and 4. Stages 3 and 4 are also called delta or slow-wave sleep and represent the deepest sleep in humans. The length of this deep delta sleep increases in proportion to how long one has been awake and further increases (and become even deeper) following sleep loss or chronic sleep disturbances (as a deep "recovery" sleep). Age also has large effects on slow-wave sleep. Children have extremely large amounts of deep slow-wave sleep. Delta sleep levels peak between 3 and 6 years of age (usually at the point when children give up daytime naps), and subsequently decrease across school age, adolescence, and throughout adulthood (many older adults have no delta sleep at all). During this deep sleep (usually 1 to 3 h after going to sleep) it is extremely difficult to arouse children, and if aroused, they often appear disoriented, confused, and are cognitively slow. Confused partial arousals (including sleep walking and night terrors) usually emerge from this state.

Figure 1 shows the typical pattern and cycling of these sleep stages in a 10-year-old child. Stages 1, 2, 3, and 4 are shown as progressively lower steps on the vertical axis with REM sleep indicated by striped boxes at an intermediate level (indicating the paradoxical relationship to sleep depth). This child (sleep pattern illustrated in Fig. 1) fell briefly into stage 1, descended to stage 2, and then to stages 3 and 4 where she remained for approximately 1 hr. Just before midnight, sleep returned to stage 2 with a 30-s arousal, followed by another hour of deep stage 3 and 4. The first REM period occurred

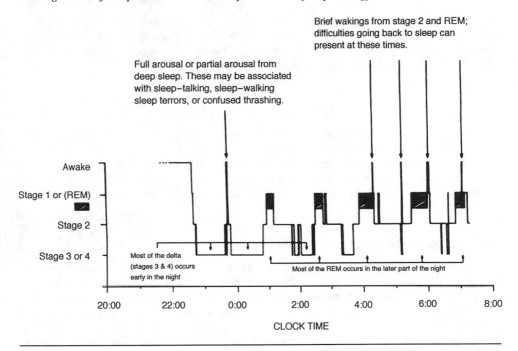

Figure 1. Sleep pattern in an early school-age child.

about 1:00 a.m. with further REM sleep periods approximately every 60 to 90 min throughout the night (with longer REM sleep periods toward early morning).

As illustrated, most of the slow-wave sleep occurs in the first 1 to 3 hr after sleep onset. Thus, most slow-wave-related disorders such as sleep terrors, sleepwalking, and partial arousals occur at this time of the night. The majority of REM sleep occurs in the second half of the night. Thus, REM-related disorders such as nightmares are more frequent in the early morning hours. Short periods of wakefulness typically occur five to seven times a night from normal sleep. Most individuals, however, quickly return to sleep after a brief adjustment in position, covers, pillows, and so forth, with no memory of the awakening.

Age-related (developmental) processes exert profound influences on sleep regulation. Total sleep decreases from 16 to 17 hr per day in the newborn period to approximately 8 hr per night by age 18 years. At age 1 year, the average child sleeps approximately 13.5 hr per 24 hr (typically 11 hr per night with another 2.5 hr of sleep obtained in two separate daytime naps). By age 3 years, the average child gets 10.5 hr of sleep each night with one 1.5-hr nap. In the United States, a typical child ceases daytime naps at about 4 to 5 years of age. It is also important to emphasize that there is considerable individual variation in sleep requirements as well as cultural influences on sleep and napping behavior (for example, daytime naps continue through adulthood in some cultures).

Maturational changes also influence sleep architecture and stage distribution. There is a small decrease in the amount of REM sleep and a significant drop-off in (stages 3 and 4) delta sleep, particularly during adolescence. Changes in sleep regulation during adolescence are complex. Adolescents demonstrate greater daytime sleepiness that is not simply a result of inadequate sleep, because this occurs in adolescents even if they obtain as much sleep as they did prior to puberty (Carskadon et al., 1980). Despite this apparent increased physiologic need for sleep near puberty, there is substantial evidence that many adolescents frequently get significantly *less* sleep than prepubertal children. A number of studies indicate that during high school ages, a substantial number of adolescents appear chronically sleep deprived and often demonstrate a wide range of daytime symptoms of inadequate sleep including fatigue, irritability, emotional lability, difficulty concentrating, and falling asleep in class (Carskadon et al., 1989; Carskadon & Mancuso, 1987, 1988).

SLEEP, AFFECT, AND ATTENTION

A strong empiric case can be made linking the regulation of these systems along at least three lines of evidence: (a) emotional disturbances frequently result in changes in sleep regulation, (b) disrupted or insufficient sleep can cause changes in the control of affect and attention; and (c) the neurobiology underlying the regulation of sleep overlaps to a large extent with neurobehavioral systems involved in the regulation of arousal, attention, and emotions. Each of these points and related evidence will be discussed briefly.

Emotional Disturbances Alter Sleep Regulation

The close relationship between emotional and sleep regulation is evident in both clinical and nonclinical populations. For most people, an experience of emotional distress—trauma, separation, personal loss, anxiety-provoking events, etc.—is associated with at least transient disruptions in sleep (Cartwright & Wood, 1991; Hall, Dahl, Dew, & Reynolds, in press). This association is so strong in common experience that most individuals experiencing insomnia are asked by friends and family: "Is something bothering you or distressing you that you can't sleep?" The most common questions by parents of children with sleep difficulties are: "Are you afraid of something? Are you upset about something that happened?" The focus of all these questions is the common experience that emotional distress underlies most transient sleep disturbances. However, even positive emotional arousal can interfere with sleep. The early stages of an intense romantic relationship or the anticipation of an exciting event such as a trip, a sporting event, or presents under the Christmas tree are also often associated with disrupted sleep.

This general link between emotional regulation and sleep regulation is even more apparent in the domain of clinical disorders of affect regulation. Disturbed sleep is so characteristic of affective disorders as to represent a major diagnostic symptom. Although the specific type and degree of sleep alteration varies across disorders, some change in sleep regulation is prominent in both unipolar and bipolar affective disorders across the lifespan (depressed children, adolescents, and throughout adulthood). Among depressed children and adolescents, 75% complain of insomnia, and 25% have symptoms of hypersomnia during the episode of depression (Ryan et al., 1987). As will be discussed later, the EEG evidence of sleep changes appear to be more subtle in young depressed subjects (Dahl et al., 1991b; Dahl & Ryan, in press); however, *subjective* changes in sleep are as prominent in early onset depression as in adult depression (Ryan et al., 1987). There are also data to suggest that sleep difficulties may predispose to the development of depression (Ford & Kammerow, 1989).

Nonetheless, sleep changes are not specific to depression. Most types of psychopathology with affective changes are also associated with altered sleep, including anxiety disorders (Mellman & Uhde, 1989), post-traumatic stress disorder (Ross, Ball, Sullivan, & Carroff, 1989), obsessive–compulsive disorder (Insel, Gillin, & Moore, 1989), schizophrenia (Zarcone & Benson, 1994), eating disorders (Benca & Casper, 1994), alcohol and substance abuse (Gillin, 1994), and Tourette's syndrome (Glaze, Frost, & Jankovic, 1983). Although the *specificity* of sleep changes with psychopathology are extensively debated, there seems little doubt that disorders of emotional regulation are strongly associated with changes in sleep.

Sleep Influences the Regulation of Emotions and Arousal

A similar relationship can be shown in the opposite direction as well. Inadequate sleep (whether from insufficient amounts of sleep or repeatedly disrupted sleep) results in alterations in affect and attention. Typically, inadequate sleep results in mood deterioration decreased arousal, difficulties with focused attention, and "tiredness." Tiredness includes at least two separate components following sleep loss: (a) "sleepiness," which is literally difficulty maintaining wakeful alertness and (b) a change in cognitive/emotional state resulting in *feeling* tired, which typically manifests as decreased motivation for tasks and goals. Irritability and a decreased threshold for anger and frustration are also often associated with sleep deprivation. However, it is often difficult to separate the mood/arousal changes from cognitive and physical symptoms secondary to sleep deprivation. (These issues and related literature will be addressed further in the next section in the context of sleep and depression.) From a developmental perspective, there are very few data on sleep deprivation in normal children. However, clinical observations are strongly supportive of the same general pattern of effects from inadequate or disrupted sleep. Whether as a result of sleep-disordered breathing (Guilleminault, Winkle, & Korobkin, 1982), late or erratic bedtimes (Dahl, Pelham, & Wierson, 1991a), medical illness (Dahl et al., 1995), or volitional sleep restriction, inadequate sleep results in increased irritability, lowered threshold for negative emotional responses, and less control of attention. Numerous authors have commented on the parallels between sleep deprivation effects in children and attention-deficit hyperactivity disorder (ADHD) symptoms (Dahl et al., 1991b; Guilleminault et al., 1982; Navelet, Anders, & Guilleminault, 1976; Picchetti & Walters, 1994). The observation that stimulant medication may improve some of these symptoms in sleep-deprived children should not be surprising since the majority of adults throughout the world use stimulants—usually coffee or tea—to help with symptoms of insufficient sleep, resulting in improved control of attention and mood.

Another clinical example of the strong link between sleep and emotional regulation in children and adolescents is observed in early onset narcolepsy. Narcolepsy syndrome is a neurologic disorder primarily affecting the ability to gate REM sleep with a frequent onset at or near puberty. Children and adolescents with narcolepsy demonstrate high comorbidity with behavioral and emotional disturbances (Dahl, Holttum, & Trubnick, 1994). In a number of cases, narcoleptic children have been misdiagnosed as having psychiatric disorders, including depression and ADHD.

These observations of extensive overlap between sleep disturbances and affective regulation do not indicate any specific cause and effect relationships between sleep changes and psychopathology. The point here is not to advocate a specific hypothesis concerning causal relationships, but primarily to emphasize the close interconnections among these systems in both nonclinical and patient samples. There are at least four alternative possibilities: (a) affective changes secondary to sleep disturbances may simply mimic or resemble psychopathologic changes through independent mechanisms; (b) sleep deprivation or disturbances may simply exacerbate pre-existing difficulties with the control of affect and/or attention; (c) sleep disturbances may contribute to the development of affective or attentional pathologies only in a subset of children with underlying vulnerabilities in these regulatory systems; and (d) the sleep disturbances may be secondary to underlying pathology in the control of arousal-related systems.

The Psychobiology of Sleep, Arousal, and Attention

The third line of evidence to link the regulation of sleep, affect, and attention comes from neurobiology. The neurobehavioral systems involved in the regulation of sleep overlap with, and are closely linked to, neural systems involved in the regulation of affect and attention. A broad description of neurobiologic structures underlying these regulatory systems is beyond the scope of the paper. For reviews of the neurobiologic basis of sleep regulation (see Chase, 1994; Jones, 1994; Siegel, 1994;

Steriade, Contreras, & Amzica, 1994). The primary tenets of this work relevant to this article include:

1. The brain regions and pathways critical for wakefulness, slow-wave sleep, REM sleep, and the cycling between states, involve complex interplay among multiple cortical and subcortical systems.

2. The synchronized EEG waves of quiet non-REM sleep, including spindles and delta waves, are closely linked to thalamocortical neural systems (Steriade et al., 1994). In addition, the thalamus appears to be the site of the blockade of synaptic transmission (during non-REM sleep) a sensory information to the cerebral cortex. Thus, this sensory information never reaches a level of cortical processing or behavioral response during deep non-REM sleep.

3. The generation of REM sleep is largely influenced by brainstem mechanisms in the pontine and medullary regions inter-acting with other brain regions (particularly areas of the forebrain) (Chase & Morales, 1994; Siegel, 1994). Additionally virtually all motor output to voluntary muscles is blocked at the level of the pons. Thus, for example, cortical signals to move the body during dream states do not create any response.

4. The gating and coordination of sleep/wake state changes includes a significant involvement of prefrontal cortex (PFC) in interactions with other cortical and subcortical systems (Horne, 1993). The role of PFC, executive control functions, and sleep will be discussed further in the section on sleep and depression.

There are numerous parallels (and direct overlap) of these sleep-related neurobiologic systems with neurobehavioral systems involved in the control of affect and attention. Again, however, each of these systems is quite complex, incompletely understood, and beyond the scope of any brief review. A few simple points can be made about the links between affective/attentional regulation with sleep/arousal regulation. Affect regulation involves a complex interplay of cortical and subcortical systems— particularly the structures in the limbic system. Cortical components include parts of the prefrontal and orbitofrontal cortex, anterior cingulate cortex and areas of hippocampal and parahippocampal cortex. Subcortical components include the amygdala, septal region, portions of the thalamus, the hypothalamus, ventral areas of striatum and pallidum, basal forebrain, and part of the midbrain (the "limbic midbrain"). In parallel to the discussion of sleep regulation, research in affect regulation has also emphasized the role of thalamocortical circuits (Alexander, DeLong, & Strick, 1986) with PFC in a central role of integration and modulation (Cummings, 1993; Fuster, 1989; MacLean, 1993; Weinberger, 1993).

Similar parallels exist for the neurobiology of attentional control (e.g., see Posner, 1990; Posner & Dehaene, 1994). Attention is also a complex system involving the interplay between cortical, midbrain, and thalamic areas with many parallels to the previous discussion with regard to arousal and affect (see LaBerge, 1995 and Posner & Peterson, 1990 for recent reviews of the cognitive neuroscience perspective on attentional processing). In particular, the executive attention network (involved in voluntary or effortful control of attentional processes) has close anatomical connections and interactions with the networks involved in vigilance and arousal (Posner & Dehaene, 1994). There are numerous strong links between the control of attention and the regulation of affect and arousal, as has been presented by numerous investigators (Derryberry & Reed, 1994; Derryberry & Tucker, 1994; LaBerge, 1995; Posner & Dahaene, 1994; Rothbart, Posner, & Rosicky, 1994; Vogt, Finch, & Olson, 1992). Another general theme across the discussion of interactions among these regulatory systems, is the role of frontal lobe development in relation to the highest level of integration and modulation of these systems (Cummings, 1993; Diamond, 1990; Goldman-Rakic, 1988; Pennington & Welsh, 1995; Rothbart et al., 1994).

In addition to the general neurobiologic overlap of cortical/subcortical interactions across these regulatory systems, one specific structure deserves mention, the lucus coeruleus (LC). The LC has been strongly linked to sleep regulation (Osaka & Matsumara, 1994), control of vigilance and arousal (Aston-Jones, Rajkowski, Kubiak, & Alexinsky, 1994), the mediation of stress responses (Valentino, Page, Van Bockstaele, & Aston-Jones, 1992), and dysregulation relevant to affective disorders (Curtis & Valentino, 1994; Kitayama et al., 1994).

To summarize briefly to this point, there appears to be very strong evidence to support the following tenets: (a) there are multiple close links between brain systems involved in the regulation of sleep and those involved in the regulation of affect and attention, (b) the process of going to sleep involves a dramatic decrease or cessation of vigilance, and thus appears to be strongly influenced by a general framework of safety versus threat, and (c) there are significant maturational and developmental changes in these systems and in the interrelationships among systems.

Clinical Vignettes

Complex links between sleep and the regulation of affect, attention, and vigilance can be further illustrated by considering some clinical cases.

Case 1. Sleep disturbances in a young child presenting with out-of-control behavior and emotional distress

> *AB, a 16-month-old girl, was brought in by her mother for chronic difficulties with night waking. For months, AB would awaken 1 to 4 times each night and would often require hours of interaction and struggles with her parents to get back to sleep. She was also resistant to daytime naps (except when falling asleep during car rides). In other aspects of her health, growth, and development she was completely normal. Her waking daytime behavior, however, showed extreme irritability, fussiness and very low tolerance for frustration. She cried frequently, showed extreme distress to any blocked goal, and was difficult to console when upset or crying. Her attention span was very short and she often changed activities rapidly. AB's sleep difficulties responded well to a behavioral program focused on self-comforting and graduated extinction of parental involvement at sleep onset (see Durand & Mindell, 1990; Blampied & France, 1993). The total amount of sleep increased from a baseline of 8 hr per 24 to 13 hr sleep per 24 hr in the month following treatment. The change in daytime behavior was described as dramatic by multiple family members. Most notable were the decreases in negative and distressed emotions, and an improved attention span. She was more easily consoled when upset, and was a more pleasant, happy child with a dramatic increase in positive social interactions. Multiple family members described her as "a totally different child," using phrases like "taming the monster."*

The main clinical point illustrated in this case is that insufficient or inadequate sleep contributes to increased irritability, easy frustration, and difficulties with focused attention.

Case 2. Sleep disturbance presenting with depressive symptomatology

> *CD was a 14-year-old boy brought in for evaluation of depressed mood, lethargy, fatigue, loss of interest in activities, and significant deterioration in school performance. CD also had complained of 1 year of extreme difficulty falling asleep at night and on further evaluation, was found to be obtaining about 6 hr of sleep per night. Based on the symptoms of difficulty with*

sleep, depressed mood, loss of interest in activities, and worsened school performance, CD was thought to have a major depressive disorder. However, when CD's insomnia was effectively treated and the total amount of night time sleep increased to 9 hr per night, he showed a significant improvement in depressive symptoms.

The clinical point illustrated in this case is that insufficient sleep in the adolescent can result in mood deterioration, decreased energy, loss of interest in activities, and can mimic or exacerbate affective disorder symptomatology. However, this is a complex clinical issue, because children and adolescents with a major depressive disorder also complain frequently about sleep disturbances (Ryan et al., 1987).

Case 3. Sleep onset insomnia exacerbating daytime mood and behavior problems in an abused child

GH was an 11-year-old girl who had a history of sexual abuse 3 years in the past. The abuse had occurred at night time in her bed and led to traumatic associations with going to bed and going to sleep, resulting in chronic insomnia. She also showed a wide range of daytime behavioral difficulties including easy distractibility, poor focused attention, and emotional lability. Following moderately successful treatment of sleep-onset insomnia (with both behavioral and pharmacologic interventions), daytime behavioral and emotional symptoms improved significantly.

These brief clinical vignettes are presented, not to suggest that sleep changes are frequently the *cause* of childhood psychopathology, but instead to illustrate the importance of a conceptualization of arousal and affect regulation that includes sleep. Our research group has been particularly interested in this broader approach to sleep and arousal regulation in relation to child and adolescent affective disorders, which is the focus of the following section of this paper.

EEG Sleep Measures in Child and Adolescent Depression

EEG sleep changes are among the most robust psychobiologic correlates of depression demonstrating abnormalities in 90% of adult subjects with major depressive disorder (MDD; Reynolds & Kupfer, 1987). These changes include: (a) difficulty going to sleep and problems staying asleep across the night; (b) less deep delta (stage 3 and 4) sleep, especially in the first 100 min of the night; (c) reduced latency to the first REM period; and (d) an altered pattern of REM sleep with more REM and greater density of eye movements early in the night. EEG studies of child and adolescent MDD, however, have revealed a mixed picture. Despite similar subjective complaints about disturbed sleep among depressed children and adolescents (Ryan et al., 1987), objective EEG studies have not found consistent sleep changes paralleling adult MDD studies. Among the four studies of prepubertal MDD subjects that included normal controls, three found no significant group differences in any sleep variables (Dahl et al., 1991b; Puig-Antich et al., 1982; Young, Knowles, MacLean, Boag, & McConville, 1982), while one study found decreased REM latency and increased sleep latency in a sample of inpatient MDD children (Emslie, Rush, Weinberg, Rintelmann, & Roffwarg, 1990). Puig-Antich et al. (1983), reported evidence of reduced REM latency and improved sleep efficiency in depressed subjects restudied after recovery from depression compared to themselves in earlier studies. Dahl et al. (1994) found reduced REM latency in MDD children following infusion of arecoline (a cholinergic agonist) indicating sleep dysregulation at an apparently sub-threshold level among some prepubertal depressed subjects that was uncovered with the cholinergic challenge.

Among eight adolescent studies using normal control subjects (Appleboom-Fondu, Kerkhofs, & Mendlewicz, 1988; Dahl et al., 1990, in press; Emslie et al., 1994; Goetz et al., 1987; Kahn & Todd,

1990; Kutcher, Williamson, Szalai, & Marton, 1992; Lahmeyer, Poznanski, & Bellur, 1983) four of eight studies found reduced REM latency, five reported increased sleep latency, and three of eight found decreased sleep efficiency in the MDD subjects. No adolescent study has reported delta sleep changes similar to that seen in adult depression.

Taken together, these results suggest that the adult pattern of sleep abnormalities in depression occurs less frequently, or are only partially expressed in early onset depression. In further support of this concept are the results of two meta-analyses. Knowles and MacLean (1990), found that age and depression appear to interact with respect to EEG sleep changes, with the smallest differences (or no differences) at early ages. Benca, Obermeyer, Thisted, and Gillin (1992) conducted a meta-analysis, and found that among the young subjects, sleep latency was the only sleep variable that differentiated depressed from control subjects.

Interpretations of these data have focused on the role of maturational changes contributing to the infrequency of sleep abnormalities in early onset depression. Clinical factors may also contribute to the discrepancies among studies of young depressed subjects. In one adolescent study suicidality and/or inpatient status appeared to be a critical factor in the early emergence of sleep abnormalities (Dahl et al., 1990). Naylor, Greden, and Alessi (1990) found that REM latency was reduced in depressed adolescents showing psychotic features compared to nonpsychotic depressed adolescents. Severity of depression has been suggested as an important factor and has been examined in a variety of studies; however, most have not supported the concept that more severe depression is associated with EEG sleep abnormalities in young subjects. In the prepubertal study by Dahl et al. (1991b), there was a small subgroup (8 of 36 depressed children) with adult pattern sleep findings, and these individuals did show more severe depression; but they were not clinically distinct from the rest of the MDD sample. However, long-term clinical follow-up of this sample will be necessary to see if this early expression of sleep abnormality portends altered clinical course. One preliminary study of the longitudinal follow-up of depressed adolescents found that REM abnormalities during adolescence were associated with future MDD episodes (Rao et al., in press).

In the most recent study of adolescent depression by our group, a great deal of effort was extended to address central methodologic questions regarding adolescent sleep studies including: (a) controlling sleep/wake schedules rigidly with careful validation with actigraphy to ensure identical sleep schedules across inpatients, outpatients, and normal controls, (b) verifying the avoidance of caffeine, nicotine, alcohol, medications, and other substances with urine tests in the home environment, and (c) examining a multiple-night study in the sleep lab including a sleep restriction challenge to the sleep regulation system with early morning awakening. The results of that study (Dahl et al., in press), indicate that with precise control over these other sources of variance on sleep measures, REM latency was significantly reduced in the depressed sample compared to controls, and there were robust differences in sleep latency between groups. There were no signs of delta sleep differences and no evidence of altered sleep continuity after sleep onset. The sleep latency differences stood out dramatically, because they occurred across conditions. That is, the depressed adolescents took longer to fall asleep at home, in the laboratory (despite uniform control over sleep/wake schedules and total amounts of sleep), and after being partially sleep deprived. Normal adolescents responded to mild sleep deprivation with rapid sleep onset and little between-subject variability, while the depressed adolescents continued to show long sleep latencies with large variabilities among subjects. Further, subjective ratings of the adolescents' subjective feelings of tiredness and sleepiness, and staff ratings of the appearance of tiredness and sleepiness, showed that the depressed adolescents were *significantly more tired* but required twice as long to fall asleep as the control adolescents.

Integrating findings across studies, these results (including the meta-analyses) suggest that the *first sign of dysregulation of sleep in early onset depression is difficulty initiating sleep*. Developmentally, reduced REM latency appears to occur as a second level of dysregulation, particularly in a subgroup of adolescents. Delta sleep differences, which are robust in adult depression, have not been evident at younger ages. This pattern of developmental changes in sleep regulation with depression may also offer some insights into the sequence and etiology of sleep dysregulation in all depression. Along these lines, the study by Ford and Kammerow (1989) from an epidemiologic sample suggested that difficulty falling asleep may predict the new onset of depression in nondepressed adults.

One theoretical framework for these findings is that sleep is relatively protected at young ages. That is, children are very deep sleepers, and it is quite difficult to disrupt sleep at young ages (Busby & Pivik, 1983). Thus, even when there exists a level of dysregulation of the sleep/wake system associated with depression, the overall architecture of sleep may remain unchanged at young ages. With increasing age, particularly at or near adolescence, this protective aspect of sleep may decrease, uncovering underlying abnormalities. *Dysregulation in sleep and arousal may also be a pathway to dysregulation in other related systems.* The interval near sleep onset appears to represent a vulnerable transition moving from a state of waking self-control (where PFC and executive functions are relatively dominant) to a sleep state where subcortical neural systems predominate. This transition into sleep requires a balancing and coordination across multiple regulatory systems and may be more vulnerable to disruption than the actual sleep states themselves. However, if the entry into sleep is chronically disturbed, this could contribute to further disruptions in the regulation of sleep and arousal. If chronic disruption of sleep onset processes lead to other changes in arousal and affect regulation, interventions focused on sleep onset may also have broader implications relevant to these disorders. This may be particularly true in some adolescents when cognitive influences significantly disrupt these physiological systems. For example, negative ruminations or recurrent distressing thoughts or images can clearly cause limbic arousal. For some individuals who have experienced traumatic events or suffer from negative self-image and poor self-esteem, negative thoughts and images at bedtime may significantly increase arousal and disrupt the ability to go to sleep. Individual differences in tendencies toward ruminative thinking, negative cognitive styles, and experiences of stressful events may, thus, interact with these physiological systems and lead to chronic changes in sleep/wake and affective regulation. There is some preliminary evidence for a differential pattern of sleep changes in relation to stressful life events among depressed versus normal adolescents (Williamson, Ryan, Dahl, Kaufman, & Puig-Antich, in press).

INTERACTIONS ACROSS REGULATORY SYSTEMS: A MODEL FOCUSED ON PFC MATURATION

Interactions between higher cognitive functions and the regulation of sleep and affect in development, leads to a focus on PFC. PFC appears to be the most likely candidate for the complex regulatory integration at the interface of sleep/arousal, affective, and higher cognitive neurobehavioral systems. PFC also shows major maturational changes over late childhood and adolescence and into early adulthood (Huttenlocher, 1979; Jernigan & Tallal, 1990; Pennington & Welsh, 1995). The next sections will outline evidence for a PFC role in these domains of sleep/arousal regulation, affective regulation, and interactions relevant to the development affective disorders.

PFC and the Regulation of Sleep and Arousal

The frontal lobes, particularly the PFC (areas rostral and mesial to motor and premotor cortex), have been established as a center for "executive control" (reviewed in Cummings, 1993; Fuster, 1989; Weinberger, 1993). Executive control refers to higher cortical and cognitive processes involved in the modulation of attention, arousal, and *guiding goal-directed behaviors* based on schemes. However, these cognitive processes are also intricately linked to motivational and emotional circuits. The PFC is uniquely situated neuroanatomically and functionally to integrate higher cognitive processes with emotional regulation (neocortical/limbic interchange) (George, Ketter, & Post, 1994; Weinberger, 1993).

The PFC has both direct and indirect connections to the amygdala, hippocampal, parahippocampal, and cingulate areas (Fuster, 1989). It is also the major neocortical region with direct connections to the hypothalamus. As Nauta (1971), MacLean (1990) and Weinberger (1993) have pointed out, *the PFC is the most compelling place for complex interplay between cognitive and emotional processing*. The PFC appears to play a "gating" role, using a cognitive scheme to inhibit or initiate specific effectors or behaviors based on both internal factors (e.g., drives and emotions) and external factors (e.g., social context and environment). One classic example of PFC function is the inhibition of context-inappropriate behaviors, that is, recognizing that remembering the "rules" relevant to a specific situation and conducting behaviors accordingly. A second well-established PFC function is the ability to anticipate or prepare a behavioral response in advance of its initiation. *The basic framework is the use of cognitive schemes, social context, and future likelihoods to mediate impulses, drives, and limbic-driven behaviors to the appropriate times and places* (context), consistent with long-term (cognitive) goals (Fuster, 1989). In integrating a wide array of basic and clinical data, Fuster has emphasized the *temporal* domain of influence of PFC. Temporal here does *not* mean circadian timing, but instead the ability to *anticipate, delay*, or *initiate* effector responses based on cognitive and social context input. Said another way, PFC is central to the *temporal modulation* in connecting a drive or impulse to a specific behavior, utilizing cognitive inputs (such as cognitive appraisal or social context). Thus, the term "gating" an output from limbic and subcortical inputs is an appropriate metaphor for this PFC function. It appears likely that gating the subcortical drive to go to sleep also involves some PFC role as well.

Recently, Horne (1993) reviewed and integrated information implicating a *PFC role in sleep regulation* as follows: (a) PFC has the highest regional cerebral metabolic rate (rCMR) in relaxed wakefulness, but the lowest rCMR during sleep; (b) the waking EEG is of higher frequency over PFC than any other area of the context; (c) coherence measures of EEG indicate PFC is a focus for human slow-wave sleep and probably accounts for age-related changes in slow-wave sleep; and (d) total *sleep deprivation causes a pattern of deficits parallel to PFC neuropsychologic anomalies*, which are reversed after recovery sleep.

This fourth point regarding sleep deprivation warrants further discussion. The strongest effect of sleep deprivation is a weakening or diminution of goal directed behaviors. Literally, being "tired" is a subjective sense of difficulty initiating and maintaining behaviors related to long-term goals or effortful tasks. These deficits can be reversed by increasing extrinsic rewards (e.g., monetary), by fear, or acute threat, whereby subjects can temporarily recruit greater effort to offset the effects of sleep deprivation. Further, there is a roughly linear relationship, with longer sleep deprivation causing greater impairment in goal-directed behavior, requiring more compensatory effort or greater extrinsic rewards to offset tiredness. Clearly, goal directed, motivated behaviors are heavily influenced by PFC/executive control, particularly when the goals are abstract or complex. Moreover, more specific neuropsychological assessments (Horne, 1988, 1993; Horne & Pettit, 1985), have shown that frontal tasks that require complex, divergent, or creative thinking—all prefrontal functions—show the most pronounced sleep deprivation deficits and the least buffering by increased subjective effort. Horne has reviewed other data for PFC impairment with sleep deprivation, including evidence for increased distractibility and decreased emotionality of speech. Other evidence shows contingent negative variation (CNV) of frontal generated waves to be abolished by total sleep deprivation (Naitoh, Johnson, & Lubin, 1971; Herscovitch, Stuss, & Broughton, 1980). There is also evidence for sleep deprivation deterioration of an imbedded figures test (Blackgrove, Alexander, & Horne, 1991), which is believed to be PFC related (Kolb & Wishaw, 1985). Horne also reviewed a study showing dramatic impairment of small group performance in a real-world test (involving novel military planning exercises; Banderet, Stokes, Francesconi, Kowal, & Naitoh, 1981). In the Banderet et al. study, young military recruits worked in small, highly motivated teams in strategic tasks during extended sleep deprivation. All teams were forced to withdraw prior to the end of the experiment (following 48 hr of sleep deprivation) because of an inability to perform tactically as a group. (In contrast, most studies of individual subjects find only modest deficits in cognitive performance following similar periods of sleep deprivation in laboratory situations.) Horne summarized this evidence as showing that only certain types of complex tasks (involving PFC) show large deficits after sleep deprivation. In the model presented in this article, this idea is extended to the hypothesis that tasks requiring the *integration of cognitive challenges with social and emotional regulation* (such as would be necessary to perform challenging maneuvers in small groups as in the Banderet study) are *particularly prone to sleep deprivation impairment*. That is, the highest level of integration (cognitive, social, and emotional processing) places the greatest modulatory demands on the PFC and is most sensitive to sleep deprivation effects. Consider a real-world example of a complex cognitive task, such as writing a grant proposal in a sleep-deprived state: If alone in a quiet setting, the ability to perform well for many hours can be achieved with no sleep through increased effort and willful concentration. However, add to these cognitive tasks a difficult emotional situation or challenging social interactions, and the sleep-related deficits are likely to become quite apparent. The point is that the ability to *balance* cognitive and emotional challenges is likely to show the greatest sensitivity to sleep deprivation effects consistent with this model.

A second common observation regarding human sleep deprivation is *variability* or *lability in emotional responses*. These changes fit common experience regarding sleep deprivation: a general "disinhibition," such as periods of "silliness," loss of inhibitions, and erratic, impulsive behaviors. For example, quoted in Horne (1993): sleep-deprived adults "periodically became hysterical and inane and did very childish things, ran wild, racing around the tables and upsetting things." Bliss, Clark, and West (1959) reported episodes of giddy, childlike, uninhibited behaviors among sleep-deprived adults. Sleep deprivation (or inadequate or disrupted night time sleep) in children has also been associated with decreased executive control, with daytime behaviors ("crankiness") reflecting impulsivity, distractibility, and emotional lability, in some cases resembling ADHD (Dahl et al., 1991a).

In summary, it appears that the most parsimonious explanation for sleep deprivation effects follows closely with Horne's presentation (1993): Human sleep deprivation impairs primary PFC functions resulting in less executive control. This translates into decreased goal directed behaviors and diminished cognitive modulation of drives, impulses, and emotions. The highest or most complex level of waking integration, such as simultaneous cognitive, emotional, and social challenges, appears to be most sensitive to sleep deprivation effects.

PFC and Affective Regulation

There is extensive literature indicating *functional asymmetry regarding the valence of emotions*. Right frontal cortex appears to have a specialized role in negative or avoidant emotional responses such as fear, disgust, and sadness, and the left frontal cortex appears to be activated in association with positive or approach emotions such as joy and happiness. Briefly, some of the data in support of these concepts are presented below:

1. *Review of stroke data* shows damage specifically located to the left anterior region of the cortex strongly associated with depressive symptoms (Lipsey, Robinson, Pearlson, Rao, & Price, 1983; Robinson, Kubos, Starr, Reo, & Price, 1984; Stark-stein, Robinson, & Price, 1987). Conversely, damage to homologous regions in the right frontal cortex is associated with indifference or euphoric behavior (Starkstein et al., 1989, 1990).

2. Based on the finding that conjugate lateral eye movements are mediated by frontal eye fields (causing the eyes to gaze toward the less active hemisphere), Heller designed a study instructing school-aged children to draw "happy pictures" and "sad pictures" and examined the placement of the figures on a blank page. Consistent with her predictions, children displaced the figures significantly to the left side of the page specifically when drawing sad pictures (Heller, 1990).

3. Recent work in the rhesus monkey also found lateralized frontal EEG during fear conditions that was reversed by benzodiazapines in parallel to human studies (Davidson, 1992).

4. *Imaging studies in depressed adults* have found decreased metabolism in the left frontal region in at least five studies (Baxter et al., 1985, 1989; Martinot et al., 1990; Dubé, Dobkin, Bowler, Thase, & Kupfer, 1993). Two studies found left frontal lobe activity correlates inversely with the severity of depression in adults (Baxter et al., 1989; Drevets, Videen, MacLeod, Haller, & Raichle, 1992). Normalization of left prefrontal activity following treatment has been reported (Baxter et al., 1989; Dubé et al., 1993); however, other results have failed to find evidence for decreased left frontal activity (Gur et al., 1984; Uytdenhoef et al., 1983).

5. *EEG evidence in depressed adults* shows that during awake, resting, eyes-closed condition, depressed subjects have greater right frontal activation compared to left frontal regions (Henriques & Davidson, 1990, 1991). Increased activity in right frontal regions (relative to left) correlated with increased severity of depression (Perris & Monakhov, 1979).

6. *EEG studies in normal adults* have revealed a remarkably consistent pattern associating greater left frontal hemisphere activity with positive or approach-related emotions and right frontal hemisphere with negative or withdrawal-related emotions. (a) When emotionally arousing films were presented to one hemisphere (by restricting visual fields), subjects rated the disturbing films initially seen by the right hemisphere as more terrifying and showed larger heart rate responses; conversely, greater heart rate responses to the enjoyable films occurred with left hemisphere viewing (Dimond & Farrington, 1977). (b) Self-rating of emotions of happiness and sadness in response to faces presented to the left and right hemisphere showed parallel patterns (Davidson, 1984). (c) Resting frontal EEG asymmetries predicted altered threshold of response to positive and negative film viewing consistent with the model (Wheeler, Davidson, & Tomarken, 1993; Tomarken, Davidson, Wheeler, & Doss, 1992). (d) Positive mood in normal subjects watching movie scenes was associated with increased relative left frontal activation while negative mood was associated with high relative right activation. (e) In a study of university students, hypnotically induced depression was associated with high EEG activation of right frontal areas and students who described themselves as characteristically depressed showed greater right than left frontal EEG activation (Tucker, Stenslie, Roth, & Shearer, 1981).

7. *EEG measures in infants and children* also show strong evidence consistent with this pattern of frontal asymmetry in emotional regulation (see Davidson, 1994; Dawson, Hessl, & Frey, 1994; Fox, Calkins, & Bell, 1994 for reviews and discussion of this area). Davidson and Fox (1989) found that R > L frontal EEG at baseline in infants predicted crying response to maternal separation. Studies by Dawson, Grofer Klinger, Panagiotides, Hill, and Spieker (1992a) replicated and extended these findings in 21-month-old toddlers, finding clear evidence of frontal (but not parietal) asymmetries in the expected directions in relation to maternal separation responses. Further, Dawson et al. recorded and scored facial expressions and showed that sad and angry faces were associated with greater right frontal activation; neutral faces were associated with balanced frontal EEG; and happy faces were associated with greater left activation. In a subsequent study, Dawson, Panagiotides, Grofer Klinger, and Hill (1992b) also examined frontal and parietal EEG activity in 13 infants of depressed

mothers and 14 infants of non-depressed mothers during baseline and emotion-eliciting conditions. Control infants revealed L > R frontal activation during a "peek-a-boo" play condition, whereas *infants of depressed mothers failed to show any hemispheric activation during this condition*. Further, the infants of depressed mothers showed another unusual pattern of response: L > R frontal activation during maternal separation (control infants demonstrated R > L frontal patterns when mother leaves the room consistent with a negative emotional experience). Preliminary data from "anxious and shy" children also show greater relative right frontal activation at rest (Davidson, 1993).

8. *Abnormal EEG asymmetry in adolescent suicide attempters* was reported by Graae et al. (1993). These investigations found a striking difference in resting EEG alpha asymmetry between suicidal adolescents and control adolescents. (R > L activation was associated with suicidality.)

In summary, although a full critical review of these studies exceeds space limitations in this paper (for excellent reviews see Heller, 1990; Davidson, 1994; Dawson et al., 1994), there is strong support for the basic concept that negative emotions (or "withdrawal-related negative affect") are associated with relative R > L frontal activation.

The Effects of Sleep Deprivation on Affective Disorders

There appears to be a *complex bidirectional relationship between the control of sleep and mood:* (a) emotional disturbances often disrupt sleep patterns; and (b) disrupted or insufficient sleep can also cause deterioration of mood, with associated tiredness, lethargy, and a tendency to be irritable and easily frustrated. Paradoxically, however, depressed subjects deprived of sleep often report activation and improvement of mood. More than 60 published studies with nearly 2,000 subjects *have documented that 50 to 60% of adults with depression experience a significant antidepressant response when deprived of sleep*, with more than 75% of these responders shooing relapse of depression following recovery sleep (reviewed in Wu & Bunney, 1990). There are a number of speculations as to the psychophysiologic mechanism of antidepressant response from sleep deprivation in depressed subjects. One theory proposes a depressogenic substance released during sleep in depressed subjects (Wu & Bunney, 1990). Another theory posits a sleep deprivation correction of a circadian abnormality associated with depression (Wehr, Wirz-Justice, & Goodwin, 1979), and a third hypothesis is based on an antidepressant effect (or substance) associated with prolonged waking (Borbely & Wirz-Justice, 1982). There is some preliminary evidence in support of each of these theories, but no consensus as to the mechanism of these paradoxical effects. There are very few data addressing sleep deprivation in early onset depression. King, Baxter, Stuber, and Fish (1987), reported a single case study of sleep deprivation providing an immediate antide-pressant response following one night of sleep restriction in a 12-year-old prepubertal boy. Detrinis, Harris, and Allen (1990) in a published abstract reported encouraging results from a pilot study using partial sleep deprivation comparing depressed children to ADHD children. The only published study in depressed adolescents (Naylor et al., 1993) reported significant improvement in mood in a small sample ($n = 4$) of "severely depressed" (defined as Hamilton Depression rating ≥ 15) adolescents following one night of total sleep deprivation (a total of 36 to 38 hr without sleep). The contrast groups in that study included four subjects with "mild depression" (Hamilton ≤ 15) and three psychiatric controls (one separation anxiety, one bulimic, one anorectic). The contrast groups showed either no improvement or significant worsening of mood following sleep deprivation.

In summary, sleep deprivation normally results in tiredness and instability of mood, however, many depressed subjects show improvements in mood and arousal following sleep deprivation. There is very little information in children and adolescents, but evidence suggests that at least some depressed adolescents show mood improvement with significant sleep deprivation.

CONCEPTUAL INTEGRATION OF SLEEP DEPRIVATION, PFC, DEPRESSION, AND DEVELOPMENT

If PFC function is chronically imbalanced (R > L) toward negative affect in depression, and sleep deprivation diminishes PFC influences over other brain regions, then, what happens when depressed patients are sleep deprived? How might the interaction of two negative processes produce a positive change in mood and activity? One possibility may be best illustrated by examining a vignette example of this level of processing: A depressed subject has an impulse to telephone an old friend. This impulse is processed cognitively at the level of PFC in a *complex temporal set*, which includes a review of *past* experiences (memories and associations related to the friend and initiating phone conversations, etc.), *projected* against *future likelihoods*—will the friend be home? will she want to talk? will the experience be good? The gating of a behavioral response (acting on the impulse to call) hinges on the balance of positive likelihoods (e.g., imagining the good feelings of talking with the friend) against the negative likelihoods (e.g., fears of rejection or pessimistic images about the interaction). Given the *negative cognitive distortions* associated with depression (Garber, Weiss, & Shanley, 1993), this past–future integration and projection of *future likelihoods may be biased by pessimism and inhibit actions in a depressed patient*. Thus, using this example, an *inhibition* of this temporal set processing at PFC with sleep deprivation could release the behavior (the impulse to call) by decreasing the relative influence of the pessimistically biased PFC processing. The transient release of behaviors linked to drives and impulses would resemble clinical improvement in a depressed subject. Biologic drives (e.g., appetite, libido) may show an analogous release or disinhibition during sleep deprivation. Said another way, one aspect of PFC temporal processing is the ability to consciously and subconsciously scan future possibilities (and their accompanying emotions) to modulate the behavioral response to drives and impulses. The other side of this coin is the scanning and remembering of *past* similar experiences and accompanying emotions. If these processes (future and past scanning) are skewed in depression toward negative affect (associated with right frontal cortex activation) and result in *chronic behavioral inhibition at the level of PFC*, then sleep deprivation could cause a transient release of drives, impulses, and behavioral responses. This model would also appear convergent with cognitive-behavioral theories of child and adolescent depression. In particular, the work of Nolen-Hoeksema, Girgus, and Seligman (1992) emphasizes the interaction of negative life events, pessimistic explanatory styles, and helpless behaviors in social and achievement settings. We have also been intrigued by the appearance of "anticipatory anhedonia" in adolescent depression (Dahl & Ryan, unpublished results). That is, many depressed adolescents have great difficulties *initiating* activities because they do not anticipate a good experience, but if "taken" to a party or "encouraged" into an activity, can have enjoyable experiences. However, over time, such a pattern could lead to social withdrawal, and perhaps more pervasive anhedonia.

Finally, it is important to *re-emphasize the developmental framework*. The ability to modulate or suppress emotions and drives based on cognitive influences is clearly a major aspect of normal development across childhood and adolescence (Kopp, 1989, 1992). Similarly, the ability to *disrupt* subcortical regulation through higher cortical influences may parallel this development and thus contribute to maturational variance in the expression of sleep abnormalities in depression. Developmental studies of PFC indicate that these regions are late developing with significant changes in frontal lobe executive function across child and adolescent development (Levin & Benton, 1991; Pennington & Welsh, 1995; Welsh, Pennington, & Groisser, 1991). There also appear to be significant neurobiologic changes in PFC occurring near puberty (Chugani, Phelps, & Mazziotta, 1987; Huttenlocher, 1979). Together, these suggest the possibility of relatively sensitive periods in development regarding the interface between higher cognitive processing and the regulation of sleep, arousal, and affect. The particular experiences and patterns of response during key maturational changes at this cognitive–emotional interface may have long-term influences on these regulatory systems.

OVERVIEW

These are complex, interacting systems, and a variety of alternative models may fit the relatively limited data available. Any concise version of one model will necessarily contain some weakly supported speculations. However, as a means of illustrating how these interacting systems may relate to the development of affective pathology, one such overview will be briefly summarized:

1. *Early in development, the sleep/arousal system is relatively protected from the arousal influences of frontal cortical and higher cognitive processing.* That is, the subcortical elements of sleep/arousal regulation are relatively dominant over PFC/cognitive influences and less likely to show acute disruptions as a result of cognitive processing of affective or threatening stimuli. From the perspective of evolutionary biology, it is possible that in the ancestral environment it was not as adaptively significant for young children to make individual judgments of safety/threat prior to going to sleep, because caretakers and other adult members of the social group performed this monitoring function.

2. *Some individuals appear to have biased cognitive processing of affective stimuli, resulting in a lower threshold for arousal responses toward potentially threatening stimuli, and probably a greater risk for anxiety and affective disorders.* This bias toward negative or withdrawal emotion is: (a) associated with functional asymmetry in frontal cortex and (b) evident very early in development as reflected by the studies of Dawson et al. (1994), Davidson et al. (1994) and Fox et al. (1994). This negative bias in emotional processing may reflect a genetic vulnerability (low threshold for negative or withdrawal responses, such as the behavioral inhibition model described by Kagan, Reznick, & Snidman, 1987) and/or negative early experiences during critical periods of early maturation of affective systems. Asymmetries in prefrontal cortex activation may reflect these alterations in cognitive emotional processing; particularly when integrating past experiences projected into future likelihoods, as a means of gating or modulating the initiation of behavioral responses.

3. *Maturational changes during childhood and adolescence result in increased influence of higher cognitive (PFC) modulation relative to other cortical or subcortical systems.* These changes contribute to greater executive control over drives, impulses, and emotions, but also to an increased capacity for disruption or dysregulation of lower regulatory systems secondary to cognitively mediated arousal. Chronic increases in arousal from cognitive sources (such as may occur with biased processing toward negative/threatening affective stimuli, or ruminating on distressing images) may significantly disrupt sleep and circadian regulation of low arousal states. Thus, increased vulnerability in these systems to cognitive influences across puberty is consistent with the observations that sleep and stress hormone changes associated with affective disorders become more apparent across adolescent maturation (Dahl & Ryan, in press).

4. *Sleep deprivation appears to weaken PFC influences over other brain regions.* Normally, this results in less cognitively motivated, goal-directed behaviors and less cognitive modulation of drives, impulses, and emotions following sleep deprivation. In depressed patients, however, it is hypothesized that weakening the PFC influence may transiently release subcortical systems from the chronic interference of the biased cognitive processing of affective stimuli, contributing to the well-documented transient improvement in many clinical depressions following sleep deprivation.

5. This sleep/PFC model is also consistent with the observations that *sleep deprivation often exacerbates externalizing disorders.* Decreased cognitive modulation of drives and impulses tend to worsen these symptoms of inattention, impulsivity, and transgressions of social rules. In normal

subjects, some deterioration of mood and motivation would be predicted following sleep deprivation, because less PFC modulation would weaken the associations with future rewarding goals and past positive experiences.

CODA

It is important to acknowledge that the model as presented has not yet addressed the primary question that framed this paper: why is sleep so important during early brain development? This question requires a broader conceptual approach concerning sleep processes that will be briefly introduced.

As stated in the beginning of this article, it is not accurate to conceptualize sleep as a period when the brain is generally shut down, or simply in a resting state. A more encompassing conceptualization is that specific stages of sleep involve an active *uncoupling* or disconnection of neurobehavioral systems. This uncoupling or disconnection occurs *within* the brain, as well as *between* internal systems and the external environment. This conceptual framework fits many of the fundamental observations of sleep state changes: the essence of going into deep non-REM sleep entails the disconnection of cognitive processing from external inputs (as reviewed earlier, incoming sensory input is blocked at the level of the thalamus). REM sleep has an altered pattern of uncoupling. One of the cardinal features of REM sleep involves the disconnection of motor cortex activity from motor output (output signal transmissions are cut off at the level of the pons, preventing any behavioral expression of "acting out" when one dreams). However, there are also fundamental shifts in the coupling within the brain during sleep stages. For example, animal research has demonstrated the changes in body temperature during REM sleep are disconnected from effector outputs (for example, animals do not shiver, vasoconstrict, or change body position when their core temperature drops during REM, they simply wake up to engage the effector responses).

Numerous examples can be provided in which sleep produces an uncoupling or disconnection between systems that are tightly coupled in an alert, awake state. The question that emerges from this conceptualization is: why would specific neurobehavioral systems require periods of disconnection? One answer to this question becomes evident when one considers the oscillatory nature of much of the neural connection in coupling. That is, there is increasing evidence that neural transmission and connectivity is at least partially achieved through timing and frequency information (Singer, 1993). The rate of oscillation of one system influences its connection and/or transmission to other systems (Engel, 1994; Gray, 1994).

In a complex multi-oscillator system, with intricate interconnections on a multitude of levels, there is likely to be a need for some *recalibration or retuning within component* systems. A simple metaphor can be created by considering the instruments in a large orchestra as a complex interacting multi-oscillator system. To operate in concert for long periods of time, harmonic relationships (tuning) must be maintained within each instrument and across instruments. Tuning within an instrument cannot be accomplished during continuous playing or coupling with the other instruments in the orchestra. Similarly, retuning or recalibration within a component neurobehavioral system may require transient uncoupling or disconnection from other oscillatory systems. Although beyond the scope of this discussion, there are compelling theoretical models that build upon the importance of precise timing codes as the primary organizing principal in brain function (Singer, 1995; Joliot, Ribary, & Llinas, 1994). The basic idea is that neural systems are coupled in the time or frequency domain rather than a simple physical or spatial connection. Some specific theories for example, have emphasized a 40 cycle/s brain sweep as underlying basic consciousness and vigilant experience (Llinas & Ribary, 1993). Other investigators have emphasized frequency and coherence mechanisms as central to the *developmental* organization of the brain (Thatcher, 1994).

If sleep creates opportunities for retuning component systems, one prediction would be that sleep deprivation effects should be most apparent in daytime functions requiring complex orchestration or modulation *across* multiple component systems. Thus, in humans, the complex modulatory roles of PFC involving numerous cortical and subcortical systems would be predicted as most sensitive to sleep deprivation effects (as presented earlier).

The final arc to complete the circle, however, is the question: Why would disconnection or un-coupling be so important in the *developing* brain? During early periods of brain maturation specific brain regions are undergoing differentiation with respect to specific functions and patterns of inter-connection between differentiated systems are becoming established (see Levitt, 1995)—such pro-cesses would require the greatest amount of recalibration or retuning. (To return to the music analogy, the early playings on a new instrument require multiple retunings after very short intervals of use.)

Clearly, these general images require translation to specific neurobiological mechanisms to evaluate the relative utility of this model. If elements of the basic model are correct, however, the implications of *how* the systems become stressed or drawn into states of imbalance (or non-optimal oscillatory rela-tionships) would be as important as understanding the mechanisms of recalibration or retuning. It may also be the case that specific neurobehavioral systems with later maturation will demonstrate greater sensitivity to sleep needs during intervals of maturation secondary to the development of new patterns of interconnection and connectivity for that system. This again raises the issue of sleep and critical periods of maturational changes in these regulatory systems. For example, many of the significant changes in sleep regulation around puberty may be linked to the activation of new neurobehavioral systems involved in reproduction and related neuroendocrine changes. Although highly speculative in this general form, there are numerous features of this disconnection or uncoupling hypothesis of sleep that may warrant further investigation relevant to development and psychopathology.

REFERENCES

Alexander, G. E., DeLong, M. R., & Strick, P. L. (1986). Parallel organization of functionally segregated circuits linking basal ganglia and cortex. *Annual Review of Neuroscience, 9,* 357–381.

Anders, T., & Roffwarg, H. (1973). The effects of selective interruption and total sleep deprivation in the human newborn. *Developmental Psychobiology, 6,* 79.

Anders, T. F., Sadeh, A., & Appareddy, V. (1995). Normal sleep in neonates and children. In R. Ferber & M. Kryger (Eds.), *Principles and practice of sleep medicine in the child* (pp. 7–18). Philadelphia: Saun-ders.

Appleboom-Foundu, J., Kerkhofs, M., & Mendlewicz, J. (1988). Depression in adolescents and young adults—Polysomnographic and neuroendocrine aspects. *Journal of Affective Disorders, 14,* 35–40.

Aston-Jones, G., Rajkowski, J., Kubiak, P., & Alexinsky, T. (1994). Locus coeruleus neurons in monkey are selectively activated by attended cues in a vigilance task. *Journal of Neuroscience, 14,* 4467–4480.

Banderet, L. E., Stokes, J. W., Francesconi, R., Kowal, D. M., & Naitoh, P. (1981). Artillery teams in simulated sustained combat: Performance and other measures. In L. C. Johnson, D. I. Tepas, W. P. Colquhoun, & M. J. Colligan (Eds.), *Biological rhythms sleep and shift work* (pp. 459–479). New York: Medical & Scientific Books.

Baxter, L. R., Phelps, M. E., Maziotta, J. C., Schwartz, J. D., Gerner, R. H., Selin, G. E., & Sumida, R. M. (1985). Cerebral metabolic rates for glucose in mood disorders. *Archives of General Psychiatry, 42,* 441–447.

Baxter, L. R., Schwartz, J. M., Phelps, M. E., Mazziotta, J. C., Guze, B. H., Selin, C. E., Gerner, R. H., & Sumida, R. M. (1989). Reduction of prefrontal cortex glucose metabolism common to three types of depression. *Archives of General Psychiatry, 46,* 243–250.

Benca, R. M., & Casper, R. C. (1994). Sleep in eating disorders. In M. H. Kryger, T. Roth, & W. C. Dement (Eds.), *Principles and practice of sleep medicine* (pp. 927–933). Philadelphia: Saunders.

Benca, R. M., Obermeyer, W. H., Thisted, R. A., & Gillin, J. C. (1992). Sleep and psychiatric disorders: A meta-analysis. *Archives of General Psychiatry, 49,* 651–668.

Blackgrove, M., Alexander, C., & Horne, J. (1991). The effects of sleep deprivation on a test of field-independence. *Sleep Research, 20A,* 458.

Blampied, N. M., & France, K. G. (1993). A behavioral model of infant sleep disturbance. *Journal of Applied Behavior Analysis, 26,* 477–492.

Bliss, E. L., Clark, L. D., & West, C. D. (1959). Studies of sleep deprivation—Relationship to schizophrenia. *Archives of Neurology, 81,* 348–359.

Bonnet, M. H. (1994). Sleep deprivation. In M. H. Kryger, T. Roth, & W. C. Dement (Eds.), *Principles and practice of sleep medicine* (2nd ed., pp. 50–67). Philadelphia: Saunders.

Borbely, A. A., & Wirz-Justice, A. (1982). Sleep deprivation and depression: A hypothesis derived from a model of sleep regulation. *Human Neurobiology, 1,* 205–210.

Brain, C. K. (1981). *The hunters or the hunted.* Chicago: University of Chicago Press.

Busby, K., & Pivik, R. T. (1983). Failure of high intensity auditory stimuli to affect behavioral arousal in children during the first sleep cycle. *Pediatric Research, 17,* 802–805.

Carskadon, M. A. (1990). Adolescent sleepiness: Increased risk in a high-risk population. *Alcohol, Drugs, and Driving, 6,* 317–328.

Carskadon, M. A., Harvey, K., Duke, P., Andres, T. F., Litt, I. F., & Dement, W. C. (1980). Pubertal changes in daytime sleepiness. *Sleep, 2,* 453–60.

Carskadon, M. A., & Mancuso, J. (1987). Reported sleep habits in boarding school students: Preliminary data. *Sleep Research, 14,* 293.

Carskadon, M. A., & Mancuso, J. (1988). Daytime sleepiness in high school adolescents: Influence of curfew. *Sleep Research, 17,* 75.

Carskadon, M. A., Rosekind, M. R., Galli, J., Sohn, J., Herman, K. B., & Davis, S. S. (1989). Adolescent sleepiness during sleep restriction in the natural environment. *Sleep Research, 18,* 115.

Cartwright, R. D., & Wood, E. (1991). Adjustment disorders of sleep: The sleep effects of a major stressful event and its resolution. *Psychiatry Research, 39,* 199–209.

Chase, M. A. (1994). Sleep mechanisms. In M. H. Kryger, T. Roth, & W. C. Dement (Eds.), *Principles and practice of sleep medicine* (pp. 105–175). Philadelphia: Saunders.

Chase, M. H., & Morales, F. R. (1990). The atonia and myoclonia of active (REM) sleep. *Annual Review of Psychology, 41,* 557–584.

Chugani, H. T., Phelps, M. E., & Mazziotta, J. C. (1987). Positron emission tomography study of human brain functional development. *Annals of Neurology, 22,* 487–497.

Cicchetti, D., & Beeghly, M. (1990). *The self in transition: Infancy and childhood.* Chicago: University of Chicago Press.

Cummings, J. L. (1993). Frontal-subcortical circuits and human behavior. *Archives of Neurology, 50,* 873–880.

Curtis, A. L., & Valentino, R. J. (1994). Coretiotiapin-releasing factor neurotianouian in LC: A possible site of anti-depressant action. *Brain Research Bulletin, 35*(5–6), 581–587.

Dahl, R. E., Bernhisal-Broadbent, J., Scanlon-Holdford, S., Lupo, M., Sampson, H. A., & AlShabbout, M. (1995). Sleep disturbances in children with atopic dermatitis. *Archives of Pediatrics and Adolescent Medicine, 149,* 856–860.

Dahl, R. E., Holttum, J., & Trubnick, L. (1994). The clinical presentation of narcolepsy in children and adolescents. *Journal of the American Academy of Child and Adolescent Psychiatry, 33,* 834–841.

Dahl, R. E., Matty, M. K., Birmaher, B., AlShabbout, M., Williamson, D. E., & Ryan, N. D. (in press). Sleep onset abnormalities in depressed adolescents. *Biological Psychiatry.*

Dahl, R. E., Pelham, W. E., & Wierson, M. (1991a). The role of sleep disturbances in attention deficit disorder symptoms: A case study. *Journal of Pediatric Psychology, 16,* 229–239.

Dahl, R. E., Puig-Antich, J., Ryan, N. D., Nelson, B., Dachille, S., Cunningham, S. L., Trubnick, L., & Klepper, T. P. (1990). EEG sleep in adolescents with major depression: The role of suicidality and inpatient status. *Journal of Affective Disorders, 19,* 63–75.

Dahl, R. E., & Ryan, N. D. (in press). The psychobiology of adolescent depression. In D. Cicchetti & S. L. Toth

(Eds.), *Rochester Symposium on developmental psychopathology, Vol. VII: Adolescence: Opportunities and challenges*. Rochester, NY: University of Rochester Press.

Dahl, R. E., Ryan, N. D., Birmaher, B., Al-Shabbout, M., Williamson, D. E., Neidig, M., Nelson, B., & Puig-Antich, J. (1991b). EEG sleep measures in prepubertal depression. *Psychiatry Research, 38*, 201–214.

Dahl, R. E., Ryan, N. D., Perel, J., Birmaher, B., Al-Shabbout, M., Nelson, B., & Puig-Antich, J. (1994). Cholinergic REM induction test with arecoline in depressed children. *Psychiatry Research, 51*, 269–282.

Davidson, R. J. (1984). Affect, cognition and hemispheric specialization. In C. E. Izard, J. Kagan, & R. Zajonc (Eds.), *Emotion, cognition, and behavior* (pp. 320–365). New York: Cambridge University Press.

Davidson, R. J. (1992). Anterior cerebral asymmetry and the nature of emotion. *Brain and Cognition, 20*, 125–151.

Davidson, R. J. (1993). Cerebral asymmetry and emotion: Conceptual and methodological conundrums. *Cognition and Motion, 7*, 115–138.

Davidson, R. J. (1994). Asymmetric brain function, affective style, and psychopathology: The role of early experience and plasticity. *Development and Psychopathology, 6*, 741–758.

Davidson, R. J., & Fox, N. A. (1982). Asymmetrical brain activity discriminates between positive versus negative affective stimuli in human infants. *Science, 218*, 1235–1237.

Dawson, G., Grofer Klinger, L., Panagiotides, H., Hill, D., & Spieker, S. (1992a). Frontal lobe activity and affective behavior of infants of mothers with depressive symptoms. *Child Development, 63*, 725–737.

Dawson, G., Hessl, D., & Frey, K. (1994). Social influences on early developing biological and behavioral systems related to risk for affective disorder. *Development and Psychopathology, 6*, 759–779.

Dawson, G., Panagiotides, H., Grofer Klinger, L., & Hill, D. (1992b). The role of frontal lobe functioning in the development of self-regulatory behavior in infancy. *Brain and Cognition, 20*, 152–175.

Derryberry, D., & Reed, M. A. (1994). Attention and temperament, orienting toward and away from positive and negative signals. *Journal of Personality and Social Psychology, 66*, 1128–1139.

Derryberry, D., & Tucker, D. M. (1994). Motivating the focus of attention. In P. Niedenthal & S. Kitayama (Eds.), *The heart's eye: Emotional influences in perception and attention* (pp. 167–196). San Diego, CA: Academic Press.

Detrinis, R., Harris, J., & Allen, R. (1990). Effects of partial sleep deprivation in children with major depression and attention deficit hyperactivity disorder (ADHD). *Sleep Research, 19*, 322.

Diamond, A. (1990). Developmental time course in human infants and infant monkeys, and the neural bases of inhibitory control in reaching. In A. Diamond (Ed.), The development of and neural bases of higher cognitive functions. *Annals of the New York Academy of Sciences, 608*, 267–317.

Dijk, D. J., Brunner, D. P., & Borbely, A. A. (1991). EEG power density during recovery sleep in the morning. *Electroencephalography and Clinical Neurophysiology, 78*, 203–214.

Dimond, S., & Farrington, L. (1977). Emotional response to films shown to the right or left hemisphere of the brain measured by heart rate. *Acta Psychologica, 41*, 255–260.

Drevets, W. C., Videen, T. O., MacLeod, A. K., Haller, J. W., & Raichle, M. E. (1992). PET images of blood flow changes during anxiety: Correction. *Science, 256*, 1696.

Dubé, S., Dobkin, J. A., Bowler, K. A., Thase, M., & Kupfer, D. J. (1993). *Biological Psychiatry, 33*, 40A–47 (Abstract).

Durand, V. M., & Mindell, J. A. (1990). Behavioral treatment of multiple childhood sleep disorders: Effects on child and family. *Behavior Modification, 14*, 37–49.

Emslie, G. J., Rush, A. J., Weinberg, W. A., Rittleman, J. W., & Roffward, H. P. (1994). Sleep EEG features of adolescents with major depression. *Biological Psychiatry, 36*, 573–581.

Emslie, G. J., Rush, A. J., Weinberg, W. A., Rintelmann, J. W., & Roffwarg, H. P. (1990). Children with major depression show reduced rapid eye movement latencies. *Archives of General Psychiatry, 47*, 119–124.

Engel, A. K., Konig, P., Kreiter, A. K., & Schillen, T. B., et al. (1992). Temporal coding in the visual cortex: New vistas on integration in the nervous system. *Trends in Neuroscience, 15*, 218–226.

Ford, D. E., & Kamerow, D. B. (1989). Epidemiological studies of sleep disturbances and psychiatric disorders: An opportunity for prevention? *Journal of the American Medical Association, 262*, 1479–1484.

Fox, N. A., Calkins, S. D., & Bell, M. A. (1994). Neural plasticity and development in the first two years of life: Evidence from cognitive and socioemotional domains of research. *Development and Psychopathology, 6,* 677–696.

Fuster, J. M. (1989). *The prefrontal cortex: Anatomy, physiology, and neuropsychology of the frontal lobe* (2nd ed.). New York: Raven Press.

Garber, J., Weiss, B., & Shanley, N. (1993). Cognitions, depressive symptoms, and development in adolescents. *Journal of Abnormal Psychology, 102,* 47–57.

George, M. S., Ketter, T. A., & Post, R. M. (1994). Prefrontal cortex dysfunction in clinical depression. *Depression, 2,* 59–72.

Gillin, J. C. (1994). Sleep and psychoactive drugs of abuse and dependence. In M. H. Kryger, T. Roth, & W. C. Dement (Eds.), *Principles and practice of sleep medicine* (pp. 934–942). Philadelphia: Saunders.

Glaze, D. G., Frost, J. D., & Jankovic, J. (1983). Sleep in Gilles de la Tourette's syndrome: Disorder of arousal. *Neurology, 33,* 586.

Goetz, R., Puig-Antich, J., Ryan, N., Rabinovich, H., Ambrosini, P. J., Nelson, B., & Krawiec, V. (1987). Electroencephalographic sleep of adolescents with major depression and normal controls. *Archives of General Psychiatry, 44,* 61–68.

Goldman-Rakic, P. S. (1988). Topography of cognition: Parallel distributed networks in primate association cortex. *Annual Review of Neuroscience, 11,* 137–156.

Graae, F., Tenke, C., Bruder, G., Rotheram-Borus, M. J., Piacentini, J., Castro-Blanco, D., Leite, P., & Towey, J. (1993). *Abnormal asymmetry of EEG in female adolescent suicide attempters.* Presented at the 1993 Annual Meeting of the American Academy of Child and Adolescent Psychiatry. San Antonio, TX.

Gray, C. M., Engel, A. K., Konig, P., & Singer, W. (1992). Synchronization of oscillatory neuronal responses in cat striate cortex: Temporal properties. *Visual Neuroscience, 8,* 337–347.

Guilleminault, C., Winkle, R., Korobkin, R., & Simmons, B. (1982). Children and nocturnal snoring: Evaluation of the effects of sleep related respiratory resistive load and daytime functioning. *European Journal of Pediatrics, 130,* 1165–1171.

Gur, R. E., Skolnick, B. E., Gur, R. C., Caroff, S., Rieger, W., Obrist, W. D., Younkin, D., & Reivich, M. (1984). Brain function in psychiatric disorders. II. Regional cerebral blood flow in medicated unipolar depressives. *Archives of General Psychiatry, 41,* 695–699.

Hall, M. H., Dahl, R. E., Dew, M. A., & Reynolds, C. F. (in press). Sleep patterns following major negative life events. *Directions in Psychiatry.*

Heller, W. (1990). The neuropsychology of emotion: Developmental patterns and implications for psychopathology. In N. Stein, B. I. Levanthal, & T. Trabasso (Eds.), *Psychological and biological approaches to emotion* (pp. 167–211). Hillsdale, NJ: Erlbaum.

Henriques, J. B., & Davidson, R. J. (1990). Regional brain electrical asymmetries discriminate between previously depressed subjects and healthy controls. *Journal of Abnormal Psychology, 99,* 22–31.

Henriques, J. B., & Davidson, R. J. (1991). Left frontal hypoactivation in depression. *Journal of Abnormal Psychology, 100,* 535–545.

Herscovitch, J., Stuss, D., & Broughton, R. (1980). Changes in cognitive processing following shortterm cumulative partial sleep deprivation and recovery oversleeping. *Journal of Clinical Neuropsychology, 2,* 301–319.

Horne, J. A. (1988). Sleep loss and "divergent" thinking ability. *Sleep, 11,* 528–536.

Horne, J. A. (1993). Human sleep loss and behavior implications for the prefrontal cortex and psychiatric disorder. *British Journal of Psychiatry, 162,* 413–419.

Horne, J. A., & Pettitt, A. N. (1985). High incentive effects on vigilance performance during 72 hours total sleep deprivation. *Acta Psychologica, 58,* 123–139.

Huttenlocher, P. R. (1979). Synaptic density in human frontal cortex—Developmental changes in effects of aging. *Brain Research, 163,* 195–205.

Insel, T. R., Gillin, J. C., Moore, A., Mendelson, W. B., Lowenstein, R. J., & Murphy, D. L. (1982). The sleep of patients with obsessive-compulsive disorder. *Archives of General Psychiatry, 39,* 1372–1377.

Joliot, M., Ribary, U., & Llinas, R. (1994). Human oscillatory brain activity near 40 Hz coexists with cognitive temporal binding. *Proceedings of the National Academy of Sciences of the United States of America, 91,* 11748–11751.

Jones, B. E. (1994). Basic mechanisms of sleep-wake states. In M. H. Kryger, T. Roth, & W. C. Dement (Eds.), *Principles and practice of sleep medicine* (pp. 145–162). Philadelphia: Saunders.

Kagan, J. (1981). *The second year.* Cambridge, MA: Harvard University Press.

Kagan, J., Reznick, S., & Snidman, N. (1987). Temperamental variation in response to the unfamiliar. *Perinatal Development: A Psychobiological Perspective,* 421–440.

Kahn, A. U., & Todd, S. (1990). Polysomnographic findings in adolescents with major depression. *Psychiatry Research, 33,* 313–320.

King, B. H., Baxter, L. R., Stuber, M., & Fish, B. (1987). Therapeutic sleep deprivation for depression in children. *Journal of the American Academy of Child and Adolescent Psychiatry, 26,* 928–931.

Kitayama, I., Nakamura, S., Yaga, T., Murase, S., Nomura, J., Kayahara, T., & Nakano, K. (1994). Degeneration of locus coeruleus axons in stress-induced depression model. *Brain Research Bulletin, 35,* 573–580.

Knowles, J. B., & MacLean, A. W. (1990). Age-related changes in sleep in depressed and healthy subjects. *Neuropsychopharmacology, 3,* 251–259.

Kolb, B., & Wishaw, I. Q. (1985). *Fundamentals of human neuropsychology* (2nd ed.). San Francisco: Freeman.

Kopp, C. B. (1989). Regulation of distress and negative emotions: A developmental view. *Developmental Psychology, 25,* 343–354.

Kopp, C. B. (1992). Emotional distress and control in young children. *New Directions For Child Development, 55,* 41–55.

Kutcher, S., Williamson, P., Szalai, U., & Marton, P. (1992). REM latency in endogeneously depressed adolescents. *British Journal of Psychiatry, 161,* 399–402.

LaBerge, D. (1995). *Attention processing: The brain's art of mindfulness.* Cambridge: Harvard University Press.

Lahmeyer, H. W., Poznanski, E. O., & Bellur, S. N. (1983). EEG sleep in depressed adolescents. *American Journal of Psychiatry, 140,* 1150–1153.

Lang, P. J. (1995). The emotion probe: Studies of motivation and attention. *American Psychologist, 50,* 372–385.

LeDoux, J. E. (1989). Cognitive–emotional interactions in the brain. *Cognition and Emotion, 3,* 267–290.

Levin, H. S., & Benton, A. L. (1991). *Frontal lobe function and dysfunction.* New York: Oxford University Press.

Levitt, P. (1995). Experimental approaches that reveal principles of cerebral cortical development. In M. S. Gazzaniga (Ed.), *The cognitive neurosciences* (pp. 147–163). Cambridge, MA: MIT Press.

Lipsey, J. R., Robinson, R. G., Pearlson, G. D., Rao, K., & Price, T. R. (1983). Mood change following bilateral hemisphere brain injury. *British Journal of Psychiatry, 143,* 266–273.

Llinas, R., & Ribary, U. (1993). Coherent 40-Hz oscilation characterizes dream state in humans. *Proceedings of the National Academy of Sciences of America, 90,* 2078–2081.

MacLean, P. D. (1990). The triune brain in evolution: Role in paleocerebral functions. New York: Plenum Press.

MacLean, P. D. (1993). Cerebral evolution of emotion. In M. Lewis & J. M. Haviland (Eds.), *Handbook of emotions* (pp. 67–83). New York: Guilford Press.

Martinot, J., Hardy, P., Feline, A., Huret, J., Mazoyer, B., Attar-Levy, D., Pappata, S., & Syrota, A. (1990). Left prefrontal glucose hypometabolism in the depressed state: A confirmation. *American Journal of Psychiatry, 147,* 1313–1317.

Mellman, T. A., & Uhde, T. W. (1989). Sleep panic attacks: New clinical findings and theoretical implications. *American Journal of Psychiatry, 146,* 1204–1207.

Naitoh, P., Johnson, L. C., & Lubin, A. (1971). A modification of surface negative slow potential (CNV) in the human brain after sleep loss. *Electroencephalography and Clinical Neurophysiology, 30,* 17–22.

Nauta, W. J. H. (1971). The problem of the frontal lobe: A reinterpretation. *Journal of Psychological Research, 8,* 167–187.

Navelet, Y., Anders, T. F., & Guilleminault, C. (1976). Narcolepsy in children. In C. Guilleminault, W. C. Dement, & P. Passouant (Eds.), *Narcolepsy* (pp. 171–177). New York: Spectrum.

Naylor, M., Greden, J., & Alessi, N. (1990). Plasma dexamethasone levels in children given the dexamethasone suppression test. *Biological Psychiatry, 27*, 592–600.

Naylor, M. W., King, C. A., Lindsay, K. A., Evans, T., Armelagos, J., Shain, B. N., & Greden, J. F. (1993). Sleep deprivation in depressed adolescents and psychiatric controls. *Journal of the American Academy of Child and Adolescent Psychiatry, 32*, 753–759.

Nolen-Hoeksema, S., Girgus, J. S., & Seligman, M. E. (1992). Predictors and consequences of childhood depressive symptoms: A 5-year longitudinal study. *Journal of Abnormal Psychology, 101*, 405–422.

Osaka, T., & Matsumara, H. (1994, February). Norad-renergic inputs in sleep-related neurons in the preoptic area from the locus coeruleus and the ventrolateral medulla in the rat. *Neuroscience Research, 19*, 39–50.

Parmeggiani, P. L. (1994). The autonomic nervous system in sleep. In M. H. Kryger, T. Roth, & W. C. Dement (Eds.), *Principles and practice of sleep medicine* (pp. 194–203). Philadelphia: Saunders.

Pennington, B. F., & Welsh, M. (1995). Neuropsychology and developmental psychopathology. In D. Cicchetti & D. Cohen (Eds.), *Developmental Psychopathology*. Cambridge, UK: Cambridge University Press.

Perris, C., & Monakhov, K. (1979). Depressive symptomotology and systemic structural analysis of the EEG. In J. Gruzelier & P. Flor-Henry (Eds.), *Hemisphere asymmetries of function in psycho-pathology*. Amsterdam/New York/Oxford: Elsevier/North-Holland.

Picchetti, D. L., & Walters, A. S. (1994). Attention deficit hyperactivity disorder and periodic limb movement disorder. *Sleep Research, 23*, 303.

Posner, M. I., & Dehaene, S. (1994). Attention networks. *Trends in Neuroscience, 17*, 75–79.

Posner, M. I., & Petersen, S. E. (1990). The attention system of the human brain. *Annual Review of Neuroscience, 13*, 25–42.

Puig-Antich, J., Goetz, R. R., Hanlon, C., Tabrizi, M. A., Davies, M., & Weitzman, E. (1982). Sleep architecture and REM sleep measures in prepubertal major depressives during an episode. *Archieves of General Psychiatry, 39*, 932–939.

Puig-Antich, J., Goetz, R., Hanlon, C., Tabrizi, M. A., Davies, M., & Weitzman, E. (1983). Sleep architecture and REM sleep measures in prepubertal major depressives: Studies during recovery from a major depressive episode in a drug free state. *Archives of General Psychiatry, 40*, 187–192.

Rao, U., Dahl, R. E., Ryan, N. D., Birmaher, B., Williamson, D. E., Giles, D. E., Rao, R., Kaufman, J., & Nelson, B. (in press). The relationship between longitudinal clinical course and sleep and cortisol changes in adolescent depression. *Biological Psychiatry*.

Rechtschaffen, A., Bergmann, B. M., Everson, C. A., Kushida, C. A., & Gilliland, M. A. (1989). Sleep deprivation in the rat: X. Integration and discussion of the findings. *Sleep, 12*, 68–87.

Robinson, R. G., Kubos, K. L., Starr, L. B., Reo, K., & Price, T. R. (1984). Mood disorders in stroke patients; importance of location of lesion. *Brain, 107*, 81–93.

Ross, R. J., Ball, W. A., Sullivan, K. A., & Caroff, S. N. (1989). Sleep disturbance as the hallmark of posttraumatic stress disorder. *American Journal of Psychiatry, 146*, 697–707.

Rothbart, M. K., Posner, M. I., & Rosicky, J. (1994). Orienting in normal and pathological development. *Development and Psychopathology, 6*, 635–652.

Ryan, N. D., Puig-Antich, J., Rabinovich, H., Ambrosini, P., Robinson, D., Nelson, B., & Novacenko, H. (1988). Growth hormone response to desmethylimipramine in depressed and suicidal adolescents. *Journal of the American Academy of Child and Adolescent Psychiatry, 27*, 755–758.

Ryan, N. D., Puig-Antich, J., Rabinovich, H., Robinson, D., Ambrosini, P. J., Nelson, B., & Iyengar, S. (1987). The clinical picture of major depression in children and adolescents. *Archives of General Psychiatry, 44*, 854–861.

Siegel, J. M. (1994). Brainstem mechanisms generating REM sleep. In M. H. Kryger, T. Roth, & W. C. Dement (Eds.), *Principles and practice of sleep medicine* (pp. 125–144). Philadelphia: Saunders.

Singer, W. (1993). Synchronization of cortical activity and its putative role in information processing and learning. *Annual Review of Physiology, 55,* 349–374.

Singer, W. (1995). Time as coding space in neocortical processing: A hypothesis. In M. S. Gazzaniga (Ed.), *The cognitive neurosciences* (pp. 91–104). Cambridge, MA: MIT Press.

Starkstein, S. E., Mayberg, H. S., Berthier, M. L., Fedoroff, P., Price, T. R., Dannals, R. F., Wagner, H. N., Leiguarda, R., & Robinson, R. G. (1990). Mania after brain injury: Neuroradiological and metabolic findings. *Annals of Neurology, 27,* 652–659.

Starkstein, S. E., Robinson, R. G., Honig, M. A., Parikh, R. M., Joselyn, J., & Price, T. R. (1989). Mood changes after right-hemisphere lesions. *British Journal of Psychiatry, 155,* 79–85.

Starkstein, S. E., Robinson, R. G., & Price, T. R. (1987). Comparison of cortical and subcortical lesions in the production of poststroke mood disorders. *Brain, 110,* 1045–1059.

Steriade, M., Contreras, D., & Amzica, F. (1994). Synchronized sleep oscillations and their paroxysmal developments. *Trends in Neuroscience, 17,* 199–208.

Thatcher, R. W. (1994). Psychopathology of early frontal lobe damage: Dependence on cycles of development. *Development and Psychopathology, 6,* 565–596.

Tomarken, A. J., Davidson, R. J., Wheeler, R. E., & Doss, R. C. (1992). Individual differences in anterior brain asymmetry and fundamental dimensions of emotion. *Journal of Personality and Social Psychology, 62,* 676–687.

Tucker, D. M., Stenslie, C. E., Roth, R. S., & Shearer, S. L. (1981). Right frontal lobe activation and right hemisphere performance decrement during a depressed mood. *Archives of General Psychiatry, 38,* 169–174.

Uytdenhoef, P., Portelange, P., Jacquy, J., Charles, G., Linkowski, P., & Mendlewicz, J. (1983). Regional cerebral blood flow and lateralized hemispheric dysfunction in depression. *British Journal of Psychiatry, 143,* 128–132.

Valentino, R. J., Page, M., Van Bockstaele, E., & Aston-Jones, G. (1992). Corticotropin-releasing factor innervation of the locus coeruleus region: Distribution of fibers and sources of input. *Neuroscience, 48,* 689–705.

Vogt, B. A., Finch, D. M., & Olson, C. R. (1992). Overview: Functional heterogeneity in cingulate cortex: The anterior executive and posterior evaluative regions. *Cerebral Cortex, 2,* 435–443.

Wehr, T. A., Wirz-Justice, A., & Goodwin, F. K. (1979). Phase advance of the circadian sleep-wake cycle as an antidepressant. *Science, 206,* 210–213.

Weinberger, D. R. (1993). A connectionist approach to the prefrontal cortex. *Journal of Neuropsychiatry, 5,* 241–253.

Welsh, M. C., Pennington, B. F., & Groisser, D. B. (1991). A normative-developmental study of executive function: A window of prefrontal function in children. *Developmental Neuropsychology, 7,* 131–149.

Wheeler, R. E., Davidson, R. J., & Tomarken, A. J. (1993). Frontal brain asymmetry and emotional reactivity: A biological substrate of affective style. *Psychophysiology, 30,* 82–89.

Williamson, D. E., Ryan, N. D., Birmaher, B., Dahl, R. F., Kaufman, J., Rao, U., & Puig-Antich, J. (in press). A case control family history study of depression in adolescents. *Journal of the American Academy of Child and Adolescent Psychiatry.*

Wu, J. C., & Bunney, W. E. (1990). The biological basis of an antidepressant response to sleep deprivation and relapse: Review and hypothesis. *American Journal of Psychiatry, 147,* 14–21.

Young, W., Knowles, J. B., MacLean, A. W., Boag, L., & McConville, B. J. (1982). The sleep of childhood depressives: Comparison with age-matched controls. *Biological Psychiatry, 17,* 1163–1169.

Zarcone, V. P., & Benson, K. L. (1994). Sleep and schizophrenia. In M. H. Kryger, T. Roth, & W. C. Dement (Eds.), *Principles and practice of sleep medicine* (2nd ed., pp. 914–926). Philadelphia: Saunders.

2

Infant Positive and Negative Emotionality: One Dimension or Two?

Jay Belsky, Kuang-Hua Hsieh, and Keith Crnic

*Department of Human Development and Family Studies,
Pennsylvania State University*

To determine whether one or two dimensions of infant (positive and negative) emotionality best characterized infant functioning, parental reports (10 months) and elicited emotion (12–13 months) were examined. The adequacy of 1- and 2-latent-construct measurement models were evaluated and the model consisting of separate positive and negative dimensions proved to fit the data better. The discriminant validity of the two-dimensional model was evaluated. It was found that early positivity (12–13 months) predicted later positivity (18–20 months) better than later negativity, with the reverse being true of early negativity. Results are discussed in terms of prior work on infant and adult emotionality, and implications for the study of development are considered.

The concept of temperament is widely used in the study of child development, especially during the first years of life (Kagan, 1994). Extended discussion of the influence of temperament on parent–infant interaction (for a review, see Crockenberg, 1986) and its role in the development of attachment security (e.g., Belsky & Rovine, 1987; Sroufe, 1985) and problem behavior (e.g., Bates, Maslin, & Frankel, 1985), to cite just a few well-studied topics, attests to its enduring significance as an explanatory construct. What seems particularly interesting in light of the attention that temperament has received over the past two decades is that consensus remains to be achieved regarding core definitional issues (Goldsmith et al., 1987). Whereas some such as Buss and Plomin (1984) define temperament in terms of early-emerging, biologically based, behavioral attributes that remain stable over time and place, others such as Goldsmith and Campos (1990) regard this classical view as outmoded, emphasizing instead the environmentally malleable nature of temperament.

It is not just the core definitional properties of temperament that have proven difficult to achieve agreement on. Much diversity of opinion also exists regarding the content of the construct of temperament. Whereas Buss and Plomin (1984) (see Goldsmith et al., 1987) highlight emotionality, activity, and sociability on the basis of their view that temperament maps on to later personality, other theorists and empiricists dimensionalize temperament differently. On the basis of conceptual concerns for

Reprinted with permission from Developmental Psychology, 1996, Vol. 32(2), 289–298. Copyright © 1996 by the American Psychological Association, Inc.

The research described herein was supported by a grant from the National Institute of Mental Health to Jay Belsky and Keith Crnic (MH44604).

reactivity and self-regulation, Rothbart (1986) (see Goldsmith et al., 1987) distinguished six dimensions: fear, distress to limitations, smiling and laughter, soothability, duration of orienting, and activity level. Bates, Freeland, and Lounsbury (1979), following Thomas and Chess's (1977) emphasis on behavioral style, highlighted still others (fussy/difficult, unadaptable, dull, and unpredictable).

Despite the lake of consensus regarding both the conceptual definition and the content of temperament, it is noteworthy that the measurement of emotion lies at the core of virtually all thinking about temperament. This is so irrespective of whether emotion is conceptualized descriptively—as in Matheny, Wilson, and Nuss's (1984) assessment of emotional tone and Buss and Plomin's (1984) assessment of emotionality—or evaluatively—as in Bates et al.'s (1979) focus on difficultness. In most cases, in fact, the emphasis in such temperament-based concern for emotion is on negative emotionality, as the very term *difficult* suggests. Indeed, in the Buss and Plomin (1984) system, the dimension of emotionality is assessed by items such as "child cries easily," "child gets upset easily," and "child reacts intensely when upset." In some other measurement approaches, however, emotionality encompasses both positive and negative poles of expression. In the Louisville, Kentucky, lab-based, temperament-assessment system, for example, the 9-point emotional tone rating ranges from a low score of 1, reflecting extreme upset and vigorous crying, to a high score of 9, reflecting excitement and animation (Matheny et al., 1984).

In light of this diversity of approaches to conceptualizing and measuring emotionality, it is noteworthy that research on adult personality, mood, and temperament has moved away from a bipolar conceptualization of an emotionality-based dispositional factor. Not only do psychometrically sound personality instruments reflective of the core, "Big 5" personality traits (McCrae & John, 1992) place negative emotional items (pertaining to anxiety, hostility, and depression) on the Neuroticism scale and positive emotional items reflecting warmth, joy, and happiness on the Extraversion scale (e.g., Costa & McCrae, 1985), but investigators of more transient emotional states (in contrast to personality traits) underscore the independent nature of positive and negative mood (Tellegen, 1985; Watson, 1988; Watson & Clark, 1984). Such independence has emerged in studies of adults in Japan (Watson, Clark, & Tellegen, 1984) and Russia (Balatsky & Diener, 1993), as well as in the United States. Diener, Smith, and Fujita's (1995) recent study showing (a) that a two-dimensional model of affect better fits emotion data obtained on college students than does a one-dimensional model (see also Green, Goldman, & Salovey, 1993) and (b) that the two dimensions are significantly correlated ($r = -.44$) suggests, however, that drawing dramatic contrasts between models in which positivity and negativity are either completely orthogonal or extremely inversely correlated may misrepresent the actual structure of emotion. In fact, in the work to be presented addressing this same issue with respect to infant emotionality, complete independence is unlikely to be discerned because negativity and positivity are assessed in the same situations, and thus crying in almost all cases precludes expressions of positive affectivity.

Recently, developmentalists interested in temperament have applied the two-dimension approach to the study of infant emotionality. Rothbart (1986), for example, composited subscales on her parent-report instrument to create higher order constructs of positive and negative reactivity (e.g., negative = fear + distress to limitations) to examine stability of individual differences over time and relations between maternal reports and home-based observations of infant behavior at ages 3, 6, and 9 months. Goldsmith and Campos (1990) explored the internal structure of a set of laboratory-elicited and maternal-report measures of positive and negative emotionality on a sample composed mostly of 9-month-old twins and concluded that "the relative independence of fear and pleasure provides developmental support to Tellegen's (1985) theoretical framework that views positive and negative emotionality as independent, second-order factors underlying the structure of adult personality traits" (p. 1959). Finally, Belsky, Fish, and Isabella (1991) drew directly on Tellegen's (1985) theorizing (see Belsky & Pensky, 1988) to create multimethod indices of positive and negative emotionality for a sample of infants studied at 3 and 9 months. The fact that distinctly different correlates of change in positive and negative emotionality emerged in this study of the family antecedents and attachment consequences of continuity and discontinuity in infant emotionality would seem to highlight the wisdom of not presuming that high positivity implies low negativity and of not focusing exclusively on negative emotionality. Such a view would seem to be buttressed by evidence indicating that the physiological correlates of positive and negative emotional response are distinct (Davidson, 1993).

In the current report, we seek to extend research on positive and negative emotionality, as two separable dimensions, during infancy. Whereas the work cited above with such a focus has concentrated on children 9 months of age and younger, in this investigation our emphasis is on somewhat older children, aged 10–13 months when parent-report and extensive laboratory assessments of emotionality were first obtained, and aged 18 and 20 months of age when subsequent, and more limited, emotionality measurements were made. Moreover, in attempt to assess the empirical viability of a two-dimensional approach to the study of infant emotionality, we rely on multiple indicators of positivity and negativity using the "early" (i.e., 10–13 month) emotionality data to test an a priori measurement model of infant emotionality on approximately half the available infants ($n = 65$) and then test the replicability of this model with the remaining infants ($n = 57$). Finally, in an effort to validate a two-dimensional model, we use structural equation modeling to determine, now using all infants on whom longitudinal data are available ($n = 104$), whether multiple-indicator, latent constructs of positivity and negativity measured at the end of the first year discriminantly predict positivity and negativity measured at 18 and 20 months of age. Support for a two-dimensional model would derive from evidence indicating (a) that a two-dimensional measurement model better fit the early emotionality data than a (bipolar) one-dimensional model and (b) that early positivity better predicted later positivity than later negativity, with the reverse being true of early negativity. As has been already noted, because positivity and negativity were assessed in the same emotion-eliciting situations, we did not expect the two emotionality constructs to be completely independent, though we did expect them to be separable (cf. Diener et al., 1995).

For reasons not pertaining to the study of emotionality, in this report we rely on data collected on a relatively large sample of firstborn boys. Although we cannot be certain that the results of this inquiry are generalizable to girls, to be noted is the fact that when Goldsmith and Campos (1990) undertook their analysis of the internal structure of fear and pleasure they specifically examined sex differences. Finding none, they combined samples of boys and girls. Such results pertaining to 9-month-olds certainly suggest that evidence to emerge from this investigation of boys would generalize to girls, though obviously replication is in order before any such conclusions can be drawn.

METHOD

Participants

The participants is this study were 122 firstborn sons born to maritally intact, middle- and working-class White families residing in central Pennsylvania. The families of these children have been the subject of several prior empirical reports dealing with co-parenting during the second year of life (Belsky, Crnic, & Gable, 1995; Gable, Belsky, & Crnic, 1995) and with adult personality as a predictor of observed parenting (Belsky, Crnic, & Woodworth, in press). At the time of enrollment into the study, mothers' and fathers' average ages were 29 and 31 years, respectively; mean length of marriage was 5 years, and mean years of education for both spouses was 15 years. Annual family income for the participating families ranged from less than $5,000 to almost $100,000 per year, with a mean of approximately $40,000. Families were recruited through birth announcements in the local newspaper; after the family was sent a letter introducing the research project, a phone call was made to determine a family's willingness to participate, and finally a home visit for the purpose of enrolling the family was conducted. Seventy percent of eligible families agreed to enroll and were paid for each data collection. For purposes of this report the sample was divided roughly in half; more specifically, analyses were carried out initially on 65 infants whom we expected to represent half the total sample and then on the 57 infants who were subsequently enrolled in the investigation.

Procedure and Measurements

Data presented in this article were gathered across a 10-month period, ranging from the time the child was 10 months of age until he was 20 months of age. At age 10 months, mothers and fathers completed, as part of an extensive questionnaire packet, a parent-report measure of infant temperament. When each infant was 12 and 13 months of age, mother and father, respectively, brought the child into the university laboratory for an extensive series of procedures designed to elicit positive and negative emotional reactions. At ages 18 and 20 months, mothers and fathers, respectively, returned to the laboratory with their child for a much more limited assessment of emotionality. Mothers' lab visits preceded fathers' visits because past experience indicates that fathers' involvement in the research process is frequently promoted by mothers' preceding involvement and because mother–father differences were not of concern to the research program.

Temperament report: 10 months. To assess both positive and negative emotionality, we selected Rothbart's (1981, 1986) Infant Behavior Questionnaire (IBQ), which reliably assesses six temperament dimensions, because it emphasized individual differences in emotionality and shows good psychometric qualities (Goldsmith & Rothbart, 1991; Rothbart, 1981). For maternal report of Activity Level, Smiling and Laughter, Duration of Orienting, Soothability. Fear, and Distress to Limitations, Rothbart (1981) reported mean 9- to 12-month stabilities of .68, .72, .64, .29, .61, and .65, respectively. Furthermore, IBQ scales have shown appropriate convergence with scales from other infant temperament questionnairs (Goldsmith & Rieser-Danner, 1986). In the current (total) sample, internal consistency (coefficient alphas) across mother and father reports for the six subscales ranged from .71 to .88. For purposes of the present investigation, and following Rothbart (1986), we created second-order composite variables reflecting Positive Emotionality (smiling and laughter + duration of orientation) and Negative Emotionality (fear + distress to limitations); for the total sample, across mothers and fathers, internal consistency ranged from .82 to .87.

Laboratory assessments: 12 and 13 months. The laboratory assessments carried out at 12 months (with mother) and 13 months (with father) were identical in nature and consisted of a series of six experimental probes designed to evoke infant positive and negative emotion. (a) First, the standard Strange Situation (Ainsworth, Blehar, Waters, & Wall, 1978) was administered, which involves numerous opportunities for children to express positive affect (free play and reunion episodes) and negative affect (separation episodes). (b) Following the Strange Situation, and in a separate laboratory room, parent and child were given the opportunity to engage in free play for a period of 5 min with a standard set of toys. (c) Next, a parent-positive-approach sequence was instituted, in which the parent was instructed to try to make the child smile and laugh while the child was seated in a high chair. Specifically, the parent approached the child in a series of graded steps (marked on the floor) across a distance of 3 m, endeavoring to evoke positive reactions from the child (through talking, smiling, and laughing). (d) An identical stranger-positive-approach sequence followed the parent-approach procedure, using as a stranger a woman total unfamiliar to the child (i.e., not the stranger from the Strange Situation). (e) Next, a puppet show involving hand puppets laughing and giggling and mentioning the child's name was presented to the child (still in the high chair) by two, now-familiar laboratory staff members; it lasted $1\frac{1}{2}$ min. (f) Finally, a four-episode frustration task was administered. In the first 90 s of this procedure, parent and child played together with an attractive busy-box toy, immediately after which he parent held the busy box just out of reach from the child (still seated in the high chair) for 2 min while maintaining a neutral expression and not interacting with the child. In the third episode of this procedure, the child was given the toy, but the parent refrained from interaction, maintaining a neutral posture. Finally, the parent joined the child's play for 1 min.

Separate teams of coders rated, from videotape, the extent and intensity of the positive and negative emotions expressed (in face, voice, and body) by the infant every 15 s, using 5-point scales ranging from 0 (no emotion expressed) to 4 (intense emotion expressed). Interrater agreement for emotionality coding was calculated using Cohen's kappa. Positive emotionality yielded a mean standard kappa of .82, as did negative emotionality. The intercorrelation of scores between pairs of coders exceeded .9 for both positivity and negativity.

To composite emotionality data, we undertook a series of data reduction steps. First, emotionality ratings on infant behavior during the Strange Situation were averaged within episode, yielding mean positive and mean negative emotionality scores for each child for each of the seven episodes of the Strange Situation that were coded (i.e., Episodes 2–8). Next, the emotionality ratings made every 15 s during the remainder of the laboratory procedure were averaged (separately for positivity and negativity) within free-play, mother-approach, stranger-approach, and puppet show tasks. Finally, average positive and average negative emotionality ratings were generated for each of the four phases of the frustration task (engagement, withdrawal, toy return, and reengagement). Because mean positivity scores for the middle two phases of the frustration task (toy withdrawal and toy return) were extremely low and involved minimal variation, these scores were deleted from further analyses, resulting in a total of 13 mean positive emotionality ratings and 15 mean negative emotionality ratings per child. These scores were subsequently subjected to factor analysis for purposes of data reduction; results of these analyses are presented in the Results section of this article.

Laboratory assessments: 18 and 20 months. Only a single procedure, the Strange Situation, was administered during the 18- and 20-month lab visits with the expressed purpose of assessing infant emotionality. Scoring of positivity and negativity was carried out in the same manner as at 12 and 13 months, using the same coders, making sure, though, that no coders scored the same child more than once.

RESULTS

Results of this investigation are reported in two major sections. In the first, efforts to develop and evaluate the adequacy of a two-dimensional model of infant emotionality are presented. Following this, analyses examining relations between early emotionality (end of the first year) and later emotionality (at 18 and 20 months) are presented.

Model Development and Testing

Three stages of model development and testing were carried out. First, efforts were undertaken to develop and evaluate the adequacy of a two-dimensional measurement model of infant emotionality with the first half of the sample ($n = 65$). Second, efforts were made to confirm in the second half of the sample findings resulting from the first half of the sample ($n = 57$). Finally, on finding support—via initial testing and subsequent confirmation—of a two-dimensional measurement model of emotionality, the adequacy of an alternative one-dimensional model was evaluated. All LISREL model testing utilized variance–covariance matrices (rather than correlation matrices).

Sample 1: Developing and testing a two-dimensional model. Because positive and negative emotionality were assessed in the same emotion-elicitation situations, the decision was made to separately construct positivity and negativity composite measures that could then be used in LISREL model testing. Toward this end, the mean positivity and negativity ratings generated for the various emotion-elicitation situations were subject to exploratory factor analysis, all with an eye toward creating

TABLE 1

Emotionality Factor Weights for Samples 1 and 2:
Strange Situation (SS)

Episode	SS POS12	SS POS13	SS NEG12	SS NEG13
	Sample 1			
2. M + B	.54	.31	.28	.26
3. M + B + S	.66	.57	.45	.49
4. B + S	.58	.57	.78	.69
5. M + B	.71	.74	.85	.79
6. B	.13	.27	.75	.78
7. S + B	.41	.62	.83	.84
8. M + B	.54	.68	.71	.65
	Sample 2			
2. M + B	.49	.56	−.03	.49
3. M + B + S	.50	.54	.44	.53
4. B + S	.33	.56	.79	.76
5. M + B	.69	.71	.82	.80
6. B	−.03	.40	.75	.76
7. S + B	.08	.65	.88	.85
8. M + B	.46	.30	.57	.77

Note: POS = positivity; NEG = negativity; M = mother; B = baby;
S = stranger.

composite variables that could serve as multiple indicators of separate latent constructs of positivity and negativity in a LISREL 7 measurement model. More specifically, principal-axis factor analyses were carried out on eight distinct sets of Sample 1 data in a effort to determine whether single-factor solutions were sufficient to represent the available information: (a) 12-month strange situation positivity scores, (b) 13-month strange situation positivity scores, (c) 12-month strange situation negativity scores, (d) 13-month strange situation negativity scores, (e) 12-month post-strange situation positivity scores, (f) 13-month post-strange situation positivity scores, (g) 12-month post-strange situation negativity scores, and (h) 13-month post-strange situation negativity scores. In all cases only a single eigenvalue exceeded 1.0, and in six of these cases, the loadings of individual variables on these single-factor solutions were almost uniformly high. In two cases, however, the single-factor loadings were very discrepant and clustered into two subgroups such that one subset of variables had markedly higher loadings than did a second subset of variables. In these two cases involving positive emotionality at 12 months and at 13 months in the post-strange situation episodes, the data were refactored using the principal-axis extraction method and oblique rotation in an effort to determine whether a two-factor solution might better represent the data. In both cases it appeared to, as discrepant loadings on single-factor solutions bifurcated into high loadings on two separate factors. The factor loadings for the six sets of variables that yielded single-factor solutions are presented in the top half of Tables 1 and 2, along with the loadings for the two sets of variables that yielded two-factor solutions; the latter are labeled, respectively, A and B. Thus, a total of 10 factors emerged from the exploratory analyses carried out on the eight sets of data. To create composite scores for use in subsequent analyses, we summed together variables loading at the level of .3 or higher on each factor.

The next phase of data analysis was designed to test the adequacy of a two-dimensional model of infant emotionality comprising two latent variables, one reflecting infant positivity and the other

TABLE 2

Emotionality Factor Weights for Samples 1 and 2: Post-Strange Situation (P-SS) Procedures

Situation	Positive Emotionality				Negative Emotionality	
	P-SS POS12A	P-SS POS12B	P-SS POS13A	P-SS POS13B	P-SS NEG12	P-SS NEG13
			Sample 1			
Free play	.19	.14	.12	.23	.13	.20
Parent approach	.53	.04	.75	.06	.57	.57
Stranger approach	.54	.20	.67	.17	.48	.72
Puppet show	.41	−.21	.58	−.15	.37	.58
Frustration						
Engage	.06	.43	−.06	.47	.44	.62
Withdraw	—[a]	—[a]	—[a]	—[a]	.59	.66
Toy return	—[a]	—[a]	—[a]	—[a]	.78	.77
Re-engage	−.13	.51	−.02	.48	.72	.66
			Sample 2			
Free play	−.03	.13	.00	.74	.42	.28
Parent approach	.32	−.09	.64	−.01	.37	.56
Stranger approach	.63	−.07	.72	−.02	.68	.80
Puppet show	.52	.14	.38	.14	.77	.65
Frustration						
Engage	−.27	.37	−.02	.74	.75	.86
Withdraw	—[a]	—[a]	—[a]	—[a]	.47	.56
Toy return	—[a]	—[a]	—[a]	—[a]	.73	.76
Re-engage	.21	.37	.22	.34	.80	.79

Note: POS = positivity; NEG = negativity; A = Factor 1; B = Factor 2; numerals indicate age in months.
[a]Variable not included in factor analysis.

infant negativity. Toward this end, the 10 factor analytically derived indices of positive and negative emotionality, along with the two mother-report scores and two father-report scores of positive and negative emotionality based on the IBQ, were used as multiple indicators to test a LISREL 7 measurement model with two latent factors. The latent factor Positive Emotionality included all eight positivity scores (six behavioral factors + two parent reports), and the latent factor Negative Emotionality consisted of all six negativity scores (four behavioral factors + two parent reports). Results of this analysis indicated not only that the model was a poor fit, χ^2 (76, $N = 62$) = 146.68, $p < .001$, goodness-of-fit index (GFI) = .77, root-mean-square residual (rms_R) = .13, but also that loadings for father reports of positive and negative emotionality, for the maternal positivity report, and for the second, 12-month post-strange situation positivity factor (PSSPOS12B: frustration task) were statistically nonsignificant.

An alternative measurement model was subsequently tested, deleting these three parental reports and the just-mentioned positivity factor. The chi-square value of 59.85 with 34 degrees of freedom proved significant at the .004 level (GFI = .86 rms_R = .09), indicating that the model still could be improved, even though fit had improved and all loadings were significant. Inspection of modification indices revealed that there might be a significant correlation between residuals of positive and negative emotionality ratings in the Strange Situation at 13 months, because of its large modification index of 12.34. After allowing for these residuals to be correlated, the measurement model was found to be a good fit. The chi-square value was nonsignificant (46.67, $df = 33$, $p = .06$); the GFI was above .8

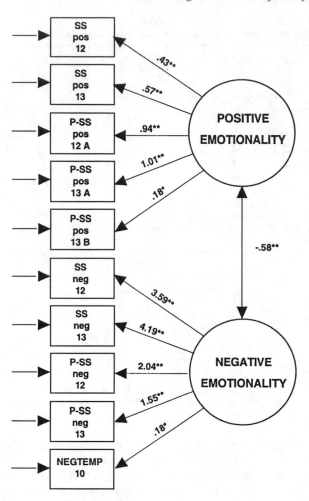

Figure 1. Two-latent-variable measurement model of infant emotionality (Sample 1, *n* = 65). SS = Strange Situation; P-SS = post-Strange Situation; NEGTEMP = maternal report of negativity; pos = positive emotionality; neg = negative emotionality; A = Factor 1; B = Factor 2; numerals indicate age in months. * $p < .05$; ** $p < .01$.

(i.e., .89), and the rms_R was below .1 (i.e., .08). In addition, only 3 of 45 standardized residuals were greater than 2.

The LISREL 7 estimates for the measurement model are presented in Fig. 1 with the correlated residual deleted. As can be seen, although a two-dimensional model of emotionality fit the data, the latent variables generated using the indicators available were by no means independent: Infants evincing high negativity evinced low positivity (and vice versa). Despite the significant association between Positive Emotionality and Negative Emotionality, it remains the case that approximately 66% of the variance in one emotionality dimension could not be explained by variation in the other emotionality dimension. Thus, although not completely orthogonal, positivity and negativity appeared to be clearly separable.

Sample 2: Confirming the two-dimensional model. In light of the fact that the two-latent factor measurement model of Positive and Negative Emotionality had to be adjusted in unanticipated ways on the basis of nonsignificant loadings for certain indicators and as a result of modification indices pertaining to originally unspecified correlated residuals, an effort was made to confirm the resulting measurement model with the second half of the sample. As a first step toward this end, the same emotionality ratings initially factored in Sample 1 (see top halves of Tables 1 and 2) were subject to an identical series of exploratory factor analyses on Sample 2 data. The results of these analyses are presented in the bottom halves of Tables 1 and 2 (to facilitate comparison with Sample 1 data). Inspection of the factor loadings reveals striking similarity across the two subsamples. Of the total of 68 loadings across 10 factors, in only four instances did a variable load substantially differently across the two sub-samples, defined as meeting the .30 cut-off in one sample but not the other. In fact, when factor loadings derived from Sample 2 were used to generate composite scores for Sample 1, the correlation between the original Sample 1 composite scores and those derived for Sample 1 using Sample 2 results ranged from .76 to .99, with a mean of .94. The same pattern of highly correlated composite scores emerged when Sample 2 composite scores were recreated using Sample 1 factor results (range = .78 to .99, $M = .94$).

In light of the similarity of factor-analytic results across the two subsamples, the next step in confirming the two-dimensional model of emotionality under consideration involved testing the equality of factor structure across two samples, that is, determining whether the estimates of factor loadings, factor intercorrelations, residuals, and the correlated residual between positive and negative emotionality ratings in the Strange Situation at 13 months in the measurement model established on Sample 1 were equivalent across the two samples. LISREL 7's procedures of multisample analyses were used by declaring the factor-loading matrix, factor intercorrelation matrix, and the residual matrix to be invariant across samples (Joreskog & Sörbom, 1989). The resulting nonsignificant chi-square value of 98.26 with 88 degrees of freedom ($p = .213$) indicated that the same factor structure and estimates held in both samples. In other words, the two-latent-factor measurement model of infant emotionality generated in Sample 1 could be confirmed in Sample 2.

Testing an alternative, one-dimensional model. Despite the fact that the two-latent-factor model of infant emotionality could be confirmed in Sample 2, the fact that the latent factors Positive Emotionality and Negative Emotionality were correlated relatively strongly raised the prospect that an alternative, one-dimensional model of emotionality might better reflect the underlying structure of the multiple indicators of infant positivity and negativity. To address this issue empirically, we used a hierarchical nested model approach using the chi-square difference test that evaluates the statistical significance of the parameters that differentiate between two competing models (Bentler & Bonett, 1980). Significant improvement in fit was found in the two-dimensional model over the one-dimensional model, $\Delta\chi^2$ (1, $N = 122$) = 26.97, $p < .0001$. Note that correlated residuals were retained in both models.

The process of comparing the one- and two-dimensional models also was reversed to determine whether the two-dimensional model would still prove a better fit if first a one-dimensional model was developed and then the nested two-dimensional model was compared to it. More specifically, an initial, poor-fitting one-dimensional model including all 10 indicators was revised on the basis of modification indices to permit two correlated residuals that resulted in a good-fitting one-dimensional model. With this one-dimensional model in hand, a two-dimensional alternative model was then tested against it with the same hierarchichal/nested model approach detailed above. Once again it was found, using the chi-square difference test that evaluates the statistical significance of the parameters that differentiates two competing models, that the two-dimensional model provided a significant improvement in fit over the one-dimensional model, $\Delta\chi^2$ (1, $N = 122$) = 8.96, $p < .01$.

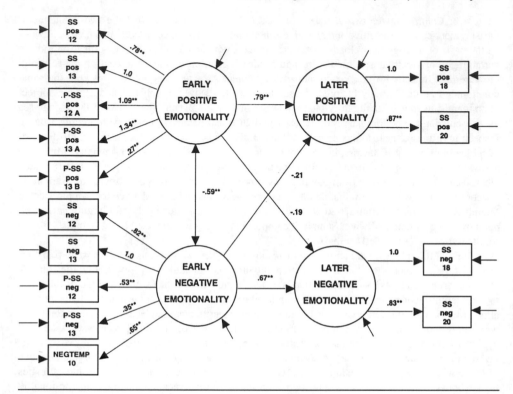

Figure 2. Structural equation model of cross-time relations between early (12/13 months) and later (18/20 months) positive and negative emotionality (*n* = 104). SS = Strange Situation; P-SS = post-Strange Situation; NEGTEMP = maternal report of negativity; pos = positive emotionality; neg = negative emotionality; A = Factor 1; B = Factor 2; numerals indicate age in months. Correlations between error terms for the same variables over time were estimated as required in a model including repeated measures. Parameter estimates of paths from early to later emotionality are standardized coefficients. The within-time relation between early positive and negative emotionality is a correlation coefficient. *$p < .05$; **$p < .01$.

Discriminant Stability and Validity of Emotionality

Having found that a two-dimensional model of infant emotionality better fit the 12- to 13-month data than did a one-dimensional model, attention was turned to validating the two dimensions discerned. Toward this end, structural equation modeling was used to determine whether cross-time linkages within emotionality constructs (earlier positivity–later positivity and earlier negativity–later negativity) were stronger than cross-time linkages between emotionality constructs (earlier positivity–later negativity and earlier negativity–later positivity). Table 3 presents the intercorrelation of all observed variables in the model along with descriptive statistics (means and standard deviations). The results of the structural equation analysis that are dipicted in Fig. 2 (with correlated residuals deleted) provide strong support for the two-dimensional model: When a latent negativity construct comprising 18- and 20-month negative emotionality scores (based on composited strange situation negativity ratings) is predicted using the earlier measured, latent constructs of negativity and positivity, it is strongly and significantly predicted by earlier negativity but not by positivity (see standard path

TABLE 3

Descriptive Statistics and Intercorrelation of Emotionality Composite Scores

Factor	1	2	3	4	5	6	7	8	9	10	11	12	13	14
1. SSPOS12														
2. SSPOS13	.36**													
3. SSNEG12	-.28**	-.34**												
4. SSNEG13	-.15	-.53**	.59**											
5. P-SSPOS12A	.30**	.26**	-.39**	-.22*										
6. P-SSPOS12B	.04	-.09	.04	.11	.03									
7. P-SSPOS13A	.20*	.32**	-.12	-.21*	.36**	.15								
8. P-SSPOS13B	.14	.18	-.17	-.11	.12	.38**	.26**							
9. P-SSNEG12	-.18	-.14	.31**	-.27**	-.26**	-.05	-.08	-.03						
10. P-SSNEG13	-.02	-.10	.08	.27**	.07	.04	-.16	-.15	.39**					
11. SSPOS18	.21*	.33**	-.23*	-.28**	.27**	.07	.35**	.16	-.03	.02				
12. SSPOS20	.26**	.32**	-.16	-.35**	.09	.02	.28**	.19	-.16	-.18	.32**			
13. SSNEG18	-.10	-.37**	.43**	.51**	-.15	.06	-.25*	-.10	.39**	.33**	-.41**	-.32**		
14. SSNEG20	-.16	-.25*	.32**	.46**	-.02	-.04	-.12	-.19	.22*	.23*	-.24*	-.50**	.58**	
M	1.15	0.86	6.44	8.12	2.40	0.25	2.08	0.34	6.06	5.59	0.92	0.83	8.64	8.57
SD	0.93	0.83	4.74	5.58	1.47	0.38	1.54	0.50	4.09	4.64	0.76	0.80	4.78	5.87

Note: SS = Strange Situation; P-SS = post-Strange Situation; POS = positivity; NEG = negativity; A = Factor 1; B = Factor 2; numerals indicate age in months.
* $p < .05$. ** $p < .01$.

coefficients). When a latent positivity construct comprising 18- and 20-month positive emotionality scores (based on composited strange situation ratings) is predicted using the earlier measured, latent constructs of negativity and positivity, it is strongly and significantly predicted by earlier positivity but not by negativity (see standardized path coefficients). Discriminant predictive validity is clearly achieved. Moreover, even though early positivity and negativity proved to be significantly associated with the full sample, they are clearly separable. Finally, it should be noted that although the overall fit of the model depicted in Fig. 2 was not of central concern (only the cross-time associations), the model fit the data reasonably well. That is, even though the chi-square value of the structural equation depicted in Fig. 2 was significant, χ^2 (67, $N = 105$) = 125.63, $p < .000$, the ratio of chi-square to degrees of freedom was 1.88 (GFI = .86, $rms_R = .08$). With large samples, some authorities assert that ratios of less than 2.0 provide better tests of fit than do pure chi-square values (Bollen, 1989; Hayduk, 1987).

DISCUSSION

It is not uncommon, when discussing temperament and personality with laypersons and developmental scholars alike, to discover that many assume emotionality to be a bipolar construct. Infants, children, and even adults who are highly irritable or more generally negative in disposition are, by definition, presumed not to be particularly happy, joyous, or enthusiastic in character. This (mis)understanding is surprising in light of an abundance of evidence in the adult mood and personality literature indicating that positivity and negativity are more independent of, than correlated with, one another (Tellegen, 1985). As was noted in our introduction, in the study of mood, positive emotion items load on one factor, and negative emotion factors load on a relatively orthogonal factor; in the study of personality, tendencies to be depressed, anxious, and hostile are central to the construct of neuroticism, whereas feelings of joy and enthusiasm are central to the construct of extraversion.

In light of Diener et al.'s (1995) recent analysis of the structure of adult affect, it appears that these observations may lead to the erroneous conclusion that negative and positive emotionality are completely independent. Addressing virtually the same fundamental question as the current study, but using adults as participants and relying on self-reports and informant reports of frequency of positive and negative emotions across days and months, these investigators found latent positivity and latent negativity constructs to be significantly and inversely correlated ($r = -.44$). They further discovered, however, that a two-dimensional model of emotion better fit the data than did a one-dimensional model, much the same way as did Green et al. (1993), who reported an extremely strong negative association (−.85) between pleasurable affect and unpleasureable affect in another study of adults. Such findings led Diener et al. (1995) to the conclusion that positive and negative affective experiences are best conceptualized as "separable" (implying a moderate degree of association), rather than as strictly independent (implying complete orthogonality) or bipolar (implying a perfect −1.0 correlation).

In the current investigation we set out to determine, in much the same way as did Diener et al. (1995), whether positive and negative emotional reactivity were better conceptualized as two separable constructs or as separate ends of a single, bipolar continuum (i.e., high negativity implies low positivity). Toward that end, we had mothers and fathers complete temperament reports on their infants when they were 10 months of age and then observed and rated positive and negative reactivity to a series of emotion-eliciting procedures in our laboratory when infants were 12 and 13 months of age. Not only did we find that a measurement model comprising two latent variables, one reflecting multiple indicators of positivity and the other multiple indicators of negativity, fit the data reasonably well after some modest modification of the model with our first 65 participants, but we also found that this two-dimensional model could be confirmed on a second sample of 57 participants. Moreover, comparisons of this two-construct model with a model reflecting a single, bipolar, emotionality construct clearly indicated that the two-construct model fit the available data better than did the single-construct model. Perhaps most significant, though, was evidence that positivity and negativity measured at the end of the first year differentially predicted positivity and negativity measured in the middle of the second year. Like Goldsmith and Campos's (1990) multimethod data gathered on 9-month-olds, these data provide strong support for a conceptualization of temperament and emotionality that distinguishes between positive and negative affectivity rather than assuming them to be opposite poles of a bipolar continuum. Given the significant inverse association (−.59) discerned between positivity and negativity with the full sample (see Fig. 2), "separable, but not strictly independent" would seem to characterize the nature of the relation between positive and negative emotionality discerned in this study of infants much as it did the relation between pleasurable and unpleasurable affect in the Diener et al. (1995) investigation of college students.

From a methodological standpoint, it seems noteworthy that the data provided by parental reports of infant temperament contributed little to the measurement model of infant positive and negative emotionality. Although this might reflect the fact that temperament reports were obtained a few months prior to eliciting emotional reactivity in the laboratory, and thus the possibility that emotionality changed over time, recent work by Seifer, Sameroff, Barrett, and Krafchuk (1994) suggests that it makes more sense to question the validity of parent reports (see also Kagan, 1994). Analysis at 8 weeks of infant temperament ratings by observers and by mothers revealed little correspondence between maternal and observer data, despite the fact that mothers rated their infants' behavior during the period when observations were made and used a questionnaire that mirrored the scoring system used by observers. In fact, Seifer et al. (1994) concluded on the basis of their extensive analysis of these two sources of data that "mothers are a poor source of information about their infants' behavioral style" (p. 1489). In light of results from the current study showing that at least one score based on maternal ratings could be included in the measurement model (i.e., difficulty), whereas this was true of no father-report scores, this conclusion would seem to apply even more strongly to fathers.

Beyond this methodological conclusion, the results of this inquiry clearly suggest that even though infant positivity and negativity are not completely independent, they do represent separable dimensions of temperament and emotionality. Fundamentally, infants who are highly positive are not necessarily very low in their negativity, and infants who are very low in their positivity are not necessarily very high in their negativity. What remains unclear on the basis of this investigation is the exact degree of independence or dependence one should expect of these two attributes of individuality. Quite conceivably, the nonindependence discerned in the current inquiry could be partly a function of the fact that positivity and negativity were scored in the same emotion-eliciting situations. The fact that a baby crying in one 15-s measurement interval is virtually unable to smile in the same interval, with the reverse being true as well, might well account for some of the interdependence observed between positivity and negativity in this study.

Actually, what becomes interesting when considered from a developmental perspective is when, how, and why these dimensions of emotionality become functionally related over time. Do positivity and negativity become more independent in adulthood because over time these constructs dissociate from one another, as a traditional developmental perspective emphasizing increasing differentiation might suggest? Or is it the case that positivity and negativity are as independent in infancy and childhood as they are in adulthood, but because of the measurement approach adopted in this investigation, they simply do not appear that way? Or might it be the case that for some children, for some reasons (biological or experiential) positivity and negativity become associated but for otheres they do not? If so, why?

Whatever the answers to these queries, the results of this inquiry highlight the utility, if not need, for thinking about infant emotionality in terms of at least two dimensions, positivity and negativity.

Such thinking stimulates thoughts about the way these distinctive dimensions go together. Some infants, after all, are likely to be high or low in both positivity and negativity, whereas others might be relatively high on one and intermediate on another. Beyond the work of Thomas and Chess (1977) highlighting the prototypic difficult child, easy child, and slow-to-warm-up child, combinations or patterns of temperament and emotionality attributes have rarely been examined, especially when it comes to investigating the consequences of temperament for parent–child interaction, for relations between siblings, or as a final example, for the development of behavior problems. Again and again, investigators tend to focus on a single dimension, typically negativity, seeming to believe that by capturing this feature of individuality, they have also captured the child's proclivity to react and behave in a positively emotional manner. This almost exclusive emphasis on negativity no doubt derives from presumptions that behavior problems that emerge later in childhood may have their origins in the negativity displayed by the infant that parents can find difficult to cope with.

It is not inconceivable that the tendency to examine temperament dimensions in isolation—or even when multiple dimensions are considered to address only their additive predictive power—may explain, at least in part, why much evidence regarding temperamental influences is so mixed. In fact, might it not be the case that Crockenberg (1986) found the evidence for an effect of infant negativity and difficultness on mother interaction so inconsistent because temperamental attributes were not considered "in context," that is, in the context of other dimensions of temperament? It is not difficult to imagine, for instance, that the effect of having a very irritable or negative infant may depend greatly on the infant's other emotional attributes. Caring for a baby, or young child, who is especially prone to distress, yet simultaneously inclined to smile and laugh a lot, is likely a quite different experience than caring for a child who is very negative and not at all positively inclined. Whereas the joy that the former child is disposed to experience and the smiles and laughs that she is inclined to emit may protect the parent from much of the stress and strain that the child's negative proclivities might engender, the parent of the latter child may experience little "protection" of this sort. One important consequence, then, of recognizing that positivity and negativity are two distinct dimensions is that it may enable us to study the effects of temperament—in this case on patterns of parenting—in ways different than we have in the past.

When the possibility is considered, as well, that positivity itself may be related to "sensation seeking" (Zuckerman, 1979) and, thereby, eventual risk taking, it becomes apparent that a two-dimensional approach to the study of infant emotionality may also affect the way relations between temperament and behavior problems are conceptualized and studied. Rather than presuming, as tends to be the case, that the origins of problem behavior lie in proneness to negative emotion, empirical inquiry that distinguishes positivity from negativity may find that either high positive emotionality by itself, or high positivity coupled with high negativity, may serve as the temperamental and emotional foundation for the development of problematic behavior.

This discussion of potential conceptual and empirical benefits that may accrue from distinguishing between positive and negative emotionality should not be read to imply that individual differences in these emotional proclivities are necessarily stable over time. Fundamentally, that is an empirical question quite distinct from the one central to this inquiry. Nevertheless, the last set of data presented in this report documents considerable stability across a 6-month period from 12–13 months to 18–20 months. This does not mean, however, that all the instability is necessarily a product of measurement error; indeed, given the features of structural equation modeling, such error is far less influential in this inquiry than is typically the case when single indicators of each construct are used to assess cross-time stability. Thus, a question that should become ever more central to the study of temperament and emotionality has to do with the conditions of stability and instability in negative and positive emotionality. Belsky et al.'s (1991) investigation of this issue across a 6-month period in the first year of life indicated that the factors and processes associated with change in one dimension were not those associated with change in the other dimension (see also Fish, Stifter, & Belsky, 1991); in fact, processes associated with declines in negativity were by no means the same (or just the inverse) of those associated with increases in negativity. (See also Maziade, Cote, Bernier, Bouitin, and Thivierge, 1989, for comparable findings from 5 months to 5 years.) Clearly, distinguishing between two dimensions of emotionality holds much promise for the study of development during infancy and early childhood years.

REFERENCES

Ainsworth, M., Blehar, M., Waters, E., & Wall, S. (1978). *Patterns of attachment.* Hillsdale, NJ: Erlbaum.

Balatsky, G., & Diener, E. (1993). Subjective well-being among Russian students. *Social Indicators Research, 28,* 21–39.

Bates, J., Freeland, C., & Lounsbury, M. (1979). Measurement of infant difficultness. *Child Development, 50,* 794–803.

Bates, J., Maslin, C., & Frankel, K. (1985). Attachment security, mother–child interaction, and temperament as predictors of behavior problem ratings at age three years. In I. Bretherton & E. Waters (Eds.), *Growing points attachment theory and research: Monographs of the Society for Research in Child Development, 50* (1–2, Serial No. 209), 167–193.

Belsky, J., Crnic, K., & Gable, S. (1995). Determinants of co-parenting in families with toddler boys. *Child Development, 66,* 629–642.

Belsky, J., Crnic, K., & Woodworth, S. (in press). Personality and parenting. *Journal of Personality.*

Belsky, J., Fish, M., & Isabella, R. (1991). Continuity and discontinuity in infant negative and positive emotionality: Family antecedents and attachment consequences. *Developmental Psychology, 27,* 421–431.

Belsky, J., & Pensky, E. (1988). Developmental history, personality and family relationships: Toward an emergent family system. In R. Hinde & J. Stevenson-Hinde (Eds.), *Relationships within families* (pp. 193–217). Oxford, UK: Oxford University Press.

Belsky, J., & Rovine, M. (1987). Temperament and attachment security in the Strange Situation: An empirical rapprochement. *Child Development, 58,* 787–795.

Bentler, P., & Bonett, D. (1980). Significance tests and goodness of fit in the analysis of covariance structures. *Psychological Bulletin, 88,* 588–606.

Bollen, K. (1989). *Structural equations with latent variables.* New York: Wiley.

Buss, A., & Plomin, R. (1984). *Temperament: Early developing personality traits.* Hillsdale, NJ: Erlbaum.

Costa, P., Jr., & McCrae, R. (1985). *The NEO personality inventory manual.* Odessa, FL: Psychological Assessment Resources.

Crockenberg, S. (1986). Are temperamental differences in babies associated with predictable differences in caregiving? In J. Lerner & R. Lerner (Eds.), *New directions for child development: Temperament and social interaction during infancy and childhood* (pp. 53–73). San Francisco: Jossey-Bass.

Davidson, R. (1993). The neuropsychology of emotion and affective style. In M. Lewis & J. Haviland (Eds.), *The handbook of emotion* (pp. 143–154). New York: Guilford Press.

Diener, E., Smith, H., & Fujita, F. (1995). The personality structure of affect. *Journal of Personality and Social Psychology, 69,* 130–141.

Fish, M., Stifter, C., & Belsky, J. (1991). Conditions of continuity and discontinuity in infant negative emotionality: Newborn to five months. *Child Development, 62,* 1525–1538.

Gable, S., Belsky, J., & Crnic, K. (1995). A descriptive account of coparenting during the child's second year. *Journal of Marriage and the Family, 57,* 609–616.

Goldsmith, H., Buss, A., Plomin, R., Rothbart, M., Thomas, A., Chess, S., Hinde, R., & McCall, R. (1987). Roundtable: What is temperament? Four approaches. *Child Development, 58,* 505–529.

Goldsmith, H., & Campos, J. (1990). The structure of temperamental fear and pleasure in infants: A psychometric perspective. *Child Development, 61*, 1944–1964.

Goldsmith, H., & Rieser-Danner, L. (1989). Variation among temperament theories and validational studies of temperament assessment. In G. A. Kohnstamm (Ed.), *Temperament discussed: Temperament and development in infancy and childhood* (pp. 1–9). Lisse, The Netherlands: Swets.

Goldsmith, H., & Rothbart, M. (1991). Contemporary instruments for assessing early temperament by questionnaire and in the laboratory. In J. Strelau & A. Angleitner (Eds.), *Explorations in temperament: Contemporary conceptualizations, measurement and methodological issues* (pp. 129–147). New York: Plenum Press.

Green, D., Goldman, S., & Salovey, P. (1993). Measurement error masks bipolarity in affect ratings. *Journal of Personality and Social Psychology, 64*, 1029–1041.

Hayduk, L. (1987). *Structural equation modeling with LISREL.* Baltimore, MD: Johns Hopkins University Press.

Joreskog, K., & Sörbom, D. (1989). *LISREL 7: A guide to the program and applications* (2nd ed.). Chicago, IL: SPSS Inc.

Kagan, J. (1994). *Galen's prophecy.* New York: Basic Books.

Matheny, A., Wilson, R., & Nuss, S. (1984). Toddler temperament: Stability across settings and over ages. *Child Development, 55*, 1200–1211.

Maziade, M., Cote, R., Bernier, H., Bouitin, P., & Thivierge, J. (1989). Significance of extreme temperament in infancy for clinical status in preschool year: II. Patterns of temperament change in implications for the appearance of disorders. *British Journal of Psychiatry, 154*, 544–551.

McCrae, R., & John, O. (1992). An introduction to the five-factor model and its applications. *Personality, 60*, 175–215.

Rothbart, M., (1981). Measurement of temperament in infancy. *Child Development, 52*, 569–578.

Rothbart, M. (1986). Longitudinal observation of infant temperament. *Developmental Psychology, 22*, 356–365.

Seifer, R., Sameroff, A., Barrett, L., & Krafchuk, E. (1994). Infant temperament measured by multiple observations and mother reports. *Child Development, 65*, 1478–1490.

Sroufe, L. A. (1985). Attachment classification from the perspective of infant–caregiver relationships and infant temperament. *Child Development, 56*, 1–14.

Tellegen, A. (1985). Structures of mood and personality and their relevance to assessing anxiety, with an emphasis on self-report. In A. Tuma & J. Maser (Eds.), *Anxiety and the anxiety disorders* (pp. 681–706). Hillsdale, NJ: Erlbaum.

Thomas, A., & Chess, S. (1977). *Temperament and development.* New York: Bruner/Mazel.

Watson, D. (1988). Intra-individual and inter-individual analyses of positive and negative affect. *Journal of Personality and Social Psychology, 54*, 1020–1030.

Watson, D., & Clark, L. (1984). Negative affectivity: The disposition to experience aversive emotional states. *Psychological Bulletin, 96*, 465–490.

Watson, D., Clark, L., & Tellegen, A. (1984). Cross-cultural convergence in the structure of mood: A Japanese replication and a comparison with U.S. findings. *Journal of Personality and Social Psychology, 47*, 127–144.

Zuckerman, M. (1979). *Sensation seeking: Beyond the optimal level of arousal.* Hillsdale, NJ: Erlbaum.

3

The Emanuel Miller Memorial Lecture 1995 Children's Relationships: Bridging the Divide Between Cognitive and Social Development

Judy Dunn

Social, Genetic and Developmental Psychiatry Centre,
Institute of Psychiatry, London

Recent research that bridges the divide between cognitive and social development in early childhood illuminates, but also sets challenges, for both fields. The implications of recent studies of children's social interactions for research on cognitive development—in particular, the development of understanding mind and emotion—are considered, then the implications of new cognitive research for understanding social development are discussed. An example of longitudinal research on children's relationships with family and friends between 2 and 7 years is described, highlighting links between individual differences in cognitive and social development.

INTRODUCTION

In a classic and illuminating study of children's social development carried out in the 1930s, Lois Barclay Murphy (1932) included a series of sensitive observations on the possible connections between the quality of children's friendships and their growing understanding of others. To make these connections, she argued, we need to look at and listen to children within their own worlds. Her attempt to bring together children's social and cognitive development raises the question of what progress we have made over the 60 years since her study in understanding how developments in these two broad domains are linked. Textbooks from the decades between the 1930s and the 1980s are notable for the divide between their presentation of cognitive development and social development. In accounts of cognitive development the child is chiefly viewed as a solitary thinker isolated from the social world, in spite of Piaget's acknowledgement of the significance of motivation and affect. And in most accounts of social development from this period the focus is also narrow, limited to a discussion of primary attachments and to the sociometrics of children's popularity within their peer group.

In the last decade or so, the picture has changed in some important ways. In particular, both research on children's relationships and studies of cognitive development that focus on children in

Reprinted with permission from *Journal of Child Psychology and Psychiatry*, 1996, Vol. 37(5), 507–518. Copyright © 1996 by the Association for Child Psychology and Psychiatry.
This research is supported by a grant from NIH (HD23158).

situations of emotional significance to them are beginning to bridge the divide, illuminating some of the connections between social and cognitive development. This research that bridges the divide not only provides clarification, but also sets challenges for both fields. On the one hand, recent studies of children's relationships present a new set of questions and research agenda for those studying children's understanding of mental states and emotion. On the other hand, the new relationship-relevant insights of cognitive developmentalists have major implications for those studying social development.

The focus of this article is on links between social and cognitive development as seen in children's relationships (not just social), in their understanding of other minds and emotions (not just cognitive). The far-reaching implications for future research are highlighted. In the first section below, the implications of recent studies of children's social interactions and relationships for ideas and research on cognitive development are considered. In the second section, the other side of the coin is considered: the implications of new cognitive research for those studying social development are discussed. In the third and final section, research on children's relationships that bridges the divide between social and cognitive development is illustrated. Although the focus will be upon young children where most research is available, the principles at issue are key throughout development. We begin with the issue of what can be learned from research on children's social relations in terms of children's growing understanding of mind and emotion.

CHILDREN'S INTERACTIONS WITH FAMILY AND FRIENDS: IMPLICATIONS FOR RESEARCH ON COGNITIVE DEVELOPMENT

The argument in the section that follows is, first, that the study of children within the context of their interactions with other family members and with their friends can illuminate the nature of their understanding of inner states and the connections between understanding other minds and action. Second, it can clarify what social processes are involved in the development of that understanding, and is especially illuminating on the development of individual differences. Third, there are important methodological lessons to be learned from this research.

Each of these three claims is considered below. Before they are discussed, some key shifts in orientation within the domain of cognitive development that have taken place over the last decades must be noted. Those that reflect an interest in the "socialization of cognition" are especially relevant to the argument of this article.

There is within cognitive psychology increasing interest in the ways in which affect influences the way that thinking proceeds (Goodnow, 1990). It is widely acknowledged now that, as Hoffman noted (see Hoffman, 1986, p. 200): Affect may initiate, terminate, accelerate, or disrupt information processing; it may determine which sector of the environment is processed and which processing modes operate; it may organize recall and influence category accessibility; it may contribute to the formation of emotionally charged schemata and categories; it may provide input for social cognition; and it may influence decision-making.

Numerous other writers have reflected recently on these connections. My point here is simply to emphasize the relevance of these general notions concerning affect for the developmental issues involved in considering children's social and intellectual growth.

There has also been a shift away from the notion of the child as a solitary thinker. This is for instance illustrated by the writing and experiments of Doise, Mugny and others in the Genevan group, on research that explores the idea that awareness of discrepancies between one's own perspective and those of another person can act as a key catalyst for cognitive change (e.g., Doise & Mugny, 1984). It is also illustrated in the increasing interest in Vygotskean accounts of cognitive development, with their strong emphasis on social interactions between more and less expert individuals working together on cognitive problems, as in the studies of Rogoff (1990). Here children are viewed as recipients of well-orchestrated enculturation on the part of "more competent" members of their culture.

A change is also evident in the new concern about the contextual validity of experimental tasks used in studies of cognitive development—especially in terms of the social situation in which children are placed in such tasks, and in the evidence for the impact of children's relations with the experimenter on their performance in these tasks (e.g., Lewis & Osborne, 1990). Perhaps most significantly, there has been a burst of interest among cognitive psychologists in children's understanding of mental life and its relation to people's behavior. It is this new work that has particular significance for those interested in children's social and emotional development (Astington, 1994; Perner, 1991; Wellman, 1990).

However, even though approaches to cognitive development are now open to criticism if they are not sensitive to the significance of the social context, and though the exciting new studies of children's understanding of mind and emotion clearly are centrally important to accounts of social development, much of the research to date appears very far from the emotional dramas of children's lives within their families and with their peers. Even the research conducted within a Vygotskean framework is chiefly limited to adult–child encounters of a didactic and emotionally neutral flavor as Goodnow has noted (Goodnow, 1990). In this first section, we consider the question of whether studies of children's interactions with their families and close friends in the emotional contexts of daily life can clarify the developmental questions at the heart of the cognitive research.

THE NATURE OF CHILDREN'S UNDERSTANDING OF MIND AND EMOTION

The nature of very young children's understanding of mind is an issue over which there is much current controversy in a remarkably rapidly growing field. Chandler, Fritz, and Hala (1989) characterized those who study children's mindreading abilities as either boosters or scoffers—depending on their willingness to attribute understanding to very young children (the boosters), or their stress on the limitations of children's capabilities (the scoffers). The distinction rests on a difference in theoretical orientation, however, it is not a trivial point that many of those who study children with naturalistic observations of their behavior and talk in their own world of family or peers are *boosters*. That is they emphasize the understanding that children show in these interactive settings. If children are observed in the heady world of shared pretend play, or the heat of battle with family or friends, many aspects of their behavior with those others appear to reflect considerable understanding of others' intentions, desires, or plans.

Of particular interest with regard to the controversies over their mindreading abilities are studies revealing the following: *teasing* which reflects some grasp of what will annoy or upset another, *jokes* that reflect some anticipation of what another will find funny, *sharing a pretend world* with another in make-believe play that involves an understanding of another's fantasy world *comforting* that reflects a grasp of what will ameliorate another's distress, or *deception*. This last, which will be briefly discussed as an example, has received much attention from theory of mind researchers, since intentional deception may involve an attempt to manipulate what another person thinks or believes.

The question of whether children of 3, 4 or 5 can and do intentionally deceive is of much current interest and dispute. Some studies in which the experimented attempts to test whether children understand the notion of deliberate deception report young children to be unable to do so (e.g., Sodian, 1991; Strichartz & Burton, 1990). In contrast, a recent study (Newton, 1994), which focused on naturally occurring incidents in which children apparently attempted to deceive other family members at home, documented a number of different kinds of deception shown by children of 3- and 4-years-old, and the circumstances in which such act appeared. There is considerable controversy among those who study deception in nonhuman primates about whether naturalistic observations of deception have established manipulation of what another thinks or believes in these animals, rather than simply the attempt to evade punishment or block intervention. It is an interesting debate, and highlights the need for caution in inferences about deception from nonverbal behavior in both human and nonhuman primates. However, conclusions about human children's deception must rest on the evidence from studies of children, and in the studies by Newton the evidence is powerful. Although Newton was admirably cautious about his interpretation of incidents of apparent deception, he drew attention both to the range of different kinds of deception engaged in, and to the circumstances in which such acts appeared.

Three points from Newton's work are particularly important in relation to the argument made here. First, the types of deception shown by 3-year-olds were similar to those of 4-year-olds, though there was an increase in frequency over age. That is, the 3-year-olds were already apparently attempting to manipulate what family members thought or expected, in the familiar and emotional circumstances of family interaction. In our own research, such episodes frequently involved false excuses for wrongdoing, or incidents in which the sibling was blamed or was falsely accused. In a typical example, one 30-month-old *reported* a transgression by her sibling to her mother, involving the (prohibited) garden hose. (This transgression had not in fact taken place, at least in the two hours preceding):

> Child: Carol's—Carol's touching a sprayer.
> Mother: Is she? [goes to look] She's not doing anything.
> Child: Carol's getting it [water] all over my hair.
> [untrue] [mother goes to look again]

In Newton's study, of particular interest are the examples of "bravado" in which children concealed their own emotion state (for instance, by denying that a punishment hurt—or claiming that they like that smack!). That is, they were apparently using deception for psychological rather than material ends, not instrumentally to avoid blame or punishment. The second point from Newton's study was that even children who failed conventional tests of mindreading (false belief tests) engaged in deception of family members. Third, Newton noted that deception often occurs "in situations of conflict when the child is in an emotionally charged state of opposition to parental control."

Such circumstances are inevitably rather different from the experimental situations in which deception has previously chiefly been studied. In a parallel way, naturalistic studies of children have reported examples of teasing, joking, comforting and shared pretend. All of these involve interactive settings that are necessarily different in emotional color, as well as in the familiarity of the interactants, from most test situations; the early stages of children's growing understanding of others' mental states are particularly vividly evident in such settings (Dunn, 1988, 1991; Reddy, 1991). To argue that we can gain a revealing perspective on the nature of children's understanding from naturalistic studies is not to deny or undervalue what, in contrast, can be learned from experimental or more formal assessments, or to gloss over the problems that naturalistic methods present—a point discussed further below. For some domains of cognitive development, for some developmental stages, and for some children, task situations can clearly be especially illuminating. The claim here is that for learning about early social understanding, naturalistic settings have a particular usefulness.

The issue of how children's emotional state relates to the development and the use of their understanding is, of course, of key theoretical interest. Relevant evidence is mixed in its implications, as research on children's arguments illustrates. Two different proposals have been made. The first is that children are more likely to use sophisticated reasoned argument in conflict when they are angry or distressed, as some studies suggest (Eisenberg, 1992; Stein & Miller, 1993). The second is, in contrast, that when they are intensely upset or angry, young children are less likely to reason maturely (e.g., Roberts & Strayer, 1987). Recent research indicates that there may well be developmental changes in the relation of intense negative emotion to reasoning. Thus, we found that 33-month-old children were, when angry or distressed, less able to draw on their reasoning abilities. In contrast, as 47-month-olds, they used reasoned argument equally often when upset or not upset—at least with their siblings (Dunn, 1995). It is possible, then, that as children's cognitive and metacognitive abilities increase they become more able to marshall their powers of argument even when angry or distressed—that they are less at the mercy of their emotions than they were as 2-year-olds. However, other findings indicated a more complex pattern of connections. Thus, differences in the affectionate quality of 47-month-olds relations with their close friends were associated with differences in their management of disputes: a high level of negative affect was associated with a failure to reason or take account of the other's perspective.

Most importantly, the findings indicate that the relations between affective state and understanding may differ for different arenas of social understanding. Thus, the children in our study were more likely to engage in causal discourse about feelings (behavior associated with later success on assessments of emotion understanding) when they were expressing negative affect than when they were expressing positive affect (Dunn & Brown, 1994). In contrast, their engagement in joint pretend play, which involves the cognitive demands of sharing an imaginary world with another, was less likely when they were upset. The general point that the various domains of social understanding should be differentiated—not only in terms of their links with affect—is one to which we will return (Dunn, 1988, 1991; Reddy, 1991).

Studies of children's conversational reference to feelings and mental states in their daily lives also provide evidence for young children's interest in and curiosity about inner states. Dramatic increases between the ages of 33 months and 40 months were found, for example, in children's reference to mental states (Brown, Donelan-McCall, & Dunn, 1996), and parallel data are reported in Bartsch and Wellman's (1995) studies of children's talk about the mind.

The significance of the social and emotional circumstances under which children perform the considerable intellectual feats of deception, teasing or shared pretend brings us to the second point concerning the implications of the study of children's relationships for understanding cognitive development: The evidence on the significance of certain social processes in the development of understanding mind and emotion.

SOCIAL PROCESSES INVOLVED IN THE DEVELOPMENT OF UNDERSTANDING

The question of what social processes might be involved in the development of social understanding is one that is generating some particularly exciting new leads. A variety of different aspects of social interaction, each of which has particular theoretical interest, are currently being studied. For instance, the potential significance of repeated experiences of sharing and negotiating a *pretend* world with another, of *arguments*, in which a child is faced with the differing perspective of another, and of various aspects of *conversation about the social world* have been studied, including talk about mental states, narrative, and causal discourse about the social world. The question of whether particular social *partners* in children's lives (parents, siblings or peers) play a distinctive role in developments in social understanding have also been studied. The results so far have drawn attention to the notable variety of social processes that are associated with the development of mindreading and emotion understanding.

Pretend

First, evidence is growing for a relationship between children's success on assessments of mindreading and emotion understanding, and their experience of joint pretend play (Astington & Jenkins, 1995; Youngblade & Dunn, 1995), and of other types of cooperative interaction (Dunn, Brown, Slomkowski, Tesla, & Youngblade, 1991). An important point from longitudinal research deserves emphasis here. The overtime correlations between social processes (such as the experience of joint pretend play) and cognitive task performance are found both from early social experience to later task performance, and vice versa. Clearly, we cannot make causal inferences about the direction of effects. It could be that the experience of sharing a pretend world fosters the understanding of others' mental states. Alternatively, it could be that children who are able to understand others' mental states and emotions make better play companions, or indeed that the associations reflect some common underlying ability. In any case, the finding that children's propensity to role enact predicted success on mindreading tests seven months later (Youngblade & Dunn, 1995) parallels data reported by Taylor, Gerow, and Carlson (1993) that 4-year-olds who were particularly inclined to engage in pretence appeared to be accelerated in their development of knowledge about the mind. It is a pattern that fits with the proposition that simulation or role taking plays a key part in the development of children's understanding of other people's and their own mental states (Harris, 1991).

Argument and Conflict

In addition to the evidence on links between experience in pretend play and sophistication in mindreading, there is also evidence for the significance of disputes and argument. Newton's (1994) emphasis on conflict as the setting for the relatively sophisticated instances of deception documented in his study (Newton, 1994) is echoed by studies of disputes and conflict, such as those of Stein and her colleagues on the significance of argumentative exchanges between mothers and their children, and between siblings and friends in the development of understanding (Stein & Miller, 1993). Children's styles of conflict management—specifically the extent to which they take account of the point of view of others in negotiating—are also correlated over time with their social understanding as assessed experimentally (Slomkowski & Dunn, 1992). How far it is the heightened salience and the affective quality of disputes, and how far it is the "meeting of minds" that contribute to the potential for fostering understanding is clearly an important topic for future research.

Conversations About the Social World

Studies of children's conversations have provided an illuminating window on their early and rapidly growing interest in and curiosity about inner states, as already noted. There is also accumulating evidence that differences in children's participation in such conversations are linked to differences in the sophistication and maturity of their early understanding, and that certain features of such conversations may be of particular developmental significance. Thus, engagement in conversations about feelings and causal talk was linked to later success on emotion understanding tasks (Dunn, Brown, & Beardsall, 1989; Dunn & Brown, 1993), and talk about mental states to success on mindreading tasks (Brown et al., 1996).

There is an interesting convergence here between the evidence from naturalistic studies and from experimental approaches. Appleton and Reddy (1996) for instance have shown that children's success at theory of mind tasks can be greatly enhanced through training interventions involving conversations (including interactive recall of the events, and positive elaboration of the children's answers). It was the provision of conversational opportunities and explanation within discussion—rather than presentation of counter-evidence—that was key to the children's success on the mindreading tasks. The authors argue that "understanding of false belief is itself a joint (discursive) construction rather than an individual (solitary logical) one. Thus, conversations are intrinsic to the understanding of false belief, not merely an external aid." Siegal and Peterson (1995), building on evidence that profoundly deaf children fail theory of mind tests, have argued that the children's problems stem from their lack of experience of conversations about mental states.

However, the data on causal conversations from our Pennsylvanian study draw attention to a key caveat here (Dunn & Brown, 1993). This concerns the importance of the pragmatics of the conversation under scrutiny. The analyses showed that the correlations with later mindreading ability were not with a simple measure of frequency of participation in mother–child conversation about cause, but rather, with causal conversations in certain pragmatic settings. Thus, children whose mothers' causal talk was chiefly in the context of controlling them did poorly on the assessment of emotion understanding later, while those whose mothers' causal talk was in the context of shared play, comforting or joking were most successful on the sociocognitive measures. It is clearly important not just to examine the content of talk, but also to examine what the interlocutors are trying to do in the conversation—the "contexts of practice" to which Bruner (1983) has drawn our attention in studies of language acquisition.

The general lesson here is that what is important in such conversations is not simply an effectively neutral "meeting of minds," with the child being exposed to another's point of view or to new information or rationale. Rather, the quality of the relationship between child and interlocutor as it is reflected in these exchanges—the emotional and pragmatic nature of the interaction—is also key. This claim goes beyond the argument that conversation is important in fostering mindreading because it highlights differences between conversational partners in information and attitudes (see e.g., Harris, in press). What is needed now is clarification of which aspects of conversation may be significant in the growth of mindreading; the evidence to date suggests that pragmatics and affect should be included in the list of candidates.

Narrative is another aspect of conversations that on theoretical grounds has been viewed as a potentially important process through which the development of understanding of mind and emotion may be influenced (Bruner, 1990). The power of narrative to hold children's interest is evident from early in the second year, and it is a striking feature of children's talk about other people and about themselves. Their sensitivity to narrative is intriguing and instructive. Persuasive arguments have been made that we account for our own actions and for the ways that others act principally in terms of narrative stories or drama, and that narrative images are powerful in generating particular selves in particular cultures. Bruner (1990) and Feldman (1992) have emphasized that patterns of narration support or scaffold the kind of metacognition about intentions that lies at the heart of the notion of "theories of mind." Indeed, developmental studies report that increases in narrative comments coincide with the appearance of comments on mental states and feelings states, and with causal conversations about psychological issues (Dunn, 1988). However, it is important to note that a focus on narratives as framing children's growing understanding of the mind does not imply that early narratives should be viewed as emotionally-neutral instances of cognitive sophistication. A striking feature of early narratives is that they are focused chiefly on socioemotional incidents (Brown, 1995). Here is a 47-month-old reporting a sequence of events to her sibling—a typically emotionally charged story:

> Child to sibling: [as she runs into the house from the garden] I came running back 'cause
> I saw two snakes and I was scared and I runned back!

There is an interesting convergence here, and also between the naturalistic data and the findings of some experimental studies investigating the relation of narrative comprehension to children's performance on false belief tasks. Lewis and his colleagues showed that when children faced with a false belief task were given the opportunity to link the events involved in the task procedures in a coherent narrative—for instance, by recounting the story involved in the false belief incident—this was enough to ensure a successful performance on the mindreading task (Lewis, Freeman, Kyriakidou, & Maridaki-Kossotaki, 1995).

The findings linking certain kinds of experience in disputes, in pretend, and in narrative to individual differences in mindreading raise a set of new questions for research. These three categories do, after all, suggest very different kinds of involvement for children: in disputes, their self-interest is closely touched, while in role play they are explicitly putting themselves in someone else's shoes, for instance. Does this imply that the sequelae and the developmental significance of engaging in argument are in important respects different from the sequelae of experiences in role play? Or are the key aspects of conflict those that involve the child being forced to take another's perspective? If so, these are not perhaps so different from the features of role play experience that are significant. These are empirical questions. They draw our attention to the next important steps in studying the different social processes implicated in the growth of mindreading.

Social Partners: The Significance of Child–Child Interaction

The question of whether particular social partners play a special role in the development of social understanding was originally raised by Piaget (1965), who argued that interaction with peers was of particular significance in the development of moral understanding. A variety of lines of evidence now show links between experience with other children and individual differences in sociocognitive development. Consider the following findings: First, children with siblings are reported to do better on mindreading tasks than those without (Perner, Ruffman, & Leekam, 1994). Second, the number of siblings that children have, and the number of kin with whom they interact daily are both reported to be positively correlated with success on mindreading tasks (Lewis et al., 1995). Lewis and his colleagues note, however, that the number of adult kin with whom children interact is also correlated with such success, and conclude that "a variety of knowledgeable members of her/his culture influence the apprentice theoretician of mind."

Third, the significance of child–child interaction was highlighted in several lines of evidence from our study following children from 2 to 7 years (Dunn et al., 1991). Two examples can serve as illustration. First, a key predictor of success on the social cognition tasks was the children's previous experience of cooperative play with their older siblings. Second, the analysis of children's talk about mental states showed that children referred to mental states strikingly more frequently when with their siblings or friends than they did with their mothers (Brown et al., 1996). Moreover, the child–child pairs were more likely to refer to shared thoughts and ideas (as opposed to their own ideas) than the mother–child dyads. The quality of the child–child relationship was important here: it was during playful cooperative interactions that the children discussed mental processes and the length of their friendship and frequency of their interaction were positively related to explicit reference to mental processes. Finally, their use of mental state terms in conversation with their friends was correlated with their performance on false belief tasks.

In summary, the studies of children's conversations, their play and their interactions with different partners are beginning to give us a clearer picture of what social processes may be implicated in the development of individual differences in mindreading and emotion understanding. But an important final point concerning such social understanding is highlighted by studies of children in their different relationships. These indicate that the same child may show very different powers of understanding-in-action within his or her different close relationships, depending on the emotional context of the relationship, and the pragmatics of the particular interaction. Observational data on children in interaction with their mothers, siblings and close friends showed that individual differences in their engagement in joint pretend play (Youngblade & Dunn, 1995), their management of conflict (Slomkowski & Dunn, 1992), and their discourse about mental states (Brown et al., 1996) were not correlated across these different partners (though each was correlated with the children's performance on standard sociocognitive assessments). That is, there was no relation between a child's participation in joint pretend play with his or her mother, with sibling and with a friend. Some engaged in elaborate role play with a friend, but not with sibling or mother; others did so with sibling but not with friend or mother, and so on. Similarly, there was no correlation between children's propensity to take account of the antagonist's inner states when in dispute with sibling, with friend or with mother. And there were no significant correlations between the frequency with which they engaged in mental state discourse with their siblings, friends or mothers. This pattern of results raises a number of further issues. It could be argued that since the indices of understanding-in-action (pretend, discourse about inner states, argument in conflict) do not correlate across social partners but do nevertheless each correlate with false-belief test performance, the test is tapping the children's "peak" performance, or some general skill, and is therefore more useful and more revealing than the naturalistic information. However, it should be noted that the interaction measures with each partner give us three important kinds of information. First, the 33-month interaction measures predict independently to the variance in the test performance measure at 40 months; that is, they tap aspects of early understanding at an age at which the children could not succeed on the task. Second, the independence reminds us that different social processes are implicated in the development of the broad capacity of mindreading assessed on the test, and gives clues as to the relative significance of interactions with siblings versus mothers. Third, the relation of these interaction measures to the affective quality of the exchange gives us information on both how children use their understanding in the context of real-life relationships, and of how the emotional context does or does not affect the marshalling of cognitive capacities.

In general, these findings suggest that it would be misleading to conceptualize individual differences in children's understanding of others' inner states solely as "within-child" characteristics, or as traits that carry over in a simple way between different social relationships. Rather, the children's understanding of their partners inner states, or at least their *use* of such understanding was crucially related to the emotional context of the interaction. This evidence provides yet another example of how important it is to frame our developmental questions in terms of both cognitive and developmental considerations.

METHODOLOGICAL ISSUES

As regards research strategies, these studies highlight three key lessons. First, it is important to include in research on understanding of mind and emotion not only formal standardized assessments, but also studies on children in real-life situations, because these have emotional significance for the children, and because the issue of familiarity between child and other may be important. The studies of deception illustrate the former point (see also Hala, Chandler, & Fritz, 1991), and studies by Knott, Lewis, and Williams (1995), of autistic children interacting with their siblings, the latter. The autistic children in the study by Knott and colleagues did engage in play with their siblings, and demonstrated social skills—a striking finding given the well-documented difficulties that autistic children have in social relations with peers. Peers are of course less familiar for autistic individuals than siblings, and perhaps less motivated to support and encourage autistic companions in play.

The lesson is that we can learn from using *both* naturalistic settings and experimental tasks, as a joint strategy. Indeed the differences in children's performance in naturalistic and experimental settings can be instructive. Thus, in Bishop and Adams (1991) study on children with specific language impairment, there was no relation between children's performance in referential communication tasks and their conversational ability. Children who were inadequate communicators in an open-ended situation, and appeared insensitive to the needs of their listener, in fact performed normally on the referential task— perhaps because of the structured nature of the situation and the instructions provided to the child.

There are undoubtedly disadvantages in the use of naturalistic settings: data from observations in such settings can be very difficult to interpret, given the tendency for many factors of interest to be intercorrelated, and the lack of experimental control. The example of the autistic children playing with their siblings (Knott et al., 1995) illustrates the problem of covariation. Was it the familiarity of the siblings, or the affective quality of their relationship, or the sensitive behavior of the older siblings that was key? We can begin to tease apart these possibilities with observational studies in the case of sibling relationships, since they differ strongly in affective quality. But there are many other instances where the rigor of experimental control is needed if we are to choose between hypotheses.

The second methodological lesson is that it is important to study children in a variety of social situations or relationships—whether by observation, interview, or task assessment. Only then we will be able to establish whether and how the affective dynamics, the familiarity, and the salience of particular social contexts influence the development of understanding, and the way children use their cognitive capabilities.

Third, the arguments and empirical evidence for the developmental significance of conversational processes in cognitive growth should be taken seriously, and a focus on discourse included in research strategies—not just because the study of conversation is revealing, but because dialogue may well be a key context in which cognitive development is fostered (see for instance Harris, in press; Scholnick & Wing, 1991, 1992).

IMPLICATIONS OF COGNITIVE RESEARCH

In the previous section, the focus was on how the study of children's social interactions could inform our understanding of cognitive development. We turn now to the other side of the coin: the issue of what those who study social development can learn from the new work on cognitive development. At the outset, a parallel with the increasing interest in the "socialization of cognition" should be noted. Among those studying social development there has been growing recognition that rapid advances in our understanding of cognitive development—such as the new research in children's social understanding—have great significance for how we view and study social relationships. A key instance is Bretherton's (1985) consideration of the importance of work on social cognition for attachment theory and research. However, much of this interest remains at a speculative level, tantalizingly far from rigorous empirical examination. In what follows—as in the previous section—we consider the implications of some of the recent cognitive work, first for ideas on the *nature* of children's relationships; second for the *processes* involved in their development; third, the *methodological implications* will be noted.

THE NATURE OF RELATIONSHIPS

Recent cognitive research has implications for how we conceptualize relationships, and what we look for in describing them. For example, the quality of our relationships is clearly importantly affected by the extent to which we understand other people's feelings, needs, and motivation. What we have learned from the cognitive research about children's understanding of and responsiveness to the feelings of others, means not only that dimensions of empathy and understanding are part of their early close relationships, but that aspects of intimacy and self-disclosure which were previously thought relevant only to the relationships of much older children may indeed be present in the close relationships of preschoolers. Recent observational research on very young children's friendships supports such a view (Howes, 1988; Corsaro, 1981; see also Gottman & Parker, 1986).

More generally, the cognitive research should alert us to the importance of looking beyond the "security" aspects of young children's relationships that have dominated studies of parent–child relationships. Aspects of adult relationships, ranging from shared humour (which presupposes understanding of what another will find funny) to manipulation of control and power within a dyadic relationship, depend on a sophisticated grasp of the other's desires, motivations, ideas and capacities. The cognitive research on young children reminds us that such dimensions may in fact also be relevant to young children's relationships. Unless we include such dimensions in our descriptive frameworks for studying relationships we will not be able to assess how far this is indeed the case.

The conceptual advances of cognitive development are particularly important in relation to our understanding of the developmental changes in children's relationships. For instance, evidence for the "lag" between children's understanding of desire and of belief, which had come from cognitive research on both normal and autistic children (Baron-Cohen, 1991; Bartsch & Wellman, 1995; Harris, Johnson, Hutton, Andrews, & Cooke, 1989) surely has implications for how the nature of children's relationships change over the second and third years. So does also the evidence for the growth in children's metacognitive abilities. Yet such changes remain to be studied in detail (see, however, Dunn, Creps, & Brown, in press, for a first step).

Perhaps most notable of all are the implications of cognitive research on children with problems such as autism, hyperactivity, or conduct disorder, for those concerned with these children's social development. A proper consideration of these issues in developmental psychopathology is beyond the scope of this article; however, the challenging ideas, the controversies, the disagreements about whether social problems are antecedent to or sequelae of these children's cognitive problems make this research clearly relevant for those interested in normal developmental processes. Will the explanatory principles established for the development of such extreme conditions as autism help us to understand the development of children who do not suffer from such problems? This remains a matter for research. It is not yet clear to what extent understanding the processes that underlie the lack of a capacity can illuminate individual differences in children who possess that capacity. But the issues such studies raise are unquestionably relevant and important (see e.g., Baron-Cohen, Tager-Flusberg, & Cohen, 1995; Hobson, 1993).

COGNITIVE PROCESSES INVOLVED IN DEVELOPING RELATIONSHIPS

Impact of Relationships Between Others

The evidence from cognitive research that children are interested in and reflect on other people's intentions, thoughts and feelings highlights how important it is for those interested in relationships to pay attention to the developmental impact on children of the relationships of those around them. Three lines of recent research highlight the associations between the quality of these other relationships and children's outcome. The first is the growing evidence for the impact of marital discord and conflict on children's development, especially their socioemotional development and adjustment (e.g., Cummings & Davies, 1994). The second is research on coparenting, which indicates that differences and disagreements between parents in the management and control of children are linked to poor outcome. This evidence that suggests children may be monitoring such disagreements and "playing off" one parent against the other even as early as the second year of life (Belsky, Crnic, & Gable, 1995; Jouriles, Murphy, Farris, Smith, & Richters, 1991).

The third line of evidence is the accumulating literature showing that differential treatment within the family affects children's later adjustment (Dunn, Stocker, & Plomin, 1990; Dunn & Plomin, 1990; McGuire, Dunn, & Plomin, 1995). We know that there are important associations here—however, we do not know how these other relationships exert their impact. The cognitive research suggests possible processes by which children may be affected, possibilities that can be explored with systematic study. These include developmental changes in attention patterns, in social comparison, and in attribution for instance.

Significance of the Peer Group

The evidence on children's interest in the inner states of others alerts us to the possibility that young children may be sensitive to the reactions and opinions of those in their peer group to an extent not fully appreciated until recently. Newton's (1994) evidence on bravado, and Gottman and Parker's (1986) evidence on gossip support such a proposition. Given the evidence on the predictive significance of children's relations with their peer groups in middle childhood (Parker & Asher, 1987), the nature of younger children's perceptions of how they are viewed by their peers, their understanding of and beliefs about their relations with the peer group to their later adjustment deserves particular attention.

Peer Collaboration

From a different tradition in cognitive developmental research, the studies of children's collaboration on cognitive tasks remind us of how broad the developmental influence of peer interaction can be (Azmitia, 1995; Damon & Phelps, 1989; Hartup, 1983; Kruger & Tomasello, 1986). The evidence for the power of the "meeting of minds" between peers for cognitive growth challenges those who study social processes to clarify what is happening between the children in such instances of cognitive advance. This research into peer collaboration has raised a host of interesting questions. How, for instance, can we explain the delayed cognitive benefits of collaboration demonstrated in the work by Howe, Tolmie, and Rodgers (1992) on children's understanding within the domain of physics? How and why do siblings and peers have unique influences on children's cognitive development (Azmitia & Hesser, 1993)?

METHODOLOGICAL IMPLICATIONS

Those of us who study social relationships have much to learn from the precision and rigor of experimental cognitive developmentalists, with the critical approach they typically take to drawing conclusions from experimental manipulations. One implication to be drawn is that we should move away from very general notions such as that of the "internal working model" of relationships— an attractive but vague notion—to try to specify more clearly the nature of what is thought to be represented in such models, and to devise tests of alternative hypotheses concerning such models. Thus, the exciting evidence for associations between attachment quality over generations, and between early attachment quality and later mindreading abilities (Fernyhough, Meins, & Russell, 1995; Fonagy, Steele, & Steele, 1991) raises a whole set of questions concerning what the nature of expectations or "representations" might be that underlie such associations. We need the precision of the cognitive developmental approach, and a rigorous testing of alternative hypotheses to begin to answer such questions. An exciting start has been made with the work of Meins, in press, testing the proposition that there are links between executive capacity and attachment (Meins & Russell, submitted).

UNDERSTANDING AND RELATIONSHIPS

In this final section, some recent research that attempts to bring together a focus on cognitive development with the study of social development is summarized. One of the implications of this and other recent research bridging the divide between studies of cognitive and social development is that a differentiated approach both to children's social understanding and to the nature and dimensions of their relationships is needed. First, it may well be a mistake to think of the development of social understanding as "all of a piece"—a point clearly made by Astington and Jenkins (1995) on the basis of their study of the connections between mindreading ability and interaction with peers (see also Lalonde & Chandler, 1995). Second, it is clearly important to differentiate the various dimensions of children's relationships; here there is much to be learned from studies in middle childhood such as that by Berndt and his colleagues (e.g., Berndt & Perry, 1986; Berndt, Hawkins, & Hoyle, 1986), and Bukowski (Bukowski & Hoza, 1989). Third, we need to examine how these different aspects of understanding and of relationships are connected over time. Already there is evidence that such a differentiated approach could be illuminating both for cognitive developmentalists and for those interested primarily in relationships. Consider the following points from our longitudinal study of children in Pennsylvania (Dunn, 1995).

First, the measures of understanding emotions and mindreading were not significantly correlated when the children were 40-months-old; that is, some children were skilled at emotion understanding, and less successful at mindreading, while others performed well on the mindreading tasks and less well on the emotion understanding assessment. Second, the sequelae of these two aspects of understanding were different. Early sophistication in emotion understanding was linked to positive perceptions of social relations with teachers and peers at school, to a mature moral sensibility at 6 and 7 years, and to particular skill at understanding mixed emotions in the school years. In contrast, early skill at mindreading was related to negative perceptions of school experiences in the first year at school, to sensitivity and self-blame in the face of teacher criticism, to skills of coordination of pretend play with another, and to negotiating strategies in conflict (Herrera & Dunn, 1995). Our examination of the children's interaction with a close friend revealed two dimensions—one of warm expressive amity, one of coordinated play and sophistication of shared pretend. The latter dimension—but not the former—was linked to the children's earlier mindreading ability.

Moreover, early differences in the target children's sociocognitive abilities were associated not only with differences in their own developmental outcomes, but with differences in the patterns of change over time in others' behavior towards them. Thus, in families in which the children showed greater understanding of emotion and other minds as 40-month-olds, their older siblings showed particularly marked increases in reflective discussion and interaction with them (Dunn et al., in press). Such differences in early social understanding were *not* related to the pattern of change in the emotional aspects of either children's or siblings' interactional behavior. A more sophisticated understanding of another family member's feelings and thoughts does not, it appears, guarantee a more rapid decrease in the expression of irritation and hostility over the next few years. This is further evidence that between siblings, greater understanding does not mean more harmony in the relationship.

Challenges

These findings are from one study, modest in scale and with obvious limitations. Yet the challenges from this and the other research described above are clear, as are the new items for the research agendas of developmentalists that they suggest. For cognitive developmentalists, the following are relevant needs: To grapple with the intractable issue of how affect is linked to cognitive change; to include examination of social context and the significance of different social partners; to assess how understanding is put to use in situations other than the context of experimental assessments; to include a differentiated approach to the investigation of social understanding, emotion understanding, executive function, memory and narrative comprehension, and their interrelations. For those studying social development, the need is for a differentiated study of dimensions of relationships, for a critical rigor in conceptualizing mental representations of relationships, and an appreciation of the nature of children's changing understanding of others in early years, and the significance of children's perceptions. To begin to understand children's relationships, which include expectations, memories, and beliefs about the other (Duck, 1989) we clearly need to be informed from cognitive research about the developmental changes in these aspects of cognition during the early years, for instance the work on memory (Fivush & Hudson, 1990).

These relations between social and cognitive development have been chiefly studied in normal children, with the key exception being research on autism. There is an urgent need for comparable attention to be paid to the nature and patterns of early connections between understanding and relationships in children with other difficulties, such as those with language delay, with anxiety problems, or described as hard-to-manage preschoolers. In each of these domains, we know that children are at risk for later problems with both social relationships and social understanding (see for instance the seminal work of Dodge and his colleagues: Dodge, 1986,1991; Dodge, Pettit, McClaskey, & Brown, 1986).

Even with the over-simple triad considered here for a relatively short period of early childhood—relationships, mindreading, emotion understanding—the challenges are considerable. And this triad clearly is too simple: one issue that has not yet been considered which should be high on our agenda concerns the cultural setting for the triad. Feldman (1992) has argued that the new interest in children's understanding of the mind has led to the specification of a new set of tasks for cognitive developmentalists, tasks which center on cultural issues. Here argument runs as follows: if the young child is not egocentric, but has access to adult interpretations, the events that the child encounters carry the interpreted meaning given to those events in their own culture. This sets a new agenda for research into cognitive development to discover the interpretations and cultural understanding of individuals at different ages. These issues are surely relevant too for social developmentalists. The question of how the meaning of different emotional experiences and the quality of relationships may differ in different cultural groups is one of great interest that is relatively unexplored, as are the links between understanding and relationships in different cultures. And these, of course, cannot properly be investigated without studying children in their own worlds. We come then full circle, with a return to Lois B. Murphy's plea that we should see and listen to children in their own worlds. Taking such a perspective makes us sensitive to the emotional force of the interactions in which children's understanding is formed, and aware that we cannot disregard the mutual influence of social and cognitive change.

REFERENCES

Appleton, M., & Reddy, V. (1996). Teaching three-year-olds to pass false-belief tests: A conversational approach. *Social Development*, in press.

Astington, J. W. (1994). *The child's discovery of the mind*. Cambridge, MA: Harvard University Press.

Astington, J. W., & Jenkins, J. M. (1995). Theory of mind development and social understanding. *Cognition and Emotion, 9*, 151–166.

Azmitia, M. (1995). Peer collaborative cognition: Theoretical, developmental and measurement issues. In P. R. Baltes & U. M. Staudinger (Eds.), *Interactive minds: Lifespan perspectives or the social foundations of cognition*. Cambridge: Cambridge University Press, in press.

Azmitia M., & Hesser, J. (1993). Why siblings are important agents of cognitive development: A comparison of siblings and peers. *Child Development, 64*, 430–444.

Baron-Cohen, S. (1991). Do people with autism understand what causes emotion? *Child Development, 62*, 385–395.

Baron-Cohen, S., Tager-Flusberg, H., & Cohen, D. J. (1995). *Understanding other minds: Perspectives from autism*. Oxford: Oxford University Press.

Bartsch, K., & Wellman, H. M. (1995). *Children talk about the mind*. Oxford: Oxford University Press.

Belsky, J., Crnic, K., & Gable, S. (1995). The determinants of coparenting in families with toddler boys: Spousal differences and daily hassles. *Child Development, 66*, 629–642.

Berndt, T. J., Hawkins, J. A., & Hoyle, S. G. (1986). Changes in friendship during a school year: Effects on children's and adolescents' impressions of friendship and sharing with friends. *Child Development, 57,* 1284–1297.

Berndt, T. J., & Perry, T. B. (1986). Children's perceptions of friendships as supportive relationships. *Developmental Psychology, 22,* 640–648.

Bishop, D. V. M., & Adams, C. (1991). What do referential tasks measure? A study of children with specific language impairment. *Applied Psycholinguistics, 12,* 199–215.

Bretherton, I. (1985). Attachment theory: Retrospect and prospect. In I. Bretherton & E. Waters (Eds.), Growing points of attachment theory and research. *Monographs of the Society for Research in Child Development, 50* (1–2), 3–35 (Series No. 209).

Brown, J. R. (1995). What happened?: Emotional experience and children's early talk about the past. Submitted.

Brown, J. R., Donelan-McCall, N., & Dunn, J. (1996). Why talk about mental states? The significance of children's conversations with friends, siblings, and mothers. *Child Development,* in press.

Bruner, J. S. (1983). *Child's talk.* Oxford: Oxford University Press.

Bruner, J. S. (1990). *Acts of meaning.* Cambridge, MA: Harvard University Press.

Bukowski, W. M., & Hoza, B. (1989). Popularity and friendship: Issues in theory, measurement, and outcome. In T. J. Berndt & G. W. Ladd (Eds.), *Peer relationships in child development* (pp. 15–45). New York: John Wiley.

Chandler, M., Fritz, A. S., & Hala, S. (1989). Small-scale deceit: Deception as a marker of two-, three-, and four-year-olds' early theories of mind. *Child Development, 60,* 1263–1277.

Corsaro, W. A. (1981). Friendship in the nursery school. In S. R. Asher & J. M. Gottman (Eds.), *The development of children's friendships* (pp. 207–241). Cambridge: Cambridge University Press.

Cummings, E. M., & Davies, P. (1994). *Children and marital conflict: The impact of dispute and resolution.* New York: Guilford Press.

Damon, W., & Phelps, E. (1989). Strategic uses of peer learning in children's education. In T. J. Berndt & G. W. Ladd (Eds.), *Peer relationships in child development* (pp. 135–157). New York: John Wiley.

Dodge, K. A. (1986). A social-information processing model of social competence in children. In M. Perlmutter (Ed.), *Minnesota symposia on child psychology* (Vol. 18, pp. 77–126). Minneapolis, MN: University of Minnesota Press.

Dodge, K. A. (1991). Emotion and social information processing. In J. Garber & K. Dodge (Eds.), *Emotion regulation* (pp. 159–181). Cambridge: Cambridge University Press.

Dodge, K. A., Pettit, G. S., McClaskey, C. L., & Brown, M. (1986). Social competence in children. *Monographs of the Society for Research in Child Development, 51* (2, Serial No. 213). Chicago: University of Chicago Press.

Doise, W., & Mugny, G. (1984). *The social development of the intellect.* Oxford: Pergamon Press.

Duck, S. (1989). Socially competent communication and relationships development. In B. H. Schneider, G. Attili, & J. Nadel (Eds.), *Social competence in developmental perspective* (pp. 91–106). Dordrecht, The Netherlands: Kluwer.

Dunn, J. (1988). *The beginning of social understanding.* Cambridge, MA: Harvard University Press.

Dunn, J. (1991). Understanding others: Evidence from naturalistic studies of children. In A. Whiten (Ed.), *Natural theories of mind* (pp. 51–61). Oxford: Blackwell Scientific Publications.

Dunn, J. (1995). Children as psychologists: The later correlates of individual differences in understanding of emotions and other minds. *Cognition and Emotion, 9,* 113–116.

Dunn, J., & Brown, J. (1993). Early conversations about causality: Content, pragmatics, and developmental change. *British Journal of Developmental Psychology, 11,* 107–123.

Dunn, J., & Brown, J. R. (1994). Affect expression in the family, children's understanding of emotions, and their interactions with others. *Merrill–Palmer Quarterly, 40,* 120–137.

Dunn, J., Brown, J., & Beardsall, L. (1989). Family talk about feeling states and children's later understanding of others' emotions. *Developmental Psychology, 27*, 448–455.

Dunn, J., Brown, J., Slomkowski, C., Tesla, C., & Youngblade, L. (1991). Young children's understanding of other people's feelings and beliefs: Individual differences and their antecedents. *Child Development, 62*, 1352–1366.

Dunn, J., Creps, C., & Brown, J. (in press). Children's family relationships between two and five: Developmental changes and individual differences. *Social Development.*

Dunn, J., & Plomin, R. (1990). *Separate lives: Why siblings are so different.* New York: Basic Books.

Dunn, J., Slomkowski, C. M., Donelan-McCall, N., & Herrera, C. (1995). Conflict understanding and relationships: Developments and differences in the preschool years. *Early Education and Development, 6*, 303–316.

Dunn, J., Stocker, C., & Plomin, R. (1990). Nonshared experiences within the family: Correlates of behavioral problems in middle childhood. *Development and Psychopathology, 2*, 113–126.

Eisenberg, A. R. (1992). Conflicts between mothers and their young children. *Merrill–Palmer Quarterly, 38*, 21–43.

Feldman, C. F. (1992). The new theory of theory of mind. *Human Development, 35*, 107–117.

Fernyhough, C., Meins, E., & Russell, J. (1995). *The influences of security of attachment on young children's understanding of other minds.* Presentation at the BPS Development Section Meeting, Glasgow.

Fivush, R., & Hudson, J. (1990). *Knowing and remembering young children.* Cambridge: Cambridge University Press.

Fonagy, P., Steele, H., & Steele, M. (1991). Maternal representations of attachment during pregnancy predict the organisation of infant–mother attachment at one year of age. *Child Development, 62*, 891–905.

Goodnow, J. J. (1990). The socialization of cognition: What's involved? In J. W. Stigler, R. A. Shweder, & G. Herdt (Eds.), *Cultural psychology* (pp. 259–286). Cambridge: Cambridge University Press.

Gottman, J. M., & Parker, J. G. (1986). *Conversations of friends: Speculations on affective development.* Cambridge: Cambridge University Press.

Hala, S., Chandler, M., & Fritz, A. S. (1991). Fledgling theories of mind: Deception as a marker of 3-year-olds, understanding of false belief. *Child Development, 62*, 83–97.

Harris, P. L. (1991). The work of the imagination. In A. Whiten (Ed.), *Natural theories of mind: The evolution, development, and simulation of everyday mindreading* (pp. 283–304). Oxford: Blackwell Scientific Publications.

Harris, P. L. (in press). Desires, beliefs and language. In P. Carruthers & P. Smith (Eds.), *Theories of theories of mind.* Cambridge: Cambridge University Press.

Harris, P. L., Johnson, C. N., Hutton, D., Andrews, G., & Cooke, T. (1989). Young children's theory of mind and emotion. *Cognition and Emotion, 3*, 379–400.

Hartup, W. W. (1983). Peer relationships. In E. M. Hetherington (Ed.), *Handbook of child psychology*, Vol. 4: Socialization, personality, and social development (pp. 103–196). New York: John Wiley.

Herrera, C., & Dunn, J. (1995). Individual differences in conflict with a friend: Associations with early social understanding. Submitted.

Hobson, R. P. (1993). *Autism and the development of mind.* Hillsdale, NJ: Lawrence Erlbaum.

Hoffman, M. L. (1986). Affect, cognition, and motivation. In R. M. Sorrentino & E. T. Higgins (Eds.), *Handbook of motivation and cognition* (pp. 244–280). New York: Guilford.

Howe, C. (1988). Peer interaction of young children. *Monographs of the Society for Research in Child Development*, Serial No. 217, 53, No. 1. Chicago: University of Chicago Press.

Howe, C., Tolmie, A., & Rodgers, C. (1992). The acquisition of conceptual knowledge in science by primary school children: Group interaction and the understanding of motion down an incline. *British Journal of Developmental Psychology, 10*, 113–130.

Jouriles, E., Murphy, C., Farris, A., Smith, D., Richters, J. Marital adjustment, parental disagreements about child rearing, and behavior problems in boys. *Child Development, 62*, 1424–1433.

Knott, F., Lewis, C., & Williams, T. (1995). Sibling interaction of children with learning disabilities: A comparison of autism and Down's syndrome. *Journal of Child Psychology and Psychiatry, 36,* 965–976.

Kruger, A. C., & Tomasello, M. (1986). Transactive discussions with peers and adults. *Developmental Psychology, 22,* 681–685.

Lalonde, C. E., & Chandler, M. J. (1995). False belief goes to school: On the social–emotional consequences of coming early or late to a first theory of mind. *Cognition and Emotion, 9,* 167–186.

Leslie, A. M. (1988). Some implications of pretense for mechanisms underlying children's theory of mind. In J. W. Astington, P. L. Harris, & D. R. Olson (Eds.), *Developing theories of mind* (pp. 19–46). Cambridge: Cambridge University Press.

Lewis, C., Freeman, N. H., Kyriakidou, C., & Maridaki-Kossotaki, K. (1995). *Social influences on false belief access: Specific contagion or general apprenticeship?* Presentation at the Biennial meeting of the Society for Research in Child Development, Indianapolis, March.

Lewis, C., & Osborne, A. (1990). Three-year-olds, problems with false belief: Conceptual deficit or linguistic artifact? *Child Development, 61,* 1514–1519.

McGuire, S., Dunn, J., & Plomin, R. (1995). Maternal differential treatment of siblings and children's behavioural problems: A longitudinal study. *Development and Psychopathology, 7,* 515–528.

Meins, E., (in press). *The social development of cognition.* Hillsdale, NJ: Lawrence Erlbaum.

Meins, E., & Russell, J. (submitted). Security and symbolic play: The relation between security of attachment and executive capacity.

Murphy, L. B. (1932). *Social behavior and child personality.* New York: Columbia University Press.

Newton, P. E. (1994). *Preschool prevarication: An investigation of the cognitive prerequisites for deception.* Unpublished Ph.D. dissertation, University of Portsmouth.

Parker, J. G., & Asher, S. R. (1987). Peer relations and later personal adjustment: Are low-accepted children 'at risk'? *Psychological Bulletin, 102,* 357–389.

Perner, J. (1991). Understanding the representational mind: Cambridge, MA: MIT Press.

Perner, J., Ruffman, T., & Leekam, S. R. (1994). Theory of mind is contagious: You catch it from your sibs. *Child Development, 65,* 1228–1238.

Piaget, J. (1965). *The moral judgement of the child.* New York: Academic Press.

Reddy, V. (1991). Playing with others, expectations: Teasing and mucking about in the first year. In A. Whiten (Ed.), *Natural theories of mind* (pp. 143–158). Oxford: Blackwell Scientific Publications.

Roberts, W., & Strayer, J. (1987). Parents' responses to the emotional distress of their children: Relations with children's competence. *Developmental Psychology, 23,* 415–422.

Rogoff, B. (1990). *Apprenticeship in thinking.* Oxford: Oxford University Press.

Scholnick, E. K., & Wing, C. S. (1991). Speaking deductively: Preschoolers, use of if in conversation and conditional inference. *Developmental Psychology, 27,* 249–258.

Scholnick, E. K., & Wing, C. S. (1992). Speaking deductively: Using conversation to trace the origins of conditional thought in children. *Merrill–Palmer Quarterly, 38,* 1–20.

Siegal, M., & Peterson, C. C. (1995). Breaking the mold: A fresh look at children's understanding of questions about lies and mistakes. *Developmental Psychology,* in press.

Slomkowski, C., & Dunn, J. (1992). Arguments and relationships within the family: Differences in children's disputes with mother and sibling. *Developmental Psychology, 28,* 919–924.

Sodian, B. (1991). The development of deception in children. *British Journal of Developmental Psychology, 9,* 173–188.

Stein, N., & Miller, C. (1993). The development of memory and reasoning skill in argumentative contexts: Evaluating, explaining, and generating evidence. In R. Glaser (Ed.), *Advances in Instructional Psychology* (Vol. 4, pp. 284–334). Hillsdale, NJ: Lawrence Erlbaum.

Strichartz, A. F., & Burton, R. V. (1990). Lies and the truth: A study of the development of the concept. *Child Development, 61,* 211–220.

Taylor, M., Gerow, L. E., & Carlson, S. M. (1993, March). *The relation between individual differences in fantasy and theory of mind.* Paper presented at the biennial meeting of the Society for Research in Child Development, New Orleans.

Wellman, H. M. (1990). *The child's theory of mind.* Cambridge, MA: MIT Press.

Youngblade, L. M., & Dunn, J. (1995). Individual differences in young children's pretend play with mother and sibling: Links to relationships and understanding of other people's feelings and beliefs. *Child Development, 66,* 1472–1492.

4

The Company They Keep: Friendships and Their Developmental Significance

Willard W. Hartup

University of Minnesota

Considerable evidence tells us that "being liked" and "being disliked" are related to social competence, but evidence concerning friendships and their developmental significance is relatively weak. The argument is advanced that the developmental implications of these relationships cannot be specified without distinguishing between having friends, the identity of one's friends, and friendship quality. Most commonly, children are differentiated from one another in diagnosis and research only according to whether or not they have friends. The evidence shows that friends provide one another with cognitive and social scaffolding that differs from what nonfriends provide, and having friends supports good outcomes across normative transitions. But predicting developmental outcome also requires knowing about the behavioral characteristics and attitudes of children's friends as well as qualitative features of these relationships.

On February 16, 1995, in the small Minnesota town of Delano, a 14-year-old boy and his best friend ambushed and killed his mother as she returned home. The circumstances surrounding this event were described in the next edition of the *Minneapolis Star Tribune* (February 18, 1995): The boy had "several learning disabilities—including attention deficit disorder." He had been "difficult" for a long time and, within the last year, had gotten in trouble with a step-brother by wrecking a car and carrying a gun to a movie theater. The mother was described as having a wonderful relationship with her daughter but having "difficulties" with her son. The family dwelling contained guns.

Against these child, family, and ecological conditions is a significant social history: The boy was "... a lonely and unliked kid who was the frequent victim of schoolmates' taunts, jeers, and assaults. He had trouble with school work and trouble with other kids .... He was often teased on the bus and at school because of his appearance and abilities .... He got teased bad. Every day, he got teased. He'd get pushed around. But he couldn't really help himself. He was kind of skinny .... He didn't really have that many friends."

Reprinted with permission from *Child Development*, 1996, Vol. 67, 1–13. Copyright © 1996 by the Society for Research in Child Development, Inc.

Presidential address to the biennial meetings of the Society for Research in Child Development, April 1, 1995, Indianapolis, IN. The author is grateful to W. Andrew Collins, Rosemary K. Hartup, Gary W. Ladd, Brett Laursen, and Andrew F. Newcomb for their comments on this manuscript.

The boy actually had two good friends: One appears to have had things relatively well put together. But with this friend, the subject "... passed [a] gun safety course for hunting; they took the class together." The second friend (with whom the murder was committed) was a troublesome child. These two boys described themselves as the "best of friends," and spent much time together. The boys have admitted to planning the ambush (one saying they had planned it for weeks, the other for a few hours). They were armed and waiting when the mother arrived home from work. One conclusion seems relatively certain: this murder was an unlikely event until these two antisocial friends reached consensus about doing it.

An important message emerges from this incident: Child characteristics, intersecting with family relationships and social setting, cycle through peer relations in two ways to affect developmental outcome: (a) through acceptance and rejection by other children in the aggregate, and (b) through dyadic relationships, especially with friends. Considerable evidence now tells us that "being liked" by other children (an aggregate condition) supports good developmental outcome; conversely, "being disliked" (another aggregate condition) is a risk factor (Parker & Asher, 1987). But the evidence concerning friendships and their developmental significance is weak—mainly because these relationships have not been studied extensively enough or with sufficient differentiation.

On the too-rare occasions in which friendships are taken into account developmentally—either in diagnosis or research—children are differentiated merely according to whether or not they have friends. This emphasis on having friends is based on two assumptions: First, making and keeping friends requires good reality-testing and social skills; "having friends" is thus a proxy for "being socially skilled." Second, friendships are believed to be developmental wellsprings in the sense that children must suspend egoism, embrace egalitarian attitudes, and deal with conflict effectively in order to maintain them (Sullivan, 1953). On two counts, then, having friends is thought to bode well for the future.

Striking differences exist, however, among these relationships—both from child to child and companion to companion. First, enormous variation occurs in who the child's friends are: Some companions are outgoing and rarely get into trouble; others are antisocial; still others are good children but socially clumsy. These choices would seem rather obviously to contribute to socialization—not only by affecting reputations (as the adage admonishes) but through what transpires between the children. Knowing that a teenager has friends tells us one thing, but the identity of his or her friends tells us something else.

Second, friendships differ from one another qualitatively, that is, in their *content* or normative foundations (e.g., whether or not the two children engage in antisocial behavior), their *constructiveness* (e.g., whether conflict resolution commonly involves negotiation or whether it involves power assertion), their *closeness* (e.g., whether or not the children spend much time together and engage in many different activities), their *symmetry* (e.g., whether social power is vested more or less equally or more or less unequally in the two children), and their *affective substrates* (e.g., whether the relationship is supportive and secure or whether it is nonsupportive and conflict ridden). Qualitative differences in these relationships may have developmental implications in the same way that qualitative variations in adult–child relationships do (Ainsworth, Blehar, Waters, & Wall, 1978).

This essay begins, then, with the argument that one cannot describe friendships and their developmental significance without distinguishing between *having friends, the identity of the child's friends* (e.g., personality characteristics of the child's friends), and *friendship quality*. In the sections that follow, these relationship dimensions are examined separately and in turn. Three conclusions emerge: First, having friends is a normatively significant condition during childhood and adolescence. Second, friendships carry both developmental advantages and disadvantages so that a romanticized view of these relationships distorts them and what they may contribute to developmental outcome. Third, the identity of the child's friends and friendship quality may be more closely tied to individual differences than merely whether or not the child has friends.

HAVING FRIENDS

Measurement Issues

Children's friends can be identified in four main ways: (a) by asking the children, their mothers, or their teachers to name the child's friends and determining whether these choices are reciprocated; (b) by asking children to assess their liking for one another; (c) by observing the extent to which children seek and maintain proximity with one another; and (d) by measuring reciprocities and coordinations in their social interaction. Concordances among various indicators turn out to be substantial, but method variance is also considerable; the "insiders" (the children themselves) do not always agree with the "outsiders" (teachers) or the observational record (Hartup, 1992; Howes, 1989).

Some variation among measures derives from the fact that social attraction is difficult for outsiders to know about. Method variance also derives from special difficulties connected with self-reports: First, children without friends almost always can name "friends" when asked to do so (Furman, in press). Second, friendship frequently seems to investigators to be a dichotomous condition (friend vs. nonfriend), whereas variation is more continuous (best friend/good friend/occasional friend/not friend). Third, whether these categories form a Guttman scale has not been determined, although researchers sometimes assume that they do (see Doyle, Markiewicz, & Hardy, 1994). Fourth, the status of so-called unilateral or unreciprocated friendship choice is unclear. Sometimes, when children's choices are not reciprocated, social interaction differs from when friendship choices are mutual; in other respects, the social exchange does not. Unilateral friends, for example, use tactics during disagreements with one another that are different from the ones used by mutual friends but similar to those used by nonfriends (e.g., standing firm). Simultaneously, conflict *outcomes* among unilateral friends (e.g., whether interaction continues) are more similar to those characterizing mutual friends than those characterizing nonfriends (Hartup, Laursen, Stewart, & Eastenson, 1988).

Developmental Significance

The developmental significance of having friends (apart from the identity of the child's friends or the quality of these relationships) has been examined in three main ways: (a) comparing the social interaction that occurs between friends and between nonfriends, (b) comparing children who have friends with those who don't, and (c) examining the extent to which having friends moderates behavioral outcomes across certain normative transitions.

Behavior with friends and nonfriends. Behaviors differentiating friends from nonfriends have been specified in more than 80 studies (Newcomb & Bagwell, 1995); four are cited here. In the first of these (Newcomb & Brady, 1982), school-aged children were asked to explore a "creativity box" with either a friend or a classmate who was not a friend. More extensive exploration was observed among the children with their friends; conversation was more vigorous and mutually oriented; the emotional exchange was more positive. Most important, when tested individually, the children who explored the box with a friend remembered more about it afterward.

Second, Azmitia and Montgomery (1993) examined problem solving among 11-year-olds (mainly their dialogues) working on "isolation of variables" problems either with friends or acquaintances (the children were required to deduce which pizza ingredients caused certain characters in a series of stories to get sick and die). Friends spontaneously justified their suggestions more frequently than acquaintances, elaborated on their partners' proposals, engaged in a greater percentage of conflicts during their conversations, and more often checked results. Most important, the children working with friends did better than children working with nonfriends—on the most difficult versions of the task only. Clearly, "a friend in need is a friend indeed." The children's conversations were related to their problem solving through engagement in transactive conflicts. That is, task performance was facilitated to a greater extent between friends than between nonfriends by free airing of the children's differences in a cooperative, task-oriented context.

Third, we recently examined conversations between friends and nonfriends (10-year-olds) in an inner-city magnet school while the children wrote stories collaboratively on a computer (Hartup, Daiute, Zajac, & Sholl, 1995). Stories dealt with the rain forest—subject matter that the children had studied during a 6-week science project. Baseline story writing was measured with the children writing alone; control subjects *always* wrote alone. Results indicate that friends did not talk more during collaboration than nonfriends but, nevertheless, (a) engaged in more mutually oriented and less individualistic utterances; (b) agreed with one another more often (but did not disagree more readily); (c) repeated their own and the other's assertions more often; (d) posed alternatives and provided elaborations more frequently; (e) spent twice as much time as nonfriends talking about writing content, the vocabulary being used, and writing mechanics; and (f) spent less time engaged in "off-task" talk. Principal component analyses confirm that the structure of friends' talk was strongly focused on the task (i.e., the text) and was assertively collaborative—reminiscent of the dialogs used by experts and novices as discovered in other social problem-solving studies (Rogoff, 1990). Our stories themselves show that, overall, the ones collaboratively written by friends were better than the ones written by nonfriends, a difference that seems to rest on better use of Standard English rather than the narrative elements included in the text. Results suggest, overall, that the affordances of "being friends" differ from the affordances of "being acquaintances" in social problem solving (Hartup, in press).

Fourth, we examined conflict and competition among school-aged children playing a board game when they had been taught different rules (Hartup, French, Laursen, Johnston, & Ogawa, 1993). Disagreements occurred more frequently between friends than between nonfriends and lasted longer. Conflict resolution, however, differed by friendship and sex: (a) boys used assertions *without rationales* more frequently than girls—but only when friends were observed; (b) girls, on the other hand, used assertions *with rationales* more frequently than boys but, again, only with friends. Sex differences in conflict talk, widely cited in the literature (see Maccoby, 1990), thus seem to be relationship manifestations rather than manifestations of individual children.

Based on these and the other available data sets, a recent meta-analysis identified significant friend versus nonfriend effects across four broad-band categories (Newcomb & Bagwell, 1995): *positive engagement* (i.e., talk, smiling, and laughter); *conflict management* (i.e., disengagement and negotiation vs. power assertion); *task activity* (i.e., being oriented to the task as opposed to being off task); and *relationship properties* (i.e., equality in the exchange as well as mutuality and affirmation). Behaviorally speaking, friendships clearly are "communal relationships" (Clark & Mills, 1979). Reciprocity constitutes their deep structure.

Existing data suggest that four cognitive and motivational conditions afford these distinctive interactions: (a) friends know one another better than nonfriends and are thus able to communicate with one another more efficiently and effectively (Ladd & Emerson, 1984); (b) friends and nonfriends have different expectations of one another, especially concerning assistance and support (Bigelow, 1977); (c) an affective climate more favorable to exploration and problem solving exists between friends than between nonfriends—namely, a "climate of agreement" (Gottman, 1983); and (d) friends more readily than nonfriends seek ways of resolving disagreements that support continued interaction between them (Hartup & Laursen, 1992).

Unfortunately, the developmental significance of these differences is not known. Only fragmentary information tells us about short-term consequences in problem solving and behavioral regulation. Recalled events (Newcomb & Brady, 1982), deductive reasoning (Azmitia & Montgomery, 1993), conflict rates (Hartup et al., 1988), creative writing (Hartup et al., 1995), and social/moral judgments (Nelson & Aboud, 1985) are better supported by transactions with friends than by transactions with nonfriends. But only a small number of investigations exists in each case—sometimes only one. The bottom line: Process-outcome studies are badly needed to tell us whether friends engage in better scaffolding than nonfriends, or whether it only seems like they do. Once process/outcome connections are established, we can then—and only then—conclude that friendships have normative significance (i.e., that children employ their friends adaptively on a daily basis as cognitive and social resources).

Having friends versus not having friends. Does having friends contribute to developmental differentiation (i.e., contribute to individual differences)? For the answer to this question to be affirmative, children who have friends must differ from those who do not.

Cross-sectional comparisons show that, first, children who have friends are more socially competent and less troubled than children who do not; they are more sociable, cooperative, altruistic, self-confident, and less lonely (Hartup, 1993; Newcomb & Bagwell, in press). Second, troubled children (e.g., clinic-referred children) are more likely to be friendless than nonreferred control cases (Rutter & Garmezy, 1983). Friendlessness is not always assessed in the same manner in these studies, but the results are consistent: Not one data set suggests that children with friends are worse off than children who do not have them.

Although friended/friendless comparisons are consistent across data sets, the results are difficult to interpret. First, having friends in these studies usually means having good supportive friends; thus having friends is confounded with friendship quality. Second, causal direction is impossible to establish: Friendship experience may contribute to self-esteem, for example, but self-confident children may make friends more readily than less confident children.

Longitudinal studies can be more convincing concerning developmental significance. Unfortunately, few exist. Short-term studies suggest that certain benefits accrue across school transitions: First, attitudes toward school are better among kindergartners (5-year-olds) who have friends at the beginning and who maintain them than those who don't. Making new friends also predicts gains in school performance over the kindergarten year (Ladd, 1990). Second, with data collected from 10-year-olds across a 1-year interval, friendship experience enhanced self-esteem (Bukowski, Hoza, & Newcomb, 1991). Third, psychosocial disturbances have been reported less frequently when school changes occur in the company of good friends than when they don't (Berndt & Hawkins, 1991; Simmons, Burgeson, & Reef, 1988). Having friends thus seems to contribute specifically to affective outcomes across normative school transitions.

One long-term investigation (Bagwell, Newcomb, & Bukowski, 1994) raises questions, however, about "having friends" as a developmental predictor: Eleven-year-old children were identified as either friended or friendless on two separate occasions; subjects were reevaluated at 23 years of age. Having friends and sociometric status (i.e., social acceptance) *together* predicted school success, aspirations, trouble with the law, and several other outcomes. Unique contributions to adult adjustment, however, were verified only for sociometric status. And even then, when stability in the childhood adjustment measures was taken into account, neither sociometric status nor friendship predicted adult outcomes.

Comment

Overall, the developmental significance of having friends is far from clear. Social interaction between friends differs from social interaction between nonfriends, but this does not tell us much more than that these relationships are unique social entities. Correlational studies are difficult to interpret because the effects of having friends are difficult to disentangle from the effects of friendship quality. Short-term longitudinal studies suggest that having friends supports adaptation during normative transitions, but more substantial evidence is needed concerning these effects. Child differences may interact with friendship experience in relation to developmental outcome rather than being main effects. Having friends, for example, may differentiate mainly among children who are vulnerable in some way prior to the transition. Stress associated with developmental transitions is known to accentuate differences among vulnerable children to a greater extent than among nonvulnerable ones (Caspi & Moffitt, 1991). Similarly, developmental interventions often have greater effects on vulnerable than on nonvulnerable individuals (see Crockenberg, 1981).

THE IDENTITY OF THE CHILD'S FRIENDS

We turn now to the identity of the child's friends. Several questions can be asked: With whom does the child become friends? Can the identity of a child's friends be forecast from what we know about the child? What is the developmental significance of the company a child keeps?

Who Are Children's Friends?

Consider, first, that children make friends on the basis of common interests and common activities. Common ground is a sine qua non in friendship relations throughout childhood and adolescence, suggesting that friends ought to be similar to one another in abilities and outlook. Folklore sometimes suggests that "opposites attract," but this notion has not found general support in the empirical literature. The weight of the evidence suggests that, instead, "Beast knows beast; birds of a feather flock together" (Aristotle, *Rhetoric*, Book 11).

Similarities between friends, however, vary from attribute to attribute, in most cases according to *reputational salience* (i.e., according to the importance of an attribute in determining the child's social reputation). Considerable evidence supports this "reputational salience hypothesis": Behavior ratings obtained more than 60 years ago by Robert Challman (1932) showed that social cooperation (an attribute with considerable reputational salience) was more concordant among friends than nonfriends; intelligence (an attribute without reputational salience among young children) was not. Among boys, physical activity (reputationally salient among males) was more similar among friends than nonfriends. Among girls, attractiveness of personality and social network size (both more reputationally salient among females than among males) were more similar among friends than nonfriends.

More recent data also suggest that behavioral concordances among school-aged children and their friends are greater than among children and nonfriends (Haselager, Hartup, Van Lieshout, & Riksen-Walraven, 1995). Peer ratings were obtained in a large number of fifth-grade classrooms centering on three constructs: prosocial behavior, antisocial behavior, and social withdrawal (shyness). First, friends were more similar to one another than nonfriends within each construct cluster (i.e., mean difference scores were significantly smaller). Second, correlations between friends were greater for antisocial behavior (i.e., fighting, disruption, and bullying) than for prosocial behavior (i.e., cooperation, offering help to others) or social withdrawal (i.e., shyness, dependency, and being victimized). These differences may reflect differences among these three attributes in reputational salience: Fighting, for example, is more consistently related to reputation than either cooperation or shyness (Coie, Dodge, & Kupersmidt, 1990). Our results also show important sex differences: (a) Friends were more similar to one another among girls than among boys in both prosocial and antisocial behavior (see also Cairns & Cairns, 1994), and (b) friends were more similar among boys than among girls in shyness. These gender variations are consistent with the reputational salience hypothesis, too: Being kind to others and being mean to them have greater implications for girls' social reputations than boys', whereas shyness/withdrawal has more to do with boys' reputations than girls' (Stevenson-Hinde & Hinde, 1986).

Concordance data from other studies are consistent with the reputational salience notion: Among adolescents, friends are most similar to one another in two general areas: (a) school-related attitudes, aspirations, and achievement (Epstein, 1983; Kandel, 1978b) and (b) normative activities such as smoking, drinking, drug use, antisocial behavior, and dating (Dishion, Andrews, & Crosby, 1995; Epstein, 1983; Kandel, 1978b; Tolson & Urberg, 1993). Sexual activity among adolescents is also consistent with the reputational salience hypothesis. Among girls (both African-American and white) in the United States, friends have been found to be similar in sexual behavior and attitudes, even when age and antisocial attitudes are taken into account. Among boys, however, sexual activity (especially engaging in sexual intercourse) was not concordant (Billy, Rodgers, & Udry, 1984). The authors argue that sexual activity is more closely related to social reputation among adolescent girls than it is among boys, thus accounting for the gender differences in the results.

Still other investigators, employing the social network as a unit of analysis, have discovered that members of friendship networks are concordant on such salient dimensions as sports, academic activities, and drug use (Brown, 1989). Antisocial behavior also distinguishes social networks from one another beginning in middle childhood (Cairns, Cairns, Neckerman, Gest, & Garieppy, 1988).

Friendship Concordances: Sources and Developmental Implications

Similarities between friends are one thing, but where do they come from and where do they lead? Developmental implications cannot be specified without understanding that these similarities derive from three sources: (a) *sociodemographic conditions* that bring children into proximity with one another; (b) *social selection* through which children construct relationships with children who are similar to themselves rather than different; and (c) *mutual socialization* through which children become similar to their friends by interacting with them.

Sociodemographic conditions. Demographic conditions determine the neighborhoods in which children live, the schools in which they enroll, and the classes they attend. Concordances among children and their friends in socioeconomic status, ethnicity, and chronological age thus derive in considerable measure from social forces that constrain the "peer pool" and the child's access to it. One should not underestimate, however, the extent to which some of these concordances derive from the children's own choices. Among children attending schools that are mixed-age, mixed-race, and mixed socioeconomically, friends are still more similar to one another in these attributes than nonfriends are (Goldman, 1981; McCandless & Hoyt, 1961).

Selection. Some similarities among friends derive from the well-known tendency among human beings (not alone among the various species) for choosing close associates who resemble themselves. Recent studies confirm that the similarity-attraction hypothesis applies to children: Among elementary school children who began an experimental session as strangers, differential attraction was evident in some groups (40%). Within them, more social contact occurred between preferred than between nonpreferred partners, and correlations were higher between preferred than nonpreferred partners in sociability and the cognitive maturity of their play (Rubin, Lynch, Coplan, Rose-Krasnor, & Booth, 1994).

But friendship selection is embedded in assortative processes occurring in larger social networks. Dishion and his colleagues (Dishion, Patterson, & Griesler, 1994) believe that these network concordances emerge through a process called "shopping" in which children and adolescents construct relationships that maximize interpersonal payoffs. Children are not believed to choose friends who are similar to themselves on a rational basis so much as on an experiential one. Accordingly, relationships become established when they "feel right." Similar individuals cleave to one another more readily than dissimilar individuals because they are more likely to find common ground in both their activities and their conversations. Antisocial children are thus most likely to make friends with other antisocial children and, in so doing, their common characteristics merge to create a "dyadic antisocial trait." Similarly, soccer players or musicians make friends, merge themselves dyadically, and set the stage for becoming even more similar to one another.

Selection thus acts simultaneously to determine the identity of the child's friends through two interlocking processes: (a) similarity and attraction occurring within dyads, and (b) assortative network formation occurring within groups. These processes undoubtedly combine differently from child to child in affecting developmental outcome: Cooperative, friendly, nonaggressive children can choose friends resembling themselves from a wide array of choices; antisocial children can also choose their friends on the basis of similarity and attraction—but frequently from a more restricted range of social alternatives.
Mutual socialization. What behavioral outcomes stem from mutual socialization? The weight of the evidence suggests, first, that children and their friends who ascribe to conventional norms move further over time in the direction of normative behavior (Ball, 1981; Epstein, 1983; Kandel & Andrews, 1986). But does antisocial behavior increase over time among children in antisocial networks? Does troublesome behavior escalate among children—especially into criminal activity—through membership in these networks? Answers to these questions have been surprisingly difficult to provide, especially since children perceive their friends as exerting more pressure toward desirable than toward undesirable conduct (Brown, Clasen, & Eicher, 1986). Nevertheless, increases in undesirable behavior through antisocial friends among children who are themselves at risk for antisocial behavior is now relatively well documented (Ball, 1981; Berndt & Keefe, 1992; Dishion, 1990; Dishion et al., 1994). Conversely, "desisting" is forecast as strongly by a turning away from antisocial friends as by any other variable (Mulvey & Aber, 1988).

What occurs on a day-to-day basis between aggressive children and their friends? Jocks and their friends? "Brains" and their friends? One guesses that children model normative behaviors *for* their friends and simultaneously receive reinforcement *from* them. Antisocial children, for example, are known to engage in large amounts of talk with their friends—talk that is deviant even when the children are being videotaped in the laboratory (Dishion et al., 1994, 1995). Ordinary children talk a lot with their friends, too, but the content is not generally as deviant (Newcomb & Bagwell, 1995). Antisocial children use coercion with one another (Dishion et al., 1995); ordinary children, on the other hand, are freewheeling with their criticisms and persuasion but are less likely to be coercive (Berndt & Keefe, 1992; Hartup et al., 1993). Finally, one guesses that friends support one another in seeking environments that support their commonly held worldviews, although not much is known about this.

Other results show that selection *combines* with socialization to effect similarity between friends. Kandel (1978a) studied changes over the course of a year in drug use, educational aspirations, and delinquency in early adolescence, discovering that similarity stemmed from both sources in approximately equal amounts. Relative effects, however, vary according to the norms and the children involved (see Hartup, 1993).

Comment

Children and their friends are similar to one another, especially in attributes with reputational salience. One must acknowledge that effects sizes are modest and that friends are not carbon copies of one another. One must also acknowledge that the reputational salience hypothesis has never been subjected to direct test and it needs to be. Nevertheless, the identity of the child's friends is a significant consideration in predicting developmental outcome. Friends may be generally intimate, caring, and supportive, thus fostering good developmental prognosis. At the same time, the activities in which they support one another (the relationship *content*) may be extremely deviant, suggesting an altogether different prognosis.

FRIENDSHIP QUALITY

Conceptual and Measurement Issues

Qualitative assessment of child and adolescent friendships currently involves two main strategies: (a) *dimensional analysis* through which one determines whether certain elements are present or absent in the social interaction between friends (e.g., companionship, intimacy, conflict, or power asymmetries), and (b) *typological* or *categorical* analysis through which one identifies patterns in social interaction believed to be critical to social development and adaptation (Furman, in press).

Dimensional assessment. Most current dimensional assessments are based on "provisions" or "features" that children mention when talking about these relationships (Berndt & Perry, 1986; Bukowski, Hoza, & Boivin, 1994; Furman & Adler, 1982; Furman & Buhrmester, 1985; Parker & Asher, 1993); most instruments tap five or six domains. Domain scores, however, are correlated with one another (Berndt & Perry, 1986; Parker & Asher, 1993), and most factor analyses yield two-factor solutions. Both Berndt (in press) and Furman (in press) argue that "positive" and "negative" dimensions adequately describe most dimensional assessments, although some data sets suggest that more elaborate solutions are warranted (e.g., Ladd, Kochenderfer, & Coleman, in press).

Typological assessment. Typological assessment is evolving slowly since the functional significance of friendships remains uncertain. Can one, for example, regard friendships as attachments? Probably not. No one has demonstrated that "the secure base phenomenon," so common among children and their caregivers, constitutes the functional core of children's friendships. Friends have been shown to be secure bases in one or two instances (Ipsa, 1981; Schwartz, 1972), but one is not overwhelmed with the evidence that children and their friends are bound to one another as attachment objects. Children describe their relationships with friends differently from their relationships with their caregivers—as *more* companionable, intimate, and egalitarian and, simultaneously, as *less* affectionate and reliable (Furman & Buhrmester, 1985). For these reasons, some writers describe friendships as affiliative relationships rather than attachments (Weiss, 1986). The challenge, then, is to describe what good-quality affiliative relationships are.

One new classification system has been devised on the basis of family systems theory (Shulman, 1993). Well-functioning friendships are considered to be balanced between closeness and intimacy, on the one hand, and individuality, on the other. The family systems model suggests three friendship types: *interdependent* ones, with cooperation and autonomy balanced; *disengaged* ones, in which friends are disconnected in spite of their efforts to maintain proximity with one another; and *consensus-sensitive* or *enmeshed* relationships, in which agreement and cohesion are maximized. Empirical data are based largely on children's interactions in a cooperative task adapted from family systems research (Reiss, 1981) and document the existence of interdependent and disengaged relationships—a promising beginning. Once again, however, caution should be exercised: Friendship networks may not revolve around the same equilibrative axes as families do.

DEVELOPMENTAL SIGNIFICANCE

Cross-sectional studies. Among the various qualitative dimensions, *support* (positivity) and *contention* (negativity) have been examined most extensively in relation to child outcomes. Support is positively correlated with school involvement and achievement (Berndt & Hawkins, 1991; Cauce, 1986) and negatively correlated with school-based problems (Kurdek & Sinclair, 1988); positively correlated with popularity and good social reputations (Cauce, 1986); positively correlated with self-esteem (Mannarino, 1978; McGuire & Weisz, 1982; Perry, 1987) and psychosocial adjustment (Buhrmester, 1990) as well as negatively correlated with identity problems (Papini, Farmer,

Clark, Micke, & Barnett, 1990) and depression—especially among girls (Compas, Slavin, Wagner, & Cannatta, 1986). Results are thus consistent but, once again, impossible to interpret. We cannot tell whether supportive relationships contribute to the competence of the individual child or vice versa. *Longitudinal studies.* Longitudinal studies dealing with friendship quality (positive vs. negative) emphasize school attitudes, involvement, and achievement. Studying children across the transition from elementary to junior high school, Berndt (1989) measured the size of the friendship network, friendship stability, and self-reported friendship quality (positivity) as well as popularity, attitudes toward school, and achievement. First, network size was negatively related to friendship support as reported by the children, suggesting that children recognize what researchers have been slow to learn, namely, that friendships are not all alike. Second, several nonsignificant results are illuminating: Neither number of friends nor friendship stability contributed to changes in school adjustment—either across the school transition or across the first year in the new school. School adjustment was relatively stable across the transition and was related to friendship stability cross-sectionally but not with earlier adjustment factored out. Third, the self-rated supportiveness of the child's friends, assessed shortly after entrance to the new school, predicted increasing popularity and increasingly positive attitudes toward classmates over the next year, suggesting that positive qualities in one's friendship relations support a widening social world in new school environments.

Other investigations focus on friendship qualities as predictors of school adaptation within the school year. Among 5-year-olds enrolled in kindergarten (Ladd et al., in press), for example, those having friendships characterized by "aid" and "validation" improved in school attitudes over the year with initial attitudes toward school factored out. Perceived conflict in friendships, on the other hand, predicted increasing forms of school maladjustment, especially among boys, including school loneliness and avoidance as well as school liking and engagement.

One other investigation (Berndt & Keefe, 1992) focused on both positive and negative friendship qualities and their correlations across time with school adjustment and self-esteem among adolescents (Berndt & Keefe, 1992). Students with supportive, intimate friendships became increasingly involved with school, while those who considered their friendships to be conflict-ridden and rivalrous became increasingly disruptive and troublesome. Friendship quality was not correlated with changes in self-esteem, possibly because self-esteem was relatively stable from the beginning to the end of the year. Additional analyses (Berndt, in press) suggest that developmental prediction is better for the negative dimensions in these relationships than the positive ones.

Other investigators have examined the interactions between stress and social support as related to behavioral outcome. With elementary school children, increases in peer support over several years predict both increasingly better adaptation and better grade point averages (Dubow, Tisak, Causey, Hryshko, & Reid, 1991). Other results, however, suggest that support from school personnel was associated with decreases in distress across a 2-year period but not support from friends (controlling for initial adjustment). Regression models showed that, actually, school grades predicted changes in friends' support rather than the reverse (DuBois, Felner, Brand, Adan, & Evans, 1992). Among adolescents, however, results are more complex: Windle (1992) reported that, among girls, friend support is positively correlated with alcohol use but negatively correlated with depression (with initial adjustment levels factored out). Among boys, friendship support is associated with outcome depending on stress levels: When stress is high, friend support encourages both alcohol use and depression; when stress is low or moderate, both alcohol use and depression are associated with having *nonsupportive* friends.

The dissonances encountered in these results would be reduced considerably were the identity of the children's friends to be known. Children and adolescents with behavior difficulties frequently have friends who themselves are troublesome (Dishion et al., 1995). These friends may provide one another with emotional support, but the interactions that occur between them may not be the same as those occurring between non-troubled children and their friends. Knowing who the child's friends are might account for the empirical anomalies.

Other difficulties in accounting for these results derive from the fact that the referents used in measuring social support in these studies (except in Berndt's work) consisted of friendship networks (the child's "friends") rather than a "best friend." And still other complications arise from the use of one child's assessments of relationship qualities (the subject's) when the evidence suggests that discrepancies between partners may correlate more strongly with adjustment difficulties than the perceptions of either partner alone (East, 1991). Nevertheless, these studies provide tantalizing tidbits suggesting that friendship quality bears a causal relation to developmental outcome.

Comment

What kinds of research are needed to better understand the developmental implications of friendship quality? One can argue that we are not urgently in need of crosstime studies narrowly focused on friendships and their vicissitudes. Rather, we need comprehensive studies in which interaction effects rather than main effects are emphasized and that encompass a wide range of variables as they cycle through time: (a) measures of the child, including temperament and other relevant early characteristics; (b) measures of early relationships, especially their affective and cognitive qualities; (c) measures of early success in encounters with relevant institutions, especially the schools; (d) status and reputation among other children (sociometric status); *and*, (e) friendship measures that simultaneously include whether a child has friends, who the child's friends are, and what these relationships are like.

Coming close to this model are recent studies conducted by the Oregon Social Learning Center (e.g., Dishion et al., 1994; Patterson, Reid, & Dishion, 1992). Child characteristics and family relations in early childhood have not been examined extensively by these investigators, but their work establishes linkages between coerciveness and monitoring within parent–child and sibling relationships, on the one hand, and troublesomeness and antisocial behavior among school-aged boys on the other. These studies also establish that poor parental discipline and monitoring predict peer rejection and academic failures, and that these conditions, in turn, predict increasing involvement with antisocial friends. Among children with these early histories, the immediate connection to serious conduct difficulties in adolescence now seems to be friendship with another deviant child. Exactly these conditions existed in the social history of that Minnesota teenager who, together with his best friend, killed his mother early in 1995.

CONCLUSION

Friendships in childhood and adolescence would seem to be developmentally significant—both normatively and differentially. When children have friends, they use them as cognitive and social resources on an everyday basis. Normative transitions and the stress carried with them seem to be better negotiated when children have friends than when they don't, especially when children are at risk. Differential significance, however, seems to derive mainly from the identity of the child's friends and the quality of the relationships between them. Supportive relationships between socially skilled individuals appear to be developmental advantages, whereas coercive and conflict-ridden relationships are developmental disadvantages, especially among antisocial children.

Nevertheless, friendship and its developmental significance may vary from child to child. New studies show that child characteristics interact with early relationships and environmental conditions, cycling in turn through relations with other children to determine behavioral outcome (Hartup & Van Lieshout, 1995). The work cited in this essay strongly suggests that friendship assessments deserve greater attention in studying these developmental pathways than they are currently given. These assessments, however, need to be comprehensive. Along with knowing whether or not children have friends, we must know who their friends are and the quality of their relationships with them.

REFERENCES

Ainsworth, M. D. S., Blehar, M. C., Waters, E., & Wall, S. (1978). *Patterns of attachment: A psychological study of the Strange Situation.* Hillsdale, NJ: Erlbaum.

Azmitia, M., & Montgomery, R. (1993). Friendship, transactive dialogues, and the development of scientific reasoning. *Social Development, 2,* 202–221.

Bagwell, C., Newcomb, A. F., & Bukowski, W. M. (1994). *Early adolescent friendship as a predictor of adult adjustment: A twelve year follow-up investigation.* Unpublished manuscript, University of Richmond.

Ball, S. J. (1981). *Beachside comprehensive.* Cambridge: Cambridge University Press.

Berndt, T. J. (1989). Obtaining support from friends during childhood and adolescence. In D. Belle (Ed.), *Children's social networks and social supports* (pp. 308–331). New York: Wiley.

Berndt, T. J. (in press). Exploring the effects of friendship quality on social development. In W. M. Bukowski, A. F. Newcomb, & W. W. Hartup (Eds.), *The company they keep: Friendships in childhood and adolescence.* Cambridge: Cambridge University Press.

Berndt, T. J., & Hawkins, J. A. (1991). *Effects of friendship on adolescents' adjustment to junior high school.* Unpublished manuscript, Purdue University.

Berndt, T. J., & Keefe, K. (1992). Friends' influence on adolescents' perceptions of themselves in school. In D. H. Schunk & J. L. Meece (Eds.), *Students' perceptions in the classroom* (pp. 51–73). Hillsdale, NJ: Erlbaum.

Berndt, T. J., & Perry, T. B. (1986). Children's perceptions of friendship as supportive relationships. *Developmental Psychology, 22,* 640–648.

Bigelow, B. J. (1977). Children's friendship expectations: A cognitive developmental study. *Child Development, 48,* 246–253.

Billy, J. O. G., Rodgers, J. L., & Udry, J. R. (1984). Adolescent sexual behavior and friendship choice. *Social Forces, 62,* 653–678.

Brown, B. B. (1989). The role of peer groups in adolescents' adjustment to secondary school. In T. J. Berndt & G. W. Ladd (Eds.), *Peer relationships in child development* (pp. 188–215). New York: Wiley.

Brown, B. B., Clasen, D. R., & Eicher, S. A. (1986). Perceptions of peer pressure, peer conformity dispositions, and self-reported behavior among adolescents. *Developmental Psychology, 22,* 521–530.

Buhrmester, D. (1990). Intimacy of friendship, interpersonal competence, and adjustment during preadolescence and adolescence. *Child Development, 61,* 1101–1111.

Bukowski, W. M., Hoza, B., & Boivin, M. (1994). Measuring friendship quality during pre- and early adolescence: The development and psychometric properties of the Friendship Qualities Scale. *Journal of Personal and Social Relationships, 11,* 471–484.

Bukowski, W. M., Hoza, B., & Newcomb, A. F. (1991). *Friendship, popularity, and the "self" during early adolescence.* Unpublished manuscript, Concordia University, Montreal.

Cairns, R. B., & Cairns, B. D. (1994). *Lifelines and risks.* Cambridge: Cambridge University Press.

Cairns, R. B., Cairns, B. D., Neckerman, H. J., Gest, S., & Garieppy, J.-L. (1988). Peer networks and aggressive behavior: Peer support or peer rejection? *Developmental Psychology, 24,* 815–823.

Caspi, A., & Moffitt, T. E. (1991). Individual differences are accentuated during periods of social change: The sample case of girls at puberty. *Journal of Personality and Social Psychology, 61,* 157–168.

Cauce, A. M. (1986). Social networks and social competence: Exploring the effects of early adolescent friendships. *American Journal of Community Psychology, 14,* 607–628.

Challman, R. C. (1932). Factors influencing friendships among preschool children. *Child Development, 3,* 146–158.

Clark, M. S., & Mills, J. (1979). Interpersonal attraction in exchange and communal relationships. *Journal of Personality and Social Psychology, 37,* 12–24.

Coie, J. D., Dodge, K. A., & Kupersmidt, J. B. (1990). Peer group behavior and social status. In S. R. Asher & J. D. Coie (Eds.), *Peer rejection in childhood* (pp. 17–59). Cambridge: Cambridge University Press.

Compas, B. E., Slavin, L. A., Wagner, B. A., & Cannatta, K. (1986). Relationship of life events and social support with psychological dysfunction among adolescents. *Journal of Youth and Adolescence, 15,* 205–221.

Crockenberg, S. B. (1981). Infant irritability, mother responsiveness, and social support influences on the security of mother–infant attachment. *Child Development, 52,* 857–865.

Dishion, T. J. (1990). The peer context of troublesome child and adolescent behavior. In P. Leone (Ed.), *Understanding troubled and troublesome youth.* Newbury Park, CA: Sage.

Dishion, T. J., Andrews, D. W., & Crosby, L. (1995). Antisocial boys and their friends in early adolescence: Relationship characteristics, quality, and interactional process. *Child Development, 66,* 139–151.

Dishion, T. J., Patterson, G. R., & Griesler, P. C. (1994). Peer adaptations in the development of antisocial behavior: A confluence model. In L. R. Huesmann (Ed.), *Current perspectives on aggressive behavior* (pp. 61–95). New York: Plenum.

Doyle, A. B., Markiewicz, D., & Hardy, C. (1994). Mothers' and children's friendships: Intergenerational associations. *Journal of Social and Personal Relationships, 11,* 363–377.

DuBois, D. L., Felner, R. D., Brand, S., Adan, A. M., & Evans, E. G. (1992). A prospective study of life stress, social support, and adaptation in early adolescence. *Child Development, 63,* 542–557.

Dubow, E. F., Tisak, J., Causey, D., Hryshko, A., & Reid, G. (1991). A two-year longitudinal study of stressful life events, social support, and social problem-solving skills: Contributions to children's behavioral and academic adjustment. *Child Development, 62,* 583–599.

East, P. L. (1991). The parent–child relationships of withdrawn, aggressive, and sociable children: Child and parent perspectives. *Merrill–Palmer Quarterly, 37,* 425–444.

Epstein, J. L. (1983). Examining theories of adolescent friendship. In J. L. Epstein & N. L. Karweit (Eds.), *Friends in school* (pp. 39–61). San Diego: Academic Press.

Furman, W. (in press). The measurement of friendship perceptions: Conceptual and methodological issues. In W. M. Bukowski, A. F. Newcomb, & W. W. Hartup (Eds.), *The company they keep: Friendships in childhood and adolescence.* Cambridge: Cambridge University Press.

Furman, W., & Adler, T. (1982). *The Friendship Questionnaire.* Unpublished manuscript, University of Denver.

Furman, W., & Buhrmester, D. (1985). Children's perceptions of the personal relationships in their social networks. *Developmental Psychology, 21,* 1016–1022.

Goldman, J. A. (1981). The social interaction of preschool children in same-age versus mixedage groupings. *Child Development, 52,* 644–650.

Gottman, J. M. (1983). How children become friends. *Monographs of the Society for Research in Child Development, 48*(3, Serial No. 201).

Hartup, W. W. (1992). Friendships and their developmental significance. In H. McGurk (Ed.), *Childhood social development* (pp. 175–205). Gove, UK: Erlbaum.

Hartup, W. W. (1993). Adolescents and their friends. In B. Laursen (Ed.), *Close friendships in adolescence* (pp. 3–22). San Francisco: Jossey-Bass.

Hartup, W. W. (in press). Cooperation, close relationships, and cognitive development. In W. M. Bukowski, A. F. Newcomb, & W. W. Hartup (Eds.), *The company they keep: Friendships in childhood and adolescence.* Cambridge: Cambridge University Press.

Hartup, W. W., Daiute, C., Zajac, R., & Sholl, W. (1995). *Collaboration in creative writing by friends and nonfriends.* Unpublished manuscript, University of Minnesota.

Hartup, W. W., French, D. C., Laursen, B., Johnston, K. M., & Ogawa, J. (1993). Conflict and friendship relations in middle childhood: Behavior in a closed-field situation. *Child Development, 64,* 445–454.

Hartup, W. W., & Laursen, B. (1992). Conflict and context in peer relations. In C. H. Hart (Ed.), *Children on playgrounds: Research perspectives and applications* (pp. 44–84). Albany: State University of New York Press.

Hartup, W. W., Laursen, B., Stewart, M. I., & Eastenson, A. (1988). Conflict and the friendship relations of young children. *Child Development, 59*, 1590–1600.

Hartup, W. W., & Van Lieshout, C. F. M. (1995). Personality development in social context. In J. T. Spence (Ed.), *Annual Review of Psychology, 46*, 655–687.

Haselager, G. J. T., Hartup, W. W., Van Lieshout, C. F. M., & Riksen-Walraven, M. (1995). *Friendship similarity in middle childhood as a function of sex and sociometric status.* Unpublished manuscript, University of Nijmegen.

Howes, C. (1989). Peer interaction of young children. *Monographs of the Society for Research in Child Development, 53*(Serial No. 217).

Ipsa, J. (1981). Peer support among Soviet day care toddlers. *International Journal of Behavioral Development, 4*, 255–269.

Kandel, D. B. (1978a). Homophily, selection, and socialization in adolescent friendships. *American Journal of Sociology, 84*, 427–436.

Kandel, D. B. (1978b). Similarity in real-life adolescent pairs. *Journal of Personality and Social Psychology, 36*, 306–312.

Kandel, D. B., & Andrews, K. (1986). Processes of adolescent socialization by parents and peers. *International Journal of the Addictions, 22*, 319–342.

Kurdek, L. A., & Sinclair, R. J. (1988). Adjustment of young adolescents in two-parent nuclear, stepfather, and mother-custody families. *Journal of Consulting and Clinical Psychology, 56*, 91–96.

Ladd, G. W. (1990). Having friends, keeping friends, making friends, and being liked by peers in the classroom: Predictors of children's early school adjustment? *Child Development, 61*, 1081–1100.

Ladd, G. W., & Emerson, E. S. (1984). Shared knowledge in children's friendships. *Developmental Psychology, 20*, 932–940.

Ladd, G. W., Kochenderfer, B. J., & Coleman, C. C. (in press). Friendship quality as a predictor of young children's early school adjustment. *Child Development.*

Maccoby, E. E. (1990). Gender and relationships: A developmental account. *American Psychologist, 45*, 513–520.

Mannarino, A. P. (1978). Friendship patterns and self-concept development in preadolescent males. *Journal of Genetic Psychology, 133*, 105–110.

McCandless, B. R., & Hoyt, J. M. (1961). Sex, ethnicity and play preferences of preschool children. *Journal of Abnormal and Social Psychology, 62*, 683–685.

McGuire, K. D., & Weisz, J. R. (1982). Social cognition and behavior correlates of preadolescent chumship. *Child Development, 53*, 1478–1484.

Mulvey, E. P., & Aber, M. S. (1988). Growing out of delinquency: Development and desistance. In R. Jenkins & W. Brown (Eds.), *The abandonment of delinquent behavior: Promoting the turn-around.* New York: Praeger.

Nelson, J., & Aboud, F. E. (1985). The resolution of social conflict between friends. *Child Development, 56*, 1009–1017.

Newcomb, A. F., & Bagwell, C. (1995). Children's friendship relations: A meta-analytic review. *Psychological Bulletin, 117*, 306–347.

Newcomb, A. F., & Bagwell, C. (in press). The developmental significance of children's friendship relations. In W. M. Bukowski, A. F. Newcomb, & W. W. Hartup (Eds.), *The company they keep: Friendship in childhood and adolescence.* Cambridge: Cambridge University Press.

Newcomb, A. F., & Brady, J. E. (1982). Mutuality in boys' friendship relations. *Child Development, 53*, 392–395.

Papini, D. R., Farmer, F. F., Clark, S. M., Micke, J. C., & Barnett, J. K. (1990). Early adolescent age and gender differences in patterns of emotional self-disclosure to parents and friends. *Adolescence, 25*, 959–976.

Parker, J. G., & Asher, S. R. (1987). Peer relations and later personal adjustment: Are low-accepted children at risk? *Psychological Bulletin, 102*, 357–389.

Parker, J. G., & Asher, S. R. (1993). Friendship and friendship quality in middle childhood: Links with peer group acceptance and feelings of loneliness and social dissatisfaction. *Developmental Psychology, 29*, 611–621.

Patterson, G. R., Reid, J. B., & Dishion, T. J. (1992). *Antisocial boys.* Eugene, OR: Castalia.

Perry, T. B. (1987). *The relation of adolescent self-perceptions to their social relationships.* Unpublished doctoral dissertation, University of Oklahoma.

Reiss, D. (1981). *The family's construction of reality.* Cambridge, MA: Harvard University Press.

Rogoff, B. (1990). *Apprenticeship in thinking.* New York: Oxford University Press.

Rubin, K. H., Lynch, D., Coplan, R., Rose–Krasnor, L., & Booth, C. L. (1994). "Birds of a feather . . .": Behavioral concordances and preferential personal attraction in children. *Child Development, 65*, 1778–1785.

Rutter, M., & Garmezy, N. (1983). Developmental psychopathology. In E. M. Hetherington (Ed.), P. H. Mussen (Series Ed.), *Handbook of child psychology: Vol. 4. Socialization, personality, and social development* (pp. 775–911). New York: Wiley.

Schwartz, J. C. (1972). Effects of peer familiarity on the behavior of preschoolers in a novel situation. *Journal of Personality and Social Psychology, 24*, 276–284.

Shulman, S. (1993). Close friendships in early and middle adolescence: Typology and friendship reasoning. In B. Laursen (Ed.), *Close friendships in adolescence* (pp. 55–72). San Francisco: Jossey-Bass.

Simmons, R. G., Burgeson, R., & Reef, M. J. (1988). Cumulative changes at entry to adolescence. In M. Gunnar & W. A. Collins (Eds.), *Minnesota symposia on child psychology* (Vol. 21, pp. 123–150). Hillsdale, NJ: Erlbaum.

Stevenson-Hinde, J., & Hinde, R. A. (1986). Changes in associations between characteristics and interaction. In R. Plomin & J. Dunn (Eds.), *The study of temperament: Changes, continuities and challenges* (pp. 115–129). Hillsdale, NJ: Erlbaum.

Sullivan, H. S. (1953). *The interpersonal theory of psychiatry.* New York: Norton.

Tolson, J. M., & Urberg, K. A. (1993). Similarity between adolescent best friends, *Journal of Adolescent Research, 8*, 274–288.

Weiss, R. S. (1986). Continuities and transformations in social relationships from childhood to adulthood. In W. W. Hartup & Z. Rubin (Eds.), *Relationships and development* (pp. 95–110). Hillsdale, NJ: Erlbaum.

Windle, M. (1992). A longitudinal study of stress buffering for adolescent problem behaviors. *Developmental Psychology, 28*, 522–530.

5

Children's Treatment by Peers: Victims of Relational and Overt Aggression

Nicki R. Crick and Jennifer K. Grotpeter
University of Illinois at Urbana–Champaign

Past research on peer victimization has focused on maltreatment through overtly aggressive behaviors. Although a relational form of aggression has been identified in recent research, studies of the victims of relational aggression have not yet been conducted. The present research was designed as a first attempt to address this issue. Four goals were pursued (n = 474; third- to sixth-grade children): (a) development of a self-report measure of victimization through relational and overt aggression; (b) assessment of the relation between overt victimization and relational victimization; (c) assessment of gender, grade, and sociometric status group differences in victimization; and (d) evaluation of the relation between victimization and social–psychological adjustment. Results showed that the newly developed victimization measure had favorable psychometric properties and that most of the identified victims were the targets of either relational or overt aggression, but not both. Further, rejected children were more relationally and overtly victimized than their better accepted peers, and boys were more overtly victimized than girls. Finally, relational victimization, overt victimization, and the lack of prosocial treatment by peers were all significantly related to social–psychological adjustment difficulties (e.g., depression, loneliness).

Although hundreds of studies have been conducted on aggressive children in the past few decades (see Achenbach, McConaughy, & Howell, 1987; Berkowitz, 1993; Crick & Dodge, 1994; Parke & Slaby, 1983, for reviews), relatively little attention has been paid to the children who serve as the targets of peers' aggressive acts. The potentially negative impact of peer victimization on children's development has been well documented in a few recent studies, which have shown victimization to be related to peer rejection and other serious adjustment difficulties (Bjorkqvist, Ekman, & Lagerspetz, 1982; Boulton & Underwood, 1992; Olweus, 1978, 1984, 1991; Perry, Kusel, & Perry, 1988). These studies highlight the importance of a research focus on the targets, as well as the perpetrators, of aggressive acts.

Reprinted with permission from *Development and Psychopathology*, 1996, Vol. 8, 367–380. Copyright © 1996 by the Cambridge University Press.

This research was funded by grants from the University of Illinois Research Board and the United States Department of Agriculture to the first author. Portions of this study were presented at the meeting of the Society for Research in Child Development, March, 1993, New Orleans. The participation of the Decatur Illinois School District in this research is gratefully acknowledged. Special thanks to Maureen A. Bigbee and the anonymous reviewers for their comments on an earlier draft of this manuscript.

To date, research on peer victimization has focused on maltreatment through overt forms of aggression (e.g., hitting, name calling, verbal threats). Study of this form of peer maltreatment is important; however, recent studies demonstrate that it does not capture the full range of harmful behaviors that children direct toward their peers. Specifically, a relationally oriented form of aggression has been recently identified that, in contrast to overt aggression, harms others through hurtful manipulation of or damage to their peer relationships (e.g., spreading mean rumors about a peer; retaliating against a peer by purposefully excluding her from one's social group) (Crick 1995; Crick & Grotpeter, 1995; Grotpeter & Crick, in press). A recent study of children's perceptions of aggression has shown that both boys and girls consider relationally aggressive behaviors to be hostile and relatively frequent aggressive events, particularly for those situations in which the aggressors are girls (Crick, Bigbee, & Howes, in press). Further, results of a second study indicate that relationally aggressive social events are more distressful for girls than boys (Crick, 1995). These findings suggest that study of relational victimization may provide information about aversive peer experiences that are particularly salient to girls. Generation of this information is important given that the majority of past research has focused on overt victimization and the study of boys, an approach that has yielded relatively little information about peer maltreatment among girls (for a review, see Olweus, 1993). As a first step toward addressing this gap in our knowledge, the present research was designed to identify the victims of relationally aggressive attacks and to assess the characteristics of these victims.

An additional goal of this research was to assess gender and sociometric status differences in treatment by peers. These two characteristics have been shown in past studies to be important correlates of overt victimization. Specifically, previous studies of overt victimization have shown that boys and rejected children are more victimized than are girls and nonrejected children, respectively (Boulton & Underwood, 1992; Perry et al., 1988; Olweus, 1978, 1984, 1991, 1993). We hypothesized that relationally victimized children would be similar to overtly victimized children in terms of their peer status (i.e., rejected). Although the form of maltreatment varies for the two groups of victimized children, both groups are the targets of extremely negative behavior and, thus, similar social standing in the peer group seemed likely. If so, relationally victimized children (and overtly victimized children) may be at risk for the future developmental difficulties that have been shown to be related to peer rejection (e.g., school failure, criminality, mental health problems; for a review, see Parker & Asher, 1987).

We also hypothesized that, in contrast to overt victimization that has been shown in past research to be more characteristic of boys than of girls (see Olweus, 1993, for a review), gender differences in relational victimization would be either negligible or would be biased in favor of girls (i.e., with girls being more relationally victimized than boys). By the time children reach school age, sanctions against boys overtly aggressing toward girls are typically well established. Because boys initiate the majority of overtly aggressive acts (Block, 1983; Parke & Slaby, 1983), it is likely that these events involve primarily boy-to-boy interactions, an hypothesis supported by the reports of children (Crick et al., in press; Olweus, 1993). In contrast to overt aggression, relational aggression is exhibited more often by girls than boys (Cairns, Cairns, Neckerman, Ferguson, & Gariepy, 1989; Crick & Grotpeter, 1995; Lagerspetz, Bjorkvist, & Peltonen, 1988) and, according to children's reports, is directed toward both boys and girls (Crick, et al., in press). Thus, we hypothesized that relationally aggressive events would involve both boys and girls as victims (i.e., resulting in either no gender differences in relational victimization or girls reporting higher levels than boys).

Another goal we had for this research was to assess children's positive treatment from peers, in addition to peer victimization, so that a more thorough and balanced evaluation of children's social experiences could be achieved than in past studies. Although previous investigators of children's peer treatment have focused solely on children's negative experiences (e.g., getting pushed or shoved by other children; Olweus, 1993; Perry et al., 1988), it seems likely that a lack of positive experiences (e.g., not receiving help from peers when it is needed) may also play an important role in children's development. For example, some children may not be confronted by aversive social events in the peer group (e.g., being the target of aggressive acts), but instead may face a peer environment that is characterized by a lack of support or even benign neglect. Even if this treatment is not motivated by malicious intent on the part of peers, it may leave these children without important instrumental and emotional resources for receiving help, coping with social or emotional difficulties, or making friends. We sought in this research to assess whether positive, prosocial treatment from peers would emerge as an important and unique aspect of children's social experiences, in addition to victimization. If so, it may be important in future intervention research to identify and assist children who lack positive peer treatment, as well as those who experience negative treatment (i.e., victimization).

To address the research goals described above, our first task was to develop a reliable measure of children's treatment by peers. Past approaches to the assessment of victimization (i.e., peer maltreatment) have most often involved either peer nominations (Bjorkqvist et al., 1982; Perry et al., 1988; Schwartz, 1993) or self-reports (Boulton & Underwood, 1992; Olweus, 1978, 1984, 1991; Perry et al., 1988). We used self-report in this study because we were most interested in children's (as opposed to peers') perceptions of their treatment by others. The importance of considering the child's perspective in studies of peer relations has been well established in recent research (e.g., Asher, Hymel, & Renshaw, 1985; Asher & Wheeler, 1985; Crick & Ladd, 1993; Hymel & Franke, 1985). Another advantage to self-report, as compared with peer report, is that it allows children to report incidences of victimization that occur outside the immediate classroom and by provocateurs who are not classmates. This is important given that a considerable proportion of victimization episodes (38–50%) have been shown to occur outside the immediate school peer group (e.g., with older peers, with younger peers, etc.) (Boulton & Underwood, 1982; Olweus, 1991). Finally, self-report was of interest because our intent was to assess whether children distinguish between relational and overt forms of victimization or whether they view their own treatment by peers in more general terms (e.g., "good" treatment versus "bad" treatment). In past studies, victimization has been assessed with items that are nonspecific to a particular form of aggression (e.g., the Perry et al., 1988, measure included items such as "kids do mean things to him" and "kids try to hurt his feelings," items that can be associated with several forms of aggression). To assess whether children distinguish between two specific forms of victimization, a new victimization measure was developed and used in this research. This self-report measure, the Social Experience Questionnaire (SEQ), was designed to specifically assess both overt victimization (e.g., getting pushed or shoved by a peer) and relational victimization (e.g., having a peer spread lies about you in the peer group), in addition to more positive aspects of children's social experiences (i.e., being the target of peers' prosocial acts).

The final issue addressed in this research concerned the relation between victimization and social–psychological adjustment. Little research has been conducted in this area to date, even on overt victimization (see Perry et al., 1988), and much of the research that does exist has been hampered by assessment limitations (e.g., the use of one-item scales to assess psychological adjustment; Boulton & Underwood, 1982) and by the study of boys only (e.g., Olweus, 1993; Schwartz, Dodge, & Coie, 1993). Our goal was to assess aspects of adjustment that are relevant to victimization and accompanying social difficulties for both boys and girls, using well-established measures with favorable psychometric properties. Aspects of adjustment included were depression, loneliness, and social anxiety/avoidance. Depression was included because past research has demonstrated a significant link between this aspect of adjustment and overt victimization for boys (Olweus, 1993). However, this link has not yet been studied for samples of overtly victimized girls or relationally victimized children. Loneliness and social anxiety/avoidance were included because past research has shown these indices to reflect important aspects of children's emotional adjustment in peer contexts (e.g., for reviews see Asher, Parkhurst, Hymel, & Williams, 1990; Hymel & Franke, 1985). Each aspect of social–psychological adjustment was assessed with instruments that have been widely used in previous studies and that have been shown to be reliable and valid for use with children (e.g., Asher, Hymel, & Renshaw, 1984; Asher & Wheeler, 1985; Crick & Ladd, 1993; Franke & Hymel, 1984; Kovacs, 1985). We hypothesized that both forms of victimization, relational and overt, would be positively related to indices of social–psychological adjustment problems, and that prosocial treatment would be negatively related to these indices (it is important to note that our assessments of maladjustment were intended as indicators of relative difficulty within a normative sample, not as clinical evaluations of pathology).

METHOD

Participants

A total of 474 third- to sixth-grade children from four public schools in a moderately sized midwestern town participated as subjects. The sample included 123 third (62 girls and 61 boys), 124 fourth (55 girls and 69 boys), 122 fifth (54 girls and 68 boys), and 105 sixth graders (54 girls and 51 boys; additional data for this sample are described in Crick & Grotpeter, 1995; Crick et al., in press). Approximately 37.6% of the sample was African American, 60.1% was European American, and 2.3% represented other ethnic groups. The socioeconomic status of the sample was estimated to be lower class to lower middle class. Each subject had parental consent to participate in the study (parental consent was more than 82%).

Assessment of Peer Treatment

Victimization and positive peer treatment were both measured with the Social Experience Questionnaire (SEQ), a self-report instrument designed specifically for use in this study. The SEQ consisted of three subscales, each of which contained five items: relational victimization, overt victimization, and receipt of prosocial acts. Items were generated based on a peer-nomination measure of aggression developed in prior research, which included subscales for relational aggression, overt aggression, and prosocial behavior (e.g., Crick & Grotpeter, 1995; Crick, 1995; Grotpeter & Crick, in press). Items from the aggression instrument were reworded to make them appropriate for self-report, and to make them appropriate for assessing peer treatment rather than social behavior. Specifically, the relational victimization subscale of the SEQ assessed children's reports of the frequency with which their peers attempt to harm, or threaten to harm, their peer relationships (e.g., How often does another kid say they won't like you unless you do what they want you to do?). The overt victimization subscale assessed children's reports of the frequency with which other children attempt to harm or threaten to harm their physical well-being (e.g., How often do you get hit by another kid at school?). The prosocial receipt subscale assessed how often subjects were the targets of peers' helping, caring, or supporting acts (e.g., How often does another kid give you help when you need it?). Possible responses to each item ranged from 1 = *never* to 5 = *all the time*.

Assessment of Social–Psychological Adjustment
Loneliness. The Asher and Wheeler (1985) loneliness scale, a measure with demonstrated reliability and validity (e.g., Asher & Wheeler, 1985; Asher & Williams, 1987; Crick & Ladd, 1993) was used to assess children's feelings of loneliness and social dissatisfaction. This scale consists of 16 items that assess loneliness at school (e.g., I don't have anyone to play with at school) and 8 filler items (e.g., I like playing board games a lot). Possible responses to each item range from 1 = *not at all true about me* to 5 = *always true about me*. Children's responses to the loneliness items were summed yielding

total scores that could range from 16 (low loneliness) to 80 (high loneliness). Cronbach's alpha for children's responses to the loneliness scale in this sample was .91.

Depression. The Children's Depression Inventory (CDI) was used to assess children's feelings and symptoms of depression (Kovacs, 1985). This measure consists of 27 items, all of which assess depression. Each item consists of three related statements, and children respond by selecting the one statement that best fits how they feel (e.g., I am sad once in a while vs. I am sad many times vs. I am sad all the time). Items are scored from 0 to 2, with higher scores indicating more evidence of depression. Two modifications were made to this instrument prior to its use in this study. First, two items were dropped from the measure due to sensitive content (i.e., an item that focused on suicidal ideation and an item concerned with self-hate). Second, five positively toned filler items that were neutral in content were added to the instrument (e.g., I like music videos a lot vs. I like music videos a little vs. I do not like music videos) in an attempt to balance the negative tone of the CDI items and to avoid negative response sets. Children's responses to the depression items (not the filler items) were summed to yield total depression scores that could range from 0 to 50. Cronbach's alpha for children's responses to the 25 depression items was .85 for this sample.

Social anxiety and avoidance. The Franke and Hymel (1984) social anxiety scale, an instrument with demonstrated reliability and validity (e.g., Franke & Hymel, 1984; Crick & Ladd, 1993), was used to assess social anxiety and social avoidance. This instrument's two subscales, social anxiety (e.g., I usually feel nervous when I meet someone for the first time.) and social avoidance (e.g., I often try to get away from all the other kids.), each consist of six items. Possible responses to each item range from $1 = not\ at\ all\ true\ about\ me$ to $5 = always\ true\ about\ me$. Children's responses to the items were summed for each subscale yielding total scores that could range from 6 (low anxiety/avoidance) to 30 (high anxiety/avoidance). Cronbach's alpha for children's responses to the social anxiety and social avoidance scales was .69 and .74, respectively.

Sociometric assessment. A peer sociometric (i.e., nominations of liked and disliked peers; Coie, Dodge, & Coppotelli, 1982) was administered to assess children's peer status. The number of nominations children received from peers for these items was standardized within each classroom. The positive and negative sociometric nominations children received from their classmates were used to identify five sociometric status groups—popular, average, neglected, rejected, and controversial children—using the procedure described by Coie and Dodge (1983; except for those in the average group, who were identified using the criteria described by Coie et al., 1982). First, children's standardized scores for the liked (Zp) and disliked (Zn) items were used to create two new variables, social preference ($Zp - Zn$) and social impact ($Zp + Zn$). Next, children's scores for each of these two variables were again standardized within each classroom. The standardized scores for social impact, social preference, number of positive nominations, and number of negative nominations were used to determine each child's social status group according to the following criteria: (a) Popular children received a social preference score greater than 1.0, a positive nomination score greater than 0, and a negative nomination score less than 0; (b) Average children received a social preference score less than .5 and greater than $-.5$; (c) Neglected children received a social impact score of less than -1.0, a positive nomination score of less than 0, and a negative nomination score less than 0; (d) Rejected children received a social preference score less than -1.0, a negative nomination score greater than 0, and a positive nomination score less than 0; and (e) Controversial children received a social impact score greater than 1.0, a negative nomination score greater than 0, and a positive nomination score greater than 0. This algorithm resulted in the identification of 61 popular, 152 average, 66 neglected, 52 rejected, and 25 controversial status children. The remaining children were unclassified (i.e., because the Coie et al. procedures do not allow for classification of all children) and, thus, they were excluded from subsequent analyses that included sociometric status as a factor.

Administration Procedures

The previously described instruments were completed by subjects during two 60-min assessment sessions (session A and session B) conducted within children's classrooms. These sessions were conducted by the authors, who employed standardized procedures. During each session, children were trained in the use of the response scales prior to administration of the instruments. Also, each item of every instrument was read aloud by the administrator and repeated as necessary to ensure understanding of item content. Administration assistants were also available to answer children's questions. The order in which sessions A and B were administered to classrooms was determined randomly. For each classroom, the two administrations occurred approximately 1 week apart.

During session A, children completed the peer sociometric, the Asher and Wheeler (1985) loneliness scale, the Franke and Hymel (1984) social anxiety scale, and an instrument that was not part of this study. The peer sociometric was always administered first (to help ensure that children would not be focused on the nominations they gave to others at the end of the session), however, the order of the loneliness and social anxiety scales was determined randomly. During session B, children completed the SEQ, the CDI (Kovacs, 1985), and three additional instruments that were not part of this study. The five instruments included in session B were presented to children in a random order.

RESULTS

To address our research objectives, four sets of analyses were conducted. The goal of the first set of analyses was to evaluate the psychometric properties of the peer treatment measure (SEQ), as well as to assess the relation between overt and relational victimization. The goals of the second and third sets of analyses were to assess gender, grade, and peer status differences in peer treatment. Finally, the goal of the fourth set was to assess the relation between peer treatment and social-psychological adjustment.

Psychometric Properties of the Social Experience Questionnaire

To assess whether relational victimization, overt victimization, and receipt of prosocial acts would emerge as separate aspects of peer treatment, a principal-components factor analysis with varimax rotation of the factors was conducted on children's responses to the SEQ. This analysis yielded the three predicted factors: (a) relational victimization (eigenvalue = 4.5), which accounted for 34.9% of the variation; (b) overt victimization (eigenvalue = 2.0), which accounted for 15.6% of the variation; and (c) receipt of prosocial acts (eigenvalue = 1.1), which accounted for 8.2% of the variation. A factor loading of .40 was used as the criterion for determining substantial crossloadings (Appelbaum & McCall, 1983; Tabachnick & Fidell, 1983). Based on this criterion, two of the overt victimization items ("being yelled at and called mean names" and "being told that you will be beaten up if you don't submit to a peer") loaded on both the overt and the relational victimization scales and, thus, were dropped from the SEQ.[1] Consequently, the overt victimization scale in

---

[1] These two items were originally included in the overt victimization subscale for both conceptual and empirical reasons. Specifically, they were included because the verbally aggressive behaviors reflected in these items have been considered to be important aspects of overt aggression in past research (e.g., see Parke & Slaby, 1983, for a review), and because past studies have shown empirically that these behaviors are significantly related to physical aggression, but not to relational aggression. For example, factor analyses of measures with these types of aggressive items have shown that they load on factors that include overt/physical aggression rather than factors that include relational aggression (Crick & Grotpeter, 1995; Grotpeter & Crick, in press). However, because these items met the criteria that we typically use (and that has been proposed by statisticians, e.g., Appelbaum & McCall, 1983) to identify crossloading items (approximately .40) for this particular sample, we deleted these items from the overt victimization subscale in this study. Thus, it is important to note that the overt victimization scale refers to being the target of physical aggression only in this research.

TABLE 1
Factor Loadings for Factor Analysis of Social Experience Questionnaire

Item	Factor		
	Relational	Overt	Prosocial
Left out on purpose when it's time to play or do an activity	.66		
A kid who is mad at them gets back at them by not letting them be in their group anymore	.69		
Has lies told about them to make other kids not like them anymore	.80		
A kid tells them they won't like them unless they do what the kid says	.67		
A kid tries to keep others from liking them by saying mean things about them	.75		
Gets hit		.81	
Gets pushed or shoved		.79	
Gets kicked or has hair pulled		.69	
Gets help from another kid when needs it			.68
Gets cheered up by another kid when sad or upset			.75
Another kid does something that makes them feel happy			.72
Another kid says something nice to them			.73
Another kid lets them know they care about them			.67

Note: All other factor loadings were less than .30 except for one item with a loading of .37.

this research reflected the degree to which children were the targets of physical aggression only. Factor loadings for the resulting three scales were relatively high, ranging from .66 to .81 (see Table 1).

Total scores were computed by summing each child's scores for the items within each scale. This procedure resulted in total scores that could range from 3 to 15 for the overt victimization scale and from 5 to 25 for the relational victimization and prosocial recipient scales. To aid with the comparison of children's scores across the three scales, average scale scores were computed and these scores were used in subsequent analyses (i.e., these scores could range from 1 to 5 for each of the three scales). Computation of Cronbach's alpha showed all three scales to be highly reliable ($\alpha = .80, .78$, and $.77$ for the relational victimization, overt victimization, and prosocial recipient scales, respectively).

The relation between overt and relational victimization was further assessed with a correlation coefficient, $r = .57$, $p < .01$. In addition, to assess whether distinct groups of relationally versus overtly victimized children could be identified, children's overt victimization scores (OVIC) and relational victimization scores (RVIC) were used to identify extreme groups of victimized and nonvictimized children. Children with scores one standard deviation above the sample means for OVIC, RVIC, or both were considered victimized, and the remaining children were considered nonvictimized. Four groups of children were identified: (a) nonvictimized (RVIC and OVIC both low); (b) overtly victimized (RVIC low, OVIC high); (c) relationally victimized (RVIC high, OVIC low); and (d) overtly and relationally victimized (RVIC high, OVIC high). This procedure resulted in the classification of 359 nonvictimized children (182 boys and 177 girls), 36 overtly victimized children (25 boys and 11 girls), 37 relationally victimized children (20 boys and 17 girls), and 42 overtly plus relationally victimized children (22 boys and 20 girls). Thus, of the 115 children classified as victimized in this sample, 73 of the victims (63.5%) were identified as experiencing either relational victimization or overt victimization, but not both.

TABLE 2
Average Victimization and Prosocial Recipient Scores by Gender

	Relational Victimization	Overt Victimization	Target of Prosocial Acts
Boys	2.27 ± 0.9	2.33 ± 1.0	3.09 ± 0.9
Girls	2.27 ± 0.9	2.12 ± 0.9*	3.55 ± 0.8***

Note: Values are mean ± SD.
$*p < .05$; $***p < .001$.

Gender and Grade Differences in Treatment by Peers

To assess gender and age-related grade differences in children's treatment by peers, a 2 (Sex) × 2 (Grade: Third/Fourth vs. Fifth/Sixth) multivariate analysis of variance (MANOVA) was conducted in which children's relational victimization scores, overt victimization scores, and prosocial recipient scores served as the dependent variables (see Table 2 for cell means and standard deviations by gender). This analysis yielded a significant multivariate main effect for gender, $F(3, 468) = 15.8$, $p < .001$. Univariate ANOVAs showed that girls reported significantly more prosocial treatment from peers than did boys, $F(1, 470) = 39.7$, $p < .001$. Further, as hypothesized, boys reported significantly more overt victimization than did girls, $F(1, 470) = 6.0$, $p < .05$.

Peer Status Group Differences in Treatment by Peers

To assess peer status differences in children's treatment by peers, a 5 (Sociometric Status Group) one-way multivariate analysis of variance (MANOVA) was conducted in which children's relational victimization, overt victimization, and receipt of prosocial acts scores served as the variates (see Table 3 for cell means and standard deviations). This analysis yielded a significant multivariate effect of sociometric status group, $F(12, 921) = 3.0$, $p < .001$. Additionally, significant univariate effects of sociometric status group were obtained for relational victimization, $F(4, 350) = 7.2$, $p < .001$; overt victimization, $F(4, 350) = 2.5$, $p < .05$; and prosocial recipient, $F(4, 350) = 3.3$, $p < .01$. Student Newman–Keuls post hoc tests ($p < .05$) of children's relational victimization scores revealed that rejected children reported significantly more relational victimization than did all other status groups. Further, average status children reported significantly more relational victimization than did popular, controversial, and neglected status children. Analyses of children's overt victimization scores showed that rejected children reported significantly more overt victimization than did popular and controversial status children. Finally, post hoc analyses of children's prosocial recipient scores

TABLE 3
Average Victimization and Prosocial Recipient Scores by Sociometric Status Group

Status Group	Relational Victimization	Overt Victimization	Target of Prosocial Acts
Popular	1.94 ± 0.7[a]	2.03 ± 1.0[a]	3.54 ± 0.7[a]
Average	2.39 ± 0.9[b]	2.25 ± 1.0[ab]	3.25 ± 0.9[ab]
Neglected	2.11 ± 0.8[a]	2.24 ± 0.9[ab]	3.31 ± 0.8[ab]
Rejected	2.69 ± 1.1[c]	2.54 ± 1.1[b]	3.06 ± 0.8[b]
Controversial	2.03 ± 0.8[a]	2.01 ± 0.9[a]	3.50 ± 0.8[ab]

Note: Values are mean ± SD. Different superscripts denote statistically significant mean differences ($p < .05$) among the sociometric status groups.

TABLE 4
R^2 and R^2 Change for Regression Equations Predicting Social–Psychological Adjustment from Negative
Treatment by Peers

Dependent Variable (Social–Psychological Adjustment Indices)	Relational Victimization Entered at Step 1		Overt Victimization Entered at Step 1	
	R^2 for Overt Victimization	R^2 Change for Relational Victimization	R^2 for Relational Victimization	R^2 Change for Overt Victimization
Loneliness	.10***	.14***	.24***	.00
Depression	.11***	.07***	.17***	.01**
Social anxiety	.03***	.04***	.07**	.00
Social avoidance	.04***	.05***	.09***	.00

Note: The r^2 change values for relational victimization represent the proportion of variation in maladjustment accounted for by relational victimization beyond that accounted for by overt victimization. In contrast, the r^2 change values for overt victimization represent the proportion of variation in maladjustment accounted for by overt victimization beyond that accounted for by relational victimization.
** $p < .01$; *** $p < .001$.

revealed that popular children reported being the recipients of prosocial acts significantly more often than did rejected children.

Treatment by Peers and Social–Psychological Adjustment

Negative treatment by peers: Relational and overt *victimization*. To assess the relation between victimization and social–psychological adjustment and to evaluate the relative contribution of overt and relational victimization to the prediction of concurrent adjustment, two sets of hierarchical multiple regression analyses were conducted. In these analyses, children's loneliness, depression, social anxiety, and social avoidance scores served as the dependent variables, and children's overt and relational victimization scores (the continuous scores, not the extreme-group classifications) served as the independent variables.[2]

In the first set of equations, children's overt victimization scores were entered at Step 1, and their relational victimization scores were entered at Step 2. This allowed for an assessment of the degree to which relational victimization added unique information to overt victimization in the prediction of maladjustment (refer to Table 4 for r^2 and r^2 change values). Results of step one analyses showed that overt victimization was significantly related to loneliness, $F(1, 436) = 49.9$, $p < .001$; depression, $F(1, 436) = 52.8$, $p < .001$; social anxiety, $F(1, 436) = 14.7$, $p < .001$; and social avoidance, $F(1, 436) = 19.6$, $p < .001$. Further, results of Step 2 analyses showed that relational victimization added significantly to the prediction of loneliness, $F(2, 435)$ change $= 82.0$, $p < .001$; depression, $F(2, 435)$ change $= 37.1$, $p < .001$; social anxiety, $F(2, 435)$ change $= 18.4$, $p < .001$; and social avoidance, $F(2, 435)$ change $= 23.9$, $p < .001$. These findings provide evidence that relational victimization provides unique information about these aspects of children's social–psychological adjustment, information that is not provided by overt victimization alone.

---

[2] These regression analyses were also computed separately for boys and girls. Results showed that, for girls, the pattern of findings was the same as that reported in the text for the whole sample. For boys, a few deviations from the findings reported in the text were obtained. Specifically, in contrast to the findings reported for the whole sample, relational victimization did not add to overt victimization in the prediction of social anxiety for boys. Further, overt victimization did not add to relational victimization in the prediction of depression, but it did add to relational victimization in the prediction of social anxiety.

TABLE 5
R^2 Change and R^2 Total for Regression Equations Predicting
Social–Psychological Adjustment from Positive and
Negative Treatment by Peers

Dependent Variable (Social–Psychological Adjustment Indices)	R^2 Change for Positive Treatment	R^2 Total for Positive and Negative Treatment
Loneliness	.05***	.30***
Depression	.05***	.23***
Social anxiety	.00	.08***
Social avoidance	.05***	.14***

Note: The r^2 change values for target of prosocial acts represent the proportion of variation in maladjustment accounted for by being the recipient of prosocial acts beyond that accounted for by victimization (i.e., prosocial recipient scores were added to the equation *after* relational and overt victimization scores were already in the equation). The r^2 total values represent the total proportion of variation in maladjustment accounted for by all three predictors (i.e., relational victimization plus overt victimization plus being the target of prosocial acts).
*** $p < .001$.

In the second set of equations, children's relational victimization scores were entered at Step 1, and their overt victimization scores were entered at Step 2. This allowed for an assessment of the degree to which overt victimization added unique information to relational victimization in the prediction of maladjustment (refer to Table 4 for r^2 and r^2 change values). Results of Step 1 analyses showed that relational victimization was significantly related to loneliness, $F(1, 436) = 140.1$, $p < .001$; depression, $F(1, 436) = 86.2$, $p < .001$; social anxiety, $F(1, 436) = 33.2$, $p < .001$; and social avoidance, $F(1, 436) = 43.8$, $p < .001$. Further, results of Step 2 analyses showed that overt victimization added significantly to the prediction of depression, $F(2, 435)$ change $= 6.9$, $p < .01$, but not to the prediction of loneliness, social anxiety, and social avoidance.

The contribution of positive treatment by peers. To assess whether positive treatment by peers (i.e., being the recipient of prosocial acts) would contribute uniquely to negative peer treatment (i.e., overt and relational victimization) in the prediction of social–psychological adjustment, children's prosocial recipient scores were added as predictors to the regression equations previously described (see Table 4 for a summary of the prior analyses).[2] Specifically, these scores were added in a third prediction step, after both forms of victimization had already been included in the equations (see Table 5 for r^2 change values). Results of these analyses revealed that positive peer treatment added significantly to victimization in the prediction of loneliness, $F(3, 434)$ change $= 31.7$, $p < .001$; depression, $F(3, 434)$ change $= 26.3$, $p < .001$; and social avoidance, $F(3, 434)$ change $= 25.9$, $p < .001$, indicating that the lack of positive peer treatment was associated with adjustment problems.

DISCUSSION

Results of this study provide additional support for the importance of overt victimization, the type of peer maltreatment that has been the focus of pervious studies. These findings also demonstrate that, although overt victimization is a highly salient and significant aspect of children's peer treatment, it does not capture the full range of harmful or neglectful events that children sometimes experience as part of their peer interactions. Specifically, these findings provide the first evidence of the validity and significance of a relational form of peer victimization. Further, they highlight the importance of positive aspects of children's peer treatment. Taken together, these findings emphasize the need to move beyond the assessment of overt victimization in studies of peer maltreatment, to include other aspects of negative peer treatment (e.g., relational victimization), as well as positive aspects of children's peer experiences (e.g., being the target of peers' prosocial acts).

A number of the findings from this study provide support for the validity of relational victimization as a related, but different, form of peer maltreatment than overt victimization (assessed as physical aggression in this study). Although these two forms of peer maltreatment were shown to be positively correlated (i.e., $r = .57$), the magnitude of this correlation was considerably less than would be predicted based on findings from past research. For example, in past studies of proactive and relative aggression, two behaviors that have also been considered relatively distinct, obtained correlations have been in the .7 to .8 range (Crick & Dodge, in press; Dodge & Coie, 1987; Price & Dodge, 1989). And, in the only previous study to evaluate the relation between two different forms of peer victimization (i.e., verbal and physical victimization), the obtained correlation was $r = .76$ (Perry et al., 1988). Thus, based on past evidence, the association between relational and overt victimization obtained in this research was relatively moderate in magnitude, a degree of association that is consistent with viewing relational and overt victimization as different indices of peer maltreatment. Other evidence from this research provides more direct support for this hypothesis, however. For example, the factor analysis of the SEQ (i.e., the peer treatment measure) yielded separate factors for each form of victimization. Further, the identification of extreme groups of victimized children revealed that, although some children reported high levels of maltreatment through both relational and overt forms of aggression, it was also possible to identify distinct groups of children who were victimized by one form of aggression only (i.e., relationally or overtly victimized children). In fact, the majority of victimized children (64%) experienced either relational or overt victimization, but *not* both. These findings indicate that, rather than viewing their negative social experiences in broad, general terms (e.g., as aversive or "bad"), children distinguish between the two hypothesized forms of victimization to some degree. In general, these findings indicate that the exclusive focus on overt victimization in past research has: (a) limited our understanding of the full range of aversive events experienced by children within their peer groups; and (b) prevented identification of a substantial percentage of children who are victimized by their peers, those who are relationally, but not overtly, victimized (8% in this sample).

The importance of relational victimization was further supported by the findings from the social–psychological adjustment assessments. These assessments revealed that, similar to overt victimization, relational victimization was significantly related to social–psychological distress (e.g., loneliness, depression). These findings are correlational in nature, however, they are consistent with the hypothesis that exposure to relational aggression is significantly damaging and harmful for children (i.e., relational victimization may lead to psychological distress). Some empirical support for this direction of effect has been obtained in a longitudinal study of overt victimization conducted by Olweus (1993). In this research, boys identified as overtly victimized in grade school were depressed as adults, even though they were no longer being victimized. Troy and Sroufe (1987) have offered an alternative hypothesis regarding the temporal relation between adjustment and victimization. Specifically, these authors have suggested that victims may exhibit an anxious vulnerability that attracts or invites hostile attacks from aggressive peers (i.e., emotional maladjustment may trigger aggressive attacks). Both of these hypotheses seem plausible. In fact, the temporal relation between adjustment and victimization may be bidirectional. If so, victimized children may be caught in a self-perpetuating cycle in which: (a) maltreatment leads to emotional difficulties for the victim, (b) the resultant distress that the child experiences makes peers believe that he or she is an easy mark, (c) the peers' views of the child result in heightened levels of victimization, and (d) the child's distress is exacerbated, etc. It will be important to address in future research the extent to which relational victimization is elicited by characteristics or behaviors of the victim (e.g., engaging in behaviors that are annoying to peers), characteristics of the attacker (e.g., being a bully), or situational factors (e.g., being at the wrong place at the wrong time).

Analyses of the relative contribution of relational and overt victimization to the prediction of adjustment showed that, for msot of the adjustment indices, relational victimization provided unique information about adjustment, whereas overt victimization did not. This may indicate that, in general, relational victimization is more strongly related to maladjustment than is overt victimization. However, the obtained pattern of associations suggests a second explanation, that the two forms of victimization are differentially related to some adjustment outcomes. For example, in this study, both forms of victimization provided unique information about depression, a fairly general type of maladjustment that is characterized by a range of problems including somatic complaints, emotional difficulties, eating or sleeping problems, etc. However, relational victimization, but not overt, provided unique information about social anxiety, social avoidance, and loneliness. In contrast to depression, these adjustment problems are fairly specific to relationship or social contexts and, thus, perhaps it is to be expected that they would be most strongly related to relational rather than overt victimization (i.e., because relational victimization involves damage to one's relationships). Additional research is needed that assesses the specificity of each form of peer maltreatment for predicting particular adjustment outcomes.

In addition to demonstrating the importance of negative peer treatment in children's lives, findings from this study also provide initial evidence for the significance of positive peer treatment. Analyses of the relation between peer treatment and social–psychological adjustment revealed that the lack of prosocial treatment by peers significantly predicted adjustment difficulties beyond that which could be accounted for by victimization. Although past investigators have focused solely on the role of negative treatment in children's adjustment (e.g., Olweus, 1993; Perry et al., 1988), these findings suggest that children's social adjustment may depend on the degree to which they obtain helpful, caring responses from peers, in addition to the degree to which they successfully avoid aggressive overtures. It appears that a more comprehensive view of children's peer treatment is needed (i.e., relative to that employed in past research) if we are to understand fully the role that social experiences play in children's social and emotional adjustment.

Assessment of gender differences in victimization showed that, consistent with past research (e.g., Boulton & Underwood, 1992), boys reported significantly more overt victimization than did girls. In contrast, no gender differences were obtained for relational victimization, indicating that girls were just as likely as boys to report experiencing this form of peer maltreatment. These findings suggest that assessment of relational victimization, in addition to overt victimization, may provide more information about girls' victimization than the assessment of overt victimization alone. Further, assessment of relational victimization may be particularly important to the study of girls' social difficulties given recent evidence that girls feel more emotionally distressed by relationally aggressive events than do boys (Crick, 1995).

The results of this study suggest a number of directions for future research. First, because this study included self-reports of victimization only, development of new measures that will allow for assessment of relational victimization by multiple informants seems warranted. Multiple informants such as peers, teachers, parents, in addition to the children themselves, can provide a more thorough assessment of victimization within a variety of contexts than assessment utilizing one informant only (see Achenbach et al., 1987, for a similar argument concerning assessment of childhood aggression). Second, evaluation of the relation between relational victimization and relational aggression seems important to determine whether the lack of a significant relation between aggression and victimization that has been demonstrated in past research for overt forms of aggressive behavior (Perry et al., 1988) also holds for relationally aggressive behaviors. Third, as has been discussed by Perry et al. (1988) regarding overt victimization, assessment of the social-information-processing mechanisms associated with relational victimization may also be a fruitful avenue for future research endeavors. Given the abusive and aversive behaviors that relationally and overtly victimized children suffer at the hands of their peers, it seems likely that these children may develop inaccurate or nonnormative views of social interaction. For example, they may develop hostile attributional biases (i.e., inaccurate, negative views of peers' intent), or they may develop negative outcome expectations for initiation of peer interaction (due to their negative and rejecting experiences with peers). Fourth, future research attention should be directed toward understanding the relation between verbal aggression (e.g., verbal insults) and physical aggression to determine whether these behaviors reflect a single form of aggression (i.e., overt aggression) or should be considered as independent forms. We are currently pursuing all of these objectives in our research.

In sum, this research provides evidence that the study of relational victimization contributes significantly to our understanding of children's day to day social difficulties in the peer group. Future research attention should be directed toward the study of factors that contribute to this form of victimization, as well as an assessment of the implications of this type of maltreatment for children's development.

REFERENCES

Achenbach, T. M., McConaughy, S. H., & Howell, C. T. (1987). Child/adolescent behavioral and emotional problems: Implications of cross-informant correlations for situational specificity. *Psychological Bulletin, 87*, 213–232.

Appelbaum, M. I., & McCall, R. B. (1983). Design and analysis in developmental psychology. In P. H. Mussen (Ed.), *Handbook of child psychology* (4th ed., Vol. 1), W. Kessen (Vol. Ed.), *History, theory and methods* (pp. 415–471). New York: Wiley.

Asher, S. R., Hymel, S., & Renshaw, P. D. (1984). Loneliness in children. *Child Development, 55*, 1457–1464.

Asher, S. R., Parkhurst, J. T., Hymel, S., & Williams, G. A. (1990). Peer rejection and loneliness in childhood. In S. R. Asher & J. D. Coie (Eds.), *Peer rejection in childhood* (pp. 253–273). New York: Cambridge University Press.

Asher, S. R., & Wheeler, V. A. (1985). Children's loneliness: A comparison of rejected and neglected peer status. *Journal of Consulting and Clinical Psychology, 53*, 500–505.

Berkowitz, L. (1993). *Aggression: Its causes, consequences, and control.* New York: Academic Press.

Bjorkqvist, K., Ekman, K., & Lagerspetz, K. (1982). Bullies and victims: Their ego picture, ideal ego picture, and normative ego picture. *Scandinavian Journal of Psychology, 23*, 307–313.

Block, J. H. (1983). Differential premises arising from differential socialization of the sexes: Some conjectures. *Child Development, 54*, 1335–1354.

Boulton, M. J., & Underwood, K. (1992). Bully/victim problems among middle school children. *British Journal of Educational Psychology, 62*, 73–87.

Cairns, R. B., Cairns, B. D., Neckerman, H. J., Ferguson, L. L., & Gariepy, J. L. (1989). Growth and aggression: 1. Childhood to early adolescence. *Developmental Psychology, 25*, 320–330.

Coie, J. D., & Dodge, K. A. (1983). Continuities and changes in children's social status: A five-year longitudinal study. *Merrill–Palmer Quarterly, 29*, 261–282.

Coie, J. D., Dodge, K. A., & Coppotelli, H. (1982). Dimensions and types of social status: A cross-age perspective. *Developmental Psychology, 18*, 557–570.

Crick, N. R. (1995). Relational aggression: The role of intent attributions, feelings of distress, and provocation type. *Development and Psychopathology, 7*, 313–322.

Crick, N. R., & Dodge, K. A. (1994). A review and reformulation of social information-processing mechanisms in children's social adjustment. *Psychological Bulletin, 115*, 74–101.

Crick, N. R., & Dodge, K. A. (in press). Social information-processing mechanisms in proactive and reactive aggression. *Child Development*.

Crick, N. R., & Grotpeter, J. K. (1995). Relational aggression, gender, and social–psychological adjustment. *Child Development, 66*, 710–722.

Crick, N. R., & Ladd, G. W. (1993). Children's perceptions of their peer experiences: Attributions, loneliness, social anxiety, and social avoidance. *Developmental Psychology, 29*, 244–254.

Crick, N. R., Bigbee, M., & Howes, C. (in press). Gender differences in children's normative beliefs about aggression: How do I hurt thee? Let me count the ways. *Child Development*.

Dodge, K. A., & Coie, J. D. (1987). Social information-processing factors in reactive and proactive aggression in children's peer groups. *Journal of Personality and Social Psychology, 53*, 1146–1158.

Franke, S., & Hymel, S. (May, 1984). Social anxiety in children: The development of self-report measures. Paper presented at the biennial meeting of the University of Waterloo Conference on Child Development, Waterloo, Ontario, Canada.

Grotpeter, J. K., & Crick, N. R. (in press). Relational aggression, overt aggression, and friendship. *Child Development*.

Hymel, S. R., & Franke, S. (1985). Children's peer relations: Assessing self-perceptions. In B. H. Schneider, K. H. Rubin, & J. E. Ledingham (Eds.), *Children's peer relations: Issues in assessment and intervention* (pp. 75–92). New York: Springer Verlag.

Kovacs, M. (1985). The children's depression inventory. *Psychopharmacology Bulletin, 21*, 995–998.

Lagerspetz, K. M. J., Bjorkqvist, K., & Peltonen, T. (1988). Is indirect aggression more typical of females? Gender differences in aggressiveness in 11- to 12-year-old children. *Aggressive Behavior, 14*, 403–414.

Olweus, D. (1978). *Aggression in the schools: Bullies and whipping boys*. Washington, DC: Hemisphere.

Olweus, D. (1984). Aggressors and their victims: Bullying at school. In N. Frude & H. Gault (Eds.), *Disruptive behaviors in schools* (pp. 57–76). New York: Wiley.

Olweus, D. (1993). *Bullying at school: What we know and what we can do*. Oxford: Blackwell.

Olweus, D. (1991). Bully/victim problems among schoolchildren: Basic facts and effects of a school based intervention program. In D. J. Peplar & K. H. Rubin (Eds.), *The development and treatment of childhood aggression* (pp. 411–448). Hillsdale, NJ: Erlbaum.

Parke, R. D., & Slaby, R. G. (1983). The development of aggression. In P. H. Mussen (Series Ed.) & M. Hetherington (Vol. Ed.), *Handbook of child psychology* (4th ed., Vol. 4, pp. 547–642).

Parker, J., & Asher, S. R. (1987). Peer acceptance and later personal adjustment: Are low-accepted children "at-risk?" *Psychological Bulletin, 102*, 357–389.

Perry, D. G., Kusel, S. J., & Perry, L. C. (1988). Victims of peer aggression. *Developmental Psychology, 24*, 807–814.

Price, J. M., & Dodge, K. A. (1989). Reactive and proactive aggression in childhood: Relations to peer status and social context dimensions. *Journal of Abnormal Child Psychology, 17*, 455–471.

Schwartz, D., Dodge, K. A., & Coie, J. D. (1993). The emergence of chronic peer victimization in boys' play groups. *Child Development, 64*, 1755–1772.

Schwartz, D. (March, 1993). *Antecedents of aggression and peer victimization: A prospective study*. Paper presented at the meeting of the Society for Research in Child Development, New Orleans, LA.

Tabachnick, B. G., & Fidell, L. S. (1983). *Using multivariate statistics*. New York: Harper & Row.

Troy, M., & Sroufe, L. A. (1987). Victimization among preschoolers: Role of attachment relationship history. *Journal of the American Academy of Child and Adolescent Psychiatry, 26*, 166–172.

Part II

INTELLIGENCE AND LEARNING

The papers in this section address various aspects of intelligence and learning. The first two papers are reviews, and the last two are empirical studies.

There has always been controversy over the meaning of *intelligence*. The first paper is an excellent review of the field of intelligence. The paper reviews concepts of intelligence, the stability and predictability of intelligence test scores, the heritability of intelligence, environmental effects on intelligence, and group differences in intelligence test scores.

The American Psychological Association created a task force to write this paper after the publication of *The Bell Curve*. *The Bell Curve*, a book that was widely cited in the popular press, made statements about race and IQ that many people in the scientific community felt were biased misinterpretations of studies. Thus, a decision was made that an unbiased paper on the intelligence literature would be worthwhile. The major topics presented are concepts of intelligence, intelligence tests and their correlates, genes and individual differences, environmental effects on intelligence, and group differences.

Neisser et al. begin by reviewing the various theories of intelligence from Spearman's single-factor "g" theory to Gardner's and Sternberg's theories of multiple intelligences. Of interest here is the notion that intelligence tests measure a limited range of skills. The basic characteristics, including stability, of test scores are summarized. The predictability of IQ to both academic and life outcomes is reviewed. Factors considered are years of education, social status and income, and social outcomes. Environmental effects reviewed include both social (culture, schooling, family) and biological (e.g., nutrition, lead, alcohol) variables. Group differences are considered for both gender and ethnicity. Neisser et al. acknowledge that there are group differences in overall mean IQ scores. However, as predictors of school performance, a primary purpose of IQ tests, the tests are not biased. The authors conclude that there is no generally accepted explanation for group differences.

The data presented here are not new; nonetheless, the paper is of significant interest because it interprets many studies that have often been misinterpreted for political purposes and because it synthesizes a vast literature.

The second paper in this section focuses on the low end of the intelligence spectrum, summarizing recent genetic findings on mental retardation. Advances in molecular genetics have enhanced the study of genotype to phenotype manifestation. Siminoff and colleagues use these findings to describe the mechanisms involved in various disorders of retardation, including Down syndrome, fragile X, other X-linked mental retardation, sex chromosome anomalies, Prader-Willi and Angelman syndromes, phenylketonuria, and autism.

One important point that Siminoff et al. make is that the distinction between familial and pathological retardation is not as simple as has been proposed. People with mild retardation have been classified as "familial," meaning that they are functioning within the lower end of the normal spectrum, based on the polygenetic transmission of intelligence. However, a substantial minority of mildly retarded individuals have identifiable causes, such as epilepsy or cerebral palsy.

The authors describe other topics, including the variation in IQ within genetic disorders and the variation in social adaptation within the low-IQ group. Then, the specific disorders are described and the variations in genetic transmission are detailed. For example, not everyone who inherits the defective fragile-X chromosome has the clinical manifestations of the syndrome. This paper describes

93

the phenotype of each syndrome and the complex process of transmission and expression of genotype. The paper concludes by discussing the implications of the new genetic research on prenatal and population screening and genetic counseling. In all, this is an extremely comprehensive update of mental retardation and genetics.

The next two papers in this section are empirical studies on learning problems. Maugham and Hagell present longitudinal data on adults who were either poor or normal readers when first studied in middle childhood. They differentiate between "generally backward readers"—those who were 28 months below age expectation but the reading was not discrepant with cognitive ability—and "specifically retarded readers"—those whose reading was 28 months below age and IQ expectations. Persons with IQ below 70 were eliminated from the study. A comparison group of 73 participants without severe reading difficulties was included for a total of three groups. Data were collected from childhood (age 10), adolescence (age 14), and early adulthood (mean age 27–28 years). The rather detailed results section indicates differences among the men in independent living, with 20% of poor readers still residing with their family of origin. Women who were poor readers had more relationship failures than did adequate readers. The study is unique in that it followed a community (school-based) sample rather than a clinical sample. It also included two groups of poor readers, not just one. It is rare that studies present the long-term implications of childhood learning difficulties.

The next paper suggests that there may be a way to prevent the long-term results of learning difficulties for some children. Tallal and colleagues present two training studies for children with language-learning impairments. Approximately 3% to 6% of children are estimated to have language-learning impairments. The authors found in their previous work that many of these children could not identify fast elements in ongoing speech. For example, the sounds *ba* and *da* are hard to discriminate in ongoing speech. In Study 1, after 4 weeks of listening to acoustically modified (slowed) speech, the 7 children's language test performance scores, originally 1 to 3 years below age level, improved by approximately 2 years. Study 2 included a treatment group and a control group to determine that the effects were due to the acoustically modified speech. The children in the training group were given language exercises and computer games with acoustically modified speech. The control group received the same training with unmodified speech. Both groups improved, but the treatment group improved significantly more. Listening to modified speech for 6 weeks resulted in the children's being better able to process normal speech sounds. The improvement in temporal processing using modified speech generalized to unmodified natural speech. Tallal et al. suggest that the rapid change in receptive language processing indicates that the children were considerably more language competent than they were able to demonstrate.

This paper presents a fascinating and significant innovation in the field of language and learning impairments. Rather than teaching strategies to compensate for processing difficulties, the brain's way of processing information was altered. Further studies are underway, and those results may shed light on questions such as these: what is the optimum training time, are there changes in reading achievement, and which groups of language-impaired children benefit most?

6

Intelligence: Knowns and Unknowns

Ulric Neisser (Chair)
Emory University

Gwyneth Boodoo
Educational Testing Service, Princeton, New Jersey

Thomas J. Bouchard, Jr.
University of Minnesota, Minneapolis

A. Wade Boykin
Howard University

Nathan Brody
Wesleyan University

Stephen J. Ceci
Cornell University

Diane F. Halpern
California State University, San Bernardino

John C. Loehlin
University of Texas, Austin

Robert Perloff
University of Pittsburgh

Robert J. Sternberg
Yale University

Susana Urbina
University of North Florida

Reprinted with permission from *American Psychologist*, 1996, Vol. 51(2), 77–101. Copyright © 1996 by the American Psychological Association, Inc.

This is a "Report of a Task Force Established by the American Psychological Association."

The Task Force appreciates the contributions of many members of the APA Board of Scientific Affairs (BSA) and the APA Board for the Advancement of Psychology in the Public Interest (BAPPI), who made helpful comments on a preliminary draft of this report. We also wish to acknowledge the indispensable logistical support of the APA Science Directorate during the preparation of the report itself.

In the fall of 1994, the publication of Herrnstein and Murray's book The Bell Curve *sparked a new round of debate about the meaning of intelligence test scores and the nature of intelligence. The debate was characterized by strong assertions as well as by strong feelings. Unfortunately, those assertions often revealed serious misunderstandings of what has (and has not) been demonstrated by scientific research in this field. Although a great deal is now known, the issues remain complex and in many cases still unresolved. Another unfortunate aspect of the debate was that many participants made little effort to distinguish scientific issues from political ones. Research findings were often assessed not so much on their merits or their scientific standing as on their supposed political implications. In such a climate, individuals who wish to make their own judgments find it hard to know what to believe. Reviewing the intelligence debate at its meeting of November 1994, the Board of Scientific Affairs (BSA) of the American Psychological Association (APA) concluded that there was urgent need for an authoritative report on these issues—one that all sides could use as a basis for discussion. Acting by unanimous vote, BSA established a Task Force charged with preparing such a report. Ulric Neisser, Professor of Psychology at Emory University and a member of BSA, was appointed Chair. The APA Board on the Advancement of Psychology in the Public Interest, which was consulted extensively during this process, nominated one member of the Task Force; the Committee on Psychological Tests and Assessment nominated another; a third was nominated by the Council of Representatives. Other members were chosen by an extended consultative process, with the aim of representing a broad range of expertise and opinion. The Task Force met twice, in January and March of 1995. Between and after these meetings, drafts of the various sections were circulated, revised, and revised yet again. Disputes were resolved by discussion. As a result, the report presented here has the unanimous support of the entire Task Force.*

CONCEPTS OF INTELLIGENCE

Individuals differ from one another in their ability to understand complex ideas, to adapt effectively to the environment, to learn from experience, to engage in various forms of reasoning, to overcome obstacles by taking thought. Although these individual differences can be substantial, they are never entirely consistent: A given person's intellectual performance will vary on different occasions, in different domains, as judged by different criteria. Concepts of "intelligence" are attempts to clarify and organize this complex set of phenomena. Although considerable clarity has been achieved in some areas, no such conceptualization has yet answered all the important questions and none commands universal assent. Indeed, when two dozen prominent theorists were recently asked to define intelligence, they gave two dozen somewhat different definitions (Sternberg & Detterman, 1986). Such disagreements are not cause for dismay. Scientific research rarely begins with fully agreed definitions, though it may eventually lead to them.

This first section of our report reviews the approaches to intelligence that are currently influential, or that seem to be becoming so. Here (as in later sections) much of our discussion is devoted to the dominant *psychometric* approach, which has not only inspired the most research and attracted the most attention (up to this time) but is by far the most widely used in practical settings. Nevertheless, other points of view deserve serious consideration. Several current theorists argue that there are many different "intelligences" (systems of abilities), only a few of which can be captured by standard psychometric tests. Others emphasize the role of culture, both in establishing different conceptions of intelligence and in influencing the acquisition of intellectual skills. Developmental psychologists, taking yet another direction, often focus more on the processes by which all children come to think intelligently than on measuring individual differences among them. There is also a new interest in the neural and biological bases of intelligence, a field of research that seems certain to expand in the next few years.

In this brief report, we cannot do full justice to even one such approach. Rather than trying to do so, we focus here on a limited and rather specific set of questions:

- What are the significant conceptualizations of intelligence at this time? (First section)

- What do intelligence test scores mean, what do they predict, and how well do they predict it? (Second section)

- Why do individuals differ in intelligence, and especially in their scores on intelligence tests? Our discussion of these questions implicates both genetic factors (Third section) and environmental factors (Fourth section).

- Do various ethnic groups display different patterns of performance on intelligence tests, and if so what might explain those differences? (Fifth section)

- What significant scientific issues are presently unresolved? (Sixth section)

Public discussion of these issues has been especially vigorous since the 1994 publication of Herrnstein and Murray's *The Bell Curve*, a controversial volume which stimulated many equally controversial reviews and replies. Nevertheless, we do not directly enter that debate. Herrnstein and Murray (and many of their critics) have gone well beyond the scientific findings, making explicit recommendations on various aspects of public policy. Our concern here, however, is with science rather than policy. The charge to our Task Force was to prepare a dispassionate survey of the state of the art: To make clear what has been scientifically established, what is presently in dispute, and what is still unknown. In fulfilling that charge, the only recommendations we shall make are for further research and calmer debate.

The Psychometric Approach

Ever since Alfred Binet's great success in devising tests to distinguish mentally retarded children from those with behavior problems, psychometric instruments have played an important part in European and American life. Tests are used for many purposes, such as selection, diagnosis, and evaluation. Many of the most widely used tests are not intended to measure intelligence itself but some closely related construct: scholastic aptitude, school achievement, specific abilities, etc. Such tests are especially important for selection purposes. For preparatory school, it's the SSAT; for college, the SAT or ACT; for graduate school, the GRE; for medical school, the MCAT; for law school, the LSAT; for business school, the GMAT. Scores on intelligence-related tests matter, and the stakes can be high. *Intelligence tests.* Tests of intelligence itself (in the psychometric sense) come in many forms. Some use only a single type of item or question; examples include the Peabody Picture Vocabulary Test (a measure of children's verbal intelligence) and Raven's Progressive Matrices (a nonverbal, untimed test that requires inductive reasoning about perceptual patterns). Although such instruments are useful for specific purposes, the more familiar measures of general intelligence—such as the Wechsler tests and the Stanford-Binet—include many different types of items, both verbal and nonverbal. Test-takers may be asked to give the meanings of words, to complete a series of pictures, to indicate which of several words does not belong with the others, and the like. Their performance can then be scored to yield several subscores as well as overall score.

By convention, overall intelligence test scores are usually converted to a scale in which the mean is 100 and the standard deviation is 15. (The standard deviation is a measure of the variability of the distribution of scores.) Approximately 95% of the population has scores within two standard deviations of the mean, i.e., between 70 and 130. For historical reasons, the term "IQ" is often used to describe scores on tests of intelligence. It originally referred to an "Intelligence Quotient" that was formed by dividing a so-called mental age by a chronological age, but this procedure is no longer used.

Intercorrelations among tests. Individuals rarely perform equally well on all the different kinds of items included in a test of intelligence. One person may do relatively better on verbal than on spatial items, for example, while another may show the opposite pattern. Nevertheless, subtests measuring different abilities tend to be positively correlated: people who score high on one such subtest are likely to be above average on others as well. These complex patterns of correlation can be clarified by factor analysis, but the results of such analyses are often controversial themselves. Some theorists (e.g., Spearman, 1927) have emphasized the importance of a general factor, g, which represents what all the tests have in common; others (e.g., Thurstone, 1938) focus on more specific group factors such as memory, verbal comprehension, or number facility. As we shall see in the second section, one common view today envisages something like a hierarchy of factors with g at the apex. But there is no full agreement on what g actually means: it has been described as a mere statistical regularity (Thomson, 1939), a kind of mental energy (Spearman, 1927), a generalized abstract reasoning ability (Gustafsson, 1984), or an index measure of neural processing speed (Reed & Jensen, 1992).

There have been many disputes over the utility of IQ and g. Some theorists are critical of the entire psychometric approach (e.g., Ceci, 1990; Gardner, 1983; Gould, 1978), while others regard it as firmly established (e.g., Carroll, 1993; Eysenck, 1973; Herrnstein & Murray, 1994; Jensen, 1972). The critics do not dispute the stability of test scores, nor the fact that they predict certain forms of achievement—especially school achievement—rather effectively (see the second section). They do argue, however, that to base a concept of intelligence on test scores alone is to ignore many important aspects of mental ability. Some of those aspects are emphasized in other approaches reviewed below.

Multiple Forms of Intelligence

Gardner's theory. A relatively new approach is the theory of "multiple intelligences" proposed by Howard Gardner in his book *Frames of Mind* (1983). Gardner argues that our conceptions of intelligence should be informed not only by work with "normal" children and adults but also by studies of gifted persons (including so-called "savants"), of virtuosos and experts in various domains, of valued abilities in diverse cultures, and of individuals who have suffered selective forms of brain damage. These considerations have led him to include musical, bodily kinesthetic, and various forms of personal intelligence in the scope of his theory along with more familiar linguistic, logical-mathematical, and spatial abilities. (Critics of the theory argue, however, that some of these are more appropriately described as special talents than as forms of "intelligence.")

In Gardner's view, the scope of psychometric tests includes only linguistic, logical, and some aspects of spatial intelligence; other forms have been almost entirely ignored. Even in the domains on which they are ostensibly focused, the paper-and-pencil format of most tests rules out many kinds of intelligent performance that matter a great deal in everyday life, such as giving an extemporaneous talk (linguistic) or being able to find one's way in a new town (spatial). While the stability and validity of performance tests in these new domains are not yet clear, Gardner's argument has attracted considerable interest among educators as well as psychologists.

Sternberg's theory. Robert Sternberg's (1985) triarchic theory proposes three fundamental aspects of intelligence—analytic, creative, and practical—of which only the first is measured to any significant extent by mainstream tests. His investigations suggest the need for a balance between analytic intelligence, on the one hand, and creative and especially practical intelligence on the other. The distinction between analytic (or "academic") and practical intelligence has also been made by others (e.g., Neisser, 1976). Analytic problems, of the type suitable for test construction, tend to (a) have been formulated by other people, (b) be clearly defined, (c) come with all the information needed to solve them, (d) have only a single right answer, which can be reached by only a single method, (e) be disembedded from ordinary experience, and (f) have little or no intrinsic interest. Practical problems, in contrast, tend to (a) require problem recognition and formulation, (b) be poorly defined, (c) require information seeking, (d) have various acceptable solutions, (e) be embedded in and require prior everyday experience, and (f) require motivation and personal involvement.

One important form of practical intelligence is *tacit knowledge*, defined by Sternberg and his collaborators as "action-oriented knowledge, acquired without direct help from others, that allows individuals to achieve goals they personally value" (Sternberg, Wagner, Williams, & Horvath, 1995, p. 916). Questionnaires designed to measure tacit knowledge have been developed for various domains, especially business management. In these questionnaires, the individual is presented with written descriptions of various work-related situations and asked to rank a number of options for dealing with each of them. Measured in this way, tacit knowledge is relatively independent of scores on intelligence tests; nevertheless it correlates significantly with various indices of job performance (Sternberg & Wagner, 1993; Sternberg et al., 1995). Although this work is not without its critics (Jensen, 1993; Schmidt & Hunter, 1993), the results to this point tend to support the distinction between analytic and practical intelligence.

Related findings. Other investigators have also demonstrated that practical intelligence can be relatively independent of school performance or scores on psychometric tests. Brazilian street children, for example, are quite capable of doing the math required for survival in their street business even though they have failed mathematics in school (Carraher, Carraher, & Schliemann, 1985). Similarly, women shoppers in California who had no difficulty in comparing product values at the supermarket were unable to carry out the same mathematical operations in paper-and-pencil tests (Lave, 1988). In a study of expertise in wagering on harness races, Ceci and Liker (1986) found that the reasoning of the most skilled handicappers was implicitly based on a complex interactive model with as many as seven variables. Nevertheless, individual handicappers' levels of performance were not correlated with their IQ scores. This means, as Ceci as put it, that "the assessment of the experts' intelligence on a standard IQ test was irrelevant in predicting the complexity of their thinking at the racetrack" (1990, p. 43).

Cultural Variation

It is very difficult to compare concepts of intelligence across cultures. English is not alone in having many words for different aspects of intellectual power and cognitive skill (*wise, sensible, smart, bright, clever, cunning...*); if another language has just as many, which of them shall we say corresponds to its speakers' "concept of intelligence"? The few attempts to examine this issue directly have typically found that, even within a given society, different cognitive characteristics are emphasized from one situation to another and from one subculture to another (Serpell, 1974; Super, 1983; Wober, 1974). These differences extend not just to conceptions of intelligence but also to what is considered adaptive or appropriate in a broader sense.

These issues have occasionally been addressed across subcultures and ethnic groups in America. In a study conducted in San Jose, California, Okagaki and Sternberg (1993) asked immigrant parents from Cambodia, Mexico, the Philippines, and Vietnam—as well as native-born Anglo-Americans and Mexican Americans—about their conceptions of child-rearing, appropriate teaching, and children's intelligence. Parents from all groups except Anglo-Americans indicated that such characteristics as motivation, social skills, and practical school skills were as or more important than cognitive characteristics for their conceptions of an intelligent first-grade child.

Heath (1983) found that different ethnic groups in North Carolina have different conceptions of intelligence. To be considered as intelligent or adaptive, one must excel in the skills valued by one's own group. One particularly interesting contrast was in the importance ascribed to verbal versus nonverbal communication skills—to saying things explicitly as opposed to using and understanding gestures and facial expressions. Note that while both these forms of communicative skill have their uses, they are not equally well represented in psychometric tests.

How testing is done can have different effects in different cultural groups. This can happen for many reasons. In one study, Serpell (1979) asked Zambian and English children to reproduce patterns in three different media: wire models, pencil and paper, or clay. The Zambian children excelled in the wire medium to which they were most accustomed, while the English children were best with pencil and paper. Both groups performed equally well with clay. As this example shows, differences in familiarity with test materials can produce marked differences in test results.

Developmental Progressions

Piaget's theory. The best-known developmentally-based conception of intelligence is certainly that of the Swiss psychologist Jean Piaget (1972). Unlike most of the theorists considered here, Piaget had relatively little interest in individual differences. Intelligence develops—in all children—through the continually shifting balance between the assimilation of new information into existing cognitive structures and the accommodation of those structures themselves to the new information. To index the development of intelligence in this sense, Piaget devised methods that are rather different from conventional tests. To assess the understanding of "conservation," for example (roughly, the principle that material quantity is not affected by mere changes of shape), children who have watched water being poured from a shallow to a tall beaker may be asked if now there is more water than before. (A positive answer would suggest that the child has not yet mastered the principle of conservation.) Piaget's tasks can be modified to serve as measures of individual differences; when this is done, they correlate fairly well with standard psychometric tests (for a review see Jensen, 1980).

Vygotsky's theory. The Russian psychologist Lev Vygotsky (1978) argued that all intellectual abilities are social in origin. Language and thought first appear in early interactions with parents, and continue to develop through contact with teachers and others. Traditional intelligence tests ignore what Vygotsky called the "zone of proximal development," i.e., the level of performance that a child might reach with appropriate help from a supportive adult. Such tests are "static," measuring only the intelligence that is already fully developed. "Dynamic" testing, in which the examiner provides guided and graded feedback, can go further to give some indication of the child's latent potential. These ideas are being developed and extended by a number of contemporary psychologists (Brown & French, 1979; Feuerstein, 1980; Pascual-Leone & Ijaz, 1989).

Biological Approaches

Some investigators have recently turned to the study of the brain as a basis for new ideas about what intelligence is and how to measure it. Many aspects of brain anatomy and physiology have been suggested as potentially relevant to intelligence: the arborization of cortical neurons (Ceci, 1990), cerebral glucose metabolism (Haier, 1993), evoked potentials (Caryl, 1994), nerve conduction velocity (Reed & Jensen, 1992), sex hormones (see the fourth section), and still others (cf. Vernon, 1993). Advances in research methods, including new forms of brain imaging such as PET and MRI scans, will surely add to this list. In the not-too-distant future it may be possible to relate some aspects of test performance to specific characteristics of brain function.

This brief survey has revealed a wide range of contemporary conceptions of intelligence and of how it should be measured. The psychometric approach is the oldest and best established, but others also have much to contribute. We should be open to the possibility that our understanding of intelligence in the future will be rather different from what it is today.

INTELLIGENCE TESTS AND THEIR CORRELATES

The correlation coefficient, r, can be computed whenever the scores in a sample are paired in some way. Typically this is because each individual is measured twice: he or she takes the same test on two occasions, or takes two different tests, or has both a test score and some criterion measure such as grade point average or job performance. (In the third section we consider cases where the paired scores are those of two different individuals, such as twins or parent and child.) The value of r measures the degree of relationship between the two sets of scores in a convenient way, by assessing how well one of them (computationally it doesn't matter which one) could be used to predict the value of the other. Its sign indicates the direction of relationship: when r is negative, high scores on one measure predict low scores on the other. Its magnitude indicates the strength of the relationship. If $r = 0$, there is no relation at all; if r is 1 (or -1), one score can be used to predict the other score perfectly. Moreover, the square of r has a particular meaning in cases where we are concerned with predicting one variable from another. When $r = .50$, for example, r^2 is .25: this means (given certain linear assumptions) that 25% of the variance in one set of scores is predictable from the correlated values of the other set, while the remaining 75% is not.

Basic Characteristics of Test Scores
Stability. Intelligence test scores are fairly stable during development. When Jones and Bayley (1941) tested a sample of children annually throughout childhood and adolescence, for example, scores obtained at age 18 were correlated $r = .77$ with scores that had been obtained at age 6 and $r = .89$ with scores from age 12. When scores were averaged across several successive tests to remove short-term fluctuations, the correlations were even higher. The mean for ages 17 and 18 was correlated $r = .86$ with the mean for ages 5, 6, and 7, and $r = .96$ with the mean for ages 11, 12, and 13. (For comparable findings in a more recent study, see Moffitt, Caspi, Harkness, & Silva, 1993.) Nevertheless, IQ scores do change over time. In the same study (Jones & Bayley, 1941), the average change between age 12 and age 17 was 7.1 IQ points; some individuals changed as much as 18 points.

It is possible to measure the intelligence of young infants in a similar way? Conventional tests of "infant intelligence" do not predict later test scores very well, but certain experimental measures of infant attention and memory—originally developed for other purposes—have turned out to be more successful. In the most common procedure, a particular visual pattern is shown to a baby over and over again. The experimenter records how long the infant subject looks at the pattern on each trial; these looks get shorter and shorter as the baby becomes "habituated" to it. The time required to reach a certain level of habituation, or the extent to which the baby now "prefers" (looks longer at) a new pattern, is regarded as a measure of some aspect of his or her information-processing capability.

These habituation-based measures, obtained from babies at ages ranging from three months to a year, are significantly correlated with the intelligence test scores of the same children when they get to be 2- or 4- or 6-years-old (for reviews see Bornstein, 1989; Columbo, 1993; McCall & Garriger, 1993). A few studies have found such correlations even at ages 8 or 11 (Rose & Feldman, 1995). A recent meta-analysis, based on 31 different samples, estimates the average magnitude of the correlations at about $r = .36$ (McCall & Garriger, 1993). (The largest r's often appear in samples that include "at risk" infants.) It is possible that these habituation scores (and other similar measures of infant cognition) do indeed reflect real cognitive differences, perhaps in "speed of information processing" (Columbo, 1993). It is also possible, however, that—to a presently unknown extent—they reflect early differences in temperament of inhibition.

It is important to understand what remains stable and what changes in the development of intelligence. A child whose IQ score remains the same from age 6 to age 18 does not exhibit the same performance throughout that period. On the contrary, steady gains in general knowledge, vocabulary, reasoning ability, etc. will be apparent. What does *not* change is his or her score in comparison to that of other individuals of the same age. A 6-year-old with an IQ of 100 is at the mean of 6-year-olds; an 18-year-old with that score is at the mean of 18-year-olds.

Factors and g. As noted in the first section, the patterns of intercorrelation among tests (i.e., among different kinds of items) are complex. Some pairs of tests are much more closely related than others, but all such correlations are typically positive and form what is called a "positive manifold." Spearman (1927) showed that in any such manifold, some portion of the variance of scores on each test can be mathematically attributed to a "general factor," or *g*. Given this analysis, the overall pattern of correlations can be roughly described as produced by individual differences in *g* plus differences in the specific abilities sampled by particular tests. In addition, however, there are usually patterns of intercorrelation among groups of tests. These commonalities, which played only a small role in Spearman's analysis, were emphasized by other theorists. Thurstone (1938), for example, proposed an analysis based primarily on the concept of group factors.

While some psychologists today still regard *g* as the most fundamental measure of intelligence (e.g., Jensen, 1980), others prefer to emphasize the distinctive profile of strengths and weaknesses present in each person's performance. A recently published review identifies over 70 different abilities that can be distinguished by currently available tests (Carroll, 1993). One way to represent this structure is in terms of a hierarchical arrangement with a general intelligence factor at the apex and various more specialized abilities arrayed below it. Such a summary merely acknowledges that performance levels on different tests are correlated; it is consistent with, but does not prove, the hypothesis that a common factor such as *g* underlies those correlations. Different specialized abilities might also be correlated for other reasons, such as the effects of education. Thus, while the *g*-based factor hierarchy is the most widely accepted current view of the structure of abilities, some theorists regard it as misleading (Ceci, 1990). Moreover, as noted in first section, a wide range of human abilities— including many that seem to have intellectual components—are outside the domain of standard psychometric tests.

Tests as Predictors

School performance. Intelligence tests were originally devised by Alfred Binet to measure children's ability to succeed in school. They do in fact predict school performance fairly well: the correlation between IQ scores and grades is about .50. They also predict scores on school achievement tests, designed to measure knowledge of the curriculum. Note, however, that correlations of this magnitude account for only about 25% of the overall variance. Successful school learning depends on many personal characteristics other than intelligence, such as persistence, interest in school, and willingness to study. The encouragement for academic achievement that is received from peers, family, and teachers may also be important, together with more general cultural factors (see the fifth section).

The relationship between test scores and school performance seems to be ubiquitous. Wherever it has been studied, children with high scores on tests of intelligence tend to learn more of what is taught in school than their lower-scoring peers. There may be styles of teaching and methods of instruction that will decrease or increase this correlation, but none that consistently eliminates it has yet been found (Cronbach & Snow, 1977).

What children learn in school depends not only on their individual abilities but also on teaching practices and on what is actually taught. Recent comparisons among pupils attending school in different countries have made this especially obvious. Children in Japan and China, for example, know a great deal more math than American children even though their intelligence test scores are quite similar (see the fifth section). This difference may result from many factors, including cultural attitudes toward schooling as well as the sheer amount of time devoted to the study of mathematics and how that study is organized (Stovenson & Stigier, 1992). In principle it is quite possible to improve the school learning of American children—even very substantially—without changing their intelligence test scores at all.

Years of education. Some children stay in school longer than others; many go on to college and perhaps beyond. Two variables that can be measured as early as elementary school correlate with the total amount of education individuals will obtain: test scores and social class background. Correlations between IQ scores and total years of education are about .55, implying that differences in psychometric intelligence account for about 30% of the outcome variance. The correlations of years of education with social class background (as indexed by the occupation/education of a child's parents) are also positive, but somewhat lower.

There are a number of reasons why children with higher test scores tend to get more education. They are likely to get good grades, and to be encouraged by teachers and counselors; often they are placed in "college preparatory" classes, where they make friends who may also encourage them. In general, they are likely to find the process of education rewarding in a way that many low-scoring children do not (Rehberg & Rosenthal, 1978). These influences are not omnipotent: some high-scoring children do drop out of school. Many personal and social characteristics other than psychometric intelligence determine academic success and interest, and social privilege may also play a role. Nevertheless, test scores are the best single predictor of an individual's years of education.

In contemporary American society, the amount of schooling that adults complete is also somewhat predictive of their social status. Occupations considered high in prestige (e.g., law, medicine, even corporate business) usually require at least a college degree—16 or more years of education—as a condition of entry. It is partly because intelligence test scores predict years of education so well that they also predict occupational status—and, to a smaller extent, even income (Herrnstein & Murray, 1994; Jencks, 1979). Moreover, many occupations can only be entered through professional schools which base their admissions at least partly on test scores: the MCAT, the GMAT, the LSAT, etc. Individual scores on admission-related tests such as these are certainly correlated with scores on tests of intelligence.

Social status and income. How well do IQ scores (which can be obtained before individuals enter the labor force) predict such outcome measures as the social status or income of adults? This question is complex, in part because another variable also predicts such outcomes: namely, the socioeconomic status (SES) of one's parents. Unsurprisingly, children of privileged families are more likely to attain high social status than those whose parents are poor and less educated. These two predictors (IQ and parental SES) are by no means independent of one another; the correlation between them is around .33 (White, 1982).

One way to look at these relationships is to begin with SES. According to Jencks (1979), measures of parental SES predict about one-third of the variance in young adults' social status and about one-fifth of the variance in their income. About half of this predictive effectiveness depends on the fact that the SES of parents also predicts children's intelligence test scores, which have their own predictive value for social outcomes; the other half comes about in other ways.

We can also begin with IQ scores, which by themselves account for about one-fourth of the social status variance and one-sixth of the income variance. Statistical controls for parental SES eliminate only about a quarter of this predictive power. One way to conceptualize this effect is by comparing the occupational status (or income) of adult brothers who grew up in the same family and hence have the same parental SES. In such cases, the brother with the higher adolescent IQ score is likely to have the higher adult social status and income (Jencks, 1979). This effect, in turn, is substantially mediated by education: the brother with the higher test scores is likely to get more schooling, and hence to be better credentialled as he enters the workplace.

Do these data imply that psychometric intelligence is a major determinant of social status or income? That depends on what one means by "major." In fact, individuals who have the same test scores may differ widely in occupational status and even more widely in income. Consider for a moment the distribution of occupational status scores for all individuals in a population, and then consider the conditional distribution of such scores for just those individuals who test at some given IQ. Jencks (1979) notes that the standard deviation of the latter distribution may still be quite large; in some cases it amounts to about 88% of the standard deviation for the entire population. Viewed from this perspective, psychometric intelligence appears as only one of a great many factors that influence social outcomes.

Job performance. Scores on intelligence tests predict various measures of job performance: supervisor ratings, work samples, etc. Such correlations, which typically lie between $r = .30$ and $r = .50$, are partly restricted by the limited reliability of those measures themselves. They become higher when r is statistically corrected for this unreliability: in one survey of relevant studies (Hunter, 1983), the mean of the corrected correlations was .54. This implies that, across a wide range of occupations, intelligence test performance accounts for some 29% of the variance in job performance.

Although these correlations can sometimes be modified by changing methods of training or aspects of the job itself, intelligence test scores are at least weakly related to job performance in most settings. Sometimes IQ scores are described as the "best available predictor" of that performance. It is worth noting, however, that such tests predict considerably less than half the variance of job-related measures. Other individual characteristics—interpersonal skills, aspects of personality, etc.—are probably of equal or greater importance, but at this point we do not have equally reliable instruments to measure them.

Social outcomes. Psychometric intelligence is negatively correlated with certain socially undesirable outcomes. For example, children with high test scores are less likely than lower-scoring children to engage in juvenile crime. In one study, Moffitt, Gabrielli, Mednick, and Schulsinger (1981) found a correlation of $-.19$ between IQ scores and number of juvenile offenses in a large Danish sample; with social class controlled, the correlation dropped to $-.17$. The correlations for most "negative outcome" variables are typically smaller than .20, which means that test scores are associated with less than 4% of their total variance. It is important to realize that the causal links between psychometric ability and social outcomes may be indirect. Children who are unsuccessful in—and hence alienated from— school may be more likely to engage in delinquent behaviors for that very reason, compared to other children who enjoy school and are doing well.

In summary, intelligence test scores predict a wide range of social outcomes with varying degrees of success. Correlations are highest for school achievement, where they account for about a quarter of the variance. They are somewhat lower for job performance, and very low for negatively valued outcomes such as criminality. In general, intelligence tests measure only some of the many personal characteristics that are relevant to life in contemporary America. Those characteristics are never the only influence on outcomes, though in the case of school performance they may well be the strongest.

Test Scores and Measures of Processing Speed

Many recent studies show that the speeds with which people perform very simple perceptual and cognitive tasks are correlated with psychometric intelligence (for reviews see Ceci, 1990; Deary,

1995; Vernon, 1987). In general, people with higher intelligence test scores tend to apprehend, scan, retrieve, and respond to stimuli more quickly than those who score lower.

Cognitive correlates. The modern study of these relations began in the 1970s, as part of the general growth of interest in response time and other chronometric measures of cognition. Many of the new cognitive paradigms required subjects to make same/different judgments or other speeded responses to visual displays. Although those paradigms had not been devised with individual differences in mind, they could be interpreted as providing measures of the speed of certain information processes. Those speeds turned out to correlate with psychometrically-measured verbal ability (Hunt, 1978; Jackson & McClelland, 1979). In some problem solving tasks, it was possible to analyze the subjects' overall response times into theoretically motivated "cognitive components" (Sternberg, 1977); component times could then be correlated with test scores in their own right.

Although the size of these correlations is modest (seldom accounting for more than 10% of the variance), they do increase as the basic tasks were made more complex by requiring increased memory or attentional capacity. For instance, the correlation between paired associate learning and intelligence increases as the pairs are presented at faster rates (Christal, Tirre, & Kyllonen, 1984).

Choice reaction time. In another popular cognitive paradigm, the subject simply moves his or her finger from a "home" button to one of eight other buttons arranged in a semicircle around it; these are marked by small lights that indicate which one is the target on a given trial (Jensen, 1987). Various aspects of the choice reaction times obtained in this paradigm are correlated with scores on intelligence tests, sometimes with values of r as high as $-.30$ or $-.40$ (r is negative because higher test scores go with shorter times). Nevertheless, it has proved difficult to make theoretical sense of the overall pattern of correlations, and the results are still hard to interpret (cf. Brody, 1992; Longstreth, 1984).

Somewhat stronger results have been obtained in a variant of Jensen's paradigm devised by Frearson and Eysenck (1986). In this "odd-man-out" procedure, three of the eight lights are illuminated on each trial. Two of these are relatively close to each other while the third is more distant; the subject must press the button corresponding to the more isolated stimulus. Response times in this task show higher correlations with IQ scores than those in Jensen's original procedure, perhaps because it requires more complex forms of spatial judgment.

Inspection time. Another paradigm for measuring processing speed, devised to be relatively independent of response factors, is the method of "inspection time" (IT). In the standard version of this paradigm (Nettelbeck, 1987; Vickers, Nettelbeck & Wilson, 1972), two vertical lines are shown very briefly on each trial, followed by a pattern mask; the subject must judge which line was shorter. For a given subject, IT is defined as the minimum exposure duration (up to the onset of the mask) for which the lines must be displayed if he or she is to meet a preestablished criterion of accuracy—e.g., nine correct trials out of ten.

Inspection times defined in this way are consistently correlated with measures of psychometric intelligence. In a recent meta-analysis, Kranzler and Jensen (1989) reported an overall correlation of $-.30$ between IQ scores and IT; this rose to $-.55$ when corrected for measurement error and attenuation. More recent findings confirm this general result (e.g., Bates & Eysenck, 1993; Deary, 1993). IT usually correlates best with performance subtests of intelligence; its correlation with verbal intelligence is usually weaker and sometimes zero.

One apparent advantage of IT over other chronometric methods is that the task itself seems particularly simple. At first glance, it is hard to imagine that any differences in response strategies or stimulus familiarity could affect the outcome. Nevertheless, it seems that they do. Brian Mackenzie and his colleagues (e.g., Mackenzie, Molloy, Martin, Lovegrove, & McNicol, 1991) discovered that some subjects use apparent-movement cues in the basic IT task while others do not; only in the latter group is IT correlated with intelligence test scores. Moreover, standard IT paradigms require an essentially spatial judgment; it is not surprising, then, that they correlate with intelligence tests which emphasize spatial ability. With this in mind, Mackenzie et al. (1991) devised a *verbal* inspection time task based on Posner's classical same-letter/different-better paradigm (Posner, Boies, Eichelman, & Taylor, 1969). As predicted, the resulting ITs correlated with verbal but not with spatial intelligence. It is clear that the apparently simple IT task actually involves complex modes of information processing (cf. Chaiken, 1993) that are as yet poorly understood.

Neurological measures. Recent research has begun to explore what seem to be still more direct indices of neural processing. Reed and Jensen (1992) have used measures based on visual evoked potentials (VEP) to assess what they call "nerve conduction velocity" (NCV). To estimate that velocity, distance is divided by time: each subject's head length (a rough measure of the distance from the eye to the primary visual cortex) is divided by the latency of an early component (N70 or P100) of his or her evoked potential pattern. In a study with 147 college-student subjects, these NCVs correlated $r = .26$ with scores on an unspeeded test of intelligence. (A statistical correction for the restricted range of subjects raised the correlation to .37.) Other researchers have also reported correlations between VEP parameters and intelligence test scores (Caryl, 1994). Interestingly, however, Reed and Jensen (1993) reported that their estimates of "nerve conduction velocity" were *not* correlated with the same subjects' choice reaction times. Thus, while we do not yet understand the basis of the correlation between NCV and psychometric intelligence, it is apparently not just a matter of overall speed.

Problems of interpretation. Some researchers believe that psychometric intelligence, especially *g*, depends directly on what may be called the "neural efficiency" of the brain (Eysenck, 1986; Vernon, 1987). They regard the observed correlations between test scores and measures of processing speed as evidence for their view. If choice reaction times, inspection times, and VEP latencies actually do reflect the speed of basic neural processes, such correlations are only to be expected. In fact, however, the observed patterns of correlation are rarely as simple as this hypothesis would predict. Moreover, it is quite possible that high- and low-IQ individuals differ in other ways that affect speeded performance (cf. Ceci, 1990). Those variables include motivation, response criteria (emphasis on speed vs. accuracy), perceptual strategies (cf. Mackenzie et al., 1991), attentional strategies, and— in some cases—differential familiarity with the material itself. Finally, we do not yet know the direction of causation that underlies such correlations. Do high levels of "neural efficiency" promote the development of intelligence, or do more intelligent people simply find faster ways to carry out perceptual tasks? Or both? These questions are still open.

THE GENES AND INTELLIGENCE

In this section of the report we first discuss individual differences generally, without reference to any particular trait. We then focus on intelligence, as measured by conventional IQ tests or other tests intended to measure general cognitive ability. The different and more controversial topic of group differences will be considered in fifth section.

We focus here on the relative contributions of genes and environments to individual differences in particular traits. To avoid misunderstanding, it must be emphasized from the outset that gene action always involves an environment—at least a biochemical environment, and often an ecological one. (For humans, that ecology is usually interpersonal or cultural.) Thus, all genetic effects on the development of observable traits are potentially modifiable by environmental input, though the practicability of making such modifications may be another matter. Conversely, all environmental effects on trait development involve the genes or structures to which the genes have contributed. Thus, there is always a genetic aspect to the effects of the environment (cf. Plomin & Bergeman, 1991).

Sources of Individual Differences

Partitioning the variation. Individuals differ from one another on a wide variety of traits: familiar examples include height, intelligence, and aspects of personality. Those differences are often of considerable social importance. Many interesting questions can be asked about their nature and origins. One such question is the extent to which they reflect differences among the genes of the individuals involved, as distinguished from differences among the environments to which those individuals have been exposed. The issue here is not whether genes and environments are both essential for the development of a given trait (this is always the case), and it is not about the genes or environment of any particular person. We are concerned only with the observed variation of the trait across individuals in a given population. A figure called the "heritability" (h^2) of the trait represents the proportion of that variation that is associated with genetic differences among the individuals. The remaining variation ($1 - h^2$) is associated with environmental differences and with errors of measurement. These proportions can be estimated by various methods described below.

Sometimes special interest attaches to those aspects of environments that family members have in common (for example, characteristics of the home). The part of the variation that derives from this source, called "shared" variation or c^2, can also be estimated. Still more refined estimates can be made: c^2 is sometimes subdivided into several kinds of shared variation; h^2 is sometimes subdivided into so-called "additive" and "nonadditive" portions (the part that is transmissible from parent to child vs. the part expressed anew in each generation by a unique patterning of genes.) Variation associated with correlations and statistical interactions between genes and environments may also be identifiable. In theory, any of the above estimates may vary with the age of the individuals involved.

A high heritability does not mean that the environment has no impact on the development of a trait, or that learning is not involved. Vocabulary size, for example, is very substantially heritable (and highly correlated with general psychometric intelligence) although every word in an individual's vocabulary is learned. In a society in which plenty of words are available in everyone's environment— especially for individuals who are motivated to seek them out—the number of words that individuals actually learn depends to a considerable extent on their genetic predispositions.

Behavior geneticists have often emphasized the fact that individuals can be active in creating or selecting their own environments. Some describe this process as active or reactive genotype– environment correlation (Plomin, DeFries, & Loehlin, 1977). (The distinction is between the action of the organism in selecting its own environment and the reaction of others to its gene-based traits.) Others suggest that these forms of gene–environment relationship are typical of the way that genes are normally expressed, and simply include them as part of the genetic effect (Roberts, 1967). This is a matter of terminological preference, not a dispute about facts.

How genetic estimates are made. Estimates of the magnitudes of these sources of individual differences are made by exploiting natural and social "experiments" that combine genotypes and environments in informative ways. Monozygotic (MZ) and dizygotic (DZ) twins, for example, can be regarded as experiments of nature. MZ twins are paired individuals of the same age growing up in the same family who have all their genes in common; DZ twins are otherwise similar pairs who have only half their genes in common. Adoptions, in contrast, are experiments of society. They allow one to compare genetically unrelated persons who are growing up in the same family as well as genetically related persons who are growing up in different families. They can also provide information about genotype–environment correlations: in ordinary families genes and environments are correlated because the same parents provide both, whereas in adoptive families one set of parents provides the genes and another the environment. An experiment involving both nature and society is the study of monozygotic twins who have been reared apart (Bouchard, Lykken, McGue, Segal, & Tellegen, 1990; Pedersen, Plomin, Nesselroade, & McClearn, 1992). Relationships in the families of monozygotic twins also offer unique possibilities for analysis (e.g., Rose, Harris, Christian, & Nance, 1979).

Because these comparisons are subject to different sources of potential error, the results of studies involving several kinds of kinship are often analyzed together to arrive at robust overall conclusions. (For general discussions of behavior genetic methods, see Plomin, DeFries, & McClearn, 1990, or Hay, 1985.)

Results for IQ Scores

Parameter estimates. Across the ordinary range of environments in modern Western societies, a sizable part of the variation in intelligence test scores is associated with genetic differences among individuals. Quantitative estimates vary from one study to another, because many are based on small or selective samples. If one simply combines all available correlations in a single analysis, the heritability (h^2) works out to about .50 and the between-family variance (c^2) to about .25 (e.g., Chipuer, Rovine, & Plomin, 1990; Loehlin, 1989). These overall figures are misleading, however, because most of the relevant studies have been done with children. We now know that the heritability of IQ changes with age: h^2 goes up and c^2 goes down from infancy to adulthood (McCartney, Harris, & Bernieri, 1990; McGue, Bouchard, Iacono, & Lykken, 1993). In childhood h^2 and c^2 for IQ are of the order of .45 and .35; by late adolescence h^2 is around .75 and c^2 is quite low (zero in some studies). Substantial environmental variance remains, but it primarily reflects within-family rather than between-family differences.

These adult parameter estimates are based on a number of independent studies. The correlation between MZ twins reared apart, which directly estimates h^2, ranged from .68 to .78 in five studies involving adult samples from Europe and the United States (McGue et al., 1993). The correlation between unrelated children reared together in adoptive families, which directly estimates c^2, was approximately zero for adolescents in two adoption studies (Loehlin, Horn, & Willerman, 1989; Scarr & Weinberg, 1978) and .19 in a third (the Minnesota transracial adoption study: Scarr, Weinberg, & Waldman, 1993).

These particular estimates derive from samples in which the lowest socioeconomic levels were under-represented (i.e., there were few very poor families), so the range of between-family differences was smaller than in the population as a whole. This means that we should be cautious in generalizing the findings for between-family effects across the entire social spectrum. The samples were also mostly White, but available data suggest that twin and sibling correlations in African American and similarly selected White samples are more often comparable than not (Loehlin, Lindzey, & Spuhler, 1975).

Why should individual differences in intelligence (as measured by test scores) reflect genetic differences more strongly in adults than they do in children? One possibility is that as individuals grow older their transactions with their environments are increasingly influenced by the characteristics that they bring to those environments themselves, decreasingly by the conditions imposed by family life and social origins. Older persons are in a better position to select their own effective environments, a form of genotype–environment correlation. In any case, the popular view that genetic influences on the development of a trait are essentially frozen at conception while the effects of the early environment cumulate inexorably is quite misleading, at least for the trait of psychometric intelligence.

Implications. Estimates of h^2 and c^2 for IQ (or any other trait) are descriptive statistics for the populations studied. (In this respect they are like means and standard deviations.) They are outcome measures, summarizing the results of a great many diverse, intricate, individually variable events and processes, but they can nevertheless be quite useful. They can tell us how much of the variation in a given trait the genes and family environments explain, and changes in them place some constraints on theories of how this occurs. On the other hand, they have little to say about specific mechanisms, i.e., about how genetic and environmental differences get translated into individual physiological and psychological differences. Many psychologists and neuroscientists are actively studying such processes; data on heritabilites may give them ideas about what to look for and where or when to look for it.

A common error is to assume that because something is heritable it is necessarily unchangeable. This is wrong. Heritability does not imply immutability. As previously noted, heritable traits can depend on learning, and they may be subject to other environmental effects as well. The value of h^2 can change if the distribution of environments (or genes) in the population is substantially altered. On the other hand, there can be effective environmental changes that do not change heritability at all. If the environment relevant to a given trait improves in a way that affects all members of the population equally, the mean value of the trait will rise without any change in its heritability (because the differences among individuals in the population will stay the same). This has evidently happened for height: the heritability of stature is high, but average heights continue to increase (Olivier, 1980). Something of the sort may also be taking place for IQ scores—the so-called "Flynn effect" discussed in the fourth section.

In theory, different subgroups of a population might have different distributions of environments or genes and hence different values of h^2. This seems not to be the case for high and low IQ levels, for which adult heritabilities appear to be much the same (Saudino, Plomin, Pedersen, & McClearn, 1994). It is also possible that an impoverished or suppressive environment could fail to support the development of a trait, and hence restrict individual variation. This could affect estimates of h^2, c^2, or both, depending on the details of the process. Again (as in the case of whole populations), an environmental factor that affected every member of a subgroup equally might alter the group's mean without affecting heritabilities at all.

Where the heritability of IQ is concerned, it has sometimes seemed as if the findings based on differences between group means were in contradiction with those based on correlations. For example, children adopted in infancy into advantaged families tend to have higher IQs in childhood than would have been expected if they had been reared by their birth mothers; this is a mean difference implicating the environment. Yet at the same time their individual resemblance to their birth mothers persists, and this correlation is most plausibly interpreted in genetic terms. There is no real contradiction: the two findings simply call attention to different aspects of the same phenomenon. A sensible account must include both aspects: there is only a single developmental process, and it occurs in individuals. By looking at means or correlations one learns somewhat different but compatible things about the genetic and environmental contributions to that process (Turkheimer, 1991).

As far as behavior genetic methods are concerned, there is nothing unique about psychometric intelligence relative to other traits or abilities. Any reliably measured trait can be analyzed by these methods, and many traits including personality and attitudes have been. The methods are neutral with regard to genetic and environmental sources of variance: if individual differences on a trait are entirely due to environmental factors, the analysis will reveal this. These methods have shown that genes contribute substantially to individual differences in intelligence test performance, and that their role seems to increase from infancy to adulthood. They have also shown that variations in the unique environments of individuals are important, and that between-family variation contributes significantly to observed differences in IQ scores in childhood although this effect diminishes later on. All these conclusions are wholly consistent with the notion that both genes and environment, in complex interplay, are essential to the development of intellectual competence.

ENVIRONMENTAL EFFECTS ON INTELLIGENCE

The "environment" includes a wide range of influences on intelligence. Some of those variables affect whole populations, while others contribute to individual differences within a given group. Some of them are social, some are biological; at this point some are still mysterious. It may also happen that the proper interpretation of an environmental variable requires the simultaneous consideration of genetic effects. Nevertheless, a good deal of solid information is available.

Social Variables

It is obvious that the cultural environment—how people live, what they value, what they do—has a significant effect on the intellectual skills developed by individuals. Rice farmers in Liberia are good at estimating quantities of rice (Gay & Cole, 1967); children in Botswana, accustomed to story-telling, have excellent memories for stories (Dube, 1982). Both these groups were far ahead of American controls on the tasks in question. On the other hand, Americans and other Westernized groups typically outperform members of traditional societies on psychometric tests, even those designed to be "culture-fair."

Cultures typically differ from one another in so many ways that particular differences can rarely be ascribed to single causes. Even comparisons between subpopulations can be difficult to interpret. If we find that middle-class and poor Americans differ in their scores on intelligence tests, it is easy to suppose that the environmental difference has caused the IQ difference (i.e., that growing up in the middle class produces higher psychometric intelligence than growing up poor). But there may also be an opposite direction of causation: individuals can come to be in one environment or another because of differences in their own abilities. Waller (1971) has shown, for example, that adult sons whose IQ scores are above those of their fathers tend to have higher social-class status than those fathers; conversely, sons with IQ scores below their fathers' tend to have lower social-class status. Since all the subjects grew up with their fathers, the IQ differences in this study cannot have resulted from class-related differences in childhood experience. Rather, those differences (or other factors correlated with them) seem to have had an influence on the status that they achieved. Such a result is not surprising, given the relation between test scores and years of education reviewed in the second section.

Occupation. In the second section, we noted that intelligence test scores predict occupational level, not only because some occupations require more intelligence than others but also because admission to many professions depends on test scores in the first place. There can also be an effect in the opposite direction, i.e., workplaces may affect the intelligence of those who work in them. Kohn and Schooler (1973), who interviewed some 3,000 men in various occupations (farmers, managers, machinists, porters, etc.), argued that more "complex" jobs produce more "intellectual flexibility" in the individuals who hold them. Although the issue of direction of effects was not fully resolved in their study—and perhaps not even in its longitudinal follow-up (Kohn & Schooler, 1983)—this remains a plausible suggestion.

Among other things, Kohn and Schooler's hypothesis may help us understand urban/rural differences. A generation ago these were substantial in the United States, averaging about 6 IQ points or 0.4 standard deviations (Terman & Merrill, 1937; Seashore, Wesman, & Doppelt, 1950). In recent years the difference has declined to about 2 points (Kaufman & Doppelt, 1976; Reynolds, Chastain, Kaufman, & McLean, 1987). In all likelihood this urban/rural convergence primarily reflects environmental changes: a decrease in rural isolation (due to increased travel and mass communications), an improvement in rural schools, the greater use of technology on farms. All these changes can be regarded as increasing the "complexity" of the rural environment in general or of farm work in particular. (However, processes with a genetic component—e.g., changes in the selectivity of migration from farm to city—cannot be completely excluded as contributing factors.)

Schooling. Attendance at school is both a dependent and an independent variable in relation to intelligence. On the one hand, children with higher test scores are less likely to drop out and more likely to be promoted from grade to grade and then to attend college. Thus, the number of years of education that adults complete is roughly predictable from their childhood scores on intelligence tests. On the other hand, schooling itself changes mental abilities, including those abilities measured on psychometric tests. This is obvious for tests like the SAT that are explicitly designed to assess school learning, but it is almost equally true of intelligence tests themselves.

The evidence for the effect of schooling on intelligence test scores takes many forms (Ceci, 1991). When children of nearly the same age go through school a year apart (because of birthday-related admission criteria), those who have been in school longer have higher mean scores. Children who attend school intermittently score below those who go regularly, and test performance tends to drop over the summer vacation. A striking demonstration of this effect appeared when the schools in one Virginia county closed for several years in the 1960s to avoid integration, leaving most Black children with no formal education at all. Compared to controls, the intelligence-test scores of these children dropped by about 0.4 standard deviations (6 points) per missed year of school (Green, Hoffman, Morse, Hayes, & Morgan, 1964).

Schools affect intelligence in several ways, most obviously by transmitting information. The answers to questions like "Who wrote Hamlet?" and "What is the boiling point of water?" are typically learned in school, where some pupils learn them more easily and thoroughly than others. Perhaps at least as important are certain general skills and attitudes: systematic problem-solving, abstract thinking, categorization, sustained attention to material of little intrinsic interest, and repeated manipulation of basic symbols and operations. There is no doubt that schools promote and permit the development of significant intellectual skills, which develop to different extents in different children. It is because tests of intelligence draw on many of those same skills that they predict school achievement as well as they do.

To achieve these results, the school experience must meet at least some minimum standard of quality. In very poor schools, children may learn so little that they fall farther behind the national IQ norms for every year of attendance. When this happens, older siblings have systematically lower scores than their younger counterparts. This pattern of scores appeared in at least one rural Georgia school system in the 1970s (Jensen, 1977). Before desegregation, it must have been characteristic of many of the schools attended by Black pupils in the South. In a study based on Black children who had moved to Philadelphia at various ages during this period, Lee (1951) found that thier IQ scores went up more than half a point for each year that they were enrolled in the Philadelphia system.

Interventions. Intelligence test scores reflect a child's standing relative to others in his or her age cohort. Very poor or interrupted schooling can lower that standing substantially; are there also ways to raise it? In fact many interventions have been shown to raise test scores and mental ability "in the short run" (i.e., while the program itself was in progress), but long-run gains have proved more elusive. One noteworthy example of (at least short-run) success was the Venezuelan Intelligence Project (Herrnstein, Nickerson, de Sanchez, & Swets, 1986), in which hundreds of seventh-grade children from underprivileged backgrounds in that country were exposed to an extensive, theoretically based curriculum focused on thinking skills. The intervention produced substantial gains on a wide range of tests, but there has been no follow-up.

Children who participate in "Head Start" and similar programs are exposed to various school-related materials and experiences for 1 or 2 years. Their test scores often go up during the course of the program, but these gains fade with time. By the end of elementary school, there are usually no significant IQ or achievement-test differences between children who have been in such programs and controls who have not. There may, however, be other differences. Follow-up studies suggest that children who participated in such programs as preschoolers are less likely to be assigned to special education, less likely to be held back in grade, and more likely to finish high school than matched controls (Consortium for Longitudinal Studies, 1983; Darlington, 1986; but see Locurto, 1991).

More extensive interventions might be expected to produce larger and more lasting effects, but few such programs have been evaluated systematically. One of the most successful is the Carolina Abecedarian Project (Campbell & Ramey, 1994), which provided a group of children with enriched environments from early infancy through preschool and also maintained appropriate controls. The test scores of the enrichment-group children were already higher than those of controls at age two; they were still some 5 points higher at age 12, seven years after the end of the intervention. Importantly, the enrichment group also outperformed the controls in academic achievement.

Family environment. No one doubts that normal child development requires a certain minimum level of responsible care. Severely deprived, neglectful, or abusive environments must have negative effects on a great many aspects—including intellectual aspects—of development. Beyond that minimum, however, the role of family experience is now in serious dispute (Baumrind, 1993; Jackson, 1993; Scarr, 1992, 1993). Psychometric intelligence is a case in point. Do differences between children's family environments (within the normal range) produce differences in their intelligence test performance? The problem here is to disentangle causation from correlation. There is no doubt that such variables as resources of the home (Gottfried, 1984) and parents' use of language (Hart & Risley, 1992, in press) are correlated with children's IQ scores, but such correlations may be mediated by genetic as well as (or instead of) environmental factors.

Behavior geneticists frame such issues in quantitative terms. As noted in the third section, environmental factors certainly contribute to the overall variance of psychometric intelligence. But how much of that variance results from differences between families, as contrasted with the varying experiences of different children in the same family? Between-family differences create what is called "shared variance" or c^2 (all children in a family share the same home and the same parents). Recent twin and adoption studies suggest that while the value of c^2 (for IQ scores) is substantial in early childhood, it becomes quite small by late adolescence.

These findings suggest that differences in the life styles of families—whatever their importance may be for many aspects of children's lives—make little long-term difference for the skills measured by intelligence tests. We should note, however, that low-income and non-White families are poorly represented in existing adoption studies as well as in most twin samples. Thus, it is not yet clear whether these surprisingly small values of (adolescent) c^2 apply to the population as a whole. It remains possible that, across the full range of income and ethnicity, between-family differences have more lasting consequences for psychometric intelligence.

Biological Variables

Every individual has a biological as well as a social environment, one that begins in the womb and extends throughout life. Many aspects of that environment can affect intellectual development. We now know that a number of biological factors—malnutrition, exposure to toxic substances, various prenatal and perinatal stressors—result in lowered psychometric intelligence under at least some conditions.

Nutrition. There has been only one major study of the effects of prenatal malnutrition (i.e., malnutrition of the mother during pregnancy) on long-term intellectual development. Stein, Susser, Saenger, and Marolla (1975) analyzed the test scores of Dutch 19-year-old males in relation to a wartime famine that had occurred in the winter of 1944–1945 just before their birth. In this very large sample (made possible by a universal military induction requirement), exposure to the famine had no effect on adult intelligence. Note, however, that the famine itself lasted only a few months; the subjects were exposed to it prenatally but not after birth.

In contrast, prolonged malnutrition during childhood does have long-term intellectual effects. These have not been easy to establish, in part because many other unfavorable socioeconomic conditions are often associated with chronic malnutrition (Ricciuti, 1993; but cf. Sigman, 1995). In one intervention study, however, preschoolers in two Guatemalan villages (where undernourishment is common) were given ad-lib access to a protein dietary supplement for several years. A decade later, many of these children (namely, those from the poorest socioeconomic levels) scored significantly higher on school-related achievement tests than comparable controls (Pollitt, Gorman, Engle,

Martorell, & Rivera, 1993). It is worth noting that the effects of poor nutrition on intelligence may well be indirect. Malnourished children are typically less responsive to adults, less motivated to learn, and less active in exploration than their more adequately nourished counterparts.

Although the degree of malnutrition prevalent in these villages rarely occurs in the United States, there may still be nutritional influences on intelligence. In studies of so-called "micronutrients," experimental groups of children have been given vitamin/mineral supplements while controls got placebos. In many of these studies (e.g., Schoenthaler, Amos, Eysenck, Peritz, & Yudkin, 1991), the experimental children showed testscore gains that significantly exceeded the controls. In a somewhat different design, Rush, Stein, Susser, and Brody (1980) gave dietary supplements of liquid protein to pregnant women who were thought to be at risk for delivering low birth-weight babies. At one year of age, the babies born to these mothers showed faster habituation to visual patterns than did control infants. (Other research has shown that infant habituation rates are positively correlated with later psychometric test scores: Columbo, 1993.) Although these results are encouraging, there has been no long-term follow-up of such gains.

Lead. Certain toxins have well-established negative effects on intelligence. Exposure to lead is one such factor. In one long-term study (Baghurst et al., 1992; McMichael et al., 1988), the blood lead levels of children growing up near a lead smelting plant were substantially and negatively correlated with intelligence test scores throughout childhood. No "threshold dose" for the effect of lead appears in such studies. Although ambient lead levels in the United States have been reduced in recent years, there is reason to believe that some American children—especially those in inner cities—may still be at risk from this source (cf. Needleman, Geiger, & Frank, 1985).

Alcohol. Extensive prenatal exposure to alcohol (which occurs if the mother drinks heavily during pregnancy) can give rise to fetal alcohol syndrome, which includes mental retardation as well as a range of physical symptoms. Smaller "doses" of prenatal alcohol may have negative effects on intelligence even when the full syndrome does not appear. Streissguth, Barr, Sampson, Darby, and Martin (1989) found that mothers who reported consuming more than 1.5 oz of alcohol daily during pregnancy had children who scored some 5 points below controls at age four. Prenatal exposure to aspirin and antibiotics had similar negative effects in this study.

Perinatal factors. Complications at delivery and other negative perinatal factors may have serious consequences for development. Nevertheless, because they occur only rarely, they contribute relatively little to the population variance of intelligence (Broman, Nichols, & Kennedy, 1975). Down's syndrome, a chromosomal abnormality that produces serious mental retardation, is also rare enough to have little impact on the overall distribution of test scores.

The correlation between birth weight and later intelligence deserves particular discussion. In some cases low birth weight simply reflects premature delivery; in others, the infant's size is below normal for its gestational age. Both factors apparently contribute to the tendency of low-birth-weight infants to have lower test scores in later childhood (Lubchenko, 1976). These correlations are small, ranging from .05 to .13 in different groups (Broman et al., 1975). The effects of low birth weight are substantial only when it is very low indeed (less than 1,500 g). Premature babies born at these very low birth weights are behind controls on most developmental measures; they often have severe or permanent intellectual deficits (Rosetti, 1986).

Continuously Rising Test Scores

Perhaps the most striking of all environmental effects is the steady worldwide rise in intelligence test performance. Although many psychometricians had noted these gains, it was James Flynn (1984, 1987) who first described them systematically. His analysis shows that performance has been going up ever since testing began. The "Flynn effect" is now very well documented, not only in the United

States but in many other technologically advanced countries. The average gain is about 3 IQ points per decade—more than a full standard deviation since, say, 1940.

Although it is simplest to describe the gains as increases in population IQ, this is not exactly what happens. Most intelligence tests are "restandardized" from time to time, in part to keep up with these very gains. As part of this process the mean score of the new standardization sample is typically set to 100 again, so the increase more or less disappears from view. In this context, the Flynn effect means that if 20 years have passed since the last time the test was standardized, people who now score 100 on the new version would probably average about 106 on the old one.

The sheer extent of these increases is remarkable, and the rate of gain may even be increasing. The scores of 19-year-olds in the Netherlands, for example, went up more than 8 points—over half a standard deviation—between 1972 and 1982. What's more, the largest gains appear on the types of tests that were specifically designed to be free of cultural influence (Flynn, 1987). One of these is Raven's Progressive Matrices, an untimed nonverbal test that many psychometricians regard as a good measure of *g*.

These steady gains in intelligence test performance have not always been accompanied by corresponding gains in school achievement. Indeed, the relation between intelligence and achievement test scores can be complex. This is especially true for the Scholastic Aptitude Test (SAT), in part because the ability range of the students who take the SAT has broadened over time. That change explains some portion—not all—of the prolonged decline in SAT scores that took place from the mid-1960s to the early 1980s, even as IQ scores were continuing to rise (Flynn, 1984). Meanwhile, however, other more representative measures show that school achievement levels have held steady or in some cases actually increased (Herrnstein & Murray, 1994). The National Assessment of Educational Progress (NAEP), for example, shows that the average reading and math achievement of American 13- and 17-year-olds improved somewhat from the early 1970s to 1990 (Grissmer, Kirby, Berends, & Williamson, 1994). An analysis of these data by ethnic group, reported in the fifth section, shows that this small overall increase actually reflects very substantial gains by Blacks and Latinos combined with little or no gain by Whites.

The consistent IQ gains documented by Flynn seem too large to result from simple increases in test sophistication. Their cause is presently unknown, but three interpretations deserve our consideration. Perhaps the most plausible of these is based on the striking cultural differences between successive generations. Daily life and occupational experience both seem more "complex" (Kohn & Schooler, 1973) today than in the time of our parents and grandparents. The population is increasingly urbanized; television exposes us to more information and more perspectives on more topics than ever before; children stay in school longer; and almost everyone seems to be encountering new forms of experience. These changes in the complexity of life may have produced corresponding changes in complexity of mind, and hence in certain psychometric abilities.

A different hypothesis attributes the gains to modern improvements in nutrition. Lynn (1990) points out that large nutritionally based increases in height have occurred during the same period as the IQ gains: perhaps there have been increases in brain size as well. As we have seen, however, the effects of nutrition on intelligence are themselves not firmly established.

The third interpretation addresses the very definition of intelligence. Flynn himself believes that real intelligence—whatever it may be—cannot have increased as much as these data would suggest. Consider, for example, the number of individuals who have IQ scores of 140 or more. (This is slightly above the cutoff used by L. M. Terman, 1925, in his famous longitudinal study of "genius.") In 1952, only 0.38% of Dutch test takers had IQs over 140; in 1982, scored by the same norms, 9.12% exceeded this figure! Judging by these criteria, the Netherlands should now be experiencing "a cultural renaissance too great to be overlooked" (Flynn, 1987, p. 187). So also should France, Norway, the United States, and many other countries. Because Flynn (1987) finds this conclusion implausible or absurd, he argues that what has risen cannot be intelligence itself but only a minor sort of "abstract problem solving ability." The issue remains unresolved.

Individual Life Experiences

Although the environmental variables that produce large differences in intelligence are not yet well understood, genetic studies assure us that they exist. With a heritability well below 1.00, IQ must be subjected to substantial environmental influences. Moreover, available heritability estimates apply only within the range of environments that are well-represented in the present population. We already know that some relatively rare conditions, like those reviewed earlier, have large negative effects on intelligence. Whether there are (now equally rare) conditions that have large positive effects is not known.

As we have seen, there is both a biological and a social environment. For any given child, the social factors include not only an overall cultural/social/school setting and a particular family but also a unique "microenvironment" of experiences that are shared with no one else. The adoption studies reviewed in the third section show that family variables—differences in parenting style, in the resources of the home, etc.—have smaller long-term effects than we once supposed. At least among people who share a given SES level and a given culture, it seems to be unique individual experience that makes the largest environmental contribution to adult IQ differences.

We do not yet know what the key features of those microenvironments may be. Are they biological? Social? Chronic? Acute? Is there something especially important in the earliest relations between the infant and its caretakers? Whatever the critical variables may be, do they interact with other aspects of family life? Of culture? At this point we cannot say, but these questions offer a ferile area for further research.

GROUP DIFFERENCES

Group means have no direct implications for individuals. What matters for the next person you meet (to the extent that test scores matter at all) is that person's own particular score, not the mean of some reference group to which he or she happens to belong. The commitment to evaluate people on their own individual merit is central to a democratic society. It also makes quantitative sense. The distributions of different groups inevitably overlap, with the range of scores within any one group always wider than the mean differences between any two groups. In the case of intelligence test scores, the variance attributable to individual differences far exceeds the variance related to group membership (Jensen, 1980).

Because claims about ethnic differences have often been used to rationalize racial discrimination in the past, all such claims must be subjected to very careful scrutiny. Nevertheless, group differences continue to be the subject of intense interest and debate. There are many reasons for this interest: some are legal and political, some social and psychological. Among other things, facts about group differences may be relevant to the need for (and the effectiveness of) affirmative action programs. But while some recent discussions of intelligence and ethnic differences (e.g., Herrnstein & Murray, 1994) have made specific policy recommendations in this area, we will not do so here. Such recommendations are necessarily based on political as well as scientific considerations, and so fall outside the scope of this report.

Besides European Americans ("Whites"), the ethnic groups to be considered are Chinese and Japanese Americans, Hispanic Americans ("Latinos"), Native Americans ("Indians"), and African Americans ("Blacks"). These groups (we avoid the term "race") are defined and self-defined by social conventions based on ethnic origin as well as on observable physical characteristics such as skin color. None of them are internally homogeneous. Asian Americans, for example, may have roots in many different cultures: not only China and Japan but also Korea, Laos, Vietnam, the Philippines, India, and Pakistan. Hispanic Americans, who share a common linguistic tradition, actually differ along many cultural dimensions. In their own minds they may be less "Latinos" than Puerto Ricans, Mexican Americans, Cuban Americans, or representatives of other Latin cultures. "Native American" is an even more diverse category, including a great many culturally distinct tribes living in a wide range of environments.

Although males and females are not ethnic or cultural groups, possible sex differences in cognitive ability have also been the subject of widespread interest and discussion. For this reason, the evidence relevant to such differences is briefly reviewed in the next section.

Sex Differences

Most standard tests of intelligence have been constructed so that there are no overall score differences between females and males. Some recent studies do report sex differences in IQ, but the direction is variable and the effects are small (Held, Alderton, Foley, & Segall, 1993; Lynn, 1994). This overall equivalence does not imply equal performance on every individual ability. While some tasks show no sex differences, there are others where small differences appear and a few where they are large and consistent.

Spatial and quantitative abilities. Large differences favoring males appear on visual-spatial tasks like mental rotation and spatiotemporal tasks like tracking a moving object through space (Law, Pellegrino, & Hunt, 1993; Linn & Petersen, 1985). The sex difference on mental rotation tasks is substantial: a recent meta-analysis (Masters & Sanders, 1993) puts the effect size at $d = 0.9$. (Effect sizes are measured in standard deviation units. Here, the mean of the male distribution is nearly one standard deviation above that for females.) Males' achievement levels on movement-related and visual-spatial tests are relevant to their generally better performance in tasks that involve aiming and throwing (Jardine & Martin, 1983).

Some quantitative abilities also show consistent differences. Females have a clear advantage on quantitative takes in the early years of school (Hyde, Fennema, & Lamon, 1990), but this reverses sometime before puberty; males then maintain their superior performance into old age. The math portion of the Scholastic Aptitude Test shows a substantial advantage for males ($d = 0.33$–0.50), with many more males scoring in the highest ranges (Benbow, 1988; Halpern, 1992). Males also score consistently higher on tests of proportional and mechanical reasoning (Meehan, 1984; Stanley, Benbow, Brody, Dauber, & Lupkowski, 1992).

Verbal abilities. Some verbal tasks show substantial mean differences favoring females. These include synonym generation and verbal fluency (e.g., naming words that start with a given letter), with effect sizes ranging from $d = 0.5$ to 1.2 (Gordon & Lee, 1986; Hines, 1990). On an average females score higher in the college achievement tests in literature, English composition, and Spanish (Stanley, 1993); they also excel at reading and spelling. Many more males than females are diagnosed with dyslexia and other reading disabilities (Sutaria, 1985), and there are many more male stutterers (Yairi & Ambrose, 1992). Some memory tasks also show better performance by females, but the size (and perhaps even the direction) of the effect varies with the type of memory being assessed.

Causal factors. There are both social and biological reasons for these differences. At the social level there are both subtle and overt differences between the experiences, expectations, and gender roles of females and males. Relevant environmental differences appear soon after birth. They range from the gender-differentiated toys that children regularly receive to the expectations of adult life with which they are presented, from gender-differentiated household and leisure activities to assumptions about differences in basic ability. Models that include many of these psychosocial variables have been successful in predicting academic achievement (Eccles, 1987).

Many biological variables are also relevant. One focus of current research is on differences in the sizes or shapes of particular neural structures. Numerous sexually dimorphic brain structures have now been identified, and they may well have implications for cognition. There are, for example, sex-related differences in the sizes of some portions of the corpus callosum; these differences are correlated with verbal fluency (Hines, Chiu, McAdams, Bentler, & Lipcamon, 1992). Recent brain imaging studies have found what may be differences in the lateralization of language (Shaywitz et al., 1995). Note that such differences in neural structure could result from differences in patterns of life experience as well as from genetically driven mechanisms of brain development; moreover, brain development and experience may have bidirectional effects on each other. This research area is still in a largely exploratory phase.

Hormonal influences. The importance of prenatal exposure to sex hormones is well established. Hormones influence not only the developing genitalia but also the brain and certain immune system structures (Geschwind & Galaburda, 1987; Halpern & Cass, 1994). Several studies have tested individuals who were exposed to abnormally high androgen levels in utero, due to a condition known as congenital adrenal hyperplasia (CAH). Adult CAH females score significantly higher than controls on tests of spatial ability (Resnick, Berenbaum, Gottesman & Bouchard, 1986); CAH girls play more with "boys' toys" and less with "girls' toys" than controls (Berenbaum & Hines, 1992).

Other experimental paradigms confirm the relevance of sex hormones for performance levels in certain skills. Christiansen and Knussman (1987) found testosterone levels in normal males to be correlated positively (about .20) with some measures of spatial ability and negatively (about −.20) with some measures of verbal ability. Older males given testosterone show improved performance on visual-spatial tests (Janowsky, Oviatt, & Orwoll, 1994). Many similar findings have been reported, though the effects are often nonlinear and complex (Gouchie & Kimura, 1991; Nyborg, 1984). It is clear that any adequate model of sex differences in cognition will have to take both biological and psychological variables (and their interactions) into account.

Mean Scores of Different Ethnic Groups

Asian Americans. In the years since the Second World War, Asian Americans—especially those of Chinese and Japanese extraction—have compiled an outstanding record of academic and professional achievement. This record is reflected in school grades, in scores on content-oriented achievement tests like the SAT and GRE, and especially in the disproportionate representation of Asian Americans in many sciences and professions. Although it is often supposed that these achievements reflect correspondingly high intelligence test scores, this is not the case. In more than a dozen studies from the 1960s and 1970s analyzed by Flynn (1991), the mean IQs of Japanese and Chinese American children were always around 97 or 98; none was over 100. Even Lynn (1993), who argues for a slightly higher figure, concedes that the achievements of these Asian Americans far outstrip what might have been expected on the basis of their test scores.

It may be worth noting that the interpretation of test scores obtained by Asians in Asia has been controversial in its own right. Lynn (1982) reported a mean Japanese IQ of 111 while Flynn (1991) estimated it to be between 101 and 105. Stevenson et al. (1985), comparing the intelligence-test performance of children in Japan, Taiwan, and the United States, found no substantive differences at all. Given the general problems of cross-cultural comparison, there is no reason to expect precision or stability in such estimates. Nevertheless, some interest attaches to these particular comparisons: they show that the well-established differences in school achievement among the same three groups (Chinese and Japanese children are much better at math than American children) do not simply reflect differences in psychometric intelligence. Stevenson, Lee, and Stigler (1986) suggest that they result from structural differences in the schools of the three nations as well as from varying cultural attitudes toward learning itself. It is also possible that spatial ability—in which Japanese and Chinese obtain somewhat higher score than Americans—plays a particular role in the learning of mathematics.

One interesting way to assess the achievements of Chinese and Japanese Americans is to reverse the usual direction of prediction. Data from the 1980 census show that the proportion of Chinese Americans employed in managerial, professional, or technical occupations was 55% and that of Japanese was 46%. (For Whites, the corresponding figure was 34%.) Using the well-established correlation between intelligence test scores and occupational level, Flynn (1991, p. 99) calculated the mean IQ that a hypothetical White group "would have to have" to predict the same proportions of upper-level employment. He found that the occupational success of these Chinese Americans—whose mean IQ was in fact slightly below 100—was what would be expected of a White group with an IQ of almost 120! A similar calculation for Japanese Americans shows that their level of achievement matched that of Whites averaging 110. These "overachievements" serve as sharp reminders of the limitations of IQ-based prediction. Various aspects of Chinese American and Japanese American culture surely contribute to them (Schneider, Hieshima, Lee, & Plank, 1994); gene-based temperamental factors could conceivably be playing a role as well (Freedman & Freedman, 1969).

Hispanic Americans. Hispanic immigrants have come to America from many countries. In 1993, the largest Latino groups in the continental United States were Mexican Americans (64%), Puerto Ricans (11%), Central and South Americans (13%), and Cubans (5%) (U.S. Bureau of the Census, 1994). There are very substantial cultural differences among these nationality groups, as well as differences in academic achievement (Duran, 1983; United States National Commission for Employment Policy, 1982). Taken together, Latinos make up the second largest and the fastest growing minority group in America (Davis, Haub, & Willette, 1983; Eyde, 1992).

In the United States, the mean intelligence test scores of Hispanics typically lie between those of Blacks and Whites. There are also differences in the patterning of scores across different abilities and subtests (Hennessy & Merrified, 1978; Lesser, Fifer, & Clark, 1965). Linguistic factors play a particularly important role for Hispanic Americans, who may know relatively little English. (By one estimate, 25% of Puerto Ricans and Mexican Americans and at least 40% of Cubans speak English "not well" or "not at all", Rodriguez, 1992). Even those who describe themselves as bilingual may be at a disadvantage if Spanish was their first and best-learned language. It is not surprising that Latino children typically score higher on the performance than on the verbal subtests of the English-based Wechsler Intelligence Scale for Children—Revised (WISC-R; Kaufman, 1994). Nevertheless, the predictive validity of Latino test scores is not negligible. In young children, the WISC-R has reasonably high correlations with school achievement measures (McShane & Cook, 1985). For high school students of moderate to high English proficiency, standard aptitude tests predict first-year college grades about as well as they do for non-Hispanic Whites (Pennock-Roman, 1992).

Native Americans. There are a great many culturally distinct North American Indian tribes (Driver, 1969), speaking some 200 different languages (Leap, 1981). Many Native Americans live on reservations, which themselves represent a great variety of ecological and cultural settings. Many others presently live in metropolitan areas (Brandt, 1984). Although few generalizations can be appropriate across so wide a range, two or three points seem fairly well established. The first is a specific relation between ecology and cognition: the Inuit (Eskimo) and other groups that live in the arctic tend to have particularly high visual-spatial skills. (For a review, see McShane & Berry, 1988.) Moreover, there seem to be no substantial sex differences in those skills (Berry, 1974). It seems likely that this represents an adaptation—genetic or learned or both—to the difficult hunting, traveling, and living conditions that characterize the arctic environment.

On the average, Indian children obtain relatively low scores on test of verbal intelligence, which are often administered in school settings. The results is a performance-test/verbal-test discrepancy similar to that exhibited by Hispanic Americans and other groups whose first language is generally not English.

Moreover, many Indian children suffer from chronic middle-ear infection (otitis media), which is "the leading identifiable disease among Indians since record-keeping began in 1962" (McShane & Plas, 1984a, p. 84). Hearing loss can have marked negative effects on verbal test performance (McShane & Plas, 1984b).

African Americans. The relatively low mean of the distribution of African American intelligence test scores has been discussed for many years. Although studies using different tests and samples yield a range of results, the Black mean is typically about one standard deviation (about 15 points) below that of Whites (Jensen, 1980; Loehlin et al., 1975; Reynolds et al., 1987). The difference is largest on those tests (verbal or nonverbal) that best represent the general intelligence factor *g* (Jensen, 1985). It is possible, however, that this differential is diminishing. In the most recent restandardization of the Stanford-Binet test, the Black/White differential was 13 points for younger children and 10 points for older children (Thorndike, Hagen, & Sattler, 1986). In several other studies of children since 1980, the Black mean has consistently been over 90 and the differential has been in single digits (Vincent, 1991). Larger and more definitive studies are needed before this trend can be regarded as established.

Another reason to think the IQ mean might be changing is that the Black/White differential in *achievement* scores has diminished substantially in the last few years. Consider, for example, the mathematics achievement of 17-year-olds as meaured by the National Assessment of Educational Progress (NAEP). The differential between Black and White scores, about 1.1 standard deviations as recently as 1978, had shrunk to .65 *SD* by 1990 (Grissmer et al., 1994) because of Black gains. Hispanics showed similar but smaller gains; there was little change in the scores of Whites. Other assessments of school achievement also show substantial recent gains in the performance of minority children.

In their own analysis of these gains, Grissmer et al. (1994) cite both demographic factors and the effects of public policy. They found the level of parents' education to be a particularly good predictor of children's school achievement; that level increased for all groups between 1970 and 1990, but most sharply for Blacks. Family size was another good predictor (children from smaller families tend to achieve higher scores); here too, the largest change over time was among Blacks. Above and beyond these demographic effects, Grissmer et al. believe that some of the gains can be attributed to the many specific programs, geared to the education of minority children, that were implemented during that period.

Test bias. It is often argued that the lower mean scores of African Americans reflect a bias in the intelligence tests themselves. This argument is right in one sense of "bias" but wrong in another. To see the first of these, consider how the term is used in probability theory. When a coin comes up heads consistently for any reason it is said to be "biased," regardless of any consequences that the outcome may or may not have. In this sense the Black/White score differential is ipso facto evidence of what may be called "outcome bias." African Americans are subject to outcome bias not only with respect to tests but along many dimensions of American life. They have the short end of nearly every stick: average income, representation in high-level occupations, health and health care, death rate, confrontations with the legal system, and so on. With this situation in mind, some critics regard the test score differential as just another example of a pervasive outcome bias that characterizes our society as a whole (Jackson, 1975; Mercer, 1984). Although there is a sense in which they are right, this critique ignores the particular social purpose that tests are designed to serve.

From an educational point of view, the chief function of mental tests is as *predictors* (see the second section). Intelligence tests predict school performance fairly well, at least in American schools as they are now constituted. Similarly, achievement tests are fairly good predictors of performance in college and postgraduate settings. Considered in this light, the relevant question is whether the tests have a "predictive bias" against Blacks. Such a bias would exist if African American performance on the criterion variables (school achievement, college GPA, etc.) were systematically higher than the same subjects' test scores would predict. This is not the case. The actual regression lines (which show the mean criterion performance for individuals who got various scores on the predictor) for Blacks do not lie above those for Whites; there is even a slight tendency in the other direction (Jensen, 1980; Reynolds & Brown, 1984). Considered as predictors of future performance, the tests do not seem to be biased against African Americans.

Characteristics of tests. It has been suggested that various aspects of the way tests are formulated and administered may put African Americans at a disadvantage. The language of testing is a standard form of English with which some Blacks may not be familiar; specific vocabulary items are often unfamiliar to Black children; the tests are often given by White examiners rather than by more familiar Black teachers; African Americans may not be motivated to work hard on tests that so clearly reflect White values; the time demands of some tests may be alien to Black culture. (Similar suggestions have been made in connection with the test performance of Hispanic Americans. e.g., Rodriguez, 1992.) Many of these suggestions are plausible, and such mechanisms may play a role in particular cases. Controlled studies have shown, however, that none of them contributes substantially to the Black/White differential under discussion here (Jensen, 1980; Reynolds & Brown, 1984; for a different view see Helms, 1992). Moreover, efforts to devise reliable and valid tests that would minimize disadvantages of this kind have been unsuccessful.

Interpreting Group Differences

If group differences in test performance do not result from the simple forms of bias reviwed above, what is responsible for them? The fact is that we do not know. Various explanations have been proposed, but none is generally accepted. It is clear, however, that these differences—whatever their origin—are well within the range of effect sizes that can be produced by environmental factors. The Black/White differential amounts to one standard deviation or less, and we know that environmental factors have recently raised mean test scores in many populations by at least that much (Flynn, 1987: see the fourth section). To be sure, the "Flynn effect" is itself poorly understood: it may reflect generational changes in culture, improved nutrition, or other factors as yet unknown. Whatever may be responsible for it, we cannot exclude the possibility that the same factors play a role in contemporary group differences.

Socioeconomic factors. Several specific environmental/cultural explanations of those differences have been proposed. All of them refer to the general life situation in which contemporary African Americans find themselves, but that situation can be described in several different ways. The simplest such hypothesis can be framed in economic terms. On an average, Blacks have lower incomes than Whites; a much higher proportion of them are poor. It is plausible to suppose that many inevitable aspects of poverty—poor nutrition, frequently inadequate prenatal care, lack of intellectual resources—have negative effects on children's developing intelligence. Indeed, the correlation between "socioeconomic status" (SES) and scores on intelligence tests is well-known (White, 1982).

Several considerations suggest that this cannot be the whole explanation. For one thing, the Black/White differential in test scores is not eliminated when groups or individuals are matched for SES (Loehlin et al., 1975). Moreover, the data reviewed in the fourth section suggest that—if we exclude extreme conditions—nutrition and other biological factors that may vary with SES account for relatively little of the variance in such scores. Finally, the (relatively weak) relationship between test scores and income is much more complex than a simple SES hypothesis would suggest. The living conditions of children result in part from the accomplishments of their parents: If the skills measured by psychometric tests actually matter for those accomplishments, intelligence is affecting SES rather than the other way around. We do not know the magnitude of these various effects in various populations, but it is clear that no model in which "SES" directly determines "IQ" will do.

A more fundamental difficulty with explanations based on economics alone appears from a different perspective. To imagine that any simple income- and education-based index can adequately describe the situation of African Americans is to ignore important categories of experience. The sense of belonging to a group with a distinctive culture—one that has long been the target of oppression—and the awareness or anticipation of racial discrimination are profound personal experiences, not just aspects of socioeconomic status. Some of these more deeply rooted differences are addressed by other hypotheses, based on caste and culture.

Caste-like minorities. Most discussions of this issue treat Black/White differences as aspects of a uniquely "American dilemma" (Myrdal, 1944). The fact is, however, that comparably disadvantaged groups exist in many countries: the Maori in New Zealand, scheduled castes ("untouchables") in India, non-European Jews in Israel, the Burakumin in Japan. All these are "caste-like" (Ogbu, 1978) or "involuntary" (Ogbu, 1994) minorities. John Ogbu distinguishes this status from that of "autonomous" minorities who are not politically or economically subordinated (like Amish or Mormons in the United States), and from that of "immigrant" or "voluntary" minorities who initially came to their new homes with positive expectations. Immigrant minorities expect their situations to improve; they tend to compare themselves favorably with peers in the old country, not unfavorably with members of the dominant majority. In contrast, to be born into a caste-like minority is to grow up firmly convinced that one's life will eventually be restricted to a small and poorly-rewarded set of social roles.

Distinctions of caste are not always linked to perceptions of race. In some countries lower- and upper-caste groups differ by appearance and are assumed to be racially distinct; in others they are not. The social and educational consequences are the same in both cases. All over the world, the children of caste-like minorities do less well in school than upper-caste children and drop out sooner. Where there are data, they have usually been found to have lower test scores as well.

In explaining these findings, Ogbu (1978) argues that the children of caste-like minorities do not have "effort optimism," i.e., the conviction that hard work (especially hard schoolwork) and serious commitment on their part will actually be rewarded. As a result they ignore or reject the forms of learning that are offered in school. Indeed, they may practice a sort of cultural inversion, deliberately rejecting certain behaviors (such as academic achievement or other forms of "acting White") that are seen as characterstic of the dominant group. While the extent to which the attitudes described by Ogbu (1978, 1994) are responsible for African American test scores and school achievement has not been empirically established, it does seem that familiar problems can take on quite a different look when they are viewed from an international perspective.

African American culture. According to Boykin (1986, 1994), there is a fundamental conflict between certain aspects of African American culture on the one hand and the implicit cultural commitments of most American schools on the other. "When children are ordered to do their own work, arrive at their own individual answers, work only with their own materials, they are being sent cultural messages. When children come to believe that getting up and moving about the classroom is inappropriate, they are being sent powerful cultural messages. When children come to confine their "learning" to consistently bracketed time periods, when they are consistently prompted to tell what they know and not, how they feel, when they are led to believe that they are completely responsible for their own success and failure, when they are required to consistently put forth considerable effort for effort's sake on tedious and personally irrelevant tasks … then they are pervasively having cultural lessons imposed on them" (1994, p. 125).

In Boykin's view, the combination of construction and competition that most American schools demand of their pupils conflicts with certain themes in the "deep structure" of African American culture. That culture includes an emphasis on such aspects of experience as spirituality, harmony, movement, verve, affect, expressive individualism, communalism, orality, and a socially defined time perspective (Boykin, 1986, 1994). While it is not shared by all African Americans to the same degree, its accessibility and familiarity give it a profound influence.

122 *Annual Progress in Child Psychiatry and Development*

The result of this cultural conflict, in Boykin's view, is that many Black children become alienated from both the process and the products of the education to which they are exposed. One aspect of that process, now an intrinsic aspect of the culture of most American schools, is the psychometric enterprise itself. He argues (Boykin, 1994) that the successful education of African American children will require an approach that is less concerned with talent sorting and assessment, more concerned with talent development.

One further factor should not be overlooked. Only a single generation has passed since the Civil Rights movement opened new doors for African Americans, and many forms of discrimination are still all too familiar in their experience today. Hard enough to bear in its own right, discrimination is also a sharp reminder of a still more intolerable past. It would be rash indeed to assume that those experiences, and that historical legacy, have no impact on intellectual development.

The genetic hypothesis. It is sometimes suggested that the Black/White differential in psychometric intelligence is partly due to genetic differences (Jensen, 1972). There is not much direct evidence on this point, and what little there is fails to support the genetic hypothesis. One piece of evidence comes from a study of the children of American soldiers stationed in Germany after the Second World War (Eyferth, 1961): there was no mean difference between the test scores of those children whose fathers were White and those whose fathers were Black. (For a discussion of possible confounds in this study, see Flynn, 1980.) Moreover, several studies have used blood-group methods to estimate the degree of African ancestry of American Blacks; there were no significant correlations between those estimates and IQ scores (Loehlin, Vandenberg, & Osborne, 1973; Scarr, Pakstis, Katz, & Barker, 1977).

It is clear from the third section that genes make a substantial contribution to individual differences in intelligence test scores, at least in the White population. The fact is, however, that the high heritability of a trait within a given group has no necessary implications for the source of a difference between groups (Loehlin et al., 1975). This is now generally understood (e.g., Herrnstein & Murray, 1994). But even though no such implication is *necessary*, some have argued that a high value of h^2 makes a genetic contribution to group differences more *plausible*. Does it?

That depends on one's assessment of the actual difference between the two environments. Consider Lewontin's (1970) well-known example of seeds from the same genetically variable stock that are planted in two different fields. If the plants in field X are fertilized appropriately while key nutrients are withheld from those in field Y, we have produced an entirely environmental group difference. This example works (i.e., h^2 is genuinely irrelevant to the differnetial between the fields) because the differences between the effective environments of X and Y are both large and consistent. Are the environmental and cultural situations of American Blacks and Whites also substantially and consistently different—different enough to make this a good analogy? If so, the within-group heritability of IQ scores is irrelevant to the issue. Or are those situations similar enough to suggest that the analogy is inappropriate, and that one can plausibly generalize from within-group heritabilities? Thus, the issue ultimately comes down to a personal judgment: How different are the relevant life experiences of Whites and Blacks in the United States today? At present, this question has no scientific answer.

SUMMARY AND CONCLUSIONS

Because there are many ways to be intelligent, there are also many conceptualizations of intelligence. The most influential approach, and the one that has generated the most systematic research, is based on psychometric testing. This tradition has produced a substantial body of knowledge, though many questions remain unanswered. We know much less about the forms of intelligence that tests do not easily assess: wisdom, creativity, practical knowledge, social skill, and the like.

Psychometricians have successfully measured a wide range of abilities, distinct from one another and yet intercorrelated. The complex relations among those abilities can be described in many ways.

Some theorists focus on the variance that all such abilities have in common, which Spearman termed *g* ("general intelligence"); others prefer to describe the same manifold with a set of partially independent factors; still others opt for a multifactorial description with factors hierarchically arranged and something like *g* at the top. Standardized intelligence test scores ("IQs"), which reflect a person's standing in relation to his or her age cohort, are based on tests that tap a number of different abilities. Recent studies have found that these scores are also correlated with information processing speed in certain experimental paradigms (choice reaction time, inspection time, evoked brain potentials, etc.), but the meaning of those correlations is far from clear.

Intelligence test scores predict individual differences in school achievement moderately well, correlating about .50 with grade point average and .55 with the number of years of education that individuals complete. In this context the skills measured by tests are clearly important. Nevertheless, population levels of school achievement are not determined solely or even primarily by intelligence or any other individual-difference variable. The fact that children in Japan and Taiwan learn much more mathematics than their peers in America, for example, can be attributed primarily to differences in culture and schooling rather than in abilities measured by intelligence tests.

Test scores also correlate with measures of accomplishment outside of school, e.g., with adult occupational status. To some extent those correlations result directly from the tests' link with school achievement and from their roles as "gatekeepers." In the United States today, high test scores and grades are prerequisites for entry into many careers and professions. This is not quite the whole story, however: a significant correlation between psychometric intelligence and occupational status remains even when measures of education and family background have been statistically controlled. There are also modest (negative) correlations between intelligence test scores and certain undesirable behaviors such as juvenile crime. Those correlations are necessarily low: all social outcomes result from complex causal webs in which psychometric skills are only one factor.

Like every trait, intelligence is the joint product of genetic and environmental variables. Gene action always involves a (biochemical or social) environment; environments always act via structures to which genes have contributed. Given a trait on which individuals vary, however, one can ask what fraction of that variation is associated with differences in their genotypes (this is the *heritability* of the trait) as well as what fraction is associated with differences in environmental experience. So defined, heritability (h^2) can and does vary from one population to another. In the case of IQ, h^2 is markedly lower for children (about .45) than for adults (about .75). This means that as children grow up, differences in test scores tend increasingly to reflect differences in genotype and in individual life experience rather than differences among the families in which they were raised.

The factors underlying that shift—and more generally the pathways by which genes make their undoubted contributions to individual differences in intelligence—are largely unknown. Moreover, the environmental contributions to those differences are almost equally mysterious. We know that both biological and social aspects of the environment are important for intelligence, but we are a long way from understanding how they exert their effects.

One environmental variable with clear-cut importance is the presence of formal schooling. Schools affect intelligence in many ways, not only by transmitting specific information but by developing certain intellectual skills and attitudes. Failure to attend school (or attendance at very poor schools) has a clear negative effect on intelligence test scores. Preschool programs and similar interventions often have positive effects, but in most cases the gains fade when the program is over.

A number of conditions in the biological environment have clear negative consequences for intellectual development. Some of these—very important when they occur—nevertheless do not contribute much to the population variance of IQ scores because they are relatively rare. (Perinatal complications are one such factor.) Exposure to environmental lead has well-documented negative effects; so too does prenatal exposure to high blood levels of alcohol. Malnutrition in childhood is another negative factor for intelligence, but the level at which its effects become significant has not been clearly established. Some studies suggest that dietary supplements of certain micronutrients can produce gains even in otherwise well-nourished individuals, but the effects are still controversial and there has been no long-term follow-up.

One of the most striking phenomena in this field is the steady worldwide rise in test scores, now often called the "Flynn effect." Mean IQs have increased more than 15 points—a full standard deviation—in the last 50 years, and the rate of gain may be increasing. These gains may result from improved nutrition, cultural changes, experience with testing, shifts in schooling or child-rearing practices, or some other factor as yet unknown.

Although there are no important sex differences in overall intelligence test scores, substantial differences do appear for specific abilities. Males typically score higher on visual-spatial and (beginning in middle childhood) mathematical skills; females excel on a number of verbal measures. Sex hormone levels are clearly related to some of these differences, but social factors presumably play a role as well. As for all the group differences reviewed here, the range of performance within each group is much larger than the mean difference between groups.

Because ethnic differences in intelligence reflect complex patterns, no overall generalization about them is appropriate. The mean IQ scores of Chinese and Japanese Americans, for example, differ little from those of Whites though their spatial ability scores tend to be somewhat higher. The outstanding record of these groups in terms of school achievement and occupational status evidently reflects cultural factors. The mean intelligence test scores of Hispanic Americans are somewhat lower than those of Whites, in part because Hispanics are often less familiar with English. Nevertheless, their test scores, like those of African Americans, are reasonably good predictors of school and college achievement.

African American IQ scores have long averaged about 15 points below those of Whites, with correspondingly lower scores on academic achievement tests. In recent years the achievement-test gap has narrowed appreciably. It is possible that the IQ-score differential is narrowing as well, but this has not been clearly established. The cause of that differential is not known: it is apparently not due to any simple form of bias in the content or administration of the tests themselves. The Flynn effect shows that environmental factors can produce differences of at least this magnitude, but that effect is mysterious in its own right. Several culturally-based explanations of the Black/White IQ differential have been proposed; some are plausible, but so far none has been conclusively supported. There is even less empirical support for a genetic interpretation. In short, no adequate explanation of the differential between the IQ means of Blacks and Whites is presently available.

It is customary to conclude surveys like this one with a summary of what has been established. Indeed, much is now known about intelligence. A near-century of research, most of it based on psychometric methods, has produced an impressive body of findings. Although we have tried to do justice to those findings in this report, it seems appropriate to conclude on a different note. In this contentious arena, our most useful role may be to remind our readers that many of the critical questions about intelligence are still unanswered. Here are a few of those questions:

1. Differences in genetic endowment contribute substantially to individual differences in (psychometric) intelligence, but the pathway by which genes produce their effects is still unknown. The impact of genetic differences appears to increase with age, but we do not know why.

2. Environmental factors also contribute substantially to the development of intelligence, but we do not clearly understand what those factors are or how they work. Attendance at school is certainly important, for example, but we do not know what aspects of schooling are critical.

3. The role of nutrition in intelligence remains obscure. Severe childhood malnutrition has clear negative effects, but the hypothesis that particular "micronutrients" may affect intelligence in otherwise adequately-fed populations has not yet been convincingly demonstrated.

4. There are significant correlations between measures of information-processing speed and psychometric intelligence, but the overall pattern of these findings yields no easy theoretical interpretation.

5. Mean scores on intelligence tests are rising steadily. They have gone up a full standard deviation in the last 50 years or so, and the rate of gain may be increasing. No one is sure why these gains are happening or what they mean.

6. The differential between the mean intelligence test scores of Blacks and Whites (about one standard deviation, although it may be diminishing) does not result from any obvious biases in test construction and administration, nor does it simply reflect differences in socioeconomic status. Explanations based on factors of caste and culture may be appropriate, but so far have little direct empirical support. There is certainly no such support for a genetic interpretation. At present, no one knows what causes this differential.

7. It is widely agreed that standardized tests do not sample all forms of intelligence. Obvious examples include creativity, wisdom, practical sense, and social sensitivity; there are surely others. Despite the importance of these abilities we know very little about them: how they develop, what factors influence that development, how they are related to more traditional measures.

In a field where so many issues are unresolved and so many questions unanswered, the confident tone that has characterized most of the debate on these topics is clearly out of place. The study of intelligence does not need politicized assertions and recriminations; it needs self-restraint, reflection, and a great deal more research. The questions that remain are socially as well as scientifically important. There is no reason to think them unanswerable, but finding the answers will require a shared and sustained effort as well as the commitment of substantial scientific resources. Just such a commitment is what we strongly recommend.

REFERENCES

Baghurst, P. A., McMichael, A. J., Wigg, N. R., Vimpani, G. V., Robertson, E. F., Roberts, R. J., & Tong, S.-L. (1992). Environmental exposure to lead and children's intelligence at the age of seven years: The Port Pirie cohort study. *New England Journal of Medicine, 327*, 1279–1284.

Bates, T. C., & Eysenck, H. J. (1993). Intelligence, inspection time, and decision time. *Intelligence, 17*, 523–531.

Baumrind, D. (1993). The average expectable environment is not good enough: A response to Scarr. *Child Development, 64*, 1299–1317.

Benbow, C. P. (1988). Sex differences in mathematical reasoning ability in intellectually talented preadolescents: Their nature, effects, and possible causes. *Behavioral and Brain Sciences, 11*, 169–232.

Berenbaum, S. A., & Hines, M. (1992). Early androgens are related to childhood sex-typed toy preferences. *Psychological Science, 3*, 203–206.

Berry, J. W. (1974). Ecological and cultural factors in spatial perceptual development. In J. W. Berry & P. R. Dasen (Eds.), *Culture and cognition: Readings in cross-cultural psychology* (pp. 129–140). London: Methuen.

Bornstein, M. H. (1989). Stability in early mental development: From attention and information processing in infancy to language and cognition in childhood. In M. H. Bornstein & N. A. Krasnegor (Eds.), *Stability and continuity in mental development* (pp. 147–170). Hillsdale, NJ: Erlbaum.

Bouchard, T. J., Jr., Lykken, D. T., McGue, M., Segal, N. L., & Tellegen, A. (1990). Sources of human psychological differences: The Minnesota study of twins reared apart. *Science, 250*, 223–228.

Boykin, A. W. (1986). The triple quandary and the schooling of Afro-American children. In U. Neisser (Ed.), *The school achievement of minority children* (pp. 57–92). Hillsdale, NJ: Erlbaum.

Boykin, A. W. (1994). Harvesting talent and culture: African-American children and educational reform. In R. Rossi (Ed.), *Schools and students at risk* (pp. 116–138). New York: Teachers College Press.

Brandt, E. A. (1984). The cognitive functioning of American Indian children: A critique of McShane and Plas. *School Psychology Review, 13*, 74–82.

Brody, N. (1992). *Intelligence* (2nd ed.). San Diego, CA: Academic Press.

Broman, S. H., Nichols, P. L., & Kennedy, W. A. (1975). *Preschool IQ: Prenatal and early developmental correlates*. Hillsdale, NJ: Erlbaum.

Brown, A. L., & French, A. L. (1979). The zone of potential development: Implications for intelligence testing in the year 2000. In R. J. Sternberg & D. K. Detterman (Eds.), *Human intelligence: Perspective on its theory and measurement* (pp. 217–235). Norwood, NJ: Ablex.

Compbell, F. A., & Ramey, C. T. (1994). Effects of early intervention on intellectual and academic achievement: A follow-up study of children from low-income families. *Child Development, 65*, 684–698.

Carraher, T. N., Carraher, D., & Schliemann, A. D. (1985). Mathematics in the streets and in schools. *British Journal of Developmental Psychology, 3*, 21–29.

Carroll, J. B. (1993). *Human cognitive abilities: A survey of factor-analytic studies*. Cambridge, England: University of Cambridge Press.

Caryl, P. G. (1994). Early event-related potentials correlate with inspection time and intelligence. *Intelligence, 18*, 15–46.

Ceci, S. J. (1990). *On intelligence . . . more or less: A bioecological treatise on intellectual development*. Englewood Cliffs. NJ: Prentice Hall.

Ceci, S. J. (1991). How much does schooling influence general intelligence and its cognitive components? A reassessment of the evidence. *Developmental Psychology, 27*, 703–722.

Ceci, S. J., & Liker, J. (1986). A day at the races: A study of IQ, expertise, and cognitive complexity. *Journal of Experimental Psychology: General, 115*, 255–266.

Chaiken, S. R. (1993). Two models for an inspection time paradigm: Processing distraction and processing speed versus processing speed and asymptotic strength. *Intelligence, 17*, 257–283.

Chipuer, H. M., Rovine, M., & Plomin, R. (1990). LISREL modelling: Genetic and environmental influences on IQ revisited. *Intelligence, 14*, 11–29.

Christal, R. E., Tirre, W., & Kyllonen, P. (1984). Two for the money: Speed and level scores from a computerized vocabulary test. In G. Lee & T. Ulrich (Eds.), *Proceedings, Psychology in the Department of Defense, Ninth Annual Symposium* (USAFA TR 8-2). Colorado Springs, CO: U.S. Air Force Academy.

Christiansen, K., & Knussmann, R. (1987). Sex hormones and cognitive functioning in men. *Neuropsychobiology, 18*, 27–36.

Columbo, J. (1993). *Infant cognition: Predicting later intellectual functioning*. Newbury Park, CA: Sage.

Consortium for Longitudinal Studies. (1983). *As the twig is bent . . . lasting effects of preschool programs*. Hillsdale, NJ: Erlbaum.

Cronbach, L. J., & Show, R. E. (1977). *Aptitudes and instructional methods*. New York: Irvington.

Darlington, R. B. (1986). Long-term effects of preschool programs. In U. Neisser (Ed.), *The school achievement of minority children* (pp. 159–167). Hillsdale, NJ: Erlbaum.

Davis, C., Haub, C., & Willette, J. (1983). U.S. Hispanics: Changing the face of America. *Population Bulletin, 38* (No. 3).

Deary, I. J. (1993). Inspection time and WAIS-R IQ subtypes: A confirmatory factor analysis study. *Intelligence, 17*, 223–236.

Deary, I. J. (1995). Auditory inspection time and intelligence: What is the causal direction? *Developmental Psychology, 31*, 237–250.

Driver, H. E. (1969). *Indians of North America*. Chicago: University of Chicago Press.

Dube, E. F. (1982). Literacy, cultural familiarity, and "intelligence" as determinants of story recall. In U. Neisser (Ed.), *Memory observed: Remembering in natural contexts* (pp. 274–292). New York: Freeman.

Duran. R. P. (1983). *Hispanics' education and background: Prediction of college achievement.* New York: College Entrance Examination Board.

Eccles, J. S. (1987). Gender roles and women's achievement-related decisions. *Psychology of Women Quarterly, 11*, 135–172.

Eyde, L. D. (1992). Introduction to the testing of Hispanics in industry and research. In K. F. Geisinger (Ed.), *Psychological testing of Hispanics* (pp. 167–172). Washington, DC: American Psychological Association.

Eyferth, K. (1961). Leistungen verchiedener Gruppen von Besatzungskindermm Hamburg-Wechsler Intelligentztest fur Kinder (HAWIK) [The performance of different groups of occupation children in the Hamburg-Wechsler Intelligence Test for Children]. *Archive fur die gesamte Psychologie, 113*, 222–241.

Eysenck, H. (1973). *The measurement of intelligence.* Baltimore: Williams & Wilkins.

Eysenck, H. J. (1986). Inspection time and intelligence: A historical introduction. *Personality and Individual Differences, 7*, 603–607.

Feuerstein, R. (1980). *Instrumental enrichment: An intervention program for cognitive modifiability.* Baltimore: University Park Press.

Flynn, J. R. (1980). *Race, IQ, and Jensen.* London: Routledge & Kegan Paul.

Flynn, J. R. (1984). The mean IQ of Americans: Massive gains 1932 to 1978. *Psychological Bulletin, 95*, 29–51.

Flynn, J. R. (1987). Massive IQ gains in 14 nations: What IQ tests really measure. *Psychological Bulletin, 101*, 171–191.

Flynn, J. R. (1991). *Asian-Americans: Achievement beyond IQ.* Hillsdale, NJ: Erlbaum.

Frearson, W. M., & Eysenck, H. J. (1986). Intelligence, reaction time [RT], and a new "odd-man-out" RT paradigm. *Personality and Individual Differences, 7*, 807–817.

Freedman, D. G., & Freedman, N. C. (1969). Behavioral differences between Chinese-American and European-American newborns. *Nature, 224*, 1227.

Gardner, H. (1983). *Frames of mind: The theory of multiple intelligences.* New York: Basic Books.

Gay, J., & Cole, M. (1967). *The new mathematics and an old culture: A study of learning among the Kpelle of Liberia.* New York: Holt, Rhinehart & Winston.

Geschwind, N., & Galaburda, A. M. (1987). *Cerebral lateralization: Biological mechanisms, associations, and pathology.* Cambridge, MA: MIT Press.

Gordon, H. W., & Lee P. (1986). A relationship between gonadotropins and visuospatial function. *Neuropsychologia, 24*, 563–576.

Gottfried, A. W. (Ed.). (1984). *Home environment and early cognitive development: Longitudinal research.* New York: Academic Press.

Gouchie, C., & Kimura, D. (1991). The relationship between testosterone levels and cognitive ability patterns. *Psychoneuroendocrinology, 16*, 323–334.

Gould, S. J. (1978). Morton's ranking of races by cranial capacity: Unconscious manipulation of data may be a scientific norm. *Science, 200*, 503–509.

Green, R. L., Hoffman, L. T., Morse, R., Hayes, M. E., & Morgan, R. F. (1964). *The educational status of children in a district without public schools* (Cooperative Research Project No. 2321). Washington, DC: Office of Education, U.S. Department of Health, Education, and Welfare.

Grissmer, D. W., Kirby, S. N., Berends, M., & Williamson, S. (1994). *Student achievement and the changing American family.* Santa Monica, CA: RAND Corporation.

Gustafsson, J.-E. (1984). A unifying model for the structure of intellectual abilities. *Intelligence, 8*, 179–203.

Haier, R. J. (1993). Cerebral glucose metabolism and intelligence. In P. A. Vernon (Ed.), *Biological approaches to the study of human intelligence* (pp. 317–332). Norwood, NJ: Ablex.

Halpern, D. (1992). *Sex differences in cognitive abilities* (2nd ed.). Hillsdale, NJ: Erlbaum.

Halpern, D. F., & Cass, M. (1994). Laterality, sexual orientation, and immune system functioning: Is there a relationship? *International Journal of Neuroscience, 77*, 167–180.

Hart, B., & Risley, T. R. (1992). American parenting of language-learning children: Persisting differences in family-child interaction observed in natural home environments. *Developmental Psychology, 28*, 1096–1105.

Hart, B., & Risley, T. R. (in press). *Meaningful differences in the everyday experience of young American children.* Baltimore: P. H. Brookes.

Hay, D. A. (1985). *Essentials of behavior genetics.* Melbourne, Australia: Blackwell.

Heath, S. B. (1983). *Ways with words.* New York: Cambridge University Press.

Held, J. D., Alderton, D. E., Foley, P. P., & Segall, D. O. (1993). Arithmetic reasoning gender differences: Explanations found in the Armed Services Vocational Aptitude Battery (ASVAB). *Learning and Individual Differences, 5*, 171–186.

Helms, J. E. (1992). Why is there no study of cultural equivalence in standardized cognitive ability testing? *American Psychologist, 47*, 1083–1101.

Hennessy, J. J., & Merrifield, P. R. (1978). Ethnicity and sex distinctions in patterns of aptitude factor scores in a sample of urban high school seniors. *American Educational Research Journal 15*, 385–389.

Herrnstein, R. J., & Murray, C. (1994). *The bell curve: Intelligence and class structure in American life.* New York: Free Press.

Herrnstein, R. J., Nickerson R. S., de Sanchez, M., & Swets, J. A. (1986). Teaching thinking skills. *American Psychologist, 41*, 1279–1289.

Hines, M. (1990). Gonadal hormones and human cognitive development. In J. Balthazart (Ed.), *Hormones, brains and behaviors in vertebrates: 1. Sexual differentiation, neuroanatomical aspects, neurotransmitters, and neuropeptides* (pp. 51–63). Basel, Switzerland: Karger.

Hines, M., Chiu, L., McAdams, L. A., Bentler, M. P., & Lipcamon, J. (1992). Cognition and the corpus callosum: Verbal fluency, visuospatial ability, language lateralization related to midsagittal surface areas of the corpus callosum. *Behavioral Neuroscience, 106*, 3–14.

Hunt, E. (1978). Mechanics of verbal ability. *Psychological Review, 85*, 109–130.

Hunter, J. E. (1983). A causal analysis of cognitive ability, job knowledge, job performance, and supervisor ratings. In F. Landy, S. Zedeck, & J. Cleveland (Eds.), *Performance measurement and theory* (pp. 257–266). Hillsdale, NJ: Erlbaum.

Hyde, J., Fennema, E., & Lamon, S. J. (1990). Gender differences in mathematics performance: A meta-analysis. *Psychological Bulletin, 107*, 139–155.

Jackson, G. D. (1975). On the report of the Ad Hoc Committee on Educational Uses of Tests with Disadvantaged Students: Another psychological view from the Association of Black Psychologists. *American Psychologist, 30*, 88–93.

Jackson, J. F. (1993). Human behavioral genetics, Scarr's theory, and her views on interventions: A critical review and commentary on their implications for African American children. *Child Development, 64*, 1318–1332.

Jackson, M., & McClelland, J. (1979). Processing determinants of reading speed. *Journal of Experimental Psychology: General, 108*, 151–181.

Janowsky, J. S., Oviatt, S. K., & Orwoll, E. S. (1994). Testosterone influences spatial cognition in older men. *Behavioral Neuroscience, 108*, 325–332.

Jardine, R., & Martin, N. G. (1983). Spatial ability and throwing accuracy. *Behavior Genetics, 13*, 331–340.

Jencks, C. (1979). *Who gets ahead? The determinants of economic success in America.* New York: Basic Books.

Jensen, A. R. (1972). *Genetics and education.* New York: Harper & Row.

Jensen, A. R. (1977). Cumulative deficit in IQ of Blacks in the rural South. *Developmental Psychology, 13*, 184–191.

Jensen, A. R. (1980). *Bias in mental testing.* New York: Free Press.

Jensen, A. R. (1985). The nature of the black–white difference on various psychometric tests: Spearman's hypothesis. *Behavioral and Brain Sciences, 8*, 193–263.

Jensen, A. R. (1987). Individual differences in the Hick paradigm. In P. A. Vernon (Ed.), *Speed of information processing and intelligence* (pp. 101–175). Norwood, NJ: Ablex.

Jensen, A. R. (1993). Test validity: *g* vs. "tacit knowledge." *Current Directions in Psychological Science, 2*, 9–10.

Jones, H. E., & Bayley, N. (1941). The Berkeley Growth Study. *Child Development, 12*, 167–173.

Kaufman, A. S. (1994). *Intelligent testing with the WISC-III*. New York: Wiley.

Kaufman, A. S., & Doppelt, J. E. (1976). Analysis of WISC-R standardization data in terms of the stratification variables. *Child Development, 47*, 165–171.

Kohn, M. L., & Schooler, C. (1973). Occupational experience and psychological functioning: An assessment of reciprocal effects. *American Sociological Review, 38*, 97–118.

Kohn, M. L., & Schooler, C. (1983). *Work and personality: An inquiry into the impact of social stratification*. Norwood, NJ: Ablex.

Kranzler, J., & Jensen, A. R. (1989). Inspection time and intelligence: A meta-analysis. *Intelligence, 13*, 329–347.

Lave, J. (1988). *Cognition in practice*. New York: Cambridge University Press.

Law, D. J., Pellegrino, J. W., & Hunt, E. B. (1993). Comparing the tortoise and the hare: Gender differences and experience in dynamic spatial reasoning tasks. *Psychological Science, 4*, 35–40.

Leap, W. L. (1981). American Indian languages. In C. Ferguson & S. B. Heath (Eds.), *Language in the USA*. Cambridge, England: Cambridge University Press.

Lee, E. S. (1951). Negro intelligence and selective migration: A Philadelphia test of the Klineberg hypothesis. *American Sociological Review, 16*, 227–232.

Lesser, G. S., Fifer, G., & Clark, D. H. (1965). Mental abilities of children from different social-class and cultural groups. *Monographs of the Society for Research in Child Development, 30* (Whole No. 102).

Lewontin, R. (1970). Race and intelligence. *Bulletin of the Atomic Scientists, 26*, 2–8.

Linn, M. C., & Petersen, A. C. (1985). Emergence and characterization of sex differences in spatial ability: A meta-analysis. *Child Development, 56*, 1479–1498.

Locurto, C. (1991). Beyond IQ in preschool programs? *Intelligence, 15*, 295–312.

Loehlin, J. C. (1989). Partitioning environmental and genetic contributions to behavioral development. *American Psychologist, 10*, 1285–1292.

Loehlin, J. C., Horn, J. M., & Willerman, L. (1989). Modeling IQ change: Evidence from the Texas Adoption Project. *Child Development, 60*, 993–1004.

Loehlin, J. C., Lindzey, G., & Spuhler, J. N. (1975). *Race differences in intelligence*. New York: Freeman.

Loehlin, J. C., Vandenberg, S. G., & Osborne, R. T. (1973). Blood group genes and Negro–White ability differences. *Behavior Genetics, 3*, 263–270.

Longstreth, L. E. (1984). Jensen's reaction-time investigations of intelligence: A critique. *Intelligence, 8*, 139–160.

Lubchenko, L. O. (1976). *The high-risk infant*. Philadelphia: Saunders.

Lynn, R. (1982). IQ in Japan and the United States shows a growing disparity. *Nature, 297*, 222–223.

Lynn, R. (1990). The role of nutrition in secular increases in intelligence. *Personality and Individual Differences, 11*, 273–285.

Lynn, R. (1993). Oriental Americans: Their IQ, educational attainment, and socioeconomic status. *Personality and Individual Differences, 15*, 237–242.

Lynn, R. (1994). Sex differences in intelligence and brain size: A paradox resolved. *Personality and Individual Differences, 17*, 257–271.

Mackenzie, B., Molloy, E., Martin, F., Lovegrove, W., & McNicol, D. (1991). Inspection time and the content of simple tasks: A framework for research on speed of information processing. *Australian Journal of Psychology, 43*, 37–43.

Masters, M. S., & Sanders, B. (1993). Is the gender difference in mental rotation disappearing? *Behavior Genetics, 23*, 337–341.

McCall, R. B., & Garriger, M. S. (1993). A meta-analysis of infant habituation and recognition memory performance as predictors of later IQ. *Child Development, 64*, 57–79.

McCartney, K., Harris, M. J., & Bernieri, F. (1990). Growing up and growing apart: A developmental meta-analysis of twin studies. *Psychological Bulletin, 107,* 226–237.

McGue, M., Bouchard, T. J., Jr., Iacono, W. G., & Lykken, D. T. (1993). Behavioral genetics of cognitive ability: A life-span perspective. In R. Plomin & G. E. McClearn (Eds.), *Nature, nurture, & psychology* (pp. 59–76). Washington, DC: American Psychological Association.

McMichael, A. J., Baghurst, P. A., Wigg, N. R., Vimpani, G. V., Robertson, E. F., & Roberts, R. J. (1988). Port Pirie cohort study: Environmental exposure to lead and children's abilities at the age of four years. *New England Journal of Medicine, 319,* 468–475.

McShane, D. A., & Berry, J. W. (1988). Native North Americans: Indian and Inuit abilities. In S. H. Irvine & J. W. Berry (Eds.), *Human abilities of cultural context* (pp. 385–426). New York: Cambridge University Press.

McShane, D. A., & Cook, V. J. (1985). Transcultural intellectual assessment: Performance by Hispanics on the Wechsler Scales. In B. B. Wolman (Ed.), *Handbook of intelligence: Theories, measurements, and applications.* New York: Wiley.

McShane, D. A., & Plas, J. M. (1984a). Response to a critique of the McShane & Plas review of American Indian performance on the Wechsler Intelligence Scales. *School Psychology Review, 13,* 83–88.

McShane, D. A., & Plas, J. M. (1984b). The cognitive functioning of American Indian children: Moving from the WISC to the WISC-R. *School Psychology Review, 13,* 61–73.

Meehan, A. M. (1984). A meta-analysis of sex differences in formal operational thought. *Child Development, 55,* 1110–1124.

Mercer, J. R. (1984). What is a racially and culturally nondiscriminatory test? A sociological and pluralistic perspective. In C. R. Reynolds & R. T. Brown (Eds.), *Perspectives on bias in mental testing.* New York: Plenum Press.

Moffitt, T. E., Caspi, A., Harkness, A. R., & Silva, P. A. (1993). The natural history of change in intellectual performance: Who changes? How much? Is it meaningful? *Journal of Child Psychology and Psychiatry, 34,* 455–506.

Moffitt, T. E., Gabrielli, W. F., Mednick, S. A., & Schulsinger, F. (1981). Socioeconomic status, IQ, and delinquency. *Journal of Abnormal Psychology, 90,* 152–156.

Myrdal, G. (1944). *An American dilemma: The Negro problem and modern democracy.* New York: Harper.

Needleman, H. L., Geiger, S. K., & Frank, R. (1985). Lead and IQ scores: A reanalysis. *Science, 227,* 701–704.

Neisser, U. (1976). General, academic, and artificial intelligence. In L. B. Resnick (Ed.), *The nature of intelligence* (pp. 135–144). Hillsdale, NJ: Erlbaum.

Nettelbeck, T. (1987). Inspection time and intelligence. In P. A. Vernon (Ed.), *Speed of information-processing and intelligence* (pp. 295–346). Norwood, NJ: Ablex.

Nyborg, H. (1984). Performance and intelligence in hormonally different groups. In G. J. DeVries, J. DeBruin, H. Uylings, & M. Cormer (Eds.), *Progress in brain research* (Vol. 61, pp. 491–508). Amsterdam: Elsevier Science.

Ogbu, J. U. (1978). *Minority education and caste: The American system in cross-cultural perspective.* New York: Academic Press.

Ogbu, J. U. (1994). From cultural differences to differences in cultural frames of reference. In P. M. Greenfield & R. R. Cocking (Eds.), *Cross-cultural roots of minority child development* (pp. 365–391). Hillsdale, NJ: Erlbaum.

Okagaki, L., & Sternberg, R. J. (1993). Parental beliefs and children's school performance. *Child Development, 64,* 36–56.

Olivier, G. (1980). The increase of stature in France. *Journal of Human Evolution, 9,* 645–649.

Pascual-Leone, J., & Ijaz, H. (1989). Mental capacity testing as form of intellectual-developmental assessment. In R. J. Samuda, S. L. Kong et al. (Eds.), *Assessment and placement of minority students.* Toronto, Ontario, Canada: Hogrefe & Huber.

Pedersen, N. L., Plomin, R., Nesselroade, J. R., & McClearn, G. E. (1992). A quantitative genetic analysis of cognitive abilities during the second half of the life span. *Psychological Science, 3*, 346–353.

Pennock-Roman, M. (1992). Interpreting test performance in selective admissions for Hispanic students. In K. F. Geisinger (Ed.), *Psychological testing of Hispanics* (pp. 95–135). Washington, DC: American Psychological Association.

Piaget, J. (1972). *The psychology of intelligence*. Totowa, NJ: Littlefield Adams.

Plomin, R., & Bergeman, C. S. (1991). The nature of nurture: Genetic influence on "environmental" measures. *Behavioral and Brain Sciences, 14*, 373–427.

Plomin, R., DeFries, J. C., & Loehlin, J. C. (1977). Genotype-environment interaction and correlation in the analysis of human behavior. *Psychological Bulletin, 84*, 309–322.

Plomin, R., DeFries, J. C., & McClearn (1990). *Behavioral gentics: A primer* (2nd ed.). New York: Freeman.

Pollitt, E., Gorman, K. S., Engle, P. L., Martorell, R., & Rivera, J. (1993). Early supplementary feeding and cognition. *Monographs of the Society for Research in Child Development, 58* (Serial No. 235).

Posner, M. I., Boies, S. J., Eichelman, W. H., & Taylor, R. L. (1969). Retention of visual and name codes of single letters. *Journal of Experimental Psychology, 79*, 1–16.

Reed, T. E., & Jensen, A. R. (1992). Conduction velocity in a brain nerve pathway of normal adults correlates with intelligence level. *Intelligence, 16*, 259–272.

Reed, T. E., & Jensen, A. R. (1993). Choice reaction time and visual pathway conduction velocity both correlate with intelligence but appear not to correlate with each other: Implications for information processing. *Intelligence, 17*, 191–203.

Rehberg, R. A., & Rosenthal, E. R. (1978). *Class and merit in the American high school*. New York: Longman.

Resnick, S. M., Berenbaum, S. A., Gottesman, I. I., & Bouchard, T. J., Jr. (1986). Early hormonal influences on cognitive functioning in congenital adrenal hyperplasia. *Developmental Psychology, 22*, 191–198.

Reynolds, C. R., & Brown, R. T. (1984). Bias in mental testing: An introduction to the issues. In C. R. Reynolds & R. T. Brown (Eds.), *Perspectives on bias in mental testing* (pp. 1–39). New York: Plenum Press.

Reynolds, C. R., Chastain, R. L., Kaufman, A. S., & McLean, J. E. (1987). Demographic characteristics and IQ among adults: Analysis of the WAIS-R standardization sample as a function of the stratification variables. *Journal of School Psychology, 25*, 323–342.

Ricciuti, H. N. (1993). Nutrition and mental development. *Current Directions in Psychological Science, 2*, 43–46.

Roberts, R. C. (1967). Some concepts and methods in quantitative genetics. In J. Hirsch (Ed.), *Behavior-genetic analysis* (pp. 214–257). New York: McGraw-Hill.

Rodriguez, O. (1992). Introduction to technical and societal issues in the psychological testing of Hispanics. In K. F. Geisinger (Ed.), *Psychological testing of Hispanics* (pp. 11–15). Washington, DC: American Psychological Association.

Rose, S. A., & Feldman, J. (1995). The prediction of IQ and specific cognitive abilities at 11 years from infancy measures. *Developmental Psychology, 31*, 685–696.

Rose, R. J., Harris, E. L., Christian, J. C., & Nance, W. E. (1979). Genetic variance in nonverbal intelligence: Data from the kinships of identical twins. *Science, 205*, 1153–1155.

Rosetti, L. (1986). *High risk infants: Identification, assessment, and intervention*. Boston: Little Brown.

Rush, D., Stein, Z., Susser, M., & Brody, N. (1980). Outcome at one year of age: Effects on somatic and psychological measures. In D. Rush, Z. Stein, & M. Susser (Eds.), *Diet in pregnancy: A randomized controlled trial of nutritional supplements*. New York: Liss.

Saudino, K. J., Plomin, R., Pedersen, N. L., & McClearn, G. E. (1994). The etiology of high and low cognitive ability during the second half of the life span. *Intelligence, 19*, 359–371.

Scarr, S. (1992). Developmental theories for the 1990s: Development and individual differences. *Child Development, 63*, 1–19.

Scarr, S. (1993). Biological and cultural diversity: The legacy of Darwin for development. *Child Development, 64*, 1333–1353.

Scarr, S., Pakstis, A. J., Katz, S. H., & Barker, W. B. (1977). Absence of a relationship between degree of White ancestry and intellectual skills within a Black population. *Human Genetics, 39*, 69–86.

Scarr, S., & Weinberg, R. A. (1978). The influence of "family background" on intellectual attainment. *American Sociological Review, 43*, 674–692.

Scarr, S., Weinberg, R. A., & Waldman, I. D. (1993). IQ correlations in transracial adoptive families. *Intelligence, 17*, 541–555.

Schmidt, F. L., & Hunter, J. E. (1993). Tacit knowledge, practical intelligence, and job knowledge. *Current Directions in Psychological Science, 2*, 8–9.

Schneider, B., Hieshima, J. A., Lee, S., & Plank, S. (1994). East-Asian academic success in the United States: Family, school, and cultural explanations. In P. M. Greenfield & R. R. Cocking (Eds.), *Cross-cultural roots of minority child development* (pp. 332–350). Hillsdale, NJ: Erlbaum.

Schoenthaler, S. J., Amos, S. P., Eysenck, H. J., Peritz, E., & Yudkin, J. (1991). Controlled trial of vitamin–mineral supplementation: Effects on intelligence and performance. *Personality and Individual Differences, 12*, 351–362.

Seashore, H., Wesman, A., & Doppelt, J. (1950). The standardization of the Wechsler Intelligence Scale for Children. *Journal of Consulting Psychology, 14*, 99–110.

Serpell, R. (1974). *Estimates of intelligence in a rural community of Eastern Zambia: Human Development Research Unit Reports, 25*. Mimeo, Lusaka: University of Zambia.

Serpell, R. (1979). How specific are perceptual skills? A cross-cultural study of pattern reproduction. *British Journal of Psychology, 70*, 365–380.

Shaywitz, B. A., Shaywitz, S. E., Pugh, K. R., Constable, R. T., Skudlarski, P., Fulbright, R. K., Bronen, R. A., Fletcher, J. M., Shankweiler, D. P., Katz, L., & Gore, J. C. (1995). Sex differences in the functional organization of the brain for language. *Nature, 373*, 607–609.

Sigman, M. (1995). Nutrition and child development: More food for thought. *Current Directions in Psychological Science, 4*, 52–55.

Spearman, C. (1927). *The abilities of man*. New York: Macmillan.

Stanley, J. (1993). Boys and girls who reason well mathematically. In G. R. Bock & K. Ackrill (Eds.), *The origins and development of high ability*. Chichester, England: Wiley.

Stanley, J. C., Benbow, C. P., Brody, L. E., Dauber, S., & Lupkowski, A. (1992). Gender differences on eighty-six nationally standardized aptitude and achievement tests. In N. Colangelo, S. G. Assouline, & D. L. Ambroson (Eds.), *Talent development, Vol. 1: Proceedings from the 1991 Henry B. and Jocelyn Wallace National Research Symposium on Talent Development*. Unionville, NY: Trillium Press.

Stein, Z., Susser, M., Saenger, G., & Marolla, F. (1975). *Famine and human development: The Dutch hunger winter of 1944–1945*. New York: Oxford University Press.

Sternberg, R. J. (1977). *Intelligence, information processing, and analogical reasoning: The componential analysis of human abilities*. Hillsdale, NJ: Erlbaum.

Sternberg, R. J. (1985). *Beyond IQ: A triarchic theory of human intelligence*. New York: Cambridge University Press.

Sternberg, R. J. (Ed.). (1994). *Encyclopedia of human intelligence*. New York: MacMillan.

Sternberg, R. J., & Detterman, D. K. (Eds.). (1986). *What is intelligence? Contemporary viewpoints on its nature and definition*. Norwood, NJ: Ablex.

Sternberg, R. J., & Wagner, R. K. (1993). The geocentric view of intelligence and job performance is wrong. *Current Directions in Psychological Science, 2*, 1–4.

Sternberg, R. J., Wagner, R. K., Williams, W. M., & Horvath, J. A. (1995). Testing common sense. *American Psychologist, 50*, 912–927.

Stevenson, H. W., Lee, S. Y., & Stigler, J. W. (1986). Mathematics achievement of Chinese, Japanese, and American children. *Science, 231*, 693–699.

Stevenson, H. W., & Stigler, J. W. (1992). *The learning gap*. New York: Summit Books.

Stevenson, H. W., Stigler, J. W., Lee, S. Y., Lucker, G. W., Kitamura, S., & Hsu, C. C. (1985). Cognitive performance and academic achievement of Japanese, Chinese, and American children. *Child Development, 56*, 718–734.

Streissguth, A. P., Barr, H. M., Sampson, P. D., Darby, B. L., & Martin, D. C. (1989). IQ at age 4 in relation to maternal alcohol use and smoking during pregnancy. *Developmental Psychology, 25*, 3–11.

Super, C. M. (1983). Cultural variation in the meaning and uses of children's "intelligence." In J. B. Deregowski, S. Dziurawiec, & R. C. Annis (Eds.), *Explorations in cross-cultural psychology*. Lisse, The Netherlands: Swets & Zeitlinger.

Sutaria, S. D. (1985). *Specific learning disabilities: Nature and needs*. Springfield, IL: Charles C Thomas.

Terman, L. M. (1925). *Genetic studies of genius: Mental and physical traits of a thousand gifted children*. Stanford, CA: Stanford University Press.

Terman, L. M., & Merrill, M. A. (1937). *Measuring intelligence: A guide to the administration of the new revised Stanford-Binet tests of intelligence*. Boston: Houghton Mifflin.

Thomson, G. H. (1939). *The factorial analysis of human ability*. Boston: Houghton Mifflin.

Thorndike, R. L., Hagen, E. P., & Sattler, J. M. (1986). *Stanford-Binet intelligence scale: Fourth edition (Technical Manual)*. Chicago: Riverside.

Thurstone, L. L. (1938). *Primary mental abilities*. Chicago: University of Chicago Press.

Turkheimer, E. (1991). Individual and group differences in adoption studies of IQ. *Psychological Bulletin, 110*, 392–405.

United States Bureau of the Census. (1994). *The Hispanic population of the United States: March 1993* (Current Population Reports, Series P20-475). Washington, DC: Author.

United States National Commission for Employment Policy. (1982). *Hispanics and jobs: Barriers to progress* (Report No. 14). Washington, DC: Author.

Vernon, P. A. (1987). *Speed of information processing and intelligence*. Norwood, NJ: Ablex.

Vernon, P. A. (1993). *Biological approaches to the study of human intelligence*. Norwood, NJ: Ablex.

Vickers, D., Nettelbeck, T., & Wilson, R. J. (1972). Perceptual indices of performance: The measurement of "inspection time" and "noise" in the visual system. *Perception, 1*, 263–295.

Vincent, K. R. (1991). Black/White IQ differences: Does age make the difference? *Journal of Clinical Psychology, 47*, 266–270.

Vygotsky, L. S. (1978). *Mind in society: The development of higher psychological processes*. Cambridge, MA: Harvard University Press.

Waller, J. H. (1971). Achievement and social mobility: Relationships among IQ score, education, and occupation in two generations. *Social Biology, 18*, 252–259.

White, K. R. (1982). The relation between socioeconomic status and academic achievement. *Psychological Bulletin, 91*, 461–481.

Wober, M. (1974). Towards an understanding of the Kiganda concept of intelligence. In J. W. Berry & P. R. Dasen (Eds.), *Culture and cognition: Readings in cross-cultural psychology* (pp. 261–280). London: Methuen.

Yairi, E., & Ambrose, N. (1992). Onset of stuttering in preschool children: Selected factors. *Journal of Speech and Hearing Research, 35*, 782–788.

7

Mental Retardation: Genetic Findings, Clinical Implications and Research Agenda

Emily Simonoff

MRC Child Psychiatry Unit and Centre for Social, Genetic and Developmental Psychiatry, Institute of Psychiatry, London

Patrick Bolton

Department of Psychiatry, University of Cambridge

Michael Rutter

MRC Child Psychiatry Unit and Centre for Social, Genetic and Developmental Psychiatry, Institute of Psychiatry, London

The most important genetic advances in the field of mental retardation include the discovery of the novel genetic mechanism responsible for the Fragile-X syndrome, and the imprinting involved in the Prader–Willi and Angelman syndromes, but there have also been advances in our understanding of the pathogenesis of Down syndrome and phenylketonuria. Genetic defects (both single gene Mendelizing disorders and cytogenetic abnormalities) are involved in a substantial proportion of cases of mild as well as severe mental retardation, indicating that the previous equating of severe mental retardation with pathology, and of mild retardation with normal variation, is a misleading oversimplication. Within the group in which no pathological cause can be detected, behavior genetic studies indicate that genetic influences are important, but that their interplay with environmental factors, which are also important, is at present poorly understood. Research into the joint action of genetic and environmental influences in this group will be an important research area in the future.

INTRODUCTION

In the past, genetic influences in severe mental retardation were usually discussed mainly in terms of the vast number of Mendelian disorders and chromosomal abnormalities associated with it. The implicit assumption tended to be that, if there were grounds for supposing that the association represented a causal connection, that provided a sufficient explanation. It is now clear that this was a misleading oversimplification. Because single gene disorders involved no environmental component, their effects

Reprinted with permission from *Journal of Child Psychology and Psychiatry*, 1996, Vol. 37(3), 259–280. Copyright © 1996 by the Association for Child Psychology and Psychiatry.

were conceptualized in terms of categorical, deterministic effects. That is, with a Mendelizing disorder, it was considered that the genetic abnormality provided a necessary and sufficient explanation for the disorder and often the mutation operated through a single, narrowly defined, biochemical abnormality (as with phenylketonuria, PKU). The oversimplification lies in the fact that, even with single gene disorders, the effects on function tend to be pleiotropic and probabilistic, although the probabilities may approach unity in some instances (Goldsmith & Gottesman, in press). That is characteristic of the way biological mechanisms operate (Crick, 1988). With many single gene and chromosomal conditions, there is a wide range in IQ, and it is necessary to explain why mental retardation occurs in some cases and yet not in others. Similarly, many of the conditions exhibit an equally wide range in behavioral manifestations and it is necessary to account for the mechanisms underlying the behavioral variability (Bregman & Hodapp, 1991). Of course, it remains the case that there is indeed a very long list of genetic diseases associated with severe and profound retardation (see Thapar, Gottesman, Owen, Donovan, & McGuffin, 1994; Wahlström, 1990). The change is that advances in molecular genetics have both provided a better understanding of genetic mechanisms and highlighted the complexities involved in understanding the links between the abnormal gene, the gene product, and the phenotypic manifestations (see for example, Wilkie, 1994) on the various mechanisms at the DNA level that could account for dominant inheritance; also the quantum leap forward provided by the understanding of how the expansion of trinucleotide repeat sequences accounts for various puzzling features in the inheritance of several neurological and neuropsychiatric disorders (Ross, McInnis, Margolis, & Li, 1993). In this paper, we seek to draw attention both to the gains of knowledge and to the questions remaining unanswered, as we consider clinical implications.

By contrast, most past discussions of the genetic contribution to mild mental retardation have been concerned with quantification of the genetic component (the "heritability"), on the implicit assumption that the level of heritability carries important implications for the potential for environmental prevention or remediation (Jensen, 1969). Not only is this implication highly questionable, but there is a need to determine *how* the interplay between genetic and environmental factors leads to mental retardation. We will draw attention to some of the key issues.

In this article, we seek to draw attention both to the gains in knowledge and to the questions remaining unanswered, as we consider clinical implications. We first explore general conceptual issues regarding the role of genetics in mental retardation. Because there are so many conditions causing mental retardation, we will focus on several different disorders or classes of disorder—Down syndrome, Fragile-X syndrome, nonspecific X-linked mental retardation (XLMR), sex chromosome anomalies, Prader–Willi/Angelman syndrome, PKU and autism—selected for discussion because each illustrates different aspects of genetic mechanisms. We then go on to explore the ways in which genes may act in conjunction with environmental influences in mild mental retardation. Implications for genetic testing of affected individuals, as well as genetic counselling and prenatal screening, are discussed.

SOME GENETIC ISSUES AS THEY APPLY TO MENTAL RETARDATION

"Pathological" and "Familial/Subcultural" Retardation

Following Lewis (1933) and Penrose (1938, 1963) a distinction has usually been drawn between "pathological" and "familial" or "subcultural" subtypes of mental retardation, the former being equated with severe and profound retardation and the latter with mild retardation (Burack, 1990; Zigler, 1967; Zigler & Hodapp, 1986). Roberts (1952) added to this distinction by suggesting that mild mental retardation should be conceptualized as based on continuous variation, while severe mental retardation was largely categorical, being due to catastrophic effects, genetic or otherwise, overwhelming the underlying influences on continuous variation. In many respects, the demarcation is well validated (McClaren & Bryson, 1987; Moser, Ramey, & Leonard, 1990; Rutter & Gould, 1985; Scott, 1994). Thus, severely retarded individuals differ markedly from the general population in having a diminished fecundity and a much reduced life expectancy. The majority, although not all, also show gross pathological abnormalities of the brain at post-mortem (Crome, 1960; Shaw, 1987). Studies of severely retarded individuals in Sweden, England, and the United States have shown that more than a third have some known genetic abnormality, about a fifth have multiple congenital anomalies and the majority (but by no means all) of the remainder have some clear evidence of organic brain dysfunction (such as cerebral palsy or epilepsy) but without a known cause (Moser et al., 1990). The two groups also differ in family background, with the social class distribution of the severely retarded group approximating that of the general population but a much increased tendency for the mildly retarded group to come from a socially disadvantaged background. The latter are also much more likely to have a family history of mental retardation. This is evident also in the mean IQ of siblings. Thus, the American National Collaborative Perinatal Project found that, within the Caucasian sample, the siblings of probands with severe mental retardation had an average IQ whereas those of probands with mild mental retardation had a mean IQ about a standard deviation below the mean, that is intermediate between that of the proband and that of the general population. Initially, the subcultural group was thought primarily to be due to polygenic influences (Lewis, 1933) but various studies pointed to the likely role of environmental factors as well (Blackie, Forrest, & Witcher, 1975; Stein & Susser, 1960), and it is now generally accepted that both genetic and environmental factors play a role, although their relative importance is not known (Burack, 1990; Zigler & Hodapp, 1986).

Although this differentiation between two broad groups has stood the test of time, it has required modification in several respects. First, the notion that the mildly retarded group does not include pathological varieties of mental retardation has had to be modified. Several systematic studies have indicated that a substantial minority have epilepsy or cerebral palsy and/or have identifiable causes of a pathological variety; estimates have put this proportion as high as 30–50% of cases, although most are somewhat lower (Einfeld, 1984; Hagberg, Hagberg, Lewerth, & Lindberg, 1981a; Lamont & Dennis, 1988; McClaren & Bryson, 1987; Rao, 1990; Sabaratnam, Laver, Bulter, & Pembrey, 1994). Second, there are some 10% or so of cases of severe retardation that have no recognizable medical condition. That these may constitute the extreme end of the normal continuum is shown by the finding that the rate of mental retardation in siblings is much the same for all levels of IQ below 70 when there is no identifiable cause for the retardation (Herbst & Baird, 1982). Third, it has become clear that evidence is still lacking on the relative contribution of genetic and environmental factors to nonpathological varieties of mild mental retardation (a point that we discuss further below).

GENETIC AND ENVIRONMENTAL INFLUENCES ON VARIATIONS IN INTELLIGENCE WITHIN THE NORMAL RANGE

Mental retardation is often viewed as a disorder, as indicated in the pathological subgroup in the two-group subdivision. As such, methods to detect the effect of single genes, such as linkage and association strategies in conjunction with molecular biology (see Brock, 1993, for a review) have been employed to elucidate genetic influences. However, as implicit in the notion of a familial/subcultural group (Zigler, 1967), mental retardation can be seen as the extreme of the normal distribution, considered either dimensionally or as a categorical trait, by applying a threshold (usually at an IQ of 70). Under either of these models, behavior genetic strategies are used to detect genetic and environmental influences. The strategies include twin, adoption and family designs (see Simonoff, McGuffin, & Gottesman, 1994; Rutter et al., 1990, for reviews). There have been more behavior genetic studies of intelligence than of any other behavioral trait and the mass of evidence points to a heritability of about 50% (Plomin & Neiderhiser, 1991; McGue, Bouchard, Iacono, & Lykken, 1993)—that is, it indicates a powerful effect from both genetic and nongenetic influences. This conclusion, based on a large range of studies using a variety of research strategies has been challenged both by those who wish to deny the importance of genetic effects (Kamin, 1974; Schiff & Lewontin, 1986) and by those who argue that environmental effects are quite minor within the normal range of environments (Rowe, 1994; Scarr, 1992). The first group point to the limitations of genetic designs (because of the assumptions required) and the flaws in individual studies, together with various inconsistencies in the evidence. These arguments were considered by Rutter and Madge (1976) who concluded that, taken as a whole, the evidence was unequivocal in pointing to a substantial genetic effect (but also that environmental influences were important). Studies with quite different patterns of strengths and limitations all pointed in the same direction; the further evidence accumulated during the last two decades amply confirm the importance of genetic effects (see Plomin & Neiderhiser, 1991).

Those who express scepticism about the importance of environmental effects tend to place most weight on the failure to account for the 50% nongenetic effects in terms of measured environmental variables and the weak effect seen in most published evaluated interventions. It has also been found that many environmental measures are partially under genetic control and not purely environmental (Plomin & Bergeman, 1991; Plomin, 1994, 1995). Nevertheless, the findings are clearcut in demonstrating that major environmental variations *do* affect cognitive performance in children from psychosocial high risk backgrounds (Rutter, 1985, 1991). For example, Schiff and Lewontin (1986) showed that children who were born to socially disadvantaged parents and then adopted into privileged homes had an IQ some 12 points higher than their half-siblings reared by disadvantaged biological parents. Capron and Duyme's (1989) tighter cross-fostering design, based on a sample of adopted children for whom there was a marked disparity between the social levels of biologic and adoptive parents, showed the importance of both genetic and environmental influences. Both biologic parentage and home of rearing had major effects of roughly comparable strength, the latter being associated with an average difference of some dozen IQ points.

With respect to interventions, the Abecedarian program of some 5–8 years special education provision for children born to young, mostly black, socially disadvantaged women, showed a 5 point IQ advantage in relation to the control group at the 12 year follow-up (Campbell & Ramey, 1994). None of the experimental group had an IQ below 70 and 13% had an IQ in the 70–85 range, as compared with 7% and 37% respectively in the control group. Similarly, Grantham-McGregor, Powell, Walker, Chang, and Fletcher (1994) showed a 9 point IQ difference at 14 years between severely malnourished children in the West Indies who participated in a 3 year house-visiting program and controls. These studies are all relevant to the issue of environmental effects in mental retardation because they concern children from the socially disadvantaged backgrounds that carry a much increased risk of retardation. While it is clear that there are clinically meaningful environmental effects, it is also evident that persisting benefits are dependent to a large degree on continuing environmental change.

Three further issues need to be noted briefly because of their implications for genetic factors in mild mental retardation: increasing heritability with age; the changes in heritability estimates over time; and ethnic group differences in IQ.

Changes with development. Contrary to many people's expectations, genetic influences on cognition (as measured in both twin and adoption studies) tend to increase with age, both during childhood and adult life (Plomin, 1986; McCartney, Harris, & Bernieri, 1990; DeFries, Plomin, & LaBuda, 1987; Loehlin, Horn, & Willerman, 1989). IQ is viewed as a generally stable individual characteristic, with high correlations between early childhood and adolescence. However, longitudinal studies of the general population show the substantial changes in IQ, in the range of 10–20 points, although some of this is due to measurement error (Moffitt, Caspi, Harkness, & Silva, 1993). Probably three rather different processes are operative. First, there are important changes in early childhood in the mix of cognitive skills that make up overall intellectual performance (especially with respect to the role of verbal skills). Second, people shape and select their environments and to the extent that such shaping and selecting reflects genetically influenced personal characteristics, this will lead to increasing heritability with age (Scarr & McCartney, 1983). Older children and adults have more control over their environments than do very young children and that control will involve characteristics that are genetically influenced in part. Third, genetic influences tend to correlate over time more highly than do nonshared environments (Kendler, 1993) resulting in a greater cumulative effect from genetic influences than environmental ones.

Changing heritability over time. Loehlin, Willerman and Horn (1988) noted that there may have been true secular changes in heritability, with both recent estimates and those from studies prior to the 1960s higher than the 1970s and early 1980s. Although it is possible that changes over time may have taken place, perhaps as a result of variations in environmental range, the apparent changes may simply be a consequence of differences between studies in sample characteristics, age distribution or tests used. The matter is unresolved but the variations do underline the fact that heritabilities have no absolute meaning.

Ethnic differences in intelligence. In a much quoted paper, Jensen (1969) argued that because heritabilities of IQ were high in both white and black populations, the mean IQ difference between them was also likely to be primarily genetically determined, and hence that environmental enrichment programs would be of little value. It is now appreciated that there is no necessary connection between within-group and between-group heritabilities and that, in any case, a high heritability has no implications for the benefits or otherwise of new forms of intervention (Rutter & Madge, 1976; Rutter, 1991). Furthermore, as discussed above, appropriate environmental interventions *do* have meaningful effects on IQ.

VARIATION IN EFFECT ON IQ WITHIN GENETIC CONDITIONS

Much of the early work in relation to Mendelian and chromosome disorders associated with severe retardation concerned conditions with a major effect on IQ. It appeared that the mental retardation was an intrinsic part of the genetically determined medical condition. Nevertheless, even with Down syndrome, the range in IQ extends into the mildly retarded range and some individuals have an IQ within the normal range. It has become obvious that there is a need to address the question of the mechanisms involved in variations in IQ within single gene or single chromosome disorders. The variation in IQ level has come into greater prominence with genetic conditions such as the fragile-X syndrome and Williams syndrome which are about as common in mildly retarded groups as in severely retarded ones. Other conditions, in particular the sex chromosome anomalies, lead to a reduction in IQ level, but one which is generally within the average range (Ratcliffe, 1994). Molecular genetic and other biological techniques begin to make it possible to understand why such variation occurs, although knowledge to date is extremely limited. Thus, variation in DNA trinucleotide repeats does account for an unusually early age of onset of onset in Huntington's disease but it does not account for variations in progression of the disease (Kieburtz et al., 1994; Trottier, Biancalana & Mandel, 1994).

INTELLIGENCE AND SOCIAL IMPAIRMENT

There has been a tendency for clinicians to diagnose mental retardation only when an IQ below 70 is accompanied by social impairment or problems in social adaptation (Schalock et al., 1994; Tarjan et al., 1972). That leaves open, however, resolution of the important question of why there is variation in the extent to which low intelligence is accompanied by social deficits. The total population survey on the Isle of Wight showed that some two-fifths of 9–10 year old children with an IQ below 70 were being educated in ordinary schools (Rutter, Tizard & Whitmore, 1970). Those in ordinary schools were comparable to those in special schools with respect to a family history of mental retardation or reading difficulties, and were also fairly similar in social background. By contrast, those in special schools were much more likely to have a history of language delay (47% vs. 9%) and also a family history of language delay (26% vs. 4%). The special school group were also more likely to show neurodevelopmental impairment and one or other of a range of medical problems. There have been no genetic studies that have compared these two groups and it is clear that such a comparison is much needed. The factors involved with low IQ may not be synonymous with those involved with associated social deficits. This issue is also underlined by the low rates of mild mental retardation (defined in terms of those at special schools) reported from Hagberg et al. (1981a) Swedish study. The prevalence of 0.4% applied to a region with relatively high socioeconomic status and few major social problems. The possibility needs to be entertained that environmental influences play a larger role in the social deficit accompanying low IQ than they do in the distribution of intelligence as such.

MECHANISM OF PSYCHIATRIC RISK

From the Isle of Wight (Rutter et al., 1970) and Aberdeen surveys (Birch, Richardson, Baird, Horobin, & Illsley, 1970; Koller, Richardson, Katz, & McLaren, 1982) onwards, it has been clear that people with mental retardation have a substantially increased risk of developing psychiatric disorder (Borthwick-Duffy, 1994; Bregman, 1991). Interestingly, and perhaps surprisingly, this risk was increased to a roughly comparable extent in children at normal schools and at special schools in the Isle of Wight study. There are many different ways in which this risk could come about (Rutter, 1971) but there is a need to determine the extent to which the genetic factors involved in mental retardation (when defined in IQ terms) are also those underlying the associated psychiatric risk (such data are lacking). The extent to which the increased risk is mediated by mental retardation per se is also unclear. It could reflect brain pathology rather than retardation as such; it could stem from the family adversities associated with retardation; it could derive from intrinsic associations between cognition and behavioral functioning; or it could reflect the stresses of educational failure. With respect to the last two possibilities, it may be relevant that, within the general population, there is a relationship between low IQ and increased questionnaire endorsements of behavioral problems (Goodman, Simonoff, & Stevenson, 1995).

MENTAL RETARDATION AND LANGUAGE DEVELOPMENT

The strong overlap between language impairment and low IQ raises the question of the extent to which the genetic factors involved in language development and those involved in intelligence are the same or different at the extreme lower end of the distribution. Within the normal range, it appears that there are both similarities and differences (Cardon & Fulker, 1993) but it cannot be assumed that the same applies at the extreme. As noted above, it also remains to be explained why the association between language and low IQ was so much stronger in the special schools group in the Isle of Wight study.

SPECIFIC BEHAVIORAL PHENOTYPES

During recent years there has been a growing interest in what have come to be called behavioral phenotypes (Dykens, 1995; Flint & Yule, 1994). Evidence has begun to accumulate indicating that there is a greater degree of specificity in the behavioral manifestations of genetic syndromes than was at one time apparent. Thus, marked social anxiety and social/communicative deficits are particularly frequent in the fragile-X syndrome and sociable garrulity tends to be a feature of children with Williams syndrome. There is a need to account for the degree of behavioral specificity that accompanies various genetic syndromes but, equally, there is a need to account for the marked behavioral variation within such syndromes. What is different, for example, between the fragile-X individuals who show extreme social anxiety and those who show a more autistic-like pattern and why do some fragile-X individuals show neither pattern? Molecular genetic studies may be useful in elucidating such differences.

GENE–ENVIRONMENT CORRELATIONS AND INTERACTIONS

Traditionally, research sought to separate the effects of nature and nurture. What has become increasingly apparent in recent years is that the interplay between the two may represent an important part of the ways in which both operate (Plomin, 1995; Rutter, 1994; Turkheimer & Gottesman, 1991). In ordinary circumstances, parents provide their children not only with their genes but also with their rearing experiences. A so-called "passive" gene–environment correlation refers to this phenomenon. The implication is that some part of a risk that has been assumed to be environmentally mediated, may actually represent a genetic effect (Plomin & Bergeman, 1991). This is not simply as a methodological problem, the origins of a risk factor and its mode of operation have no necessary connection with one another (Rutter, 1994). Thus, it could be that genetically influenced parental characteristics play a major role in the social disadvantage that tends to accompany mild mental retardation. Even though the depriving environment has been genetically influenced it may well bring about environmentally mediated risks. It is important that we obtain a greater understanding of how this interplay between nature and nurture actually affects children's cognitive development. Indirect attempts to assess the extent of gene–environment correlation intelligence indicate that it may well account for as in as much as one-fifth of the phenotypic variance (Loehlin & DeFries, 1987).

There are two other types of gene–environment correlation that must also be taken into account (Plomin, DeFries, & Loehlin, 1977). "Evocative" or "reactive" correlations arise because the ways in which people respond to children are influenced by the children's own characteristics. It is likely that mentally retarded children elicit different responses from their parents and from their teachers than do children of normal intelligence. Those differences in interpersonal interaction may, in turn, influence their own later development. "Active" correlations arise because, as children grow older, they have an increasing control over the environments that they experience, both selecting and shaping environments. Mentally retarded children, may be less likely to spend time in cognitively enriching activities and these differences in experiences will impinge on their cognitive development.

Gene–environment interaction refers to circumstances in which genetically influenced individual characteristics affect people's responsiveness to the environments that they encounter. A dramatic example of this is provided by the condition of PKU. This is an entirely genetic disorder but the ill-effects on cognition occur because the genetic defect means that the children cannot handle the ordinary levels of phenylalanine in their diet. Dietary phenylalanine condemns those with PKU to mental retardation but has no effect on intelligence in the rest of the population. The disorder is entirely genetic but the effects arise entirely through interactions with the environment. Such examples of person–environment interactions are widespread in biology and medicine (Rutter & Pickles, 1991) but there has been little evidence of such interactions in relation to variation in intelligence as they occur within the normal range (Plomin, DeFries, & Fulker, 1988). In part this may be because most designs have rather weak power to detect interactions (see Wahlsten, 1990) and in part because interactions can only be detected if both show variance. Thus the PKU example would not be detected in an ordinary multivariate design because the damaging food substance, phenylalanine, is pervasive in all ordinary diets. In the same sort of way, although the allergic diathesis refers to a genetically influenced unusual sensitivity to allergens in the environment, this will not be evident in statistical interaction effects because such allergens are all pervasive in most environments. So far as mental retardation is concerned what is needed are genetic designs that include both appropriate measures of the environment and also analyses that are designed to test hypotheses on particular mechanisms of gene–environment interaction.

DOWN SYNDROME

Chromosomal anomalies are the single most common cause of severe mental retardation (Gustavson, Holmgren, Jonsell, & Son Blomquist, 1977; McDonald, 1973). Trisomies account for about two-thirds of cytogenetic abnormalities associated with mental retardation and, of these, Down syndrome or trisomy 21, is the most common (Hamerton, Canning, Ray, & Smith, 1975; Haspeslagh et al., 1991; Kumada, 1990).

Down syndrome occurs in about 1.5 per 1000 births (de Grouchy & Turleau, 1990). That rate underestimates the number of foetuses with trisomy 21 because many spontaneously abort. The incidence of trisomy 21 dropped during the 1960s and 1970s (Hamerton et al., 1975; Jacobs, Melville, Ratcliffe, Keay, & Syme, 1974; McGrother & Marshall, 1990; Mikkelsen, 1981); this probably mainly stemmed from a decrease in maternal age rather than termination of pregnancy following prenatal testing (Huether & Gummere, 1982). The decrease in new cases of Down syndrome has, however, been offset by the improved survival of affected individuals (Baird & Sadovnick, 1989; McGrother & Marshall, 1990), resulting in an upward shift of the age profile (Bell, Pearn, & Firnan, 1989; Huether & Gummere, 1982).

Approximately 95% of cases of Down syndrome are due to nondisjunction of chromosome 21 during meiosis and four-fifths of meiotic nondisjunction arise in the mother's germ cells (Mikkelsen, Poulsen, Grimsted, & Lange, 1980). Nondisjunction is strongly related to maternal age, the rate of Down syndrome increasing from 0.9 per 1000 live births in mothers under the age of 33, to 2.8 in mothers aged between 35 and 38, and 38 per 1000 in mothers 44 years and over (Trimble & Baird, 1978). Less certainly, there is also a possible minor paternal effect arising from the effect on spermatogenesis of environmental toxins, as suggested by the variation in risk according to the father's occupation (Olshan, Bard, & Teschke, 1989).

One in 20 cases of Down syndrome is due to a chromosomal translocation. This form of Down syndrome is unrelated to maternal age but has implications for recurrence. In cases of Down syndrome due to meiotic nondisjunction, the recurrence risk for older mothers (the majority) is no different than for any other woman of similar age; for younger mothers, it may be slightly increased to 1–2%, perhaps due to genetic factors predisposing to nondisjunction (de Grouchy & Turleau, 1990). On the other hand, recurrence risks are substantially higher for Down syndrome due to translocation, with the exact risk depending on the nature of the translocation and varying between 15% and 100%.

The cause of mental retardation in Down syndrome is unknown. The fact that translocation of chromosome 21 leads to Down syndrome has been helpful in mapping areas of the chromosome responsible for various components of the Down phenotype. It has been possible to identify "critical regions", defined as the smallest chromosomal region which, when unbalanced, gives rise to a particular phenotypic characteristic (Epstein, 1990). The characteristic features of Down syndrome, including facial, hand and cardiac abnormalities and mental retardation have been related to the more distal region of the long arm of chromosome 21. Imbalance of the more proximal region of the long arm is also associated with mental retardation, without the classical physical features of Down syndrome (Williams, Frias, McCormick, Antonarakis, & Cantu, 1990).

Such work has raised the question of how specific are the phenotypic abnormalities associated with various disorders of chromosome imbalance. All nonlethal trisomies are associated with a wide range of physical abnormalities and mental retardation (de Grouchy & Turleau, 1990). Proponents of the nonspecificity hypothesis have pointed out that there is considerable phenotypic variation among individuals affected with the same chromosomal imbalance and, furthermore, that different types of chromosomal imbalance give rise to similar phenotypic features (Blum-Hoffman, Rehder, & Langen-beck, 1987; Shapiro, 1983). They argue that the mechanism of action is one in which developmental instability is enhanced, that certain tissues, including neural tissue, are most vulnerable to this increased instability; and that the similarity in features of different trisomies reflect a commonality in the way this instability is expressed. Others have argued that each trisomy reflects a specific genetic disorder of development, in which there is considerable phenotypic variability among individuals (Epstein, 1990). Phenotypic variation is also seen in most disorders, including single gene disorders. In addition, experienced clinicians can diagnose the specific trisomy with which an individual child is affected with fairly good reliability, indicating that there are distinct clinical differences between the different trisomies. The argument will not be resolved until the gene(s) responsible for the various abnormalities in trisomy 21 are identified and their mode of action studied.

It is likely that the mechanism involves an imbalance in gene dosage. There does not appear to be any compensation for the number of genes present in the amount of protein produced; thus blood levels of gene products involved in trisomies and monosomies, respectively, are roughly 1.5 and 0.5 times the levels seen in diploid (normal) cells (Epstein, 1986). The importance of having not only the right product but also the right dose is suggested by X chromosome inactivation in females. It has been further suggested that such dosage effects might exert an important influence through specific alterations in regulatory mechanisms during development and that such abnormalities would be causative in the development of the phenotype. Recent work characterizing one of the genes in the region of chromosome 21 critical for Down syndrome has suggested homology with a gene in *Drosophila* that is expressed during embryonic development and plays a key role in midline CNS development, including the development of nerve cell precursors (Chen et al., 1995). Further work on the human gene is required, but these early findings highlight the potential importance of genes involved in the regulation of development as a factor leading to widespread abnormalities, including mental retardation.

THE FRAGILE-X SYNDROME

The fragile-X anomaly constitutes the most common cause of inherited mental retardation (Down syndrome is more frequent but is rarely inherited) and also accounts for about half of all causes of XLMR, affecting 1 in 1500–2000 males and 1 in 2000–2500 females (Kahkonen et al., 1987; Webb, Bundey, Thake, & Todd, 1986). There is a characteristic but subtle facial appearance that develops with age, including a large forehead, prominent jaw and low, protuberant ears; however, this is by no means always present. Macroorchidism, hyperextensibility of joints and sometimes mitral valve prolapse are common features. Mental retardation is usual, is generally in the mild to moderate range (i.e., 35–69), but some individuals are profoundly handicapped and others are of normal intelligence.

Lubs (1969) described the cytogenetic features of the fragile-X chromosome and suggested that the constriction on the distal portion of the long arm of the X chromosome might be a marker for a defective gene. This suggestion was not taken up until the late 1970s because a folate-deficient culture medium for chromosomes, used by Lubs but not again until the late 70s, is essential for the expression of the fragile-X site. When it was used the association between the fragile-X site and mental retardation with macroorchidism was confirmed (Giraud, Aymes, & Mattei, 1976; Harvey, Judge, & Wiener, 1977; Sutherland, 1977).

Several puzzling phenomena concerning the transmission of the fragile-X syndrome were noted in terms of what became known as Sherman's paradox (Sherman et al., 1985). About one-fifth of males known to be carrying the defect show neither cytogenetic nor clinical evidence of doing so. These men referred to as normal transmitting males, also had fewer affected male sibs than would be expected. Mendelian inheritance predicts that one-half of the male sibs would be affected but Sherman et al.'s study of over 200 pedigrees found that only 10% were. In addition, a low rate of fragile-X expression, and no physical or mental abnormalities were found in the female carriers. By contrast, about one-third of the daughters of these carrier women who inherited the defective chromosome were mentally subnormal and showed a considerably higher rate of fragile-X expression than their mothers.

None of these observations were consistent with conventional X-linked Mendelian inheritance and investigators realized that novel genetic mechanisms would be required to account for the pattern of inheritance. Both Pembrey and colleagues (Pembrey, Winter, & Davies, 1985; Winter & Pembrey, 1986) and Laird (1987) suggested mechanisms (a premutation and genomic imprinting, respectively) that could account for the findings but neither predicted the novel abnormality that was detected by molecular genetics.

In 1991, there were several simultaneous reports that the fragile-X syndrome involved a trinucleotide repeat sequence, in the region containing the FMR-1 gene (Oberle et al., 1991; Verkerk et al., 1991; Yu et al., 1991). Individuals in the general population show between 6 and 50 CGG trinucleotide repeats whereas clinically and cytogenetically normal obligate carriers, both male and female, have 50–200 repeats. This expanded sequence, also referred to as the premutation, is unstable and liable to further expansion. The full mutation, >200 repeats, is seen in the fragile-X syndrome. Although the mechanisms associated with the transition from the normal repeat sequence to the premutation are not well understood, the expansion from pre- to full mutation only occurs when the premutation passes through a female, and the expansion is related to the size of the premutation, with larger repeat sequences being at greater risk of expansion to the full mutation (Fu et al., 1992; Mulley et al., 1992b). Further molecular genetic work has shown that individuals with the full mutation do not express the FMR-1 gene (Pieretti et al., 1991), while those with the premutation do (Feng, Lakkis, Devys, & Warren, 1995), although methylation status may also play a role (Hagerman et al., 1994).

A minority of individuals with the full mutation show the features of autism, many more show slightly different social and communicative abnormalities, and a pattern of extreme social anxiety of an unusual kind appears especially characteristic, although present in only a minority (Flint & Yule, 1994; Turk, 1992). Molecular genetic methods now allow determination of whether the phenotypic variation is explicable on the basis of either the repeat sequence length or degree of methylation (see Loesch et al., 1993). The findings to date suggest that the main effect derives from nonexpression of the FMR-1 gene but that does not account for the cognitive and behavioral diversity shown by individuals with the syndrome.

The function of the FMR-1 gene is still unknown although it has been shown to be expressed in the brain and particularly in the cytoplasm of neurons (Devys, Lutz, Rouyer, Belloeq & Mandel, 1993). Its causative role in the fragile-X syndrome has been confirmed by instances of individuals demonstrating the full clinical picture of the fragile-X syndrome but without cytogenetic evidence of the fragile site. Molecular genetic examination of these individuals has demonstrated either a deletion of all (Gedeon et al., 1992) or part (Wohrle et al., 1992) of the FMR-1 gene or a missense mutation in the gene (DeBoulle et al., 1993).

The elucidation of the molecular genetic basis of the fragile-X syndrome has had important implications. In practical terms, it has led to the development of a direct molecular test for the defect that is both more accurate and less labour-intensive than the previous cytogenetic test. The ability to measure the length of the trinucleotide repeat sequence has made it possible to give potential female carriers much more precise information regarding their risk of having affected offspring (Fisch et al., 1995). It also raises queries about phenotypic consequences of the premutation. The evidence is inconclusive but it seems that carriers with the premutation are not intellectually different from controls (Reiss, Freund, Abrams, Boehm, & Kazazian, 1993; Taylor et al., 1994). The relationship of behavioral abnormalities to expansion size is less clear with one study (Sobesky, Pennington, Porter, Hull, & Hagerman, 1994) suggesting an increased rate of schizotypy in carriers with pre- and full mutations but another (Reiss et al., 1993) indicating no abnormalities in those with premutations. Further work on genotype–phenotype relationships within both the full mutation and the premutation is necessary. However, variations in the trinucleotide repeat sequence within the normal range probably have no clinical significance (Daniels et al., 1994).

In addition, the time-saving molecular methods will make it possible to consider the implementation of population-based screening programmes, if this seems appropriate (see discussion under Genetic screening). We have yet to identify the gene product and it is not known how this leads to mental retardation or to the range of associated behavioral and physical features seen, such understanding will almost certainly come within the next decade. With it, will be a model of how the absence of a single protein can disrupt normal brain development. It is possible that gene therapy will also be available to treat those with complete or relative absence of the FMR-1 protein (Palomaki & Haddow, 1993).

Since the first elucidation of the molecular genetics of fragile X, two further mutations, occurring at different nearby loci but causing an indistinguishable cytogenetic appearance have been described. The FRAX-E site is slightly distal to FRAX-A (the original mutation) and is associated with either normal intelligence (Sutherland & Baker, 1992) or mild mental retardation (Flynn et al., 1993; Mulley et al., 1995), but not with macroorchidism or the facial characteristics of the classical fragile-X syndrome (Hamel et al., 1994). It is unclear whether the FRAX-E is seen with any phenotypic abnormalities or whether the mild mental retardation seen in some cases reflects ascertainment bias. The FRAX-F site is further distal and is associated with mental retardation but no other abnormalities (Hirst et al., 1993a). The frequency of FRAX-E and FRAX-F is not known. Neither will be detected by the molecular genetic investigation for FRAX-A, highlighting the importance of maintaining cytogenetic investigations until the significance of the abnormalities is better understood. However, rapid screening tests are being developed and, if their validity is confirmed, they may provide an important way forward (Wang, Green, Bobrow, & Mathew, 1995; Willemsen et al., 1995).

One puzzle has been why the fragile-X syndrome is so common, given that affected hemizygous males and heterozygous females rarely reproduce. Sherman et al. (1985) argued for a high rate of new mutations. However, molecular analysis has failed to identify new mutations in sporadic cases. Others (Vogel, Crusio, Kovac, Fryns, & Freund, 1990) have suggested that there might be selective advantage for unaffected heterozygous carriers, but the nature of such advantage remains obscure. Recent studies have suggested that the fragile-X mutation arises from a small number of original mutations (Hirst et al., 1993b; Richards et al., 1992). A possible explanation for this apparent inconsistency was first put forward by Morton and MacPherson (1992) who suggested that several steps are involved. The mutation rate from the normal (6–50 repeats) sequence to the premutation (50–200 repeats) is low explaining the appearance of a "founder effect". However, the larger premutations become unstable at a much higher rate and, because of their propensity to develop into full mutations lead to a high rate of affected individuals occurring in apparently normal families. Recently, the loss of AGG repeats (normal in the general population) has been hypothesized as a further predisposing factor in the conversion to premutation (Snow et al., 1994).

Since the description of the expanding repeat sequence in the fragile-X syndrome, similar discoveries have been made in Huntington's disease, myotonic dystrophy, spinobulbar atrophy and spinocerebellar atrophy, all of which show some irregularities of inheritance (Ross et al., 1993). It remains to be seen how many more disorders will be found to be caused by expanding repeats. It seems that the mechanism of action of the expanded repeat may vary between disorders; in fragile X, the region is not translated into the protein whereas it may be in Huntington's Disease. It is interesting to note that all the disorders in which expanding trinucleotide repeats have been discovered are ones affecting the central nervous system but it is unclear at present whether this is merely coincidence or whether it is likely to explain other psychiatric disorders (Petronis & Kennedy, 1995).

OTHER FORMS OF X-LINKED MENTAL RETARDATION

Only about half of XLMR is accounted for by the fragile-X syndrome (Opitz, 1986). A gene map of mental retardation compiled by Wahlström in 1990 listed 503 separate disorders; 69 had been assigned to one of the 22 autosomes and 73 to the X chromosome (Wahlström, 1990). These figures illustrate the apparent importance of the X chromosome in mental retardation syndromes. It is unclear whether there are truly more genes relating to mental retardation on the X chromosome or whether such genes are more readily revealed by their characteristic pattern of inheritance and by the fact that males are hemizygous for these genes, revealing defects that would be obscured in the heterozygous state.

The pioneering population-based study of the Reeds (Reed & Reed, 1965), found a 49% excess of males and highlighted the possibility of X-linked inheritance by showing a two-fold increase in the risk of affected offspring in retarded women married to normal males, compared with retarded males married to normal females. Lehrke (1972) argued for X-linked major genes affecting intelligence in the normal range which, when mutated, would lead to mental retardation. His hypothesis was initially criticized (Anastasi, 1972) but subsequent careful examination of families, along with linkage studies, support his view.

It is likely that the majority of the male excess will be explained by X-linked disorders. A recent review by Glass (1991) showed those genes already identified to be distributed over the entire X chromosome. In some, e.g. Coffin–Lowry syndrome, Lowe syndrome and X-linked spastic paraplegia, mental retardation is just one of a number of features. In other less well-defined disorders, there is a constellation of abnormalities, of which mental retardation is a cardinal symptom, that cosegregate in affected family members. Such disorders include XLMR with hypotonia, Renpenning syndrome and XLMR with growth retardation, deafness and macrogenitalism. In still other cases, mental retardation appears to be the only abnormality; such cases are referred to as nonspecific XLMR. Linkage analysis of a number of individual families indicates clearly that nonspecific XLMR relates to more than one locus, although the number involved cannot yet be specified (see Mulley, Kerr, Stevenson, & Lubs, 1992a, for a review). Because of the lack of distinguishing phenotypic characteristics, it will be difficult to combine families a priori, making the task for linkage studies more difficult. However, rapid advances are occurring. A conference report in 1990 indicated that regional mapping for 17 XLMR disorders had been reported (Neri, Gurrieri, Gal, & Lubs, 1990). A further update in 1994 reported regional mapping for 53 disorders and gene cloning in 15 (Neri, Chiurazzi, Arena, & Lubs, 1994).

A recent report on XLMR with alpha-thalassaemia (ATR-X syndrome) has identified a mutation that is probably responsible for the disorder, which is made up of a complex phenotype of severe mental retardation, characteristic facial features, genital abnormalities and alpha-thalassaemia. Unlike many of the trisomy syndromes, in which the phenotype is complex but variable, the features of ATR-X are consistent across individuals, suggesting pleiotropic effects of a single gene. Several different mutations in the XH2 gene have been identified in families with ATR-X syndrome (Gibbons, Picketts, Villard, & Higgs, 1995), making it highly likely that the gene is responsible for the syndrome. The sequence of XH-2 indicates that it belongs to a class of genes that play various roles in cellular regulation, and the XH-2 gene may be involved in translation (from RNA to protein). A mutation in a gene involved in overall cellular regulation could explain the complex but consistent phenotype of ATR-X. While the exact role of XH2 needs further elucidation, it may provide a genetic example of how a single gene defect can have pleiotropic effects.

SEX CHROMOSOME ANOMALIES

Abnormalities in the number of sex chromosomes are generally less devastating in their effects than aneuploidies in the autosomes. Sex chromosome anomalies occur in roughly 1 in 400 live births. The most common include Turner's Syndrome (45, XO), Klinefelter's syndrome (47 XXY) and the 47 XXX and 47 XYY karyotypes. Other karyotypes, with two or more additional sex chromosomes (e.g., 48 XXXX, 49 XXXXX, 48 XXXY, 49 XXXXY) are very much more rare and also more deleterious in their effects. All four are associated with a slight decrease in IQ, as evidenced by comparison with siblings and by their higher frequency in mentally retarded populations (de la Chapelle, 1990). However, in all cases, the deficit is generally small, usually 5–20 IQ points lower than that of siblings, and most individuals have IQs in the normal range, with a few being in the mild mental retardation range and a small minority having IQs of <50.

Differential patterns of cognitive performance may depend on the type of sex chromosome anomaly. Thus, Turner's Syndrome (XO) characteristically involves a visuo-spatial deficit whereas Klinefelter's syndrome and 47 XXX are associated with speech and language disorders (Bolton & Holland, 1994; Ratcliffe, 1994). Probably, too, XYY is associated with characteristic temperamental features, such as hyperactivity, and a raised rate of behavior problems as well as a height that is usually well above average. The relative specificity of the cognitive and behavioral features associated with particular chromosomal abnormalities in general population samples suggests that genetic influences play a key note in the associations. Even so the associations are probabilistic and only of moderate strength and much has still to be learned about the causal mechanisms, including interplay with environmental factors and the role of self concepts.

PRADER–WILLI AND ANGELMAN SYNDROMES: THE IMPORTANCE OF IMPRINTING AND MICRODELETIONS

The Prader–Willi (PWS) and Angelman syndromes (AS) exemplify two phenomena likely to be increasingly important in the genetics of mental retardation: *imprinting* and *microdeletions*. At a phenotypic level, the syndromes have little in common other than mental retardation, which is usually mild in PWS and more severe in AS. However, they are linked by having loci that are very close to each other on chromosome 15, and by demonstrating imprinting (Nicholls, 1994).

Classical Mendelian inheritance does not distinguish between genes transmitted through the father or mother. However, it is necessary not only for the chromosomal complement to be diploid but also to have one set of maternal and one of paternal origin. A *complete* chromosomal complement originating from one parent is incompatible with life in humans; two paternally derived haploid sets results in a hydatidiform mole and two maternally derived sets leads to an ovarian teratoma. At least part of the imprinting process involves the extent to which the DNA is methylated, with maternally derived chromosomes having relatively over-methylated DNA, paternally derived ones relatively under-methylated. Erasure of the imprint occurs during gametogenesis and a new imprint is made with each generation. Uniparental disomy, receiving both of a particular pair of chromosomes from one parent, has been demonstrated in both humans and animals. In mice, behavioral differences depending on the chromosomal origin have been demonstrated; mice with a maternal uniparental disomy of chromosome 2 or 11 were small and under-active whereas those with a paternally derived disomy were large and relatively overactive (see Hall, 1990, for a review).

PWS is a rare disorder, whose main features include mental retardation (usually mild to moderate), obesity associated with overeating, hypogonadism and marked hypotonia in infancy. Short stature, small hands and feet, hypopigmentation are frequently noted along with and a characteristic narrow face are also common. Its prevalence has been estimated at 5–10 per 100,000 (Akefeldt, Gillberg, & Larsson, 1991; Burd, Vesely, Martsolf, & Kerbeshian, 1990; Butler, 1990). The association between PWS and chromosome 15 was first noted in the late 1970s, with the proximal region of the long arm of chromosome 15 being pinpointed (15q11–13) (Ledbetter et al., 1981). About 60% of PWS is associated with cytogenetically detectable deletions in this region, and a further 20% are due to microdeletions, sometimes associated with translocation, which can only be detected using molecular genetic techniques (Robinson et al., 1991; Trent et al., 1991). It was noted that the deletions were always from the paternal chromosome 15 (Butler, Meaney, & Palmer, 1986). Although the majority of PWS could be explained either by microscopically visible deletions or by microdeletions, a small number showed no karyotypic defect. Nicholls, Knoll, Butler, Karam, and Lalande (1989) found that, in these cases, both chromosome 15s originated from the mother; thus, no paternally-derived chromosome 15 was present. This maternal uniparental disomy accounts for about a fifth of all PWS cases (Mascari et al., 1992). At least some cases of uniparental disomy occur when there is initially a chromosome 15 trisomy, for example, two maternal chromosome 15s and one paternal, where the paternally-derived chromosome 15 is lost during early fetal life (Cassidy et al., 1992; Purvis-Smith et al., 1992). The findings of either paternal deletion in the 15q11–13 region *or* maternal uniparental disomy argue strongly that PWS is caused by the *lack* of some paternal gene(s) in this region.

AS is another chromosome 15 disorder associated with mental retardation (usually moderate to severe) but with rather different features. It is characterized by ataxia, hypotonia, jerky movements, hand-flapping, seizures and the absence of speech; facial features include a large jaw and open-mouthed expression. As in PWS, hypopigmentation compared with relatives is frequently seen. Although the syndrome was first described in 1965 (Angelman, 1965), it was not until the late 1980s that the pattern of inheritance started to become clear. The possibility of autosomal recessive inheritance was raised by studies of affected sib pairs. Then, in 1987, two cases of AS were reported to show a deletion of the proximal portion of 15q, the short arm of the chromosome (Magenis, Brown, Lacy, Budden, & LaFranchi, 1987) and the finding was confirmed in subsequent investigations. Detailed molecular examination of the deleted region indicated that it overlapped to a large extent with the region involved in PWS, although in some cases the AS deletion was larger, raising the question as to how two such different disorders could apparently be caused by the same genetic defect. A number of studies confirmed that the deleted chromosomal region was always maternal in AS as opposed to the paternal origin in PWS (Magenis et al., 1990). Subsequently, cases of paternal uniparental disomy were described; the frequency of this as a cause in AS appears to be lower than in PWS (Chan et al., 1993). The genetic mechanisms underlying PWS and AS are still not entirely resolved. It appears, however, that the syndromes are due to the lack of gene(s) very close to each other. The marked phenotypic differences appear to be due to whether the genetic material that is *absent* is of paternal or maternal origin.

The role of microdeletions in mild and severe mental retardation not associated with known medical syndromes is not known but the study by Flint and his colleagues (Flint et al., 1995) suggests that they may be found in some 1 in 20 cases, indicating the need for further study of their effects.

PHENYLKETONURIA

PKU occurs in approximately one in 10,000 individuals in Northern Europeans (DiLella & Woo, 1987; Guthrie & Susi, 1963) but with some variability within this group and considerably lower rates in other racial and ethnic groups (Scott & Cederbaum, 1990). Penrose's family studies were among the first to indicate that the inheritance was autosomal recessive (Penrose, 1935). PKU is one of the best understood examples of an inborn error of metabolism, many of which cause mental retardation as one of the consequences. It is also an example of a genetic disorder in which environmental treatment has had a striking effect on the outcome. Inborn errors of metabolism account for some 3–7% of cases of severe mental retardation (Moser et al., 1990) and, as such, are an important subgroup.

The majority of cases of PKU are due to altered function and activity of the enzyme, phenylalanine hydroxylase (PAH), and treatment involves dietary restriction of phenylalanine that must begin during early life. Early reports highlighted the impressive effects, comparing untreated sibs with those detected at birth (Smith & Wolff, 1974). More recently, it has been recognized that the IQ's of children with treated PKU may be depressed some 4–7 points below their unaffected sibs (Dobson, Williamson, Azen, & Koch, 1977; Koch, Azen, Freedman, & Williamson, 1984). In addition, while it was formerly thought to be reasonable to discontinue dietary restriction in middle childhood, there is now evidence to suggest that this may lead to a decline in intellectual performance (Holtzman, Krommal, van Doornick, Azen, & Koch, 1986; Krause et al., 1985). Now that affected individuals have received early treatment, young women have begun to reproduce and the effects of maternal PKU have been shown to include high rates of birth defects and subsequent mental retardation in offspring (Lenke & Levy, 1980). It appears that severe dietary restriction, if begun prior to conception, may ameliorate these problems.

In 1984, following a number of previously unconfirmed reports of linkage to other chromosomes, the locus for PAH was assigned to the short arm of chromosome 12 (Lidsky et al., 1984). Since that time, over 60 different mutations in the gene have been described. The mutations detected affect PAH in a number of different ways. The majority involved the substitution of a single base pair, leading to an amino acid substitution in many cases and to a nonsense mutation stopping transcription in others. Still others are splicing mutations, which alter the dinucleotide repeats that are a signal for the way in which messenger RNA is to be cut and rejoined into mature mRNA prior to polypeptide translation. *Genotype–phenotype relationships.* Given that different mutations affect the amino acid sequence and protein conformation in different ways, leading to variation in the extent to which PAH activity is reduced, researchers have asked whether there is a regular relationship between different mutations and the severity of mental retardation. Two groups found a strong association between different mutations and the degree of PAH activity (Okano et al., 1991; Svensson, von-Dobeln, Eisensmith, Hagenfeldt, & Woo, 1993). Ramus, Forrest, Pitt, Saleeba, and Cotton (1993) examined the relationship between different mutations and intellectual functioning in a group of untreated patients. In general, the level of retardation followed the reduction in enzyme activity with the exception of one family in whom the level of PAH activity should have predicted severe to profound retardation but where only mild to moderate impairment was present. Further work will be necessary to determine whether the relationship between genotype and intellectual functioning is, in fact, weaker than that with metabolic measures. If so, it would be important to know what other mechanisms were involved in determining the degree of retardation.

Variants of PKU. It is now recognized that there are important variants of "classical" PKU both reflecting less severe mutations in PAH and also mutations in other enzymes and cofactors involved in phenylalanine metabolism. The findings in PKU are typical of many single gene disorders. Population-based screening of neonates identified two forms of hyperphenylalanaemia that are clinically insignificant, benign hyperphenylalanaemia and transient hyperketonuria. In benign hyperphenylalanaemia, phenylalamine levels are raised above normal but below that seen in PKU. Such elevations do not result in mental retardation. As in PKU, specific PAH haplotypes have been identified, suggesting that the disorder is due to more benign mutations in the PAH gene (Gunter et al., 1987; Ledley, Levy, & Woo, 1986). Transient PKU, in which infants are detected because of phenylalanine levels as high as in PKU, but where the elevations do not persist, is less well described. It has been suggested that the transient increases in phenylalanine represent a response to stress but neither the metabolic nor genetic mechanism is understood (Scott & Cederbaum, 1990).

In the mid-1970s, after screening and early intervention programs were well in place, it became apparent that a small group (about 1%) of children were developing neurological and intellectual impairments despite treatment (Smith, Clayton, & Wolff, 1975). Careful study revealed that the abnormality in this group was a defect in tetrahydrobiopterin (BH_4), a cofactor not only in the hydroxylation of phenylalanine but also of tyrosine and tryptophan (Kaufman, Holtzman, Milstien, Butler, & Krumholz, 1975). Hence, treatment through reductions in phenylalamine intake still leaves abnormalities in other metabolites.

Screening and prevention. Widespread neonatal screening became possible with the advent of the Guthrie test which is a simple method to detect high levels of phenylalanine (Guthrie & Susi, 1963). Many had thought that identification of the gene and the defect in it would lead not only to more accurate detection of affected individuals but also to prenatal population screening for the carrier status. However, the large number of mutations has made this problematic. While individuals from any one particular ethnic background are likely to carry a subgroup of mutations, the individual mutations involved vary widely according to ethnic background, making it difficult to contemplate comprehensive screening in racially and ethnically varied populations (Eisensmith et al., 1992). Currently, the use of molecular genetics is restricted to families in which there is already an affected individual. In such cases, either linkage analysis or actual DNA sequencing can be used (DiLella & Woo, 1987).

Gene therapy. Severe dietary restriction to reduce phenylalanine intake continues to be the treatment for PKU. This means a very restricted diet resulting in limited compliance (Gleason, Michals, Matalon, Langenberg, & Kamath, 1992). Gene replacement therapy providing the normal PAH gene to PKU patients, constitutes a potential alternative. Current work, using a mouse model of PKU, has indicated that the PAH gene can be incorporated into hepatocytes (where PAH ordinarily functions) successfully (Cristiano, Smith, & Woo, 1993). It seems likely that the treatment will be applicable to humans and it could obviate the need for any other treatment (see Lever & Goodfellow, 1995, for an account of the current state of the art with respect to gene therapy).

AUTISM

Autism is a neurodevelopmental disorder characterized by a particular pattern of social and communicative deficits, associated with repetitive stereotyped behaviors (Lord & Rutter, 1994). As traditionally diagnosed, it occurs in some 4 children per 10,000, is much commoner in males (a ratio of 3–4:1), and is associated with mental retardation in about three quarters of cases. Usually, there are no obvious stigmata and the affected children have often been said to be physically attractive. Nevertheless, autism is associated with some increase in the rate of minor congenital anomalies and, more specifically, about a quarter of individuals with autism have a head circumference above the 97th percentile (Bailey et al., 1995; Bolton et al., 1994). Also, one-fifth to one-quarter of autistic individuals develop epilepsy, most characteristically with an onset in adolescence or early adult life. During the past decade, autism has been found to be associated with various apparently circumscribed cognitive deficits, particularly those said to reflect "theory of mind" skills (Baron-Cohen, Tager-Flusberg, & Cohen, 1993). There has been great interest in the possibility that pervasive social and behavioral abnormalities might be due to a specific cognitive abnormality. An understanding of those cognitive-behavioral connections would undoubtedly be extremely valuable in understanding the causal processes involved in autism (Bailey, Phillips, & Rutter, 1996) but, not only are there unresolved questions concerning those connections, but the relatively strong association with mental retardation remains unexplained (Rutter & Bailey, 1993).

For many years, the likelihood of major genetic influences in autism was discounted by most reviewers because there were no reported cases of vertical transmission (i.e., no cases of autism in parent and child) and because the rate of autism in siblings (2% as reported in studies up to the 1980s) was so low in absolute terms (Rutter, Silberg, & Simonoff, 1993). An appreciation that this was the wrong consideration (the key point is that this represented a 50- to 100-fold increase in risk) led to the first twin study by Folstein and Rutter in the 1970s. This pointed to a major genetic contribution and subsequent larger scale twin studies have produced an estimate of greater than 90% heritability of an underlying predisposition to autism (Bailey et al., 1995; Rutter et al., 1993), the highest for any multifactorial psychiatric disorder.

The findings, however, also revealed three other important features. First, the huge disparity between monozygotic (MZ) and dizygotic (DZ) pairs with concordance rates (60% vs. 3%), together with the marked drop off in risk from first to second degree relatives, indicated that several genes were likely to be involved. That is because although MZ pairs share all their genes and DZ pairs half their segregating genes on average, the disparity is greater for combinations of genes. Thus, DZ pairs will share only 1 in 4 of two-gene and 1 in 8 of three-gene combinations, whereas MZ pairs will share all combinations. Quantitative estimates suggest that a small number (say 3 or 4) of interacting genes is most likely to be the case (Pickles et al., in press). Second, both twin (Bailey et al., 1995) and family studies (Bolton et al., 1994; Piven et al., 1994) suggest that what is inherited is a broader range of social and cognitive deficits than represented by the handicapping condition of autism. Several studies have suggested an aggregation of affective and anxiety disorders in the families of autistic probands (Piven et al., 1991; Smalley, McCracken, & Tanguay, 1995); the aetiology of this finding remains uncertain.

It is clinically important to note that this broader phenotype occurs in individuals of normal intelligence. A key question is why autism is associated with mental retardation and epilepsy whereas the broader phenotype is not. It could reflect simply a higher "dose" of genetic risk or it could reflect an interplay with some other risk factor. Third, the pattern of findings in both the twin and family studies suggests that, in many instances, the obstetric complications sometimes associated with autism reflect the effect of a genetically abnormal foetus rather than an environmentally mediated risk. That this occurs is indicated, for example, by the well known increased rate of complications in Down syndrome. The clinical implication is that there needs to be caution in any inference that autism (or mental retardation unassociated with autism) is *due* to obstetric complications. This issue is discussed further in relation to multifactorial inheritance.

It should be added that, in addition to the idiopathic variety of autism, some one in ten cases are associated with a known medical condition, often of genetic origin (Folstein & Rutter, 1988; Rutter, Bailey, Bolton, & LeCouteur, 1994; Smalley, Asarnow, & Spence, 1988). Probably, the most common of these is the fragile-X anomaly but, contrary to some early reports, this probably account for no more than 5% of cases (Bailey et al., 1993).

GENETIC FACTORS IN IDIOPATHIC MENTAL RETARDATION
FAMILIALITY AND RECURRENCE RISK

There is abundant evidence that mild mental retardation shows a strong tendency to run in families, and that there is a much increased recurrence risk if either a parent or sib has mental retardation. Thus, Reed and Reed (1965) found that, having had one retarded child the chance of a further retarded child was 6% if both parents and their sibs were "normal", 13% if both parents were normal but one had a retarded sib, 20% if one parent was retarded, and 42% if both were retarded. Bundey, Thake, and Todd (1989) similarly reported a recurrence risk of 37% if one or both parents were affected compared with a rate of 15% if neither parent was affected; and a rate of 39% if there was an older affected sib compared with a rate of 10% if there was not. Interestingly, Bundey et al. (1989) found that the recurrence rate was markedly lower in Asian families (ca 2% compared with 20% in non-Asian families), and equally surprisingly that the recurrence risk was unaffected by whether or not the index patient had a birth weight below the tenth percentile and had been admitted to a neonatal unit or whether or not the patient had epilepsy. Other studies have found rather lower recurrence risks for nonspecific mental retardation, in the region of 5%, the risk not varying substantially by level of retardation if there is no known cause (Herbst & Baird, 1982; Turner, Collins, & Turner, 1971). These findings are relatively uninformative on whether the mediation is genetic or environmental (the increased risk from having a retarded uncle or aunt suggests the former but only weakly so in the absence of detailed information on parental qualities). Also, they should be taken as only a very approximate guide for genetic counselling in view of the crudity of the figures, the variations among studies, and their reliance on ascertainment validity.

Reed and Rich (1982) reanalyzed the Reed and Reed (1965) data, examining the size of the parent–offspring regression coefficient according to the extent to which the parental IQ was above below the mean. They found that the coefficient was greatest when the parental IQ was more than two standard deviations below the mean. Vogler and DeFries (1983) found a trend in the same direction using general population data but only when using the same groupings as Reed and Rich (i.e., with a focus on retardation in the parents rather than variations within the normal range). These findings support the idea of greater familiality, or familial recurrence, in mild rather than severe retardation.

TWIN STUDIES

The only twin studies of mild mental retardation as such involve samples that are too selective or too small for reliable quantification of genetic and environmental influences (Nichols, 1984; Rosanoff, Handy, & Plesset, 1937; Wilson & Matheny, 1976). There have been, however, a number of twin studies that have sought to determine whether heritability is higher or lower at the bottom of the IQ range (Bailey & Horn, 1986; Bailey & Revelle, 1990; Cherny, Cardon, Fulker, & DeFries, 1992; Detterman, Thompson, & Plomin, 1989; Saudino, Plomin, Pedersen, & McClearn, 1994; Thompson, Detterman, & Plomin, 1993). The findings are extremely contradictory and allow of no firm conclusions. The samples vary greatly in age, from infancy (Cherny et al., 1992) to old age (Saudino et al., 1994), the statistical techniques used rely on the assumption of normality of IQ score distribution, and in most studies there were too few subjects with an IQ below 70 for any inferences to be drawn about mental retardation. It cannot be assumed that an IQ in the 70–85 range is equivalent to an IQ below 70. Clearly there is a great need for a systematic large scale twin study of mildly retarded individuals.

The point of such a study, of course, would not lie in determining whether heritability is higher or lower at the bottom of the IQ range. Rather, the objective would be to obtain a better understanding of the mechanisms involved in the causation of mental retardation. There are six main issues requiring investigation. First, it is well established that obstetric and perinatal complications are much more frequent in the histories of mentally retarded children (Hagberg, Hagberg, Lewerth, & Lindberg, 1981b; Rao, 1990; Rutter et al., 1970). Because brain imaging studies of very low birth weight babies have shown the occurrence of periventricular ischaemia and bleeding, and because these abnormalities have been found to predict later cognitive impairment (Casaer, de Vries, & Marlow, 1991; Reynolds, in press), it is quite possible that obstetric complications represent an environmental influence that is more important with respect to mild retardation than to variations within the normal range. Although to some extent this is likely, many of the reported complications have an uncertain associations with biological risk (and do not seem to be associated with differences in recurrence risk; Bundey et al., 1989), some complications reflect a response to an abnormal foetus (Bolton & Holland, 1994), and a genetically informative design is required to test the environmental risk hypothesis. It should be added that one longitudinal study (McDermott, Coker, & McKeown, 1993) found that the associations between low birth weight and mild mental retardation were greater in younger children, and also varied with ethnicity.

Second, all studies have shown the much increased frequency with which mildly retarded children come from severely socially disadvantaged families (Birch et al., 1970; Hagberg et al., 1981a, 1981b; Rao, 1990; Rutter et al., 1970). This could represent a more important environmental risk factor than variations in social background within the middle of the normal range (see Capron & Duyme, 1989). Furthermore, the mechanisms of environmental risk may be complex; for example, low birth weight is associated with social disadvantage (Read & Stanley, 1993).

Third, it could be that genetically influenced parental mental retardation is a major cause of suboptimal rearing conditions (Keltner, 1994). Perhaps surprisingly, parental IQ is not the main feature accounting for family influences on cognitive development (see Plomin, 1995), but the situation might be very different when dealing with the lower extremes of parental IQ. Relatively little is known on qualities of the rearing environment provided by retarded parents (see Dowdney & Skuse, 1993; Tymchuk, 1992). Genetic designs examining effects on both IQ means and variance in the offspring are needed to determine the risk processes involved. In that connection it is relevant that the frequency with which the parents of mildly retarded children are both of low IQ and of low social status with associated adversities in rearing (Lamont & Dennis, 1988; Reed & Reed, 1965) may have divergent effects on means and variances. If there is reduced environmental variation, as is implied, this would lead to increased heritability estimates but also to a greater negative effect on the levels of cognitive functioning in the children. Thus, in the Milwaukee study of disadvantaged slum children, a cumulative deficit in IQ was seen only in children whose mothers had an IQ < 80 (Heber, Dever, & Conry, 1968).

Fourth, although gene–environment interactions in relation to IQ have not been evident in the normal range (see Plomin et al., 1988), they may be more important in the mental retardation range. Individual differences in response to specific environmental hazards are usual (see Rutter & Pickles, 1991) and it has been suggested that biologically damaged children may be more likely to be adversely affected by poor rearing conditions (Sameroff & Chandler, 1975). The same could apply to children who are at risk genetically.

Fifth, it is clear that in the general population as a whole, there is some tendency for people to marry someone of similar intellectual level. It may well be that this tendency for assortative mating is greater at the lower end of the IQ range, although data are lacking on this point. If so, however, it will have two consequences. First, it will lead to an artefactual underestimate of heritability in twin studies (see Rutter et al., 1990; Simonoff et al., 1994). Second, it might also lead to a greater environmental risk because each parent may be less able to compensate for limitations in the other. An extended twin plus family design with measures of the observed environment and calculation of risk ratios, as well as within-pair concordance and correlations, is needed to assess these rather different effects.

Finally, there is the balance between shared and nonshared environmental effects. In general, research findings show that shared effects on cognitive performance markedly fade in importance as children grow older, with nonshared effects increasing (Plomin, 1986). The mechanisms involved in this transition, however, remain ill-understood, and it is not known whether the same pattern applies to mild mental retardation. The transition presumably comes about because individual IQ levels change with age, because the relative importance of different specific skills for overall IQ also alters with age, and because children come to exert a greater effect on their interactions with other people. It remains to be determined, however, whether these age-related shifts apply in the same way to mentally retarded children.

MOLECULAR GENETIC STUDIES

Up to now, molecular genetic research has been mainly directed at single gene disorders but it can be applied to the study of multiple genes as they operate in multifactorial intelligence-so-called quantitative trait loci (QTL) (Plomin et al., 1994). The value of identifying QTL lies in the potential for understanding genetic risk processes and the mechanisms involved in the interplay between nature and nurture (gene–environment correlations and interactions). Because it is unlikely that any one gene will account for more than a very small amount of population variance, however, genetic markers will not be useful for identifying children at risk for mental retardation. It is important that this be appreciated in view of the important ethical concerns regarding the possible misuses of genetic findings for discriminatory practices.

INVESTIGATION OF MENTALLY RETARDED INDIVIDUALS

It is clear from the frequency with which medical conditions due to a genetic abnormality play a role in mental retardation, both mild and severe, that any adequate clinical assessment must include a systematic medical screening for such disorders. Bailey (1994) and Scott (1994) have outlined what is needed in that connection. Thus, for example, a careful medical history, combined with systematic physical inspection and testing, is essential. Inspection is crucial because an abnormal physical appearance is often most striking at the first encounter and may be diagnostic (as with Down syndrome) or at least highly suggestive (as with Williams syndrome, fragile X, PWS and AS; see Flint & Yule, 1994). The skin should be examined, using a Wood's light, for the depigmented macules that are diagnostic of tuberose sclerosis, attention should be paid to congenital anomalies and the head circumference should be measured.

Because of its importance in relation to recurrence risk for nonpathological (i.e., idiopathic and presumably multifactorial) varieties of mental retardation, a family history for both first and second degree relatives (plus cousins) should always be taken with respect to general and specific learning difficulties. A history of such difficulties is also clearly helpful in relation to recessive Mendelizing disorders and conditions such as the fragile-X anomaly.

Because some of the Mendelizing metabolic disorders are associated with severe retardation, possibly it is prudent to undertake a metabolic screen (using blood and urine samples). However, in the absence of pointers in the medical history and examination, very few such conditions are detected on a screen (McClaren & Bryson, 1987; Scott, 1994). Chromosomal examination, including the use of molecular genetic techniques to detect the fragile-X anomaly, should also be a routine in view of the frequency of their occurrence and the fact that most are not associated with any strongly diagnostic clinical characteristics. It is important to remember that fragile X is as common in mild as severe retardation, and that it affects girls almost as frequently as boys.

A somewhat more uncertain issue is whether or not to undertake karyotyping in mildly retarded children without dysmorphic features. Graham and Selikowitz (1993) found chromosomal anomalies in 4% of all children referred for developmental delay of unknown origin; the rate was 20% in those with dysmorphic features and higher in those with general retardation (5%) than in those with a specific delay (2%). Probably the pick-up rate even with the lowest risk group is sufficient to warrant routine testing on the grounds that a specific diagnosis is helpful for the individual and in some cases has implications for the family.

GENETIC SCREENING

Population Screening

Once a gene defect is identifiable at the DNA level, genetic screening for carriers, and for individuals who will develop diseases at a later age, becomes possible either for the general population or for high risk groups. At first sight that sounds a thoroughly worthwhile endeavour on the grounds that increased knowledge about specific genetic risks for individuals is bound to be helpful. Experience with disorders where that is case, however, indicates the need for caution. There is the practical problem of detection rates below 100%, as will be the case with multiple mutations (see, for example, cystic fibrosis where there are >300 mutations, the frequencies varying by ethnic group; Gilbert, 1994). Also, there is the potential problem of stigmatization of identified carriers, a major issue with recessive genes or susceptibility genes (for multifactorial disorders) that are carried by a high proportion of the population (see Gilbert, 1994; Garver & Garver, 1994; Parker, 1994). In addition, there are the ethical issues associated with loss of patient autonomy, and with the difficulties implicit in the fact that the findings on one individual will have implications for other family members who may not wish to know. Experience with diseases such as Huntington's disease and cystic fibrosis where genetic screening is possible indicates that only a minority of people for whom tests are relevant take up the option. Also, it is important to note that evidence that a person does *not* carry the gene in question is not necessarily as reassuring as one might think. Nevertheless, genetic screening is potentially very helpful in enabling people to plan their lives, and to take more rational decisions about having children. At present, the most common condition giving rise to mental retardation for which genetic screening is currently available is fragile X; however, guidelines from the American College of Medical Genetics have recommended that population screening *not* be implemented at the present time, for many of the reasons given above (Howard-Peebles et al., 1994; Pick, Howard-Pebbles, Sherman, Taylor & Wulfsberg, 1994).

PRENATAL SCREENING

Prenatal screening constitutes a particular form of genetic screening that involves its own set of issues (Brock, Rodeck, & Ferguson-Smith, 1992). Traditionally it has been used to determine whether a foetus has some genetic abnormality (such as Down syndrome) giving rise to a seriously handicapping condition, so that parents may decide whether or not to proceed with the pregnancy. Thus, ultrasound scanning can detect many conditions associated with physical defects, maternal alpha-feto-protein levels may be helpful in indicating the level of risk (and hence the desirability of direct tests—Garver, 1989), and both amniocentesis (ordinariy performed at 12–16 weeks) and chorionic villus sampling (CVS) (ordinarily performed at 10–12 weeks) allow prenatal diagnosis of chromosomal abnormalities and genetic diseases identifiable at the DNA level. CVS has the advantage of earlier diagnosis but somewhat greater problems of interpretation, especially when there is mosaicism (Smidt-Jensen et al., 1993). At first, CVS was undertaken by the transcervical route but increasingly transabdominal sampling is being used because it may involve a lower risk of fetal loss as well as being technically easier (Smidt-Jensen et al., 1992), although not all trials have shown a difference between the two methods (Jackson et al., 1992).

In recent years, two different techniques, still at the experimental stage, have become available for prenatal diagnosis. First, there is the examination of fetal cells in maternal blood (Adinolf, 1992) which has the advantage of being noninvasive. It provides a rapid method of karyotyping but at present its rather low sensitivity makes it appropriate only for low-risk screening (Evans et al., 1994). However, specificity of detection of foetal cells is improving (Bianchi et al., 1993) and both biochemical and molecular techniques can be used to detect abnormalities (Porstmann et al., 1991). Second, there is the biopsy of foetal cells at the primitive blastocyte stage, using eggs flushed out of the uterus (Edwards, 1993; Verlinsky, & Kuliev, 1993). This carries the potential advantage of allowing healthy blastocytes to be replaced in the womb, but many uncertainties remain over its utility.

It is clear that the next decade is going to see substantial advances in genetic screening. These will allow much greater precision in genetic counselling but this increase in power carries with it the need for careful concern regarding both ethical issues and psychological consequences. At present, technology for genetic screening is advancing more rapidly than the ethical and practical guidelines for its use. Work in this latter area is essential (Shapiro, 1994). In that connection, there is a fundamental difference between using genetic information to get rid of illness and altering people to promote desired (or get rid of undesired) personal characteristics (Sutton, 1995).

GENETIC COUNSELLING

As with prenatal screening, all too often genetic counselling has been viewed as a procedure designed to enable people to decide when to abort. As Pembrey (1991) emphasized, this constitutes a fundamental misunderstanding of the objectives, which are to provide individuals with an understanding of the risks so that they may decide for themselves what to do. This includes providing an appreciation of the *low* level of absolute risk when that is the case, and information on the possibility of remediation when that is possible. (For a fuller discussion, see Harper, 1994, or Skinner, 1990.) At present, the latter is rarely possible but, with the advent of gene therapy, the potential may be greater in the future.

Counselling is most straightforward in the case of Mendelizing disorders for which risks follow well understood patterns, and even more so in those for whom carrier status can be established using DNA methods. But even here, complications are introduced if there is linkage heterogeneity (as with spinal muscular atrophy) or incomplete penetrance (i.e., possession of the abnormal gene only sometimes gives rise to the disease phenotype). In these circumstances, calculations of confidence or support intervals (Leal & Ott, 1994) may be helpful in determining the degree of certainty obtainable on risk probabilities. The situation is most uncertain with multifactorial conditions even when they involve a strong genetic component (as with autism). Counselling needs to involve helping people to understand how the presence in one child of a condition that is strongly genetic may carry a low absolute risk of recurrence (because of its rarity and the need for involvement of several genes), even if that risk is greatly increased relative to the general population. In some disorders, such as autism, the phenotype in affected individuals is very variable, as are the implications for degree of handicap. For these reasons, counsellors need to have a good understanding of the clinical conditions involved, as well as of the genetics. Of course, the situation would become much more straightforward if there were unambiguous tests for the disorder (most needed in relation to the milder forms of expression) and, even more so, by the possibility of DNA diagnosis of carrier status. Advances in the next decade may well make both possible for a greater range of multifactorial disorders but, so far, possibilities are quite limited.

CONCLUSIONS

Genetic influences are important in both mild and severe mental retardation. The nature of these influences are extremely diverse and cover the full range of genetic mechanisms that are currently known. In the past decade, there has been a rapid growth in our understanding of the genetic mechanisms underlying a number of conditions associated with severe retardation, such as the fragile-X syndrome and the PWS/AS. We can expect further expansion of our knowledge in the coming decade. Despite this, the biological mechanisms by which impaired intellect occurs are poorly understood in virtually all cases. Identification of abnormal genes, or genes involving an increased risk for particular disorders, is invaluable for genetic screening and counselling, but it does little in itself to specify new, more effective and targeted modes of treatment for mental retardation. One of the challenges of the coming decades will be to translate knowledge of genetic defects into an understanding of the effects on the nervous system and the ways in which intellectual retardation is caused.

The picture is less clear in idiopathic mild mental retardation where there is a dearth of systematic genetic research. Whereas the scanty evidence available suggests that genetic effects are important, the genes involved have not been specified. There is a strong relationship between mild mental retardation and psychosocial disadvantage that needs further work to disentangle. Behaviour genetic designs employing direct measures of relevant aspects of the environment will be essential in this task. Such research may contribute an important way to targeting interventions.

REFERENCES

Adinolf, M. (1992). Breaking the blood barrier. *Nature Genetics, 1*, 316–318.

Akefeldt, A., Gillberg, C., & Larsson, C. (1991). Prader–Willi syndrome in a Swedish rural county: Epidemiological aspects. *Developmental Medicine and Child Neurology, 33*, 715–721.

Anastasi, A. (1972). Four hypotheses with a dearth of data. Response to Lehrke's "A theory of X-linkage of major intellectual traits." *American Journal of Mental Deficiency, 76*, 620–622.

Angelman, H. (1965). 'Puppet children': A report of three cases. *Developmental Medicine and Child Neurology, 7*, 681–688.

Bailey, A. (1994). Physical examination and medical investigations. In M. Rutter, E. Taylor, & L. Hersov (Eds.), *Child and adolescent psychiatry: Modern approaches* (3rd ed., pp. 79–93). Oxford: Blackwell Scientific.

Bailey, A., Bolton, P., Butler, L., LeCouteur, A., Murphy, M., Scott, S., Webb, T., & Rutter, M. (1993). Prevalence of the fragile X anomaly amongst autistic twins and singletons. *Journal of Child Psychology and Psychiatry, 34*, 673–688.

Bailey, A., LeCouteur, A., Gottesman, I., Bolton, P., Simonoff, E., Yuzda, E., & Rutter, M. (1995). Autism as a strongly genetic disorder: Evidence from a British twin study. *Psychological Medicine, 25*, 63–77.

Bailey, A. J., Phillips, W., & Rutter, M. (1996). Autism: Towards an integration of clinical, genetic, neuropsychological and neurobiological perspectives. *Journal of Child Psychology and Psychiatry, 37*, 89–126.

Bailey, J. M., & Horn, J. M. (1986). A source of variance in IQ unique to the lower-scoring monozygotic (MZ) cotwin. *Behavior Genetics, 16*, 509–516.

Bailey, J. M., & Revelle, W. (1990). Increased heritability for lower IQ levels? *Behavior Genetics, 21*, 397–404.

Baird, P. A., & Sadovnick, A. D. (1989). Life tables for Down syndrome. *Human Genetics, 82*, 291.

Baron-Cohen, S., Tager-Flusberg, H., & Cohen, D. J. (Eds.). (1993). *Understanding other minds: Perspectives from autism*. Oxford: Oxford University Press.

Bell, J. A., Pearn, J. H., & Firnan, D. (1989). Childhood deaths in Down's syndrome: Survival curves and causes of death from a population study in Queensland, Australia. *Journal of Medical Genetics, 26*, 764–768.

Bianchi, D. W., Zickwolf, G. K., Yih, M. C., Flint, A. F., Geifman, O. H., Erikson, M. S., & Williams, J. M. (1993). Erythroid-specific antibodies enhance detection of fetal nucleated erythrocytes in maternal blood. *Prenatal Diagnosis, 13*, 293–300.

Birch, H. G., Richardson, S. A., Baird, D., Horobin, G., & Illsley, R. (1970). *Mental subnormality in the community: A clinical and epidemiological study*. Baltimore: Williams and Wilkins.

Blackie, J., Forrest, A., & Witcher, G. (1975). Subcultural mental handicap. *British Journal of Psychiatry, 127,* 335–339.

Blum-Hoffman, E., Rehder, H., & Langenbeck, U. (1987). Skeletal abnormalities in trisomy 21 as an example of amplified developmental instability in chromosomal disorders: A histological study of 21 mid-trimester fetuses with trisomy 21. *American Journal of Medical Genetics, 29,* 155–160.

Bolton, P., & Holland, A. (1994). Chromosomal abnormalities. In M. Rutter, E. Taylor, & L. Hersov (Eds.), *Child and adolescent psychiatry: Modern approaches* (3rd ed., pp. 152–171). Oxford: Blackwell Scientific Publications.

Bolton, P., Macdonald, H., Pickles, A., Rios, P., Goode, S., Crowson, M., Bailey, A., & Rutter, M. (1994). A case-control family history study of autism. *Journal of Child Psychology and Psychiatry, 35,* 877–900.

Borthwick-Duffy, S. A. (1994). Epidemiology and prevalence of psychopathology in people with mental retardation. *Journal of Consulting and Clinical Psychology, 62,* 17–27.

Bregman, J. D. (1991). Current developments in the understanding of mental retardation. Part II. Psychopathology. *Journal of the American Academy of Child and Adolescent Psychiatry, 30,* 861–872.

Bregman, J. D., & Hodapp, R. M. (1991). Current developments in the understanding of mental retardation. Part I: Biological and phenomenological perspectives. *Journal of the American Academy of Child and Adolescent Psychiatry, 30,* 707–719.

Brock, D. J. H. (1993). *Molecular genetics for the clinician.* Cambridge: Cambridge University Press.

Brock, D. J. H., Rodeck, C. H., & Ferguson-Smith, M. A. (1992). *Prenatal diagnosis and screening.* Edinburgh: Churchill-Livingstone.

Bundey, S., Thake, A., & Todd, J. (1989). The recurrence risk for mild idiopathic mental retardation. *Journal of Medical Genetics, 26,* 260–266.

Burack, J. A. (1990). Differentiating mental retardation: The two-group approach and beyond. In R. M. Hodapp, J. A. Burack, & E. Zigler (Eds.), *Issues in the developmental approach to mental retardation* (pp. 27–48). Cambridge: Cambridge University Press.

Burd, L., Vesely, B., Martsolf, J., & Kerbeshian, J. (1990). Prevalence study of Prader–Willi syndrome in North Dakota. *American Journal of Medical Genetics, 37,* 97–99.

Butler, M. G. (1990). Prader–Willi syndrome: Current understanding of cause and diagnosis. *American Journal of Medical Genetics, 35,* 319–332.

Butler, M. G., Meaney, F. J., & Palmer, C. G. (1986). Clinical and cytogenetic survey of 39 individuals with Prader–Lambert–Willi syndrome. *American Journal of Medical Genetics, 23,* 793–809.

Campbell, F. A., & Ramey, C. T. (1994). Effects of early intervention on intellectual and academic achievement: A follow-up study of children from low-income families. *Child Development, 65,* 684–698.

Capron, C., & Duyme, M. (1989). Assessment of the effects of socioeconomic status on IQ in a full cross-fostering study. *Nature, 340,* 552–554.

Cardon, L. R., & Fulker, D. W. (1993). Genetics of specific cognitive abilities. In R. Plomin & G. E. McClearn (Eds.), *Nature, nurture and psychology* (pp. 99–120). Washington, DC: American Psychological Association.

Casaer, P., de Vries, L., & Marlow, N. (1991). Prenatal and perinatal risk factors for psychosocial development. In M. Rutter & P. Casaer (Eds.), *Biological risk factors for psychosocial disorders* (pp. 139–174). Cambridge: Cambridge University Press.

Cassidy, S. B., Lai, L. W., Erickson, R. P., Magnuson, L., Thomas, E., Gendron, R., & Herrmann, J. (1992). Trisomy 15 with loss of the paternal 15 as a cause of Prader–Willi syndrome due to maternal disomy. *American Journal of Human Genetics, 51,* 701–708.

Chan, C. T., Clayton-Smith, J., Chang, X. J., Buston, J., Webb, T., & Pembrey, M. E. (1993). Molecular mechanisms in Angelman syndrome: A survey of 93 patients. *Journal of Medical Genetics, 30,* 895–902.

de la Chapelle, A. (1990). Sex chromosome abnormalities. In A. E. H. Emery & D. L. Rimoin (Eds.), *Principles and practice of medical genetics* (pp. 273–300). Edinburgh: Churchill-Livingstone.

Chen, H., Chrast, R., Rossier, C., Gos, A., Antonarakis, S. E., Kudoh, J., Yamaki, A., Shindoh, N., Maeda, H., Minoshima, S., & Shimizu, N. (1995). Single-minded and Down Syndrome? *Nature Genetics, 10,* 9–10.

Cherny, S. S., Cardon, L. R., Fulker, D. W., & DeFries, J. C. (1992). Differential heritability across levels of cognitive ability. *Behavior Genetics, 22*, 153–162.

Crick, F. (1988). *What mad pursuit: A personal view of scientific discovery.* New York: Basic Books.

Cristiano, R. J., Smith, L. C., & Woo, S. L. (1993). Hepatic gene therapy: Adenovirus enhancement of receptor-mediated gene delivery. *Proceedings of the National Academy of Science (U.S.A.), 90*, 2122–2126.

Crome, L. (1960). The brain and mental retardation. *British Medical Journal, 1*, 897.

Daniels, J. K., Owen, M. J., McGuffin, P., Thompson, L., Determan, D. K., Chorney, M., Chorney, K., Smith, D., Skuder, P., Vignetti, S., McClearn, G. E., & Plomin, R. (1994). IQ and variation in the number of fragile X CGG repeats: No association in a normal sample. *Intelligence, 19*, 45–50.

DeBoulle, K., Verkerk, A. J. M. H., Reyniers, E., Vits, L., Hendrickx, J., Van Roy, B., Van Den Bos, F., de Graaff, E., Oostra, B. A., & Willems, P. J. (1993). A point mutation in the FMR-1 gene associated with fragile X mental retardation. *Nature Genetics, 3*, 31–35.

DeFries, J. C., Plomin, R., & LaBuda, M. C. (1987). Genetic stability of cognitive development from childhood to adulthood. *Developmental Psychology, 23*, 4–12.

Determan, D. K., Thompson, L. A., & Plomin, R. (1989). Differences in heritability across groups differing in ability. *Behavior Genetics, 20*, 369–384.

Devys, S., Lutz, Y., Rouyer, N., Belloeq, J.-P., & Mandel, J.-L. (1993). The FMR-1 protein is cytoplasmic, most abundant in neurons and appears normal in carriers of a fragile X premutation. *Nature Genetics, 4*, 335–340.

DiLella, A., & Woo, S. L. C. (1987). Molecular basis of phenylketonuria and its clinical applications. *Molecular Biology and Medicine, 4*, 183–192.

Dobson, J. C., Williamson, M. L., Azen, C., & Koch, R. (1977). Intellectual assessment of 111 four year old children with phenylketonuria. *Pediatrics, 60*, 822–827.

Dowdney, L., & Skuse, D. (1993). Parenting provided by adults with mental retardation. *Journal of Child Psychology and Psychiatry, 34*, 25–48.

Dykens, E. M. (1995). Measuring behavioral phenotypes: Provocations from the 'new genetics'. *American Journal of Mental Retardation, 99*, 522–532.

Edwards, R. G. (1993). *Preconception and preimplantation diagnosis of human genetic disease.* Cambridge: Cambridge University Press.

Einfeld, S. L. (1984). Clinical assessment of 4500 developmentally delayed individuals. *Journal of Mental Deficiency Research, 28*, 129–142.

Eisensmith, R. C., Okano, Y., Dasovich, M., Wang, T., Guttler, F., Lou, H., Guldberg, P., Lichter-Konecki, U., Konecki, D. S., Svensson, E., Hagenfeldt, L., Rey, F., Munnich, A., Lyonnet, S., Cockburn, F., Conner, J. M., Pembrey, M. E., Smith, I., Gitzelmann, R., Steinmann, B., Apold, J., Eiken, H. G., Giovannini, M., Riva, E., Longhi, R., Romano, C., Cerone, R., Naughten, E. R., Mullings, C., Cahalane, S., Ozalp, I., Fekete, G., Schuler, D., Berencsi, G. Y., Nasz, I., Brdicka, R., Kamaryt, J., Pijackova, A., Cabalska, B., Boszkowa, K., Schwartz, E., Kalinin, V. N., Jin, L., Charkroaborty, R., & Woo, S. L. C. (1992). Multiple origins for phenylketonuria in Europe. *American Journal of Human Genetics, 51*, 1355–1365.

Epstein, C. J. (1986). *The consequences of chromosomal imbalance: Problems, mechanisms and models.* Cambridge: Cambridge University Press.

Epstein, C. J. (1990). The consequences of chromosomal imbalance. *American Journal of Medical Genetics, 7*, 31–37(suppl.).

Evans, M. I., Ebrahim, S. A., Berry, S. M., Holzgreve, W., Isada, N. B., Quintero, R. A., & Johnson, M. P. (1994). Fluorescent in situ hybridization utilization for high-risk prenatal diagnosis: A trade-off. *American Journal of Obstetrics and Gynaecology, 171*, 1055–1057.

Feng, Y., Lakkis, L., Devys, D., & Warren, S. T. (1995). Quantitative comparison of FMRI gene expression in normal and premutation alleles. *American Journal of Human Genetics, 56*, 106–113.

Fisch, G. S., Snow, K., Thibodeau, S. N., Chalifaux, M., Holden, J. J. A., Nelson, D. L., Howard-Peebles, P. M., & Maddalena, A. (1995). The fragile X premutation in carriers and its effect on mutation size in offspring. *American Journal of Human Genetics, 56*, 1147–1155.

Flint, J., Wilkie, A. O. M., Buckle, V. J., Winter, R. M., Holland, A. J., & McDermid, H. E. (1995). The detection of subtelomeric chromosomal rearrangements in idiopathic mental retardation. *Nature Genetics, 9,* 132–139.

Flint, J., & Yule, W. (1994). Behavioural phenotypes. In M. Rutter, E. Taylor, & L. Hersov (Eds.), *Child and adolescent psychiatry: Modern approaches* (3rd ed., pp. 666–687). Oxford: Blackwell Scientific.

Flynn, G. A., Hirst, M. C., Knight, S. J. L., Macpherson, J. N., Barber, J. C. K., Flannery, A. V., Davies, K. E., & Buckle, V. J. (1993). Identification of the FRAXE fragile site in two families ascertained for X-linked mental retardation. *Journal of Medical Genetics, 30,* 97–100.

Folstein, S., & Rutter, M. (1988). Autism: Familial aggregation and genetic implications. *Journal of Autism and Developmental Disorders, 18,* 3–30.

Fu, Y.-H., Kuhl, D. P. A., Pizzuti, A., Pieretti, M., Sutcliffe, J. S., Richards, S., Verkerk, A. J. M. H., Holden, J. J. A., Fenwick, R. G., Warren, S. T., Oostra, B. A., Nelson, D. L., & Caskey, C. T. (1992). Variation of the CGG repeat at the fragile X site results in genetic instability: Resolution of the Sherman paradox. *Cell, 67,* 1047–1058.

Garver, K. L. (1989). Update on MSAFP policy statement from the American Society of Human Genetics. *American Journal of Human Genetics, 45,* 332–334.

Garver, K. L., & Garver, B. (1994). The human genome project and eugenic concerns. *American Journal of Human Genetics, 54,* 148–158.

Gedeon, A. K., Baker, E., Robinson, H., Partington, M. W., Gross, B., Korn, B., Poustka, A., Yu, S., Sutherland, G. R., & Mulley, J. C. (1992). Fragile X sydrome without CGG amplification has an FMR-1 deletion. *Nature Genetics, 1,* 341–344.

Gibbons, R. J., Picketts, D. J., Villard, L., & Higgs, D. R. (1995). Mutations in a putative global transcriptional regulator cause X-linked mental retardation with alphathalassemia (ATR-X syndrome). *Cell, 80,* 837–845.

Gilbert, F. (1994). Cystic fibrosis carrier screening: Comparability of data and uniformity of testing. *American Journal of Human Genetics, 54,* 925–927.

Giraud, F., Aymes, S., & Mattei, M. G. (1976). Constitutional chromosome breakage. *Human Genetics, 34,* 125–136.

Glass, I. A. (1991). X-linked mental retardation. *Journal of Medical Genetics, 28,* 361–371.

Gleason, L. A., Michals, K., Matalon, R., Langenberg, P., & Kamath, S. (1992). A treatment program for adolescents with phenylketonuria. *Clinical Pediatrics (Philadelphia), 31,* 331–335.

Goldsmith, H. H., & Gottesman, I. I. (1995). Heritable variability and variable heritability in developmental psychopathology. In M. F. Lenzenweger & J. Haugaard (Eds.), *Frontiers of developmental psychopathology.* New York: Oxford University Press.

Goodman, R., Simonoff, E., & Stevenson, J. (1995). The relationship of child IQ, parental IQ and sibling IQ to child behavioural deviance scores. *Journal of Child Psychology and Psychiatry, 36,* 409–425.

Graham, S. M., & Selikowitz, M. (1993). Chromosome testing in children with developmental delay in whom the aetiology is not evident clinically. *Journal of Paediatrics and Child Health, 29,* 360–362.

Grantham-McGregor, S., Powell, C., Walker, S., Chang, S., & Fletcher, P. (1994). The long-term follow-up of severely malnourished children who participated in an intervention program. *Child Development, 65,* 428–439.

de Grouchy, J., & Turleau, C. (1990). Autosomal disorders. In A. E. H. Emery & D. L. Rimoin (Eds.), *Principles and practice of medical genetics* (pp. 247–272). Edinburgh: Churchill-Livingstone.

Gunter, F., Ledley, F. D., Lidsky, A. S., DiLella, A. G., Sullivan, S. E., & Woo, S. L. C. (1987). Correlation between polymorphic DNA haplotypes at the phenylalanine hydroxylase locus and clinical phenotype of phenylketonuria. *Journal of Pediatrics, 110,* 68–71.

Gustavson, K. H., Holmgren, R., Jonsell, R., & Son Blomquist, H. K. (1977). Severe mental retardation in children in a northern Swedish county. *Journal of Mental Deficiency Research, 21,* 161–180.

Guthrie, R., & Susi, A. (1963). A simple phenylalanine method for determining phenylketonuria in large populations of newborn infants. *Pediatrics, 32,* 338–343.

Hagberg, B., Hagberg, G., Lewerth, A., & Lindberg, U. (1981a). Mild mental retardation in Swedish school children. I. Prevalence. *Acta Paediatrica Scandinavica, 70*, 441–444.

Hagberg, B., Hagberg, G., Lewerth, A., & Lindberg, U. (1981b). Mild mental retardation in Swedish school children. II. Etiological and pathogenetic aspects. *Acta Paediatrica Scandinavica, 70*, 445–452.

Hagerman, R. J., Hull, C. E., Safanda, J. F., Carpenter, I., Staley, L. W., O'Connor, R. A., Seydel, C., Mazzocco, M. M., Snow, K., & Thibodeau, S. N. (1994). High functioning fragile X males: Demonstration of an unmethylated fully expanded FMR-1 mutation associated with protein expression. *American Journal of Medical Genetics, 51*, 298–308.

Hall, J. G. (1990). Genomic imprinting: Review and relevance to human disease. *American Journal of Human Genetics, 46*, 857–873.

Hamel, B. C., Smits, A. P., de-Graaff, E., Smeets, D. F., Schoute, F., Eussen, B. H., Knight, S. J., Davies, K. E., Assman-Hulsmans, C. F., & Oostra, B. A. (1994). Segregation of FRAXE in a large family: Clinical, psychometric, cytogenetic, and molecular data. *American Journal of Human Genetics, 55*, 923–931.

Hamerton, J. L., Canning, N., Ray, M., & Smith, S. (1975). A cytogenetic survey of 14,069 newborn infants I: Incidence of chromosomal abnormalities. *Clinical Genetics, 8*, 223–243.

Harper, P. S. (1994). *Practical genetic counselling* (4th ed.). Oxford: Butterworth-Heinemann.

Harvey, J., Judge, C., & Wiener, S. (1977). Familial X-linked retardation with an X chromosome abnormality. *Journal of Medical Genetics, 14*, 46–50.

Haspeslagh, M., Fryns, J. P., Holvoet, M., Collen, G., Dierck, G., & Baeke, J. B. H. (1991). A clinical, cytogenetic and familial study of 307 mentally retarded, institutionalized adult male patients with special interest for fra(X) negative X-linked mental retardation. *Clinical Genetics, 39*, 434–441.

Heber, R., Dever, R., & Conry, J. (1968). The influence of environmental and genetic variables on intellectual development. In J. Prehm, L. A. Hamerlynck, & J. E. Crosson (Eds.), *Behavioural research in mental retardation*. Eugene, Oregon: University of Oregon School of Education.

Herbst, D. S., & Baird, P. A. (1982). Sib risks for nonspecific mental retardation in British Columbia. *American Journal of Medical Genetics, 13*, 197–208.

Hirst, M. C., Barnicoat, A. A. B., Flynn, G., Wang, Q., Daker, W., Buckle, V. J., Davies, K. E., & Bobrow, M. (1993a). The identification of a third fragile site, FRAXF, in Xq27-q28 distal to both FRAXA and FRAXE. *Human Molecular Genetics, 2*, 197–200.

Hirst, M. C., Knight, S. J. L., Christodoulou, Z., Grewal, P. K., Fryns, J. P., & Davies, K. E. (1993b). Origins of the fragile X syndrome mutation. *Journal of Medical Genetics, 30*, 647–650.

Holtzman, N. A., Krommal, R. A., van Doornick, W., Azen, C., & Koch, R. (1986). Effects of age at loss of dietary control on intellectual performance and behaviour in children with phenylketonuria. *New England Journal of Medicine, 314*, 595–598.

Howard-Peebles, P. N., Maddalena, A., Spence, W. C., Levinson, G., Fallon, L., Bick, D. P., Black, S. H., & Schulman, J. D. (1994). Fragile X screening: What is the real issue? (letter). *American Journal of Medical Genetics, 53*, 382.

Huether, C. A., & Gummere, G. R. (1982). Influence of demographic factors on annual Down's syndrome birth in Ohio 1970–1979 and the United States 1920–1979. *American Journal of Epidemiology, 115*, 846–860.

Jacobs, P. A., Melville, M., Ratcliffe, S., Keay, A. J., & Syme, J. (1974). A cytogenetic survey of 11,680 newborn infants. *Annals of Human Genetics, 37*, 359–376.

Jackson, L. G., Zachary, J. M., Fowler, S. E., Desnick, R. J., Golbus, M. S., Ledbetter, D. H., Mahoney, M. J., Pergament, E., Simpson, J. L., Black, S., Wapner, R. J., & the U.S. National Institute of Child and Human Development Chorionic-Villus Sampling and Amniocentesis Study Group (1992). A randomized comparison of transcervical and transabdominal chorionic-villus sampling. *New England Journal of Medicine, 327*, 594–598.

Jensen, A. R. (1969). How much can we boost IQ and scholastic achievement? *Harvard Educational Review, 39*, 1–123.

Kahkonen, M., Alitalo, T., Airaksinen, E., Matilamen, R., Laumiala, K., Auno, S., & Leisti, J. (1987). Prevalence of fragile X syndrome in four birth cohorts of children of school age. *Human Genetics, 30*, 234–238.

Kamin, L. J. (1974). *The science and politics of IQ*. Potomac: Erlbaum.

Kaufman, S., Holtzman, N. Z., Milstien, S., Butler, I. J., & Krumholz, A. (1975). Phenylketonuria due to deficiency of dihydropteridine reductase. *New England Journal of Medicine, 293*, 782–790.

Keltner, B. (1994). Home environments of mothers with mental retardation. *Mental Retardation, 32*, 123–127.

Kendler, K. S. (1993). Twin studies of psychiatric illness: Current status and future directions. *Archives of General Psychiatry, 50*, 905–915.

Kieburtz, K., Macdonald, M., Shih, C., Feigin, A., Steinberg, K., Bordwell, K., Zimmerman, C., Jayalakshmi, S., Sotack, J., Gusella, J., & Shoulson, I. (1994). Trinucleotide repeat length and progression of illness in Huntington's Disease. *Journal of Medical Genetics, 31*, 872–874.

Koch, R., Azen, C., Freedman, E. G., & Williamson, M. L. (1984). Paired comparisons between early treated PKU children and their matched sibling controls on intelligence and school achievement test results at eight years of age. *Journal of Inherited Metabolic Disease, 7*, 86–90.

Koller, H., Richardson, S. A., Katz, M., & McLaren, J. (1982). Behavior disturbance in childhood and the early adult years in populations who were and were not mentally retarded. *Journal of Preventative Psychiatry, 1*, 453–468.

Krause, W., Halminski, M., McDonald, M., Donohue, P., Friedes, D., & Elsas, L. (1985). Biochemical and neuropsychological effects of elevated plasma phenylalanine in patients with treated phenylketonuria. *Journal of Clinical Investigation, 75*, 40–48.

Kumada, T. (1990). A clinical and cytogenetic study of institutionalized mental retardates. *Hiroshima Journal of Medical Sciences, 39*, 39–56.

Laird, C. (1987). Proposed mechanism of inheritance and expression of the human fragile X syndrome of mental retardation. *Genetics, 117*, 587–599.

Lamont, M. A., & Dennis, N. R. (1988). Aetiology of mild mental retardation. *Archives of Disease in Childhood, 63*, 1032–1038.

Leal, S. M., & Ott, J. (1994). A likelihood approach to calculating risk support intervals. *American Journal of Human Genetics, 54*, 913–917.

Ledbetter, D. H., Riccardi, V. M., Airhard, S. D., Strobel, R. J., Keenan, B. S., & Crawford, J. D. (1981). Deletion of chromosome 15 is a cause of the Prader–Willi syndrome. *New England Journal of Medicine, 304*, 325–329.

Ledley, F. D., Levy, H. L., & Woo, S. L. C. (1986). Molecular analysis of the inheritance of phenylketonuria and mild hyperphenyalanemia in families with both disorders. *New England Journal of Medicine, 314*, 1276–1280.

Lehrke, R. (1972). A theory of X linkage of major intellectual traits. *American Journal of Mental Deficiency, 76*, 611–619.

Lenke, R. R., & Levy, H. L. (1980). Maternal phenylketonuria and hyperphenylalanemia: An international survey of the outcome of treated and untreated pregnancies. *New England Journal of Medicine, 303*, 1202–1208.

Lever, A. M. L., & Goodfellow, P. (1995). Gene therapy. *British Medical Bulletin, 51*, 1–242.

Lewis, E. O. (1933). Types of mental deficiency and their social significance. *Journal of Mental Science, 79*, 293–304.

Lidsky, A. S., Robson, K. J. H., Thirumalachary, C., Barker, P. E., Ruddle, F. H., & Woo, S. L. C. (1984). The PKU locus in man is on chromosome 12. *American Journal of Human Genetics, 36*, 527–535.

Loehlin, J. C., & DeFries, J. C. (1987). Genotype–environment correlation and IQ. *Behavior Genetics, 18*, 263–278.

Loehlin, J. C., Horn, J. M., & Willerman, L. (1989). Modeling IQ change: Evidence from the Texas Adoption Project. *Chid Development, 60*, 993–1004.

Loehlin, J. C., Willerman, L., & Horn, J. (1988). Human behavior genetics. *Annual Review of Psychology, 33*, 101–133.

Loesch, D. Z., Higgins, R., Hay, D. A., Gedeon, A. K., Mulley, J. C., & Sutherland, G. R. (1993). Genotype-relationships in fragile X syndrome: A family study. *American Journal of Human Genetics, 53*, 1064–1073.

Lord, C., & Rutter, M. (1994). Autism and pervasive developmental disorders. In M. Rutter, E. Taylor, & L. Hersov (Eds.), *Child and adolescent psychiatry: Modern approaches* (3rd ed., pp. 569–593). Oxford: Blackwell Scientific.

Lubs, H. (1969). A marker X chromosome. *American Journal of Human Genetics, 21*, 231–244.

Magenis, R. E., Brown, M. G., Lacy, D. A., Budden, S., & LaFranchi, S. (1987). Is Angelman Syndrome an alternate result of del (15) (q11q13)? *American Journal of Medical Genetics, 28*, 829–838.

Magenis, R. E., Toth-Fejel, S., Allen, L. J., Black, M., Brown, M. G., Budden, S., Cohen, R., Friedman, J. M., Kalousek, D., Zonana, J., Lacy, D., Larranchi, S., Lahr, M., Macfarlane, J., & Williams, C. P. S. (1990). Comparisons of the 15q deletions in Prader–Willi and Angelman syndromes: Specific regions, extent of deletions, parental origin and clinical consequences. *American Journal of Medical Genetics, 35*, 333–349.

Mascari, M. J., Gottlieb, W., Rogan, P. K., Butler, M. G., Waller, D. A., Armour, J. A., Jeffreys, A. J., Ladda, R. L., & Nicholls, R. D. (1992). The frequency of uniparental disomy in Prader–Willi syndrome. Implications for molecular diagnosis. *New England Journal of Medicine, 326*, 1599–61507.

McCartney, H., & Bernieri, F. (1990). Growing up and growing apart: A developmental meta-analysis of twin studies. *Psychological Bulletin, 107*, 226–237.

McClaren, J., & Bryson, S. E. (1987). Review of recent epidemiological studies of mental retardation: Prevalence, associated disorders, and etiology. *American Journal of Mental Retardation, 92*, 243–254.

McDermott, S., Coker, A. L., & McKeown, R. E. (1993). Low birthweight and risk of mild mental retardation by ages 5 and 9 to 11. *Paediatric and Perinatal Epidemiology, 7*, 195–204.

McDonald, A. P. (1973). Severely retarded children in a Quebec province: Causes and care. *American Journal of Mental Deficiency, 70*, 205–215.

McGrother, C. W., & Marshall, B. (1990). Recent trends in incidence, morbidity and survival in Down's syndrome. *Journal of Mental Deficiency Research, 34*, 49–57.

McGue, M., Bouchard, Jr. T. J., Iacono, W. G., & Lykken, D. T. (1993). Behavioral genetics of cognitive ability: A life-span perspective. In R. Plomin & G. E. McClearn (Eds.), *Nature, nurture and psychology* (pp. 59–76). Washington, DC: American Psychological Association.

Mikkelsen, M. (1981). Epidemiology of trisomy 21: Population, peri and antenatal data. In G. R. Burgio, M. Fraccaro, L. Trepolo, & U. Wolf (Eds.), *Trisomy 21*. Berlin: Springer-Verlag.

Mikkelsen, M., Poulsen, H., Grimsted, J., & Lange, A. (1980). Non-disjunction in trisomy 21: Chromosomal heteromorphisms in 110 families. *Annals of Human Genetics, 44*, 17.

Moffitt, T. E., Caspi, A., Harkness, A. R., & Silva, P. A. (1993). The natural history of change in intellectual performance. Who changes? How much? Is it meaningful? *Journal of Child Psychology and Psychiatry, 34*, 455–506.

Morton, N. E., & MacPherson, J. N. (1992). Population genetics of the fragile-X syndrome: Multiallele model of the FMR1 locus. *Proceedings of the National Academy of Science (U.S.A.), 89*, 4215–4217.

Moser, H. W., Ramey, C. T., & Leonard, C. O. (1990). Mental retardation. In A. E. H. Emery & D. L. Rimoin (Eds.), *Principles and practice of medical genetics* (2nd ed., Vol. 1, pp. 495–511). Edinburgh: Churchill-Livingstone.

Mulley, J. C., Kerr, B., Stevenson, R., & Lubs, H. (1992a). Nomenclature guidelines for X-linked mental retardation. *American Journal of Medical Genetics, 43*, 383–391.

Mulley, J. C., Yu, S., Gedeon, A. K., Turner, G., Loesch, D., Chapman, C. J., Gardner, R. J. M., Richards, R. I., & Sutherland, G. R. (1992b). Experience with direct molecular diagnosis of fragile X. *Journal of Medical Genetics, 29*, 368–374.

Mulley, J. C., Yu, S., Loesch, D. Z., Hay, D. A., Donnelly, A., Gedeon, A. K., Carbonell, P., Lopez, I., Glover, G., Gabarron, I., Yu, P. W. L., Baker, E., Haan, E. A., Hockey, A., Knight, S. J. L., Davies, K. E., Richards, R. I., & Sutherland, G. R. (1995). FRAXE and mental retardation. *Journal of Medical Genetics, 31*, 162–169.

Neri, G., Chiurazzi, P., Arena, J. F., & Lubs, H. A. (1994). XLMR genes: Update 1994. *American Journal of Medical Genetics, 51*, 542–549.

Neri, G., Gurrieri, F., Gal, A., & Lubs, H. A. (1990). XLMR genes: Update 1990. *American Journal of Medical Genetics, 38*, 186–189.

Nichols, P. L. (1984). Familial mental retardation. *Behavior Genetics, 14*, 161–170.

Nicholls, R. D. (1994). New insights reveal complex mechanisms involved in genomic imprinting. *American Journal of Human Genetics, 54*, 733–740.

Nicholls, R. D., Knoll, J. H., Butler, M. G., Karam, S., & Lalande, M. (1989). Genetic imprinting suggested by maternal heterodisomy in nondeletion Prader–Willi syndrome. *Nature, 342*, 281–285.

Oberle, I., Rousseau, F., Heitz, D., Kretz, C., Devys, D., Hanauer, A., Boue, J., Bertheas, M. F., & Mandel, J. L. (1991). Instability of a 550-base pair DNA segment and abnormal methylation in Fragile X syndrome. *Science, 252*, 1097–1102.

Okano, Y., Eisensmith, R. C., Guttler, R., Lichter-Konecki, U., Konecki, D. S., Trefz, F. K., Dasovich, M., Wang, T., Henriksen, K., Lou, H., & Woo, S. L. C. (1991). Molecular basis of phenotype heterogeneity in phenylketonuria. *New England Journal of Medicine, 324*, 1232–1238.

Olshan, A. F., Bard, P. A., & Teschke, K. (1989). Paternal occupational exposure and the risk of Down's syndrome. *American Journal of Human Genetics, 44*, 646–651.

Opitz, J. M. (1986). Editorial comment: On the gates of hell and a most unusual gene. *American Journal of Medical Genetics, 23*, 1–10.

Palomaki, G. E., & Haddow, J. E. (1993). Is it time for population-based prenatal screening for fragile X? [letter]. *Lancet, 341*, 373–374.

Parker, L. S. (1994). Bioethics for human geneticists: Models for reasoning and methods for teaching. *American Journal of Human Genetics, 54*, 137–147.

Pembrey, M. (1991). Prenatal diagnosis: Healthier, wealthier and wiser? In D. J. Roy, B. E. Wynn, & R. W. Old (Eds.), *Bioscience and society* (pp. 53–66). London: Wiley.

Pembrey, M. E., Winter, R. M., & Davies, K. E. (1985). A premutation that generates a defect at crossing over explains the inheritance of fragile X mental retardation. *American Journal of Medical Genetics, 21*, 709–717.

Penrose, L. S. (1935). Inheritance of phenylpyruvic anaemia (phenylketonuria). *Lancet, 2*, 192–194.

Penrose, L. S. (1938). *A clinical and genetic study of 1280 cases of mental defect (The Colchester Study)*. London: Medical Research Council.

Penrose, L. S. (1963). *The biology of mental defect* (2nd ed.). New York: Grune and Stratton.

Petronis, A., & Kennedy, J. L. (1995). Unstable genes—unstable mind? *American Journal of Psychiatry, 152*, 164–172.

Pick, V., Howard-Pebbles, P., Sherman, S., Taylor, A., & Wulfsberg, E. (1994). Fragile X syndrome: Diagnostic and carrier testing. Working Group of the Genetic Screening Subcommittee of the Clinical Practice Committee. American College of Medical Genetics. *American Journal of Medical Genetics, 53*, 380–3611.

Pickles, A., Bolton, P., Macdonald, H., Bailey, A., LeCouteur, A., Sim, C.-H., & Rutter, M. (1995). Latent class analysis of recurrence risks for complex phenotypes with selection and measurment error: A twin and family history study of autism. *American Journal of Human Genetics, 57*, 17–26.

Pieretti, M., Zhang, F., Fu, Y.-H., Warren, S. T., Oostra, B. A., Caskey, C. T., & Nelson, D. L. (1991). Absence of the expression of the FMR-1 gene in fragile X syndrome. *Cell, 86*, 817–822.

Piven, J. P., Chase, G. A., Landa, R., Wzorek, M., Gayle, J., Cloud, D., & Folstein, S. (1991). Psychiatric disorders in the parents of autistic individuals. *Journal of the American Academy of Child and Adolescent Psychiatry, 30*, 471–478.

Piven, J., Wzorek, M., Landa, R., Lainhart, J., Bolton, P., Chase, G. A., & Folstein, S. (1994). Personality characteristics of the parents of autistic individuals. *Psychological Medicine, 24*, 783–795.

Plomin, R. (1986). *Development, genetics, and psychology*. Hillsdale, NJ: Erlbaum.

Plomin, R. (1994). *Genetics and experience: The developmental interplay between nature and nurture.* Newbury Park, CA: Sage Publications.

Plomin, R. (1995). Genetics and children's experiences in the family. *Journal of Child Psychology and Psychiatry, 36,* 33–68.

Plomin, R., & Bergeman, C. S. (1991). The nature of nurture: Genetic influence on "environmental" measures. *Behavior and Brain Science, 14,* 373–386.

Plomin, R., DeFries, J. C., & Fulker, D. W. (1988). *Nature and nurture during infancy and early childhood.* Cambridge: Cambridge University Press.

Plomin, R., DeFries, J. C., & Loehlin, J. C. (1977). Genotype–environment interaction and correlation in the analysis of human behavior. *Psychological Bulletin, 84,* 309–322.

Plomin, R., McClearn, G. E., Smith, D. L., Vignetti, S., Chorney, M. J., Chorney, K. A., Venditti, C., Kasarda, S., Thompson, L. A., Detterman, D. K., Daniels, J. K., Owen, M., & McGuffin, P. (1994). DNA markers associated with high versus low IQ: The IQ QTL Project. *Behavior Genetics, 24,* 107–118.

Plomin, R., & Neiderhiser, J. M. (1991). Quantitative genetics, molecular genetics, and intelligence. *Intelligence, 15,* 369–387.

Porstmann, T., Wietschke, R., Cobet, G., Stamminger, G., Bollmann, R., Rogalski, V., & Pas, P. (1991). Cu/Zn superoxide dismutase quantification from fetal erythrocytes—an efficient confirmatory test for Down's syndrome after maternal serum screening and sonographic investigations. *Prenatal Diagnosis, 11,* 295–303.

Purvis-Smith, S. G., Saville, T., Manass, S., Yip, M. Y., Lam-Po-Tang, P. R., Duffy, B., Johnston, H., Leigh, D., & McDonald, B. (1992). Uniparental disomy 15 resulting from "correction" of an initial trisomy 15 [letter]. *American Journal of Human Genetics, 50,* 1348–5130.

Ramus, S. J., Forrest, S. M., Pitt, D. B., Saleeba, J. A., & Cotton, R. G. H. (1993). Comparison of genotypes and intellectual phenotype in untreated PKU patients. *Journal of Medical Genetics, 30,* 401–405.

Rao, J. M. (1990). A population-based study of mild mental handicap in children: Preliminary analysis of obstetric associations. *Journal of Mental Deficiency Research, 34,* 59–65.

Ratcliffe, S. G. (1994). The psychological and psychiatric consequences of sex chromosome abnormalities in children, based on population studies. In F. Poustka (Ed.), *Basic approaches to genetic and molecular biological developmental psychiatry* (pp. 99–122). Berlin: Quintessenz.

Read, A. W., & Stanley, F. J. (1993). Small-for-gestational-age term birth: The contribution of socio-economic, behavioral, and biological factors to recurrence. *Paediatric and Perinatal Epidemiology, 7,* 177–194.

Reed, E. W., & Reed, S. G. (1965). *Mental retardation: A family study.* Philadelphia: W. B. Saunders.

Reed, S. C., & Rich, S. S. (1982). Parent–offspring resemblances and regressions for IQ. *Behavior Genetics, 12,* 535–542.

Reiss, A. L., Freund, L., Abrams, M. T., Boehm, C., & Kazazian, H. (1993). Neurobehavioral effects of the fragile X premutation in adult women: A controlled study. *American Journal of Human Genetics, 52,* 884–894.

Reynolds, O. (1996). Causes and outcome of perinatal brain injury. In D. Magnusson (Ed.), *The life-span development of individuals: A synthesis of biological and psychological perspectives* (pp. 52–75). Barking: Keyword Publications.

Richards, R., Holman, K., Friend, K., Kremer, E., Hillen, D., Staples, A., & Brown, W. T. (1992). Evidence of founder chromosomes in fragile X syndrome. *Nature Genetics, 1,* 257–260.

Roberts, J. A. F. (1952). The genetics of mental deficiency. *Eugenics Review, 15,* 71–83.

Robinson, W. P., Bottani, A., Xie, Y. G., Balakrishman, J., Binkert, F., Machler, M., Prader, A., & Schinzel, A. (1991). Molecular, cytogenetic, and clinical investigations of Prader–Willi syndrome patients. *American Journal of Human Genetics, 49,* 1219–1234.

Rosanoff, A. J., Handy, L. M., & Plesset, I. R. (1937). The etiology of mental deficiency with special reference to its occurrence in twins. *Psychological Monograph, 216,* 1–137.

Ross, C. A., McInnis, M. G., Margolis, R. L., & Li, S.-H. (1993). Genes with triplet repeats: Candidate mediators of neuropsychiatric disorders. *Trends in Neuroscience, 16,* 254–260.

Rowe, D. C. (1994). *The limits of family influence: Genes, experience, and behavior.* New York: Guilford Publications Inc.

Rutter, M. (1971). Psychiatry. In J. Wortis (Ed.), *Mental retardation: An annual review III* (pp. 186–221). New York: Grune and Stratton.

Rutter, M. (1985). Family and school influences on behavioral development. *Journal of Child Psychology and Psychiatry, 26,* 349–368.

Rutter, M. (1991). Nature, nurture, and psychopathology: A new look at an old topic. *Development and Psychopathology, 3,* 125–136.

Rutter, M. (1994). Psychiatric genetics: Research challenges and pathways forward. *American Journal of Medical Genetics (Neuropsychiatric Genetics), 15,* 185–198.

Rutter, M., & Bailey, A. (1993). Thinking and relationships: Mind and brain (some reflections on theory of mind and autism). In S. Baron-Cohen, H. Tager-Flusberg, & D. J. Cohen (Eds.), *Understanding other minds: Perspectives from autism* (pp. 481–504). Oxford: Oxford University Press.

Rutter, M., Bailey, A., Bolton, P., & LeCouteur, A. (1994). Autism and known medical conditions: Myth and substance. *Journal of Child Psychology and Psychiatry, 35,* 311–322.

Rutter, M., Bolton, P., Harrington, R., LeCouteur, A., Macdonald, H., & Simonoff, E. (1990). Genetic factors in child psychiatric disorders—I. A review of research strategies. *Journal of Child Psychology and Psychiatry, 31,* 3–38.

Rutter, M., & Gould, M. (1985). Classification. In M. Rutter & L. Hersov (Eds.), *Child and adolescent psychiatry: Modern approaches* (2nd ed., pp. 304–321). Oxford: Blackwell Scientific.

Rutter, M., & Madge, N. (1976). *Cycles of disadvantage.* London: Heinemann Educational Books Ltd.

Rutter, M., & Pickles, A. (1991). Person–environment interaction: Concepts, mechanisms, and implications for data analysis. In T. D. Wachs & R. Plomin (Eds.), *Conceptualization and measurement of organism-environment interaction* (pp. 105–141). Washington, DC: American Psychological Association.

Rutter, M., Silberg, J., & Simonoff, E. (1993). Whither behavior genetics? A developmental psychopathology perspective. In R. Plomin & G. E. McClearn (Eds.), *Nature, nurture, and psychology* (pp. 433–456). Washington, DC: APA Books.

Rutter, M., Tizard, J., & Whitmore, K. (1970). *Education, health, and behavior.* London: Longman.

Sabaratnam, M., Laver, S., Bulter, L., & Pembrey, M. (1994). Fragile-X syndrome in North-East Essex: Towards systematic screening: Clinical selection. *Journal of Intellectual Disability Research, 38,* 27–35.

Sameroff, A. J., & Chandler, M. J. (1975). Reproductive risk and the continuum of caretaking casualty. In F. D. Horowitz (Ed.), *Review of child development research* (Vol. 4, pp. 187–244). Chicago: University of Chicago Press.

Saudino, K., Plomin, R., Pedersen, N. L., & McClearn, G. E. (1994). The etiology of high and low cognitive ability during the second half of the life span. *Intelligence, 19,* 359–371.

Scarr, S. (1992). Developmental theories for the 1990s: Development and individual differences. *Child Development, 63,* 1–18.

Scarr, S., & McCartney, K. (1983). How people create their own environments: A theory of genotype environment effects. *Child Development, 54,* 424–435.

Schalock, R. L., Stark, J. A., Snell, M. E., Coulter, D. L., Polloway, E. A., Luckasson, R., Reiss, S., & Spitalnik, D. M. (1994). The changing conception of mental retardation: Implications for the field. *Mental Retardation, 32,* 181–193.

Schiff, M., & Lewontin, R. (1986). *Education and class: The irrelevance of IQ genetic studies.* Oxford: Clarendon.

Scott, S. (1994). Mental retardation. In M. Rutter, E. Taylor, & L. Hersov (Eds.), *Child and adolescent psychiatry: Modern approaches* (3rd ed., pp. 616–646). Oxford: Blackwell Scientific.

Scott, C. R., & Cederbaum, S. D. (1990). Disorders of amino acid metabolism. In A. E. H. Emery & D. H. Rimoin (Eds.), *Principles and practice of medical genetics* (pp. 1639–1673). Edinburgh: Churchill-Livingstone.

Shapiro, B. L. (1983). Down's syndrome—a disruption of homeostasis. *American Journal of Medical Genetics, 14*, 241–269.

Shapiro, D. (1994). The ethics of genetic screening: The first report of the Nuffield Council on Bioethics: Another personal view. *Journal of Medical Ethics, 20*, 185–187.

Shaw, C. M. (1987). Correlates of mental retardation and structural changes of the brain. *Brain Development, 9*, 1–8.

Sherman, S. L., Jacobs, P. A., Morton, N. E., Froster-Iskenius, U., Howard-Peebles, P. N., Nielson, K. B., Partington, M. W., Sutherland, G. R., Turner, G., & Watson, M. (1985). Further segregation analysis of the fragile X syndrome with special reference to transmitting males. *Human Genetics, 69*, 289–299.

Simonoff, E., McGuffin, P., & Gottesman, I. I. (1994). Genetic influences on normal and abnormal development. In M. Rutter, E. A. Taylor, & L. Hersov (Eds.), *Child and adolescent psychiatry: Modern approaches* (pp. 129–151). Oxford: Blackwell Scientific Publications.

Skinner, R. (1990). Genetic counselling. In A. E. H. Emery & D. L. Rimoin (Eds.), *Principles and practice of medical genetics* (pp. 1923–1934). Edinburgh: Churchill-Livingstone.

Smalley, S., McCracken, J., & Tanguay, P. (1995). Autism, affective disorders, and social phobia. *American Journal of Medical Genetics, 50*, 19–26.

Smalley, S. L., Asarnow, R. F., & Spence, M. A. (1988). Autism and genetics: A decade of research. *Archives of General Psychiatry, 45*, 953–961.

Smidt-Jensen, S., Lind, A. M., Permin, M., Zachary, J. M., Lundsteen, C., & Philip, J. (1993). Cytogenetic analysis of 2928 CVS samples and 1075 amniocentesis from randomized studies. *Prenatal Diagnosis, 13*, 723–740.

Smidt-Jensen, S., Permin, M., Philip, J., Lundsteen, C., Zachary, J. M., Fowler, S. E., & Grunning, K. (1992). Randomised comparison of amniocentesis and transabdominal and transcervical chorionic villus sampling. *Lancet, 340*, 1237–1244.

Smith, I., Clayton, B. E., & Wolff, O. H. (1975). New variant of phenylketonuria with progressive neurological illness unresponsive to phenylalanine restriction. *Lancet, 1*, 108–111.

Smith, J., & Wolff, O. H. (1974). Natural history of phenylketonuria and early treatment. *Lancet, 2*, 540–544.

Snow, K., Tester, D. J., Kruckeberg, K. E., Schaid, D. J., & Thibodeau, S. N. (1994). Sequence analysis of the fragile X trinucleotide repeat: Implications for the origin of the fragile X mutation. *Human Molecular Genetics, 3*, 1543–1551.

Sobesky, W. E., Pennington, B. F., Porter, D., Hull, C. E., & Hagerman, R. J. (1994). Emotional and neurocognitive deficits in Fragile X. *American Journal of Medical Genetics, 51*, 378–385.

Stein, Z., & Susser, M. (1960). The families of dull children: a classification for predicting careers. *British Journal of Preventative and Social Medicine, 14*, 83–88.

Sutherland, G. R. (1977). Fragile sites on human chromosomes. Documentation of their dependence on type of tissue culture. *Science, 197*, 265–266.

Sutherland, G. R., & Baker, E. (1992). Characterisation of a new rare fragile site easily confused with the fragile X. *Human Molecular Genetics, 1*, 111–113.

Sutton, A. (1995). The new gene technology and the difference between getting rid of illness and altering people. *European Journal of Genetics and Society, 1*, 12–19.

Svensson, E., von-Dobeln, U., Eisensmith, R. C., Hagenfeldt, L., & Woo, S. L. (1993). Relation between genotype and phenotype in Swedish phenylketonuria and hyperphenylalanemia patients. *European Journal of Pediatrics, 152*, 132–139.

Tarjan, M. D., Tizard, J., Rutter, M., Bergab, M., Brooke, E., de la Cruz, F., Lin, T.-Y. Montenegro, H., Strotzka, H., & Sartorius, N. (1972). Classification and mental retardation: Issues arising in the Fifth WHO Seminar on Psychiatric Diagnosis, Classification and Statistics. *American Journal of Psychiatry, 128*, 34–35 (suppl.).

Taylor, A. K., Safanda, J. F., Fall, M. Z., Quince, C., Lang, K. A., Hull, C. E., Carpenter, I., Staley, L. W., & Hagerman, R. J. (1994). Molecular predictors of cognitive involvement in female carriers of fragile X syndrome. *Journal of the American Medical Association, 271*, 507–514.

Thapar, A., Gottesman, I. I., Owen, M. J., Donovan, M. C., & McGuffin, P. (1994). The genetics of mental retardation. *British Journal of Psychiatry, 164*, 747–758.

Thompson, L. A., Detterman, D. K., & Plomin, R. (1993). Differential heritability across groups differing in ability, revisited. *Behavior Genetics, 23*, 331–336.

Trent, R. J., Volpato, F., Smith, A., Lindeman, R., Wong, M. K., Warne, G., & Haan, E. (1991). Molecular and cytogenetic studies of the Prader–Willi syndrome. *Journal of Medical Genetics, 28*, 649–654.

Trimble, B. K., & Baird, P. A. (1978). Maternal age and Down syndrome: Age specific incidence rates by single year intervals. *Journal of Medical Genetics, 2*, 1.

Trottier, Y., Biancalana, V., & Mandel, J. L. (1994). Instability of CAG repeats in Huntington's disease: Relation to parental transmission and age of onset. *Journal of Medical Genetics, 31*, 377–382.

Turk, J. (1992). The fragile X syndrome: On the way to a behavioral phenotype. *British Journal of Psychiatry, 160*, 24–35.

Turkheimer, E., & Gottesman, I. I. (1991). Individual differences and the canalization of human behavior. *Developmental Psychology, 27*, 18–22.

Turner, G., Collins, E., & Turner, B. (1971). Recurrence risk of mental retardation in sibs. *Medical Journal of Australia, 1*, 1165–1166.

Tymchuk, A. K. (1992). Predicting adequacy of parenting by people with mental retardation. *Child Abuse and Neglect, 16*, 165–178.

Verkerk, A. J. M. H., Pieretti, M., Sutcliffe, J. S., Fu, Y.-H., Kuhl, D. P. A., Pizzuti, A., Reiner, O., Richards, S., Victoria, M. F., Zhang, F., Eussen, E. B., Van Ommen, G.-J., Blonden, L. A. J., Riggins, G. J., Chastein, J. L., Kunst, C. B., Galjaard, L. J., Caskey, C. T., Nelson, D. L., Oostra, B. A., & Warren, S. T. (1991). Identification of a gene (FMR-1) containing a CGG repeat coincident with a breakpoint cluster region exhibiting length variation in Fragile X syndrome. *Cell, 65*, 905–914.

Verlinsky, Y., & Kuliev, A. M. (1993). *Preimplantation diagnosis of genetic diseases: A new technique in assisted reproduction.* New York: Wiley-Liss.

Vogel, F., Crusio, W. E., Kovac, C., Fryns, J. P., & Freund, M. (1990). Selective advantage of the fra(x) heterozygotes. *Human Genetics, 86*, 25–32.

Vogler, G. P., & DeFries, J. C. (1983). Linearity of offspring–parent regression for general cognitive ability. *Behavior Genetics, 13*, 355–360.

Wahlsten, D. (1990). Insensitivity of the analysis of variance to heredity–environment interaction. *Behavior and Brain Sciences, 13*, 109–161.

Wahlstrom, J. (1990). Gene map of mental retardation. *Journal of Mental Deficiency Research, 34*, 11–27.

Wang, Q., Green, E., Bobrow, M., & Mathew, C. G. (1995). A rapid, non-radioactive screening test for fragile X mutations at the FRAXA and FRAXE loci. *Journal of Medical Genetics, 32*, 170–173.

Webb, T. P., Bundey, S., Thake, A., & Todd, J. (1986). The frequency of the fragile X chromosome among school-children in Coventry. *Journal of Medical Genetics, 23*, 396–399.

Wilkie, A. O. M. (1994). The molecular basis of genetic dominance. *Journal of Medical Genetics, 31*, 89–98.

Willemsen, R., Mohkamsing, S., De Vries, B., Devys, D., van den Ouweland, A., Mandel, J. L., Gaijaard, H., & Oostra, B. (1995). Rapid antibody test for fragile X syndrome. *Lancet, 345*, 1147–1148.

Williams, C. A., Frias, J. L., McCormick, M. K., Antonarakis, S. E., & Cantu, E. S. (1990). Clinical cytogenetic, and molecular evaluation of a patient with partial trisomy 21 (21q11–q22) lacking the classical Down syndrome plenotype. *American Journal of Medical Genetics, 7*, 110–114 (suppl.).

Wilson, R. S., & Matheny, Jr. A. P. (1976). Retardation and twin concordance in infant mental development: A reassessment. *Behavior Genetics, 6*, 353–358.

Winter, R. M., & Pembrey, M. E. (1986). Analysis of linkage relationships between genetic markers around the fragile X locus with special reference to daughters of normal transmitting males. *Human Genetics, 74*, 94–97.

Wohrle, D., Kotzot, D., Hirst, M. C., Manca, A., Korn, B., Schmidt, A., Barbi, G., Rott, H.-D., Poustka, A., Davies, K. E., & Steinbach, P. (1992). A microdeletion of less than 250 kb including the proximal part of the FMR-1 gene and the fragile X site, in a male with the clinical phenotype of fragile X syndrome. *American Journal of Human Genetics, 51*, 299–306.

Yu, S., Pritchard, M., Kremer, E., Lynch, M., Nancarrow, J., Baker, E., Holman, K., Mulley, J. C., Warren, S. T., Schlessinger, D., Sutherland, G. R., & Richards, R. T. (1991). Fragile X genotype characterised by an unstable region of DNA. *Science, 252*, 1179–1181.

Zigler, E. (1967). Familial mental retardation: A continuing dilemma. *Science, 155*, 292–298.

Zigler, E., & Hodapp, R. (1986). *Understanding mental retardation*. New York: Cambridge University Press.

8

Poor Readers in Adulthood: Psychosocial Functioning

Barbara Maughan

MRC Child Psychiatry Unit, Institute of Psychiatry, London

Ann Hagell

Policy Studies Institute, London

Samples of poor and normal readers were followed into early adulthood to assess the implications of childhood reading difficulties for the transition to adulthood, and for early adult psychosocial functioning. Some group differences were found in patterns of early adult transitions, and, for women only, on wider measures of early adult functioning. Global self-esteem in adulthood did not differ between the childhood reading groups, and there were few marked variations in vulnerability to later psychiatric disorder. The findings are discussed in regard to differing developmental pathways for problems in adult functioning, and the possible role of contextual changes in enabling more positive functioning for many childhood poor readers.

Tracing the course of childhood disorders and assessing the ways in which early difficulties affect children's capacities to meet the demands of new developmental periods are among the central concerns of developmental psychopathology (Cicchetti & Richters, 1993). In this article, we examine childhood reading problems from a developmental perspective of this kind. Reading disabilities are among the most common childhood disorders and show strong overlaps with emotional and behavior problems in childhood. Elevated rates of anxiety and depression have been noted in clinic samples (Livingston, 1990; Cornwell & Bawden, 1992), while epidemiologic data suggest that low achieving readers show vulnerabilities to both emotional and conduct problems (Richman, Stevenson, & Graham, 1982; Jorm, Share, Matthews, & Maclean, 1986). Specific, IQ-discrepant reading difficulties

Reprinted with Permission from *Development and Psychopathology*, 1996, Vol. 8, 457–476. Copyright © 1996 by the Cambridge University Press.

Many colleagues contributed to the various phases of this study. We thank in particular Dr. Michael Berger, and Professors William Yule and Michael Rutter, who initiated the study; Mrs. Bridget Yule, who administered the 14-year data collection; and Lesley Gulliver, Christine Groothues, Rosanna Heal, Angela Park, Christina Shearer, and Frances Winder, who interviewed with us on the adult follow-up. Many teachers provided information on the children's progress. The data collection was supported by grants from the Social Science Research Council, the Department of Education and Science, and the Medical Research Council. Finally, we are indebted to the study members themselves for their generous cooperation.

have been especially linked with disruptive behaviors: overactivity and attention deficits in early child-hood, and more overtly antisocial behavior during the middle childhood years (Hinshaw, 1992).

To date, much less is known about the implications of early reading problems, and their comor-bidities with behavioral disorders, for psychosocial functioning in adulthood. In more broadly defined learning disabled (LD) groups, the transition to adulthood appears to present considerable problems, with many LD young adults facing difficulties in achieving independent living, leading restricted social lives, and showing only limited engagement with the community (see e.g., Patton & Polloway, 1992, for an overview).

Adult social functioning and psychological well-being have been less widely examined in reading disabled samples. The evidence currently available comes primarily from clinic samples, and so may be difficult to generalize. Early small-scale studies (Balow & Blomquist, 1965; Carter, 1967; Hardy, 1968) suggested that many poor readers showed personality or social difficulties in adulthood, and recent larger scale investigations have tended to confirm that view. Bruck (1985), for example, reported that slightly more than a third of her clinic sample showed poor overall adjustment in the late teens and early twenties, with difficulties more evident for women than for men. Problem rates were higher than in a peer control group, but few suggested evidence of major psychopathology, and only 5% of subjects had recent histories of counseling or psychiatric help. The largest single problem category in the reading disabled sample was characterized as withdrawal—subjects who were depressed, sensitive, withdrawn, or worriers.

Spreen (1987), in a study of ex-attenders from a neurological clinic, reached broadly similar conclusions. Both in their late teens and mid-twenties, LD subjects scored less well than controls on personality and adjustment inventories, but few fell within a psychopathological range. In one of the few prospective studies of community-based samples, Jaklewicz (1982, 1992) reported on adult outcomes of "dyslexics" identified from the school population in Gdansk. Although a nonreferred group, the dyslexics showed high rates of birth complications and nervous system injury or disease in early childhood, raising some cautions about their representativeness. In their early twenties, more than three quarters were described as showing neurotic symptoms, with high levels of anxiety, fear, and emotional tension. Childhood dyslexics reported feelings of inferiority, distrustfulness, lack of independence in making decisions, emotional immaturity and difficulty in making social contacts. In their early thirties, however, subjects' family relationships were reported as close and supportive (Jaklewicz, 1992).

These findings suggest vulnerability to problems in psychosocial functioning for some, if not a majority, of disabled readers in adulthood. If generalizable, they raise important questions about the developmental pathways involved. Several rather different possibilities arise here. First, given the marked comorbidities between reading and behavior disorders in childhood, psychosocial problems in adult life might largely reflect continuities from earlier behavior problems. Hardy (1968), Bruck (1985), and Spreen (1987) all concluded that their samples showed *lower* rates of adjustment prob-lems in adulthood than in childhood, but none of these authors presented specific analyses of the extent to which adult difficulties reflected continuities from preexisting behavior problems. Indeed, in all of these studies measures of childhood behavior were based at least in part on retrospective reports collected in adulthood, rather than on contemporaneous childhood accounts. Ideally, prospec-tive assessments of both behavioral and cognitive problems are required if we are to tease out the contributions of these differing childhood vulnerabilities.

Other routes to poor adult functioning might reflect more direct effects of continuing literacy difficulties. Negative self-evaluations and low self-esteem might constitute particular susceptibili-ties here. In childhood, academic self-esteem covaries strongly with reading attainment (Chapman, Lambourne, & Silva, 1990), and learning disabled children's self-views seem especially sensitive to social comparisons with peers (Renick & Harter, 1989). It is less clear, however, how far processes of this kind are context-dependent, and reflect school-related stressors that may lessen once children complete their education. The school setting, with its inevitable emphasis on reading competence, seems likely to present nearly unavoidable pressures for reading disabled children at some stage in their school careers. Later in the life course, the opportunity to select working and social environments might allow for changes in the salience of academic skills problems and also in their impact on self-esteem. Studies of poor readers' educational and occupational histories suggest that many do indeed select courses and career paths with reduced literacy demands, in which interpersonal or other skills are of greater importance (see e.g., Finucci, 1986). Very little is known of the possible protective effects of strategies of this kind for self-esteem or psychological well-being. There are suggestions, however, that self-perceptions of impairment continue to be important mediators of psychological well-being in adulthood. Findings from the 1970 British birth cohort, for example, showed that young adults who performed poorly on literacy and numeracy tests were more likely than others to report depressed mood, but the highest levels of depressive affect were associated with *self*-reports of continuing literacy problems in adulthood (Ekynsmith & Bynner, 1994).

A third possibility is that later functioning may be affected by more indirect processes, whereby early reading problems act to select individuals into environments that carry increased risks of later stressors. Follow-up studies of conduct-disordered children suggest that mechanisms of this kind may play an important role in the persistence of their difficulties, whether through selection into unsupportive personal relationships (Quinton, Pickles, Maughan, & Rutter, 1993) or into adult environments involving increased exposure to life events and other adversities (Champion, Goodall, & Rutter, 1995). The role transitions of early adulthood may be of particular importance here. Typically, the period from late adolescence to early adulthood is marked by a series of major transitions—leaving school, leaving home, entering marriage or cohabitation, and the start of family formation. Choices made at these points do much to determine the occupational and interpersonal contexts, and the supports and stressors, that form the backdrop for early adult life. The timing of these transitions varies systematically by socioeconomic (SES) group and educational background (Kerckhoff, 1990) and has been shown to have long-term implications for occupational and other life chances (Hogan & Astone, 1986). To date, there has been little systematic examination of how childhood poor readers approach these transitions, although some pointers are again suggested in the British birth cohort studies. There, women reporting continuing literacy and numeracy problems in adulthood were more likely to have left work and begun family formation early in their twenties, while young men were more likely to have experienced periods of unemployment (Adult Literacy and Basic Skills Unit [ALBSU], 1987; Ekynsmith & Bynner, 1994). Both these patterns suggest the possibility of increased levels of environmental stress that, in addition to any intraindividual effects of continuing literacy problems, might also contribute to difficulties in adult functioning.

We take up these varying possibilities here, using data from a prospective follow-up in adulthood of representative samples of poor and normal readers first studied in middle childhood. We have reported else-where on these young people's academic progress in secondary school (Maughan, Hagell, Rutter, & Yule, 1994) and on specifically antisocial outcomes in adulthood (Maughan, Pickles, Hagell, Rutter, & Yule, in press). Here, we focus on broader aspects of psychosocial adjustment, beginning with patterns of early adult role transitions, then turning to assessments of social functioning in the early twenties, self-esteem, and rates of adult psychiatric disorder. In addition to general contrasts between normal and disabled readers, our sample allowed for tests of one further issue, little if at all explored in long-term studies of disabled readers to date. Both DSM-IV (American Psychiatric Association, 1994) and ICD-10 (World Health Organization, 1992) criteria for academic skills disorders require evidence of *under*achievement in reading in relation to IQ, and exclude children showing generally low reading performance assessed against age-norms alone. As Stanovich (1994) and others have argued, however, evidence for the discriminant validity of IQ-discrepant definitions of reading difficulties is far from consistent in the cognitive literature, and there have been a number of calls for the abandonment of the distinction. One area where somewhat different patterns of correlates has been noted is in terms of comorbidities with behavioral disorders. Longitudinal comparisons between age- and IQ-discrepant poor readers might thus throw valuable light on the processes involved in continuities to later difficulties in functioning. Insofar as later psychosocial problems are associated with restricted reading skills, both age- and IQ-discrepant poor readers would be expected to show similar patterns of later adjustment. If continuities from earlier behavior problems constitute an important source of later vulnerabilities, different patterns of between-group adjustment might be anticipated.

METHOD

Samples

The data were drawn from a longitudinal follow-up in early adulthood of representative samples of poor and normal readers first identified in epidemiological studies in middle childhood (Berger, Yule, & Rutter, 1975; Maughan, 1989). A two-stage screening process was used to identify poor readers and comparison subjects from all the Caucasian, English-speaking 10-year-old children ($n = 1689$) attending local authority primary schools in one inner London borough. The first stage involved the administration of National Foundation for Educational Research (NFER) group tests of nonverbal intelligence (NFER NV5) and reading (NFER SRA). In the second stage, individual psychometric testing was undertaken with (a) a randomly selected comparison group ($n = 106$) and (b) a one-in-two random sample of children scoring more than two standard deviations below the mean on the group reading tests ($n = 143$). The individual tests included the short form of the Wechsler Intelligence Scale for Children (WISC; Wechsler, 1949) and the Neale Analysis of Reading Ability (Neale, 1958), a diagnostic test of reading accuracy and comprehension. The Neale shows high reliability (0.96 and higher for accuracy scores on parallel versions of the test). Applying a regression formula to take account of WISC short form IQ (Yule, 1967; Berger et al., 1975), the poor reading sample was divided into two groups, one of low achieving *generally backward* readers, reading 28 months or more below age expectations, but whose reading was not discrepant from their general intellectual abilities ($n = 51$), and the second of IQ-discrepant, *specifically retarded* readers, reading 28 months below both age and IQ expectations ($n = 77$).

For the longitudinal analyses presented here, we needed to compare poor readers with a group without severe reading difficulties. To achieve this, three main revisions were made in the allocation of children to reading groups. First, subjects in the comparison group who met both group and individual test criteria for poor readers were reassigned to the backward ($n = 7$) or retarded ($n = 16$) reading groups as appropriate. Second, nine comparison group subjects who met one but not the other criterion for reading difficulties were excluded from the analyses, as were four subjects subsequently found to be outside the selected age group, or not to meet the ethnicity criteria. Finally, children with measured IQ scores of less than 70 were excluded, to ensure that the groups included in the follow-up analyses were all broadly within the normal ability range. After these revisions, 200 subjects were available for follow-up: 38 backward readers, 89 retarded readers, and a comparison group of 73 participants without severe reading difficulties.

Measures

The participants were followed through their secondary schooling and in early adulthood. Measures from the childhood, adolescent and early adult study waves are used here.

Childhood and adolescence. In addition to psychometric testing, the age-10 surveys included a social background questionnaire giving details of the occupation of the main family breadwinner and Rutter

B(2) teacher behavior questionnaires (Rutter, 1967). The B(2) has been extensively used as a screening questionnaire for emotional and behavioral difficulties and shows high test–retest reliability ($r = .89$). It includes 26 items, each scored on a 3-point scale ($0 = Doesn't apply$, $1 = Applies somewhat$, $2 = Certainly applies$). Total scale scores provide an index of generalized behavior disturbance, while more focused subscales highlighting conduct/oppositional problems, inattentiveness, emotional difficulties, and problems in peer relationships can be derived from subsets of items. The teacher ratings were repeated when the children were of age 14 years.

Adulthood. The subjects were recontacted and interviewed in early adulthood, at a mean age of 27–28 years. Interviews were undertaken blind to selection status and covered a range of topics: current demographic details; educational, occupational, and cohabitation/marital histories; assessments of psychosocial functioning, self-esteem, and psychiatric disorder (see below); and self-reports of current impairment in reading and writing.

Psychosocial functioning. Psychosocial functioning in early adulthood was evaluated using the Adult Personality Functioning Assessment (APFA; Hill, Harrington, Fudge, Rutter, & Pickles, 1989). The APFA assesses functioning in a range of domains (work, intimate relationships, friendships, nonspecific social contacts, everyday coping, and negotiations with officials and others) and is capable of identifying specific difficulties in particular domains, along with more pervasive problems in functioning. Unlike trait-based measures of personality functioning, the APFA depends on detailed descriptions of behaviors and ratings are made for relatively extended periods (of 5 years at the least), excluding any periods when subjects are experiencing acute psychiatric episodes. In this study, ratings were made for the period from age 21 to 25 years.

Questioning in each domain covers a range of issues. In relation to work, for example, participants are questioned on their employment histories during the selected rating period; reasons for changing or losing jobs, including dismissals; evidence of difficulties in relationships with colleagues, employers, or customers; and the frequency and extent of any periods of unemployment, lateness, or absenteeism from work. In relation to marriage/cohabitation, questioning covers relationship histories during the rating period, and the extent of shared activities, support, confiding, arguments, and violence in each relevant relationship. The interview also provides evidence on the extent of any deviance (defined as criminality, drinking problems, or episodes of psychiatric disorder) in participants' partners.

Functioning in each domain is rated on a 6-point scale, with ratings of 1 indicating exceptionally positive functioning, 2 indicating good functioning, 3 reflecting relatively minor or transient problems, and ratings of 4, 5, and 6 indicating increasing degrees of difficulty. Total scores, summed across domains, provide an assessment of overall social functioning. The APFA shows good interrater reliability, with intraclass correlations (ICCs) ranging from .65 to .88 in individual domains, and a mean ICC of .77 (Hill et al., 1989). In this study, all protocols were rated independently by two interviewers involved in the study and by at least one APFA-trained member of a separate research team. Any discordant ratings were resolved in discussion.

Psychiatric history and state. Psychiatric history was assessed using the Past History Schedule for the Present State Examination (McGuffin, Katz, & Aldrich, 1986)—a brief structured approach to eliciting details of past psychiatric contacts and episodes that shows high inter-rater agreement (kappas of 0.88 and higher, McGuffin et al., 1986). The type and severity of symptoms during any specified episode were assessed using an interview module giving systematic coverage of major areas of psychiatric symptomatology (Rutter, Cox, Tupling, Berger, & Yule, 1975). Final diagnostic ratings of the severity and type of episodes of adult disorder were made by experienced clinicians on the basis of vignettes prepared by the interviewers. An episode of disorder was rated if symptoms of clinical intensity had been present (a) for at least a 2-week period and/or had involved help seeking and (b) had involved some impairment in social functioning *or* (c) were noticeable to others in the subject's household or social circle.

Clinical ratings of personality disorder were also made from case vignettes. As only low rates of personality disorder were expected in a sample of this size, a simplified classification was used, involving two main categories: (a) "dramatic" personality disorders, including antisocial personality and borderline states; and (b) "avoidant" personality disorders. In each case, the criteria required evidence of pervasive and persistent difficulties in personality functioning for these ratings to be made.

Alcohol problems. Past and current alcohol problems were assessed using RDC criteria, based on relevant sections of the Schedule for Affective Disorders and Schizophrenia–Lifetime Version (Endicott & Spitzer, 1978).

Self-esteem. Self-esteem in adulthood was assessed using the Rosenberg self-esteem scale (Rosenberg, 1965), a 10-item Guttman scale tapping global positive and negative attitudes to the self. The scale includes items such as "On the whole I am satisfied with myself" and "I feel I do not have much to be proud of." It has been used with a wide variety of subject populations and shows good test–retest reliablity ($r = .85$). It was selected here for its focus on *global* self-statements, rather than those likely to reflect more specific responses to ongoing literacy difficulties. The Rosenberg was designed as a self-completion questionnaire; if subjects had difficulty in reading the items interviewers read them aloud.

Reading tests. Subjects completed two reading tests, the Gray Oral Reading Test (Gray, 1967), a measure of reading accuracy, and shortened versions of the Edinburgh Reading Tests (University of Edinburgh, 1977), tapping comprehension skills. These tests were selected for their capacity to cover the full range of reading skills likely to be encountered in the sample in adulthood, from early childhood grade level equivalents to competent adult reading levels. The Gray has been used in a number of follow-up studies of disabled readers (see e.g., Bruck, 1985; Finucci, Whitehouse, Isaacs, & Childs, 1984; Naylor, Felton, & Wood, 1990); alternative form reliability estimates for the original normative sample ranged from .96 to .98. Reliabilities for original versions of the Edinburgh tests were all of .95 or higher.

Tracing and Response Rates

One participant had died prior to the follow-up, and a second had sustained a severe head injury, making an interview impractical. Of the remainder, 183 (93.4%) were successfully traced, and some follow-up data collected on 160 (80.8%). Interviews were conducted with 147 participants (74.2% of those available for follow-up); a further 9 participants (4.5%) completed a postal questionnaire; and in four cases (2%) information was gained from agency records. Reading test data were obtained on 133 participants; 67.2% of the participants available for follow-up, and 90.5% of those who were interviewed. This rate is broadly comparable with rates of repeated testing achieved in previous follow-ups of reading disabled participants in adulthood (see e.g., Rodgers, 1986). Two sets of analyses were undertaken to assess the effects of subject attrition: (a) comparisons *between* the reading groups in the proportions with follow-up data available and (b) comparisons *within* each reading group, to assess the representativeness of the follow-up sample by contrast with the original groups identified in childhood.

Between-group comparisons. There were no differences between the reading groups in the proportions traced (backward readers: 94.7%, retarded readers: 92.0%; comparison group: 91.8%, $\chi^2 = 0.36$, 2 *df*, n.s.); with general follow-up data (84.2%, 79.3%, 80.8%, $\chi^2 = 0.41$, 2 *df*, n.s.); or in the proportions of those interviewed who had reading test data (86.2%, 90.2%, and 93.0%, $\chi^2 = 1.04$, 2 *df*, n.s.).

Within-group comparisons. Analyses of the representativeness of the follow-up samples within each reading group highlighted only two sets of significant differences. First, comparison group cases successfully contacted in the follow-up had shown less behavioral deviance than others on the teacher ratings at age 10 years. Second, among retarded readers, cases with full follow-up data were significantly less impaired in reading comprehension in childhood and had significantly higher verbal IQ scores than those not contacted in the follow-up. To assess the likely effects of these differences, we reweighted the data for retarded readers to reflect the original distributions within this group on the childhood measures. Results using the weighted and unweighted data were closely similar on the psychosocial outcomes of interest here. On categorical measures, the percentages rated as showing negative later outcomes never differed by more than 1.5% in the weighted and unweighted data. On continuous indicators the largest difference in mean scores was of 0.04 *SD* units. As these differences were so slight, and statistical tests are less efficient using weighted data, the original unweighted data have been reported here throughout.

RESULTS

Group Characteristics

The study took place in a relatively disadvantaged inner-city area, where the majority of the children came from lower SES backgrounds. Across the sample as a whole, 57.4% came from families in skilled work, and slightly more than 30% had parents in semi-or completely unskilled roles. The two groups of poor readers did not differ in terms of social background, but both came from lower SES backgrounds than children in the comparison group ($\chi^2 = 11.28$, 2 *df*, $p = .004$). This pattern was most marked among the girls ($\chi^2 = 8.93$, 2 *df*, $p = .012$).

Table 1 provides descriptive data for each reading group on reading and IQ levels in childhood and on mean teacher behavior ratings in late childhood and adolescence. In each case where omnibus tests for overall differences between the reading groups indicated significant differences, these were followed by planned comparisons between each possible pair of groups (backward readers vs. comparison group, retarded readers vs. comparison group, and backward vs. retarded readers).

As follows from the group definitions, the backward readers were of below average IQ and had reading test scores approximately 30 months below those in the comparison group. Retarded readers were of average performance IQ but had even more seriously depressed reading levels. There were approximately equal proportions of girls and boys in the backward reading and comparison groups, but boys outnumbered girls 3 : 1 among retarded readers. Both groups of poor reading girls, and retarded reading boys, were rated as showing high levels of behavior problems in the school setting at age 10 years. For girls, this pattern was maintained in adolescence. For boys, the behavioral profiles of the three groups showed relatively few differences at age 14 years (see Maughan et al., in press, for further details).

The poor readers' cognitive difficulties were reflected in markedly depressed examination attainments at age 16 years. More than 40% left school without any formal qualifications, by contrast with 23% of comparison group members. Of those who did achieve qualifications, the majority were at low grades. Fewer than 10% of poor readers had achieved the minimum school-leaving qualifications necessary for entry into most forms of further or higher education or into jobs with extended training opportunities; 38% of the comparison group had achieved grades of at least this level (see Maughan et al., 1994, for further details).

The Sample in Adulthood: Overview

The participants were in their late twenties, at a mean age of 27.7 years (± 1.27) at the time of the early adult follow-up. Almost three quarters still lived in greater London—the majority in

TABLE 1
Sample Characteristics

Variable	Poor Readers		Comparison Group (c) (n = 73)	Omnibus Tests			Pairwise Comparisons (p) Values		
	Backward (a) (n = 38)	Retarded (b) (n = 38)		F	df	p	a vs. c	b vs. c	a vs. b
Age 10									
Reading (years)									
Accuracy	7.66 ± 0.44	7.23 ± 0.70	10.27 ± 1.23	244.34	2, 196	<.001	<.001	<.001	.014
Comprehension	7.84 ± 0.50	7.22 ± 0.70	10.40 ± 1.36	224.85	2, 196	<.001	<.001	<.001	.001
IQ									
Verbal	86.16 ± 9.60	94.13 ± 13.35	104.46 ± 10.99	32.29	2, 196	<.001	<.001	<.001	.001
Performance	92.00 ± 8.55	103.40 ± 12.23	106.63 ± 15.14	16.63	2, 196	<.001	<.001	n.s.	<.001
Teacher behavior ratings									
Girls	5.39 ± 4.27	6.87 ± 6.03	2.88 ± 4.14	4.84	2, 71	.011	.081	.003	n.s.
Boys	5.40 ± 4.56	10.65 ± 9.69	5.10 ± 8.39	6.22	2, 123	.003	n.s.	.002	.019
Age 14									
Teacher behavior ratings									
Girls	6.07 ± 5.74	8.55 ± 6.93	2.97 ± 3.96	6.63	2, 63	.002	.073	.001	n.s.
Boys	5.35 ± 5.27	5.68 ± 6.64	4.17 ± 4.98	0.73	2, 109	n.s.	n.s.	n.s.	n.s.

Note: Values are mean ± *SD.*

TABLE 2
Tested Reading Ages in Adulthood

	Poor Readers		Comparson Group ($n = 53$)
	Backward ($n = 25$)	Retarded ($n = 55$)	
Tested reading levels (reading age equivalents)			
<12 years	28.0	38.2	0
12 years–16.9 years	52.0	38.2	3.8
≥17 years	20.0	23.6	96.2

Note: Values are in percents. $\chi^2 = 71.72$, 4 *df*, $p < .001$.

the immediate vicinity of the original study area. The remainder were spread throughout England, Scotland, and Wales. Two participants were interviewed abroad, both in the United States. Poor readers were as likely as comparison group members to have stayed in the inner city, or to have moved outside ($\chi^2 = 2.94$, 4 *df*, n.s.). By the time of the follow-up, the participants had spent an average of 11–12 years in the labor market. Youth employment options were relatively extensive at the time the study members left school, and only a quarter had faced a total of more than 6 months' unemployment during this time. More than three quarters of the participants had married or cohabited by their late twenties, and more than 40% had already experienced the breakdown of a cohabitation.[1]

Tables 2 and 3 show results from the adult reading tests, and from the participants' own reports of continued reading impairment in adulthood. For these analyses, the test results were classified into a simple three-way grouping: reading ages of below 12 years, reflecting severe continuing literacy problems; reading ages of 12 years to 16 years, 11 months, suggesting some degree of continuing impairment; and reading ages of 17 years and above, the ceiling for standardized scores on the tests. As expected, almost all comparison group members scored in the maximum score range. Scores for the poor readers showed considerable spread. About a quarter of the subjects in each group remained severely impaired in reading, and a further half still faced some continuing difficulties. The remainder, however, had achieved functionally higher reading levels in adulthood. Tested reading levels were unrelated to childhood social class among the men ($\chi^2 = 2.38$, 4 *df*, n.s.), but did show social background effects for the women ($\chi^2 = 14.47$, 4*df*, $p = .006$). A log-linear model including childhood social class continued, however, to show significant differences in adult reading levels between the childhood reading groups (χ^2 to remove 45.37, 4 *df*, $p < .001$).

Self-reports of reading difficulties in adulthood (elicited before the objective tests were administered) reflected a somewhat different pattern. Just less than half of both groups of poor readers considered that their reading difficulties had essentially resolved by the time of the adult follow-up, and less than a fifth felt that their current problems were severe. The perceived impairment associated with any given level of reading skill will, of course, vary with environmental demands: quite minor difficulties may be experienced as problematic in "literacy-intense" environments, while relatively severe problems on objective testing may nonetheless give rise to few perceived limitations in contexts with circumscribed literacy demands. The relatively positive self-reports in our sample suggest that a number of the childhood poor readers had moved into adult environments with relatively restricted literacy demands, where their problems were of limited functional significance for their day-to-day lives.

---

[1]The term *cohabitation* is used to refer to cohabiting relationships of 6 months or longer, whether or not subjects were legally married.

TABLE 3
Self-Reported Adult Reading Problems

| | Poor Readers | | Comparson Group ($n = 58$) |
	Backward ($n = 31$)	Retarded ($n = 67$)	
None	48.4	52.2	98.3
Dubious/minor	35.5	29.9	1.7
Marked	16.1	17.9	0

Note: Values are in percents. $\chi^2 = 38.25$, 4 *df*, $p < .001$.

The Transition to Adulthood: Moving to Independence

As a background to assessments of social functioning in the twenties, we began by examining the subjects' progress through the major role transitions of early adulthood: leaving home, entering cohabitations, and family formation. As outlined earlier, the capacity to achieve independent living has been noted as an area of particular concern in follow-ups of learning disabled samples (Patton & Polloway, 1992).

In this study, the great majority of sample members had left home and entered cohabitations by the time of the adult interviews. Women were somewhat more likely to have made each of these moves to independence than men (left home: 92.5% vs. 82.8%; married or cohabited: 84.6% vs. 74.2%). They were also rather more likely to have had a child (61.2% vs. 46.2%). Among the women, reading group profiles for the proportions making these various transitions were closely similar. For men, however, rather larger proportions of poor readers had remained with their families of origin. Although all but 7% of comparison group men had lived independently by their late twenties, 21% of retarded readers and 25% of men in the backward reading group had remained in their parental homes throughout. A similar pattern was evident in measures of the men's living situations at the time of the interviews. By that stage, some who had lived independently had returned to their families of origin, and 31.3% of backward readers, 38.3% of retarded readers, but only 13.8% of comparison group men were living in their parental homes. There were no differences between the two groups of poor readers on this measure, but significant differences between the combined group of poor readers and the comparison group ($\chi^2 = 3.91$, 1 *df*, $p = .048$). Achieving independent living was unrelated to childhood social background, and showed no associations with either tested or self-report reading difficulties in adulthood. It was, however, associated with measures of childhood behavior problems, and in particular with difficulties in peer relationships. Although 89.2% of men without peer problems in middle childhood had achieved independent living, only 57.9% of those with peer difficulties had done so ($\chi^2 = 8.31$, 1 *df*, $p = .004$). A logistic regression model of independent living with a dichotomous indicator of peer problems and reading group as predictors showed significant effects for peer problems only. The lack of independence shown by some male poor readers appeared to owe as much to earlier difficulties in peer relations as to reading problems per se.

Timing of Transitions

Turning to the timing of these various transitions, women were likely to have left home somewhat earlier than men (women: 19.72 years, 95% CI 19.08–20.36; men: 20.47 years, CI 19.83–21.10; $F = 1.99$, *df* 1, 135, $p = .16$), and significantly more likely to have entered cohabitations at younger ages (women: 20.21 years, CI 19.56–20.87; men: 21.29 years, CI 20.63–21.94; $F = 5.34$, *df* 1, 120,

TABLE 4
Ages at Early Adult Transitions

		Transition				
		Left Home		First Cohabitation		First Child
	n	Mean Age	*n*	Mean Age	*n*	Mean Age
Women						
Backward readers	16	19.25	15	19.60	13	21.38
Retarded readers	18	19.11	18	19.89	13	21.31
Comparison group	27	20.41	23	20.87	17	22.53
ANOVAS:						
Poor readers vs.		$F = 3.85\ (1, 59)$		$F = 2.93\ (1, 54)$		$F = 1.10\ (1, 41)$
comparison group		$p = .055$		$p = .093$		n.s.
Men						
Backward readers	11	21.00	11	21.00	8	23.25
Retarded readers	35	20.14	32	21.06	21	22.29
Comparison group s	27	20.67	23	21.74	12	22.42
ANOVAS:						
Poor readers vs.		$F = 0.23\ (1, 71)$		$F = 1.02\ (1, 64)$		$F = 0.03\ (1, 39)$
comparison group		n.s.		n.s.		n.s.

$p = .023$). Mean ages at the birth of first children show no significant gender differences (women: 21.81 years, CI 20.70–22.93; men: 22.51 years, CI 21.74–23.28).

Table 4 shows mean ages at each transition for men and women in each reading group. Men in all three reading groups who had left home, entered cohabitations, and fathered children had done so at very similar ages. For women, there were no significant differences between the two groups of poor readers, but a tendency for the combined group of poor readers to have left home, moved into cohabitations, and had their first pregnancies between 1 year and 18 months earlier than women in the comparison group.

Multiple regression analyses were used to explore other factors that might have contributed to these variations in transition timing among the women. Childhood social class was unrelated to transition timing in this largely working class sample, but the two earlier transitions—leaving home and entering cohabitations—showed strong links with school-leaving qualifications, and with the types of jobs the women entered when they first left school. Age at first cohabitation, for example, showed a clear gradient across qualification levels: women with no formal qualifications began their first cohabitation at a mean age of 19.0 years (95% CI 18.04–19.96), those with lower graded qualifications at 20.7 (19.56–21.74), and those with higher graded examinations at 21.3 years (19.89–22.70), $t = 2.62$, $p = .011$. Earlier cohabitations were also more common among women entering unskilled, practical first jobs than those who went into clerical or social/personal roles ($t = 2.32$, $p = .024$). Women with reading difficulties were much more likely to have entered unskilled work of this kind (54.1% poor readers vs. 13.3% comparison group, $\chi^2 = 10.24$, 1 df, $p = .001$). The depressed educational qualifications and limited employment options of women with histories of reading difficulties seemed the more immediate influences of their tendency to earlier cohabitation.

Psychosocial Functioning in Early Adulthood

As outlined earlier, the subjects' social functioning in early adulthood was assessed in six life domains, over a 5-year age period, aged 21 to 25 years. To give an initial impression of the extent

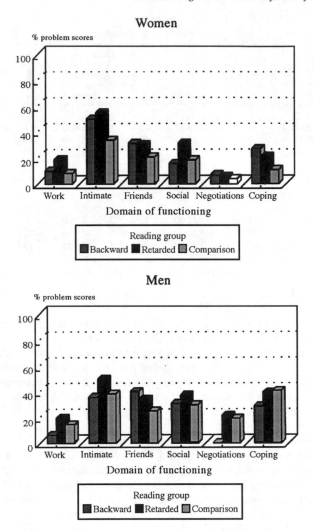

Figure 1. Psychosocial functioning in early adulthood: percentage problem scores.

of poor functioning evident in the sample, Fig. 1 shows the proportions of men and women in each reading group rated as showing problems (with Adult Personality Functioning Assessment [APFA] ratings of 4 or poorer) in each of the six domains assessed.

For both men and women, the highest levels of difficulty were in the area of intimate relationships—cohabitations, and, for those who had not cohabited, relationships with steady boy- or girlfriends. This pattern was also found in the original reliability study for the APFA (Hill et al., 1989). There were no overall gender differences in rates of problems in intimate relationships, nor in work, but in all other areas rather more men than women were rated as showing difficulties. These were most apparent on measures of day-to-day coping (women: 17.7% problem scores, men: 38.1%, $\chi^2 = 6.17$, 1 df,

TABLE 5
Psychosocial Functioning: Mean APFA Ratings Ages 21–25 Years

APFA Ratings	Poor Readers		Comparison Group (c)	Omnibus Tests			Pairwise Comparisons (p Values)		
	Backward (a)	Retarded (b)		F	df	p	a vs. c	b vs. c	a vs. b
Women	17.48 ± 4.08	18.73 ± 4.21	15.93 ± 4.60	2.93	2, 54	.062	n.s.	.021	n.s.
Men	16.69 ± 2.78	19.03 ± 4.41	18.32 ± 4.80	1.53	2, 79	n.s.	—	—	—

Note: Values are mean ± *SD*.

$p = .013$), and negotiations (women: 5.1% problem scores, men: 17.3% problem scores, $\chi^2 = 3.69$, 1 *df*, $p = .055$).

Reading group comparisons on these dichotomized scores showed no significant differences at the 5% level in any individual domain. As Fig. 1 suggests, however, there were indications that childhood poor readers—especially among the women—had functioned somewhat less well than comparison group members in a number of areas. Total APFA scores, summed across domains, provided a means of testing this.

Table 5 shows mean total APFA scores for men and women in each reading group. The raw scores were log-transformed to reduce skewness; all statistics presented are derived from analyses using the transformed scores. One-way ANOVAs (see Table 5) showed no significant reading group differences among the men, but some variations for the women. Pairwise contrasts showed that these primarily reflected higher rates of problems among retarded readers than comparison group members ($F = 5.68$, *df* 1, 54 $p = .021$).

For both men and women, early adult psychosocial functioning was unrelated to childhood social class, but was poorer among subjects who had failed to achieve independent living, and was significantly associated with teacher ratings of behavior problems in adolescence (women, $r = .363$, men, $r = .348$). Including the age 14 teacher ratings as covariates in the analyses for the women, no differences in adult functioning scores remained between retarded readers and comparison group members ($F = 1.16$, *df* 1, 48, n.s.). The poorer early adult functioning of women with IQ-discrepant reading problems seemed largely attributable to continuities from behavior difficulties already evident in their teens.

Cohabitation Breakdowns

The high rate of difficulties in intimate relationships identified in the APFA ratings led us to look in more detail at one central indicator of relationship problems: cohabitation breakdowns. As outlined earlier, more than 40% of the sample members had already experienced the breakdown of a cohabitation by their late twenties. There were no gender differences in rates of breakdown (46.3% women vs. 42.4% men, $\chi^2 = 0.06$, 1 *df*, n.s.), and no reading group differences among the men (41.7% backward readers, 45.2% retarded readers, 39.1% comparison group, $\chi^2 = 0.20$, 2 *df*, n.s.). Among the women, however, rates of breakdown were markedly elevated for those with childhood reading problems. By their late twenties, women in both poor reading groups were three times more likely to have experienced the breakdown of a cohabitation than their peers (backward readers 61.5%, retarded readers, 66.7%, comparison group, 21.7%, $\chi^2 = 9.80$, 2 *df*, $p = .007$).

Logistic regressions were used to identify other factors associated with cohabitation breakdowns among the women. Taking account of age at interview, breakdowns showed no associations with childhood social class or performance IQ. Instead, they were most strongly predicted by age at first cohabitation (early cohabitations being more likely to break down, χ^2 to remove $= 9.42$, 1 *df*, $p = .002$), with some additional effects of behavior difficulties at age 10 ($\chi^2 = 3.66$, 1 *df*, $p = .056$). In their turn, early cohabitations were associated with problems on a number of other relationship indicators: lower levels of confiding, poorer support from partners, and higher rates of partner deviance were all associated with younger ages at cohabitation. On the measure of partner support, for example, women reporting little or no support had begun cohabiting at a mean age of 18.90 years (95% CI 18.32–19.42), those reporting some, but limited or unreliable support at 19.69 years (18.05–21.34), and those in reliably supportive relationships at 21.30 years (20.19–22.41), $F = 5.63$, *df* 2, 48, $p = .006$.

These indicators of the quality of relationships were then added to the logistic regression model to predict relationship breakdowns (age at interview, age at first cohabitation, and behavior ratings at age 10 years). Partner support contributed significantly ($\chi^2 = 15.85$, 2 *df*, *sp* $< .001$), and with this included in the model, age at first cohabitation no longer showed significant effects ($\chi^2 = 1.59$, 1 *df*, n.s.). The lack of support reported by women who had entered their first cohabitations early seemed the most important contributor to their high risk of relationship breakdowns. A reduced model, excluding age at first cohabitation, was then used to test the remaining effects. Partner support remained the strongest predictor of relationship breakdown ($\chi^2 = 18.55$, 2 *df*, $p < .0001$), with indications of continuing effects of childhood behavior problems ($\chi^2 = 3.43$, 1 *df*, $p = .06$). With these effects included in the model, no significant differences between the reading groups remained ($\chi^2 = 4.28$, 2 *df*, n.s.).

Two rather different processes thus appeared to have contributed to the much heightened risk of relationship breakdowns among women with childhood reading problems. The first reflected behavioral continuities at the individual level: women with behavior problems in childhood were less likely to sustain cohabiting relationships in their early adult lives. The second route was more complex. Most immediately, it reflected a range of aspects of the women's relationships, especially lack of support from partners. Contrasts between the reading groups were striking here: where 68.2% of women in the comparison group reported definite and reliable support in their first partnerships, only 28.6% of backward readers and 26.7% of retarded readers did so. These poorer relationships were more likely to occur in early cohabitations; and, as outlined earlier, these occurred rather more frequently among poor than competent readers.

Self-Esteem

Across the sample as a whole men rated themselves significantly more positively than did women on the self-esteem scale (men: $M = 31.79$, 95% CI 30.93–32.66, women: $M = 29.57$, CI 28.60–30.54, $F = 11.64$, *df* 1, 135, $p < .001$). Table 6 shows mean Rosenberg scores for men and women in each reading group. There were no differences between the reading groups for either women or men, suggesting that a history of childhood reading problems had few implications for subjects' overall evaluations of their self-worth in adulthood. Indeed, additional tests failed to identify significant

TABLE 6
Mean Self-Esteem Scores

	Poor Readers		Comparison Group	Omnibus Tests		
	Backward	Retarded		F	df	p
Women	29.67 ± 3.79	29.19 ± 4.10	29.72 ± 3.66	0.11	2, 57	n.s.
Men	32.64 ± 2.84	31.58 ± 4.09	31.77 ± 3.80	0.33	2, 73	n.s.

Note: Values are mean $\pm$ *SD*.

associations between the Rosenberg scores and any of the behavioral, reading, or IQ scores from the childhood phases of the study or with childhood social class.

As the Rosenberg taps current self-perceptions, this lack of association with childhood indicators was not perhaps surprising. We went on to examine links with adult reading difficulties, in terms of both objective test scores and self-reported problem levels. There were no significant differences according to objectively tested reading levels for the men ($F = 0.62$, $df\ 2$, 63, n.s.), although there were some suggestions of links with current reading performance among the women ($F = 2.75$, $df\ 2$, 50, $p = .074$). Associations with the subjects' self-reports of continued reading impairment were, however, stronger especially among the women ($F = 5.21$, $df\ 2$, 57, $p = .008$). Multiple regression analyses including both test score levels and self-reports bore out the importance of perceived rather than tested reading levels for the women: only the self-report measures showed significant associations with Rosenberg scores (self-report reading impairment: $t = -3.22$, $p = .002$; adult test score: $t = -0.42$, n.s.). For the men, neither measure showed significant links with self-esteem (self-report reading impairment: $t = -0.96$, n.s.; adult test score: $t = -0.25$, n.s.).

Psychiatric Disorder

The interviews provided data on four types of psychiatric morbidity in adulthood: psychosis; episodic disorder (very predominantly anxiety and depression); alcohol problems; and personality disorders. As expected, psychosis was rare in a sample of this size. Only one participant (a woman from the retarded reading group) was known to have suffered from any psychotic illness (schizophrenia) in adulthood. Rates of other disorders were at broadly the levels expected in a community sample (Bebbington, Hurry, & Tennant, 1991) and showed anticipated patterns of gender differences. Women were two and a half times more likely than men to have experienced an episode of anxiety or depression since age 16 years (30.8% vs. 12.1%, $\chi^2 = 8.31$, 1 df, $p = .004$), while serious alcohol problems were almost exclusively confined to the men (16.5% vs. 1.6%, $\chi^2 = 9.04$, 1 df, $p = .003$). Personality disorders were also more common in men than women (8.9% vs. 1.5%), but at these low rates contrasts failed to reach significance ($\chi^2 = 2.51$, 1 df, n.s.).

Table 7 shows the proportions of women and men in each childhood reading group who had experienced the three main types of psychiatric problem. Women in the retarded reading group were somewhat more likely than those in either of the other groups to report episodes of anxiety and depression, and the only woman in the sample rated as showing a personality disorder (antisocial

TABLE 7
Rates of Adult Psychiatric Disorder

| | Poor Readers | | | | |
	Backward (W: $n = 16$) (M: $n = 14$)	Retarded (W: $n = 21$) (M: $n = 48$)	Comparison Group (W/M: $n = 29$)	χ^2 (2 df)	p
Women					
Episodic disorder	25.0	42.9	25.0	2.13	n.s.
Alcohol problems	0	0	3.6	1.31	n.s.
Personality disorder	0	5.0	0	2.29	n.s.
Men					
Episodic disorder	28.6	8.3	10.3	4.30	.12
Alcohol problems	6.7	17.0	20.7	1.43	n.s.
Personality disorder	7.1	14.6	0	4.97	.083

Note: Values are in percents.

personality) also came from this group. Among the men, episodic disorder was rather more frequent among backward readers. The only cases of personality disorder also occurred among men with reading difficulties in childhood. The one man with severe personality problems in the backward reading group showed antisocial difficulties, but the personality problems of men in the retarded reading group were very predominantly (in five of the seven cases) of an immature, avoidant kind.

For women, episodic disorder in adulthood showed few direct associations with the childhood measures available in the study. None of the age 10 reading or IQ scores showed significant links with adult psychiatric problems, and associations with childhood behavior problems and social background also failed to reach statistical significance. For the men, childhood behavior ratings emerged as more important predictors of adult disorder. Both alcohol problems and personality disorder were significantly associated with teacher behavior ratings at age 14 years (alcohol: $\chi^2 = 4.86, 1 \ df$, $p = .028$; personality disorder: $\chi^2 = 3.96, 1 \ df, p = .047$). Episodic disorder among men in the sample also showed links with self-reports of current reading difficulties. Men who perceived themselves as having continuing literacy problems were more likely to have experienced episodes of anxiety and depression ($\chi^2 = 12.20, 2 \ df, p = .002$).

DISCUSSION

This study set out to examine the implications of severe childhood reading difficulties for a range of aspects of psychosocial functioning in early adulthood. Despite the prevalence of developmental reading problems, and their well-established overlaps with behavioral and psychiatric problems in childhood, previous follow-up evidence of this kind has been limited. Existing evidence has derived very largely from clinicreferred samples, and suggested continuing difficulties for varying—and sometimes quite high—proportions of participants.

Our findings in representative samples were in many ways more positive, although they too pointed to problems for some participants in some areas, and to somewhat different patterns of vulnerability for women and men. Among the men, there were no marked differences between the reading groups on measures of social functioning, nor in terms of adult self-esteem. There were suggestions that poor readers were more vulnerable to both "avoidant" personality problems and anxiety and depression, but the clearest systematic differences among the men occurred in the area of independent living: larger proportions of poor than competent reading men were still, in their late twenties, living with their families of origin, and more appeared to have done so throughout their early adult lives. Although this pattern applied to a sizeable minority of male poor readers—just over a fifth—it was by no means typical of the group as a whole.

For women in the sample, outcomes were less positive in a number of respects. Previous studies (e.g., Bruck, 1985) have suggested that young women with histories of reading difficulties are more likely to show adjustment problems in adulthood, and our data also supported that view. Measures of social functioning in the early twenties showed higher problem levels among retarded readers than in the comparison group, and these women also appeared at some increased risk of psychiatric disorder. Probably the most striking feature of the findings, however, was the high rate of relationship break-downs among women with childhood reading problems, and their elevated risks of other relationship difficulties.

Our findings thus suggested some areas of continuing vulnerability for childhood poor readers, as well as evidence of more positive functioning. Where problems for poor readers persisted, we had hypothesized that three rather different developmental pathways might be implicated: continuities from earlier behavior problems, reactions to awareness of ongoing literacy difficulties, and more indirect influences mediated through intervening or current life circumstances. The findings suggested effects of all three pathways, differing in their importance in different domains of functioning.

Associations with childhood behavior problems were evident at a number of points in the analyses. For men, the only marked differences between poor and competent readers—in the proportions achieving independence from their families of origin—appeared to owe more to early comorbidities with problems in peer relations than to reading difficulties per se. In a similar way, later vulnerabilities to both alcohol problems and personality disorder showed links with earlier behavior problems. For women, comorbid child and adolescent behavior problems contributed both to the poorer adult social functioning of childhood retarded readers, and to the elevated risks of first partnership breakdowns.

Relationship difficulties among the women also pointed to effects of our third postulated pathway—via intervening and current life circumstances. Here, the analyses suggested a series of linkages, with early reading problems acting as forerunners to poor school-leaving qualifications and relatively undemanding—and probably unrewarding—early employment options. These in turn were associated with earlier ages at cohabitation and most proximally with unsupportive early adult relationships.

Our findings here were based on small numbers and clearly require replication. They are consistent, however, with the earlier moves to family formation noted in previous studies of young women with selfreported literacy problems in adulthood (ALBSU, 1987; Ekynsmith & Bynner, 1994). If replicated, they are also important in highlighting the implications of poor educational achievements for later psychosocial functioning among women. With other colleagues, we have recently shown how conduct disorder can elevate risks of poor intimate relationships in adulthood through processes of assortative pairing on deviance (Quinton et al., 1993). In this study, although childhood behaviors also played some part, the strongest predictors of early cohabitation and its contingent relationship difficulties were poor educational qualifications. Although limited educational credentials were, of course, an especially salient outcome in a study of reading difficulities, they are likely to occur at high rates among many disordered and disadvantaged childhood groups. Our findings suggest that they may warrant attention as mediators of childhood–adult continuities in a range of samples.

For poor readers, we had also anticipated that a history of reading problems, or awareness of continuing literacy difficulties, might influence adult functioning through effects on self-evaluations. In childhood, poor readers have consistently been found to show low academic self-esteem, although findings on global self-ratings have been more varied (see e.g., Bryan & Bryan, 1990). In adulthood, we found no evidence for long-term effects of early reading problems on global self-esteem, suggesting that a history of childhood academic skills problems need in no way presage low general self-worth in adulthood. Perceptions of current reading difficulties were, however, associated with lower self-esteem for the relatively small group who saw their skills as seriously impaired in their late twenties. Elsewhere (Hagell, 1992) we have examined these subjects' attributions for success and failure in a range of domains. Poor and competent readers did not differ in attributional style when asked to generate causes for nonreading-related failures, but did show differences when explaining reading problems. In that context, poor readers were more likely to produce explanations that indicated self-blame—internal, controllable attributions. More differentiated measures of self-esteem, reflecting a multifaceted, hierarchical model of the self-concept, such as that proposed by Marsh and Shavelson (1985), might have revealed similar group differences in academic self-esteem.

Our findings highlighted some differences, but also considerable similarities, in the adult functioning of the two groups of childhood poor readers included in the study. As we have seen, the problems faced by poor readers in some domains—most obviously those concerned with independent living for men and cohabitation problems for women—occurred at similar rates for both low and underachievers. Although current diagnostic criteria would not identify the backward readers studied here as showing academic skills disorders in childhood, these findings suggest that they too may face some long-term vulnerabilities associated with their achievement problems. The clearest pointers to difficulties more specific to underachievers arose in the measures of social functioning and episodic disorder for the women—in both instances childhood underachievers appeared to be at greatest risk. This suggests some specificity in later outcomes, most clearly associated, in the case of problems in social functioning, with difficulties that also reflected continuities from earlier behavior problems.

Set against these difficulties, the findings also revealed many areas where childhood poor readers functioned very comparably with their peers in adulthood. If replicated, this pattern suggests a more positive prognosis for later psychosocial functioning among representative groups of children with reading difficulties than reported in previous studies of referred groups. We can only speculate on the factors that may have contributed here. While improved reading skills can only have been beneficial, the analyses gave few suggestions that more positive psychosocial functioning was in any sense directly dependent on these. Instead, it seemed most likely that contextual factors, along with variations in the subjects' own perceptions of their continuing impairment, may have been among the most important influences. Our study tracked subjects from their schooling—when rates of behavioral problems were relatively high—into adulthood, when for men in particular difficulties seemed much less marked. As proposed in early commentaries on the childhood comorbidity between reading and disruptive behaviors (Rutter, Tizard, Whitmore, 1970), the sense of failure and frustration almost inevitably experienced by poor readers during schooling may well have exacerbated their difficulties at that stage. By the same token, the more wide-ranging options available to young men in particular once they left school may have played some part in enabling more positive social functioning in adulthood. Once able to select environments in adulthood, many subjects may have been able to minimize the functional implications of any ongoing literacy difficulties, and build on their other skills and talents.

Our findings must be evaluated in the light of both the strengths and the limitations of our sample for a long-term follow-up of this kind. Our study had a number of advantages: most importantly, it focused on representative samples of children with severe reading difficulties, drawn from screening a full school population, and so unaffected by referral bias. Nonreferred samples offer advantages in many contexts, but may be especially important in studies of psychosocial functioning. Children referred for special reading help may well include disproportionate numbers with associated behavior problems, which could contribute to difficulties in adult functioning. Studying an unselected sample offered the means to avoid potential biases of this kind.

Other positive features of our design concerned the inclusion of two groups of poor readers—generally reading backward and specifically reading retarded—and the availability of contemporaneous measures of behavior problems, collected in childhood. To our knowledge, no previous follow-ups of disabled readers have included measures of this kind. Set against these advantages, we must also note a number of limitations in our design. First, the sample was modest in size, especially when assessments required separate comparisons by gender. This inevitably constrained the power of some analyses to detect group differences. Some variations in outcome that failed to reach conventional levels of statistical significance in our data might thus emerge more clearly in larger groups. Second, all our subjects were drawn from a relatively disadvantaged inner-city area, where rates of reading difficulties, behavior problems, and associated family risk factors were all high, and showed higher than expected overlaps (Rutter et al., 1975; Sturge, 1982). In previous studies of poor readers, social background has shown important effects on later educational and occupational outcomes (O'Connor & Spreen, 1988). In this study, the relatively limited impact of childhood social class throughout the analyses undoubtedly reflected the restricted range of social circumstances included in the sample. These characteristics of the setting for the study may place some limitations on the generalizability of our findings. Once again, replications in other samples, especially those differing in social contexts for development, would be extremely valuable.

REFERENCES

Adult Literacy and Basic Skills Unit (ALBSU). (1987). *Literacy, Numeracy and Adults: Evidence from the National Child Development Study*. London: ALBSU.

American Psychiatric Association. (1994). *Diagnostic and Statistical Manual of Mental Disorders. 4th Ed.— DSM-IV*. Washington, DC: Author.

Balow, B., & Blomquist, M. (1965). Young adults ten to fifteen years after reading disability. *Elementary School Journal, 66*, 44–48.

Bebbington, P. E., Hurry, J., & Tennant, C. (1991). The Camberwell Community Survey: A summary of results. *Social Psychiatry and Psychiatric Epidemiology, 26*, 195–201.

Berger, M., Yule, W., & Rutter, M. (1975). Attainment and adjustment in two geographical areas II: The prevalence of specific reading retardation. *British Journal of Psychiatry, 126*, 510–519.

Bruck, M. (1985). The adult functioning of children with specific learning disability: A follow-up study. In I. Siegel (Ed.), *Advances in applied developmental psychology* (pp. 91–129). Norwood, NJ: Ablex.

Bryan, J. H., & Bryan, T. (1990). Social factors in learning disabilities: Attitudes and interactions. In G. Th. Pavlidis (Ed.), *Perspectives on Dyslexia, Vol. 2* (pp. 247–281). London: Wiley.

Carter, R. P. (1967). The adult social adjustment of retarded and non-retarded readers. *Journal of Reading, 11*, 224–228.

Champion, L., Goodall, G., & Rutter, M. (1995). Behaviour problems in childhood and stressors in early adult life: I. A twenty-year follow-up of London school children. *Psychological Medicine, 25*, 231–246.

Chapman, J. W., Lambourne, R., & Silva, P. A. (1990). Some antecedents of academic self-concept: A longitudinal study. *British Journal of Educational Psychology, 60*, 142–152.

Cicchetti, D., & Richters, J. E. (1993). Developmental considerations in the investigation of conduct disorder. *Development and Psychopathology, 5*, 331–344.

Cornwell, A., & Bawden, H. N. (1992). Reading disabilities and aggression: A critical review. *Journal of Learning Disabilities, 25*, 281–288.

Ekynsmith, C., & Bynner, J. (1994). *The basic skills of young adults: Some findings from the 1970 British cohort study*. London: ALBSU.

Endicott, J., & Spitzer, R. L. (1978). A diagnostic interview: The schedule for affective disorders and schizophrenia. *Archives of General Psychiatry, 35*, 837–844.

Finucci, J. M. (1986). Follow-up studies of developmental dyslexia and other learning disabilities. In Smith, S. D. (Ed.), *Genetics and learning disabilities* (pp. 97–121). Philadelphia: Taylor and Francis.

Finucci, J. M., Whitehouse, C. C., Isaacs, S. D., & Childs, B. (1984). Derivation and validation of a quantitative definition of specific reading disability for adults. *Developmental Medicine and Child Neurology, 26*, 143–153.

Gray, W. S. (1967). *The Gray Oral Reading Test*. Indianapolis: Bobbs–Merrill.

Hagell, A. (1992). *The social psychology of illiteracy: An attributional perspective*. Unpublished PhD thesis, University of London.

Hardy, M. I. (1968). Disabled readers: What happens to them after elementary school? *Canadian Education and Research Digest, 8*, 338–346.

Hill, J., Harrington, R., Fudge, H., Rutter, M., & Pickles, A. (1989). Adult Personality Functioning Assessment (APFA): An investigator-based standardized interview. *British Journal of Psychiatry, 155*, 24–35.

Hinshaw, S. P. (1992). Externalizing behavior problems and academic underachievement in childhood and adolescence: Causal relationships and underlying mechanisms. *Psychological Bulletin, 111*, 127–155.

Hogan, D. P., & Astone, N. M. (1986). The transition to adulthood. *American Review of Sociology, 12*, 109–130.

Jaklewicz, H. (1982). Dyslexia: Follow-up studies. *Thalamus (International Academy for Research in Learning Disabilities), 2*, 3–9.

Jaklewicz, H. (1992). Dyslexia and its consequences in the life of dyslexics. In B. Ericson (Ed.), *Aspects on*

Annual Progress in Child Psychiatry and Development

literacy: Selected papers from the 13th IRA World Congress on Reading. Linkoping, Sweden: Linkoping University.

Jorm, A. F., Share, D. L., Matthews, R., & Maclean, R. (1986). Behaviour problems in specific reading retarded and general reading backward children: A longitudinal study. *Journal of Child Psychology and Psychiatry, 27*, 33–43.

Kerckhoff, A. C. (1990). *Getting started: Transition to adulthood in Great Britain.* Boulder, CO: Westview.

Livingston, R. (1990). Psychiatric comorbidity with reading disability: A clinical study. *Advances in Learning Disabilities: A Research Annual Vol. 6, 1990* (pp. 143–155). Greenwich: JAI Press.

Marsh, H. W., & Shavelson, R. J. (1985). Self-concept: its multifaceted, hierarchical structure. *Educational Psychologist, 20*, 107–125.

Maughan, B. (1989). Growing up in the inner city: Findings from the inner London longitudinal study. *Paediatric and Perinatal Epidemiology, 3*, 195–215.

Maughan, B., Hagell, A., Rutter, M., & Yule, W. (1994). Poor readers in secondary school. *Reading and Writing: An Interdisciplinary Journal, 6*, 125–150.

Maughan, B., Pickles, A., Hagell, A., Rutter, M., & Yule, W. (in press). *Reading problems and antisocial behavior: Developmental trends in comorbidity.*

McGuffin, P., Katz, R., & Aldrich, J. (1986). Past and present state examination: The assessment of "life-time ever" psychopathology. *Psychological Medicine, 16*, 461–465.

National Foundation for Educational Research (NFER). (1970). *Manual of Instructions: Sentence Reading Tests.* Windsor: NFER.

Naylor, C. E., Felton, R. H., & Wood, F. B. (1990). Adult outcome in developmental dyslexia. In G. Th. Pavlidis (Ed.), *Perspectives on Dyslexia Vol. 2* (pp. 215–229). London: Wiley.

Neale, M. D. (1958). *Neale Analysis of Reading Ability Manual.* London: Macmillan.

O'Connor, S., & Spreen, O. (1988). The relationship between parents' socioeconomic status and education level and adult occupational and educational achievement of children with learning disabilities. *Journal of Learning Disabilities, 21*, 148–153.

Patton, J. R., & Polloway, E. A. (1992). Learning disabilities: The challenges of adulthood. *Journal of Learning Disabilities, 25*, 410–415, 447.

Quinton, D., Pickles, A., Maughan, B., & Rutter, M. (1993). Partners, peers and pathways: Assortative pairing and continuities in conduct disorder. *Development and Psychopathology, 5*, 763–783.

Renick, M. J., & Harter, S. (1989). Impact of social comparisons on the developing self-perceptions of learning disabled students. *Journal of Educational Psychology, 81*, 631–638.

Richman, N., Stevenson, J., & Graham, P. J. (1982). *Pre-school to school: A behavioural study.* London: Academic Press.

Rodgers, B. (1986). Changes in the reading attainment of adults: A longitudinal study. *British Journal of Developmental Psychology, 4*, 1–17.

Rosenberg, M. (1965). *Society and the adolescent self-image.* Princeton: Princeton University Press.

Rutter, M. (1967). A children's behaviour questionnaire for completion by teachers: Preliminary findings. *Journal of Child Psychology and Psychiatry, 8*, 1–11.

Rutter, M., Cox, A., Tupling, C., Berger, M., & Yule, W. (1975). Attainment and adjustment in two geographical areas. I. The prevalence of psychiatric disorder. *British Journal of Psychiatry, 126*, 493–509.

Rutter, M., Tizard, J., & Whitmore, K. (Eds.). (1970). *Education, Health and Behaviour.* London: Longman and Green.

Rutter, M., Yule, B., Quinton, D., Rowlands, O., Yule, W., & Berger, M. (1975). Attainment and adjustment in two geographical areas. III. Some factors accounting for area differences. *British Journal of Psychiatry, 126*, 520–533.

Spreen, O. (1987). *Learning disabled children growing up: A follow-up into adulthood.* Lisse, Netherlands: Swets & Zeitlinger.

Stanovich, K. E. (1994). Does dyslexia exist? *Journal of Child Psychology and Psychiatry, 35*, 579–596.

University of Edinburgh. (1977). *Edinburgh reading tests: Manual of instructions*. London: Hodder & Stoughton.

Wechsler, D. (1949). *Wechsler Intelligence Scale for Children (Manual)*. New York: Psychological Corporation.

World Health Organization (1992). *The ICD-10 Classification of Mental and Behavioral Disorders: Clinical Descriptions and Diagnostic Guidelines*. Geneva: Author.

Yule, W. (1967). Predicting reading ages on Neale's analysis of reading ability. *British Journal of Educational Psychology, 37*, 252–255.

9

Language Comprehension in Language-Learning Impaired Children Improved with Acoustically Modified Speech

Paula Tallal, Steve L. Miller, Gail Bedi, and Gary Byma
Center for Molecular and Behavioral Neuroscience, Rutgers University

Xiaoqin Wang, Srikantan S. Nagarajan, Christoph Schreiner, William M. Jenkins, and Michael M. Merzenich
W. M. Keck Center for Integrative Neurosciences and Coleman Laboratory, University of California, San Francisco

A speech processing algorithm was developed to create more salient versions of the rapidly changing elements in the acoustic waveform of speech that have been shown to be deficiently processed by language-learning impaired (LLI) children. LLI children received extensive daily training, over a 4-week period, with listening exercises in which all speech was translated into this synthetic form. They also received daily training with computer "games" designed to adaptively drive improvements in temporal processing thresholds. Significant improvements in speech discrimination and language comprehension abilities were demonstrated in two independent groups of LLI children.

Exposure to a specific language alters an infant's phonetic perceptions within the first months of life, leading to the setting of prototypic phonetic representations, the building block on which a child's native language develops (Kuhl, Williams, Lacerda, Stevens, & Lindblom, 1992; Eiams, Miller, & Jusczyk, 1987; Steinschneider, Arezzo, & Vaughan, 1990). Although this occurs normally without explicit instruction for the majority of children, epidemiological studies estimate that nearly 20% of children fail to develop normal speech and language when exposed to speech in their native environment (Bitchman, Nair, Clegg, & Patel, 1986; Silva, 1980; Stevenson & Richman, 1976; Williams, Darbyshive, & Vaghy, 1980). Even after all other primary sensory and cognitive deficits are accounted

Informed consent was obtained from the parent or parents of each child after the potential risks and benefits of the studies were explained. We thank the therapists who referred subjects as well as the parents and children who participated. We thank A. Rubenstein, B. Glazewski, J. Flax, C. Roesler, K. Masters, J. Reitzel, T. Delaney, and P. Johnston for assistance in subject selection, stimulus preparation, and clinical testing and T. Realpe, I. Shell, C. Kapelyan, A. Katsnelson, L. Brzustowicz, C. Brown, A. Khoury, and S. Shapack for assistance in the experimental training. Valuable comments on the manuscript by I. Creese are appreciated. We thank the Charles A. Dana Foundation for supporting the research. For more information, see http://www.ld.ucsf.edu

for, approximately 3% to 6% of children still fail to develop normal speech and language abilities (National Conf. on Learning Disabilities, 1987). Longitudinal studies have demonstrated a striking convergence between preschool language delay and subsequent reading disabilities (such as dyslexia). A broad body of research now suggests that phonological processing deficits may be at the heart of these language-learning impairments (LLIs) (Stark et al., 1994; Bishop & Adams. 1990; Catts, 1993; Liberman, Shankweiler, Fischer, & Carter, 1974; Scarborough, 1990; Torgesen, Wagner, & Rashotte, 1994; Rissman, Curtiss, & Tallal, 1990).

Tallal's earlier research has shown that rather than deriving from a primarily linguistic or cognitive impairment, the phonological and language difficulties of LLI children may result from a more basic deficit in processing rapidly changing sensory inputs (Tallal & Pievcy, 1973a). Specifically, LLI children commonly cannot identify fast elements embedded in ongoing speech that have durations in the range of a few tens of milliseconds, a critical time frame over which many phonetic contrasts are signaled (Tallal & Piercy, 1974; Tallal, 1980a; Tallal & Stark, 1982; Tallal, Stark & Mellits, 1985a; Stark & Tallal, 1988). For example, LLI children have particular difficulty in discriminating between many speech syllables, such as [ba] and [da], which are characterized by very rapid frequency changes (formant transitions) that occur during the initial few tens of milliseconds. Interestingly, LLI children are able to identify these same syllables when the rates of change of the critical formant transitions are simply synthetically extended in time by about twofold (Tallal & Piercy, 1975). A strong prediction is suggested by these findings: If the critical acoustic cues within the context of fluent, ongoing speech could be altered to be emphasized and extended in time, then the phonological discrimination and the on-line language comprehension abilities of LLI children should significantly improve.

To test this prediction, we have conducted two studies with LLI children who have been trained with the application of temporally modified speech. These same children also received training at making distinctions about fast and rapidly sequenced acoustic inputs in exercises mounted in the format of computer "games" (Merzenich et al., 1996). Modification of fluent speech was achieved by application of a two-stage processing algorithm.[1] In the first stage, the duration of the speech signal was prolonged by 50% while preserving its spectral content and natural quality. In the second processing stage, fast (3–30 Hz) transitional elements of speech were differentially enhanced by as much as 20 dB. This two-step acoustic modification process was applied to speech and language listening exercises that were recorded on audiotapes, as well as to the speech tracks of children's stories recorded on tapes and on educational CD-ROMs. The differential emphasis of fast elements also resulted in a speech envelope that was more sharply segmented. This processed speech had a staccato quality in which the fast (primarily consonant) elements were exaggerated relative to more slowly modulated elements (primarily vowels) in the ongoing speech stream. We reasoned that amplifying the fast elements should render them more salient, and thus more reliably temporally integrated, and less likely to be

---

[1]Speech modification was achieved by a two-stage processing algorithm. In the first stage, the rate of the speech signal was prolonged by 50%, while preserving its spectral content and natural quality. This time-scale modification was implemented with a digital signal processing algorithm (Portnoff, 1981). This algorithm involved computation of the short-time. Fourier transform (STFT) of the speech signal with the fast-Fourier transform (FFT), linear interpolation, and phase-modification of the STFT to the new time scale, followed by additive synthesis with the inverse-Fourier transform. In the second stage of processing, the fast transition elements were differentially amplified by as much as 20 dB. The fast transition elements of speech were defined as the 3- to 3-Hz components of the speech envelope within rate-changed narrow-band channels. This differential "emphasis" was also implemented with a digital signal processing algorithm. The modification involved band-pass filtering of the speech signal into critical-band channels, computation of the envelope within each channel, band-pass filtering of the speech envelope, modification of the narrow-band signals to carry the new band-pass envelope followed by additive synthesis of the modified speech signal from the narrow-band channels. The above-mentioned algorithm was implemented initially by using a filter-bank summation algorithm and then improved on with the overlap-add procedure and the FFT (Langhans & Strube, 1982).

subject to forward or backward masking by neighboring, slowly modulated speech elements. That sharpening of the envelope offsets the slower envelope modulation that applies for prolonged speech. Cortical plasticity experiments have indicated that a more sharply modulated form of speech should be more powerful for inducing complex signal learning (Merzenich & Jenkins, 1995).

Seven LLI children participated in a 6-week study aimed at evaluating the effect that exposure to acoustically modified speech had on speech discrimination and on-line language comprehension (see reference 10 of Merzenich et al., 1996, in this issue for subject characteristics). In week 1 (pretraining) and week 6 (posttraining), clinical benchmark scores were derived with natural, unprocessed speech by using a series of standardized speech, language, and auditory temporal processing tests.[2] In weeks 2–5 the children rotated each week through a series of 10 different listening exercises that were designed to provide consistent exposure to the acoustically modified speech. Training exercises were conducted for 3 hours a day, 5 days a week, at the laboratory, and 1 to 2 hours a day, 7 days a week as "homework" over a 4-week period. The language exercises,[3] which consisted of exposure to prerecorded, acoustically modified speech, were delivered one-on-one by trained clinicians as well as through the use of computer games (Merzenich et al., 1996) designed specifically for this study. The children also listened to stories on audio tapes or CD-ROMs that had been acoustically modified with the same computer algorithm. The goal was to have the children actively listen to the acoustically modified fluent speech in a highly consistent format, for as many hours per day as possible.

A comparison of pretraining and posttraining test performances is shown in Fig. 1. The LLI children were between 1 and 3 years behind their chronological age in speech and language development based on their pretraining test scores. After 1 month of daily training with acoustically modified speech, a repeated measures analysis of variance showed that posttraining test scores significantly improved ($F(1, 6) = 200.1, P < 0.001$) by approximately 2 years, with each of the seven LLI

---

[2]The following five tests were used as clinical benchmark measures during pretraining (week 1) and posttraining (week 6). These clinical speech and language tests were recorded with natural, unmodified speech and presented over headphones. (i) The Token Test assesses the ability to follow auditory commands of increasing length and grammatical complexity. (DiSimoni, 1978). (ii) The GFW test assesses speech-sound discrimination within words. (Goldman, Fristoe, & Woodcock, 1974). (iii) The CYCLE-R thoroughly examines comprehension of specific components of grammar (morphology and syntax) (Curtiss and Yamada, unpublished). (iv) The Computerized Repetition Test is a modification of the Repetition Test (Tallal, 1980b; Tallal & Miller, 1994). In the Repetition Test, subjects are operantly trained to press one panel on a response box after hearing stimulus 1 and a different panel for stimulus 2. Two stimuli are then presented sequentially in various combinations (that is, 1-1, 2-1, 1-2, and 2-2 with an interstimulus interval (ISI) interposed between the two tones. The subject is required to reproduce the sequence by pressing the panels in the correct order. The Computerized Repetition Test determines the threshold ISI at which sequences of two pure-tone stimuli of 150-, 75-, 40-, or 17-ms duration are perceived and reproduced with 75% accuracy. The ISIs vary from 500 to 0 ms. (v) The Soundsin-Words subtest was used to assess accuracy in speech articulation. Speech was elicited by having the child label a picture that depicted a common object or activity. (Goldman & Fristoe, 1986).

[3]The speech and language exercises were developed as games to maintain attention and motivation over the course of the study. Tape recorded syllables, words, phrases, and sentences that had been acoustically modified with the speech algorithm developed for this study were presented to the child over headphones or free field. The games included acting out commands in a Simon Says format with props; pointing to pictures or colored blocks in response to commands; repeating verbatim syllables, nonsense words, real words, or sentences; and pointing to pictures corresponding to spoken words. Throughout training, commands of increasing length and grammatical complexity were used in these games. Careful attention was given in the design of the listening exercises to ensure that foils developed for each item would focus the attention of the child on the salient aspects of speech discrimination or receptive grammar being trained. In the listening games, regardless of the accuracy of the child's response, immediate nonverbal feedback was given after each response ("thumbs up" or "thumbs down"), followed by a repetition of the item with the correct response indicated by the clinician, so the child could have a second chance to process correctly. Each child won points for cooperation throughout the training, which were tallied daily and exchanged for prizes at the end of each week.

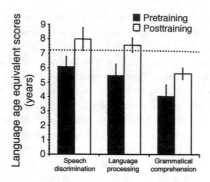

Figure 1. Performance of LLI subjects from study 1 on specific speech and language measures was obtained with natural speech before (pretraining) and after (posttraining) 4 weeks of temporal processing training and training with acoustically modified speech exercises. Measures included speech discrimination (GFW test), language processing (Token Test), and grammatical comprehension (CYCLE-R) (DiSimoni, 1978; Goldman et al., 1974; Curtiss & Yamada, unpublished; Tallal & Miller, 1994, Tallal, 1990; Goldman & Fristoe, 1986). Mean and standard error of the mean data are shown for each measure. Mean chronological age (7.3 years) is displayed as a horizontal dotted bar. Data obtained at posttraining (white bars) reflect significantly higher performance for each measure than the pretraining values (black bars) obtained 4 weeks earlier. Note that performance after training approached or exceeded that expected for normally developing children of the same chronological age.

children approaching or exceeding normal limits for their age in speech discrimination and language comprehension.

A second study was done to examine the extent to which the significant improvements in receptive speech and language abilities were replicable in an independent, larger group of LLI subjects, and the extent to which those improvements derive specifically from training with acoustically modified speech coupled with temporal processing training. Twenty-two LLI children participated (mean chronological age = 7.4 years; mean language age = 4.9 years) (see reference 13 of Merzenich et al., 1996, for subject characteristics). The design of the first 6-week study was replicated, with some minor revisions, to accommodate the larger number of subjects.[4] The children were divided into two matched groups on the basis of pretraining measures of nonverbal intelligence and receptive language abilities.[5] Both groups performed the same training exercises used in study 1. However, to assess the efficacy of the processed speech and temporal training, we presented half of the children (group A) with computer games that adaptively trained temporal processing and with language exercises recorded with acoustically modified speech. The other LLI children (group B) received

---

[4]Changes from study 1 to study 2 included (i) increasing the duration of the laboratory sessions from 3 to 3.5 hours per day, (ii) providing homework solely in the form of recorded children's stories on tape (either acoustically modified (group A) or with natural unmodified speech (group B)) instead of computer games, (iii) increasing the number of computer game formats from two to four, and (iv) modifying the ratio of clinicians to children in each training session from one-to-one to usually one-to-one, but on occasion one-to-two. The children in study 1 and group A in study 2 received computer games that adaptively trained temporal processing and phoneme perception, whereas the children in group B study 2 received the same schedule of computer game training and reinforcement, but with games that did not contain temporally or phonetically adaptive stimuli.

[5]Subjects were assigned to the two groups to minimize the differences between subjects on measures of performance IQ (PIQ) (The Psychological Corporation, 1991) reported as mean (SEM) (PIQ, group A = 96.1 (2.6), group B = 96.6 (3.3)), and receptive language performance (Token Test Age scores) reported as mean (SEM) (group A = 5.4 (0.4), group B = 6.1 (0.7)).

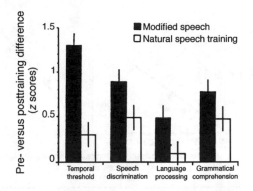

Figure 2. Difference z scores (posttraining minus pretraining) are shown for LLI subjects in study 2 who received speech and language training with either acoustically modified or natural speech. Difference z scores are presented for measures of temporal threshold, speech discrimination (GFW), language processing (Token Test), and grammatical comprehension (CYCLE-R). To facilitate group comparisons across each of the measures, we converted raw scores to z scores on the basis of the pretraining performance of all subjects on each individual test. Mean and standard error values for each measure demonstrate that significantly larger improvements were achieved by the LLI children receiving the acoustically modified speech training (black bars) as compared with the performance improvements recorded for the subjects receiving natural speech training (white bars). The temporal threshold values were converted to positive values for display purposes.

essentially the same training, but with computer games that were not temporally adaptive, and with precisely the same language exercises, but with natural, unmodified speech.

A comparison of the two treatment groups is shown in Fig. 2. A repeated measures analysis of variance comparing performance on pretraining and posttraining measures again showed that performance improved significantly from pretraining to posttraining ($F(1, 20) = 34.18$, $P < 0.001$). Furthermore, improvement made by the children in group A (who received training with temporal modification) was significantly greater ($F(1, 20) = 5.44$, $P = 0.015$, one-tailed) than that of group B.

It should be noted that the LLI children in study 1 and group A in study 2 were trained with exercises designed to improve their reception of rapidly presented and short duration nonverbal and phonetic elements (Merzenich et al., 1996) as well as speech and language training with acoustically modified speech. The measured improvement in a child's threshold for correctly segmenting and sequencing successive nonverbal auditory stimuli[6] was significantly correlated with posttraining outcome in on-line language processing (study 1, Pearson product–moment correlation co-efficient (r) $= 0.81$, $P <$ 0.05; study 2 group A, $r = 0.89$, $P < 0.01$) (Fig. 3).

It has been demonstrated that LLI children have a specific deficit in recognizing and distinguishing between brief and rapidly changing sensory events presented within the domain of tens of

---

[6]Previous studies (Tallal & Piercy, 1973a) have shown that the total signal duration of auditory stimulus patterns, as indexed by the relation between the duration and interval among stimulus elements, is critical for demonstrating the temporal processing deficits of LLI children. In the present investigation, temporal threshold values were calculated as the sum of the minimal tone durations (150-, 75-, 40-, or 17-ms tone pairs) and the average ISI based on an adaptive staircase (two-up and one-down) procedure to which subjects were able to reproduce pairs of tone sequences by pressing a response panel. A performance level of 75% or greater accuracy was required at a particular stimulus duration before a threshold would be calculated. The average pretraining thresholds by the LLI children were 491 ms in study 1 and 287 ms in study 2 (Merzenich et al., 1996). Normally developing children of a comparable age have been shown to require ISIs of less than 20 ms on this test (Rissman et al., 1990).

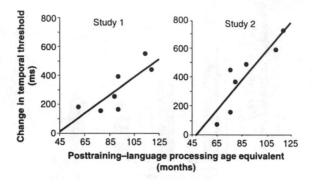

Figure 3. Relation between the improvement in temporal threshold (Tallal & Piercy, 1973a) and language processing, as measured on the Token Test, is displayed for the study 1 and study 2 children who received the temporal training and modified speech exercises. Note that data from four subjects in study 2 are not shown in this figure because they failed to reach criterion (75% or greater accuracy) at any stimulus duration either at the pre- or posttraining evaluations on the temporal threshold procedure. For study 1, $r = 0.81$; for study 2, $r = 0.89$.

milliseconds. Tallal and colleagues have hypothesized that this basic temporal processing deficit may disrupt the normal sharpening of neurally represented phonetic prototypes for the native language in LLI children, resulting in a cascade of negative effects on subsequent receptive and expressive language development—and ultimately resulting in a failure to generate the robust phonetic code that is so essential to learning to read. Although previous research has shown consistently significant correlations between the severity of nonverbal temporal processing deficits and various components of language and reading (Tallal & Piercy, 1975; Tallal, Stark, & Mellits, 1985b), these studies were unable to address issues regarding the causality, etiology, or effectiveness of remediation of LLI and temporal processing deficits.

In the current study we have demonstrated that training children with speech stimuli in which the brief, rapidly changing components have been temporally prolonged and emphasized, coupled with adaptive training exercises designed to sharpen temporal processing abilities (Merzenich et al., 1996), results in a dramatic improvement in receptive speech and language in LLI children. Longitudinal studies with LLI children have shown that these children are not only delayed in the onset of speech and language development, but progress considerably more slowly than normal children in language development, despite conventional therapeutic intervention (Rissman et al., 1990; Curtiss, Katz, & Tallal, 1992; Leonard, 1989). The results of the studies reported here are contrary to this expectation, showing that uncharacteristically rapid growth (approximately 2 years) in receptive speech and language abilities can be achieved by LLI children over a training period of only 4 weeks. We emphasize that significant improvements were demonstrated not only during training with modified speech stimuli, but also generalized to unmodified, natural speech used for pretraining and posttraining test administration. Furthermore, the gains achieved in training were substantially maintained when children were retested 6 weeks after the completion of the training study, suggesting that the perceptual and language skills of these children have been enduringly modified.[7]

---

[7]Six weeks after training was completed in study 1, six of the seven children were retested with the same battery of benchmark speech and language measures to determine the extent to which the significant gains made between pre- and posttraining were maintained, without further exposure to acoustically modified speech. The results showed that the significant improvements over pretraining baseline scores were maintained.

The degree of rapid change in receptive language processing (including receptive phonology, morphology, and syntax), shown here to result from changes made in the acoustic signal of speech and adaptive temporal training (Merzenich et al., 1996), suggests that the symptomatology of LLI children may reflect primarily bottom-up processing constraints rather than a defect in linguistic competence per se. It seems unlikely that these children learned the equivalent of approximately 2 years of language in 1 month. Rather, it appears that they had already developed considerably more language competence than they were able to demonstrate or use "on-line" under normal listening and speaking conditions. This study demonstrates that providing LLI children with access to an acoustically modified signal that they can adequately process, coupled with reducing their temporal processing deficit, achieved through adaptive training (Merzenich et al., 1996), significantly improves LLI children's subsequent processing of natural "on-line" speech. The resulting improvements in the fidelity of their speech inputs result in major and rapid improvements in their speech reception and language comprehension performance.

Preliminary studies suggest that temporal processing abilities can be assessed in the first year of life and that these abilities may predict subsequent language comprehension abilities (Benasich & Tallal, 1993; Henderson & Trehub, 1995). The LLI children participating in the current study were already 5- to 10-years old. Even greater benefits of temporal processing training coupled with exposure to acoustically modified speech during the critical period for speech and language development may be expected to be achieved from earlier intervention, as well as from a longer intervention training period. This training strategy would appear to provide a powerful basis for remediating the speech reception deficits of the many millions of LLI children and adults, as well as the deficits of aged, aphasic, and other special populations whose speech discrimination and language comprehension may be impaired because of an underlying input timing-based speech reception deficit (Gordon-Salant & Fitzgibbons, 1993; Tallal & Newcombe, 1978).

REFERENCES

Beitchman, J. H., Nair, R., Clegg, M., & Patel, P. G. (1986). *J. Speech Hear. Disord.*, *51*, 98.

Benasich, A. A., & Tallal, P. (1993). *Infant Behav. Dev.* (in Press); In P. Tallal, A. M. Galaburda, R. R. Llinas, & C. von Euler (Eds.), *Temporal information Processing in the nervous system: Special reference to Dyslexia and Dysphasia* (Vol. 682, pp. 312–314). New York: New York Academy of Science.

Bishop, D. V. M., & Adams, C. (1990). *J. Child Psychol. Psychiatry*, *31*, 1027.

Catts, H. W. (1993). *J. Speech Hear. Res.*, *36*, 948.

Curtiss, S., Katz, W., & Tallal, P. (1992). *Am. Speech Hear. Assoc.*, *35*, 373.

Curtiss, S., & Yamada, J. *Curtiss and Yamada comperhensive language evaluation receptive (CYCLE-R)*. Unpublished manuscript.

DiSimoni, F. (1978). *The token test for children*. Boston, MA: Teaching Resources Corporation.

Eimas, P. D., Miller, J. L., & Jusczyk, P. S. (1987). In S. Harnad (Ed.), *Categorical preception* (pp. 161–195). New York: Cambridge Univ. Press.

Goldman, R., & Fristoe, M. (1986). *Goldman–Fristoe test of articulation*. Circle Pines, MN: American Guidance Service.

Goldman, R., Fristoe, M., & Woodcock, R. W. (1974). *Goldman–Fristoe–Woodcock diagnostic auditory discrimination test*. Circle Pines, MN: American Guidance Service.

Gordon-Salant, S., & Fitzgibbons, P. J. (1993). *J. Speech Hear. Res.*, *36*, 1276.

Henderson, J. L., & Trehub, S. E. (1995, April). Paper presented at the 61st biennial meeting of the Society for Research in Child Development, Indianapolis, IN.

Kuhl, P. K., Williams, K. A., Lacerda, F., Stevens, K. N., & Lindblom, B. (1992). *Science*, *255*, 606.

Langhans, T., & Strube, I. I. W. (1982). *Proc. of IEE Int. Conf. on Acoustics and Speech Signal Process. 1982*, 156.

Leonard, L. B. (1989). *Appl. Psycho-linguist, 10*, 179.

Liberman, I. Y., Shankweiler, D., Fischer, R. W., & Carter, B. (1974). *J. Exp. Child Psychol., 18*, 201.

Merzenich, M. M., & Jenkins, W. M. (1995). In B. Julesz & I. Kovács (Eds.), *Maturational windows and adult cortical plasticity* (pp. 247–264). Reading, MA: Addison-Wesley.

Merzenich, M. M., et al. (1996). *Science, 271*, 77.

Proc. of the National Conf. on Learning Disabilities (1987). Bethesda, MD, 12 and 13 Jan 1987 (York, Parkton, MD, 1988).

Portnoff, M. R. (1981). *IEE Trans. Acoust. Speech Signal Process. 29*(3), 374.

Psychological Corporation (1991). *Wechsler intelligence scale for children-III*. New York.

Rissman, M., Curtiss, S., & Tallal, P. (1990). *J. Speech-Lang. Pathol. Aud., 14*, 49.

Scarborough, H. S. (1990). *Child Dev., 61*, 1728.

Silva, P. A. (1980). *Dev. Med. Child Neurol., 22*, 768.

Stark, R., & Tallal, P. (1988). *Language, speech and reading disorders in children: Neuropsychological studies.* Boston: College-Hill.

Stark, R., et al. (1984). *Ann. Dyslexia, 34*, 49.

Steinschneider, M., Arezzo, J. C., & Vaughan, H. G., Jr. (1990). *Brain Res., 519*, 158.

Stevenson, J., & Richman, N. (1976). *Dev. Med. Child Neurol., 18*, 431.

Tallal, P., (1980a). *Brain Lang. 9*, 182.

Tallal, P., (1980b). In R. Schiefelbusch (Ed.), *Non-speech language and communication* (pp. 449–467). Baltimore, MD: University Park Press.

Tallal, P., & Miller, S. (1994). *Computerized version of the Tallal repetition test*, unpublished.

Tallal, P., & Piercy, M. (1973a). *Nature, 241*, 468.

Tallal, P., & Piercy, M. (1973b). *Neuropsychologia, 11*, 389.

Tallal, P., & Piercy, M. (1974). *Neuropsychologia, 12*, 83.

Tallal, P., & Piercy, M. (1975). *Neuropsychologia, 13*, 69.

Tallal, P., & Stark, R. E. (1982). *Ann. Dyslexia, 32*, 163.

Tallal, P., Stark, R. E., & Mellits, E. D. (1985a). *Brain Lang., 25*, 314.

Tallal, P., Stark, R. E., & Mellits, E. D. (1985b). *Neuropsychologia, 23*, 527.

Tallal, P., & Newcombe, F. (1978). *Brain and Lang., 5*, 13.

Torgensen, J. K., Wagner, R. K., & Rashotte, C. A. (1994). *J. Learning Disabil., 5*, 276.

Williams, D. M., Darbyshire, J. D., & Vaghy, D. A., (1980). *J. Otolaryngol., 7* (Suppl.), 5.

Part III

CLINICAL ISSUES

The first three papers in this section address aspects of attention deficit hyperactivity disorder (ADHD). ADHD is of major clinical importance. The disorder may affect 3% to 5% of school-aged children and makes up as many as 50% of child psychiatry clinic populations. Although symptoms may change as development proceeds from the preschool years through adulthood, it is a persistent problem that can significantly affect many areas of life. It can be successfully treated, but if ignored it predisposes a child to significant psychiatric and social pathology in later life.

In the first paper, "Attention Deficit Disorder: A Review of the Past 10 Years," Cantwell provides a cogent update of current knowledge. Information is organized into the following areas: epidemiology, etiology, core clinical criteria, comorbidity, differential diagnosis and assessment, natural history, and management. As Cantwell points out, much has been learned: The clinical picture has been more precisely described, neuroimaging and family genetic studies are providing leads to possible underlying etiological factors, and psychopharmacologic and psychosocial treatment options have expanded to include multimodal treatments as interventions of choice. This comprehensive review orients the reader to recent advances in an area of considerable significance for clinicians and investigators alike.

Pharmacologic treatment is a mainstay of intervention for ADHD. Although stimulants are the most established medication used in the treatment of ADHD, as many as 30% of affected individuals may not respond to or are unable to tolerate such treatment. Although various alternative approaches have been proposed and evaluated, many questions remain as to the effectiveness, tolerability, and safety of these alternative approaches. In addition, it has become increasingly recognized that ADHD is a heterogeneous disorder with considerable comorbidity with conduct, mood, anxiety, and tic disorders, and it is not clear whether different comorbid groups respond preferentially to different psychotropic medications.

In the second paper in this section, Spencer and colleagues address these questions in the course of a review of the English-language literature on the pharmacotherapy of ADHD across the life cycle. Information is conveniently organized into separate tables for stimulants, antidepressants, antipsychotics, antihypertensives, mood stabilizers, and antianxiety drugs, with each table specifying the number of studies, dose range, number and age range of subjects, study design and duration, and response to medication. A final table summarizes information on the pharmacotherapy of ADHD, which is comorbid with conduct disorder and aggressive behavior, anxiety and depression, tics and Tourette's disorder, and mental retardation. Although the pharmacological armamentarium is large, by far the greatest proportion of existing studies are on stimulant drugs in general and methylphenidate in particular. A growing body of evidence has documented the efficacy of tricyclic antidepressants on symptoms of ADHD, but associated cardiac risks (see Wilens et al., this volume) lead to the recommendation that TCAs should be used as second-line treatment for ADHD and only after carefully weighing risks and benefits. Similar cautions are urged when considering stimulant medication for individuals with comorbid tics. Despite great progress over the past 3 decades, little is known about the treatment of ADHD in preschool children, adolescents, adults, women, and minorities or on the treatment of comorbid ADHD. Nevertheless, practitioners will find this paper a useful resource in considering pharmacological alternatives, most particularly for difficult and treatment-refractory patients.

In the next paper in this section, Spencer et al. revisit the question of whether stimulants cause growth deficits in children with ADHD. Although a number of studies have shown statistically significant associations between stimulant treatment and growth deficits in children with ADHD, uncertainties have remained as to their clinical significance and permanence. As the authors point out, studies of growth deficits in children of different ages raise complex methodological issues. They have designed a study of growth deficits in ADHD that is sensitive to issues of dysmaturity, therapeutics, comorbidity, and familiality. The earlier literature led to the expectation that children with ADHD would display growth deficits in height and weight as compared with controls. To account for these growth deficits the following competing hypotheses were examined: (a) if deficits in height are due to deficits in weight, then an association between the two is to be expected; (b) if growth deficits are due to pharmacological treatment, then they should be more marked in children who received medication; (c) if growth deficits are due to comorbid psychopathology, then these deficits would be more marked in children with comorbid disorders; (d) if growth deficits are limited to a genetic subtype of ADHD, then they should be limited to familial cases; and (e) if growth deficits are due to developmental "dysmaturity," then growth deficits would be observable during early but not late puberty.

The most striking conclusion of this carefully designed study of 245 children (132 with ADHD and 113 normal controls) who were in the age group of 6 to 17 years was that although small but statistically significant deficits in growth in height were identified in ADHD children as compared with controls, these deficits were unrelated to use of psychotropic medication. Moreover, height deficits were evident in early but not late adolescent children with ADHD, findings consistent with the hypothesis that ADHD may be associated with a temporary delay in the tempo of growth in height. If confirmed, these findings suggest that previously reported stimulant-associated height deficits in ADHD children may well be temporary pre- and early pubertal manifestations of ADHD itself and not complications of its treatment.

The next two papers in this section are concerned with the various manifestations of childhood depression. In their report on "Developmental Pathways in Depression: Multiple Meanings, Antecedents, and Endpoints," Harrington, Rutter, and Fombonne provide an overview of a program of research conducted at the Institute of Psychiatry in London that has extended over a 30-year period.

In broad outline, Harrington et al. describe how initially the research addressed basic questions of definition and measurement. Data from epidemiologic studies indicated that depressive symptoms were common in children and were a good, if nonspecific, indicator of psychological disturbance. Further study of both clinical and epidemiologic samples indicated that depressive symptoms tended to cluster together into distinct syndromes, ranging from nonspecific clusters of symptoms that were usually part of another psychopathological problem through what appeared to be distinctive depressive disorder. The validity of major depressive disorder in children was further tested in longitudinal and family-genetic studies. The results of this next investigative stage further validated the concept of major depression in children and also confirmed heterogeneity with respect to both developmental stage at time of onset and comorbidity with conduct disorder.

Harrington et al. conclude that there are probably several different kinds of depressive symptoms in children, with some being strongly linked with depressive disorders in adulthood. However, others are most probably better conceptualized as part of another psychopathological problem altogether. This article is of particular interest because of the clarity with which Harrington et al. make explicit how their thinking about childhood depression has evolved over the years, delineating how the questions raised by the findings of one set of studies influenced the design of subsequent investigations.

In the final paper in this section, "Presentation and Course of Major Depressive Disorder During Childhood and Later Years of the Life Span," Kovacs addresses the question of whether major depressive disorder (MDD) in childhood, adolescence, and adulthood represents the same diagnostic entity. The strategy used was one of the selective and targeted review of the literature. Recent publications of studies of clinically referred samples that used operational psychiatric diagnostic criteria and systematic evaluations were examined. In reviewing the literature, the author assumed that MDD—whether identified through RDC, *DSM–III*, or *DSM–III–R* criteria—was essentially the same psychopathological entity. Findings from clinical descriptive studies of individuals in the same broad developmental stage, regardless of the setting in which the patients were recruited were synthesized and substantial differences in aspects of depression across developmental stages or age groups, were attributed to age differences in the study cohorts.

Studies included both inpatients and outpatients in the age group of 6 to 80+ years. Information on six phenomenological features of the disorder was abstracted: episode number, symptom presentation, psychiatric comorbidity, recovery from index episode, recurrence of MDD, and switch to bipolar illness. When information across broad age groups was synthesized, it was found that from 90% to 100% of depressed youths were studied in their first episode of illness, regardless of setting. In contrast, only approximately one third of clinically referred patients presented in their first MDD episode among adults, as well as the elderly. Nevertheless, in comparison with adults and the elderly, youth display comparable symptom pictures, have similar rates of psychiatric comorbidity, recover somewhat faster from their index episode of MDD, have a similar recurrence rate, and are at greater risk for bipolar switch.

The results of this innovative approach to the literature leads Kovacs to conclude that although similar clinical outcomes are observable among youths and adults, they occur, in children, about 20 years earlier in the life span, suggesting that very early onset MDD is a particularly serious form of affective illness. The treatment and management of young persons with MDD is challenging and should include long-term continued monitoring and patient education as well as direct clinical care.

10

Attention Deficit Disorder: A Review of the Past 10 Years

Dennis P. Cantwell

Department of Psychiatry and Biobehavioral Sciences,
UCLA Neuropsychiatry Institute

Objective: *To summarize knowledge about attention deficit disorder in the areas of epidemiology, etiology, clinical predictors, assessments, natural history and outcome, and management.* **Method:** *A literature review of articles, books, and chapters primarily published in the past 10 years was completed. Articles presenting new information, most relevant to clinical practice, were reviewed.* **Results:** *Key findings in the areas listed above are presented.* **Conclusions:** *Major advances have been made in all areas. The clinical picture has been refined and developmental manifestations have been delineated. Patterns of comorbidity have been detailed. Various etiological factors, particularly in the biological area, have been investigated. Multimodal management has been promulgated as the treatment of choice.*

Attention deficit disorder (ADD) is one of the most important disorders that child and adolescent psychiatrists treat. It is important because it is highly prevalent, making up as much as 50% of child psychiatry clinic populations. It is a persistent problem that may change its manifestation with development from preschool through adult life. It interferes with many areas of normal development and functioning in a child's life. Untreated, it predisposes a child to psychiatric and social pathology in later life. Most importantly, it can be successfully treated.

EPIDEMIOLOGY

The figure usually given for prevalence of ADD in the general population is approximately 3% to 5% of school-age children. This figure does not take into account preschool, adolescent, and adult populations. Prevalence rates, however, vary according to the population that is sampled, the diagnostic criteria, and diagnostic instruments that are used. More recent data suggest higher figures in school-age children.

Reprinted with permission from *J. Am. Acad. Child Adolesc. Phychiatry*, 1996, Vol. 35(8), 978–987. Copyright © 1996 by the American Academy of Child and Adolescent Psychiatry.

This is the second in a series of 10-year updates in child and adolescent psychiatry. Topics are selected in consultation with the AACAP Committee on Recertification, both for the importance of new research and its clinical or developmental significance. The authors have been asked to place an asterisk before the five or six most seminal references.

Wolraich, Hannah, Pinnock, Baumgaertel, and Brown (1996) and Baumgaertel, Wolraich, and Dietrich (1995) have recently completed two epidemiological studies using *DSM-IV* criteria (American Psychiatric Association, 1994). One was conducted in Tennessee and one in Germany. Teacher information was the sole source of data in both studies. The prevalence rates for the primarily inattentive, primarily hyperactive, and combined subtypes of *DSM-IV* ADD in the Tennessee sample were 4.7%, 3.4%, and 4.4%, respectively. In the German sample the rates for the same subtypes were 9.0%, 3.9% and 4.8%, respectively.

Both in clinical and epidemiological samples the condition is much more common in males—9 to 1 in clinical samples, 4 to 1 in epidemiological samples. This suggests selective referral bias since girls may have primarily inattentive and cognitive problems and less of the aggressive/impulsive conduct symptomatology which leads to earlier referral (Baumagaertel et al., 1995; Cantwell, 1994b; Wolraich et al., 1996).

ETIOLOGY

The etiology of ADD is unknown. It is unlikely that one etiological factor leads to all cases of what we all the clinical syndrome of ADD. Most likely there is an interplay of both psychosocial and biological factors that may lead to a final common pathway of the syndrome of ADD. Thus, there are some known conditions such as fragile-X syndrome, fetal alcohol syndrome, very low birth weight children, and a very rare, genetically transmitted thyroid disorder that can present behaviorally with symptoms of ADD. However, these cases make up only a small portion of the total population of children with the diagnosis (Arnold and Jensen, 1995; Cantwell, 1994b).

Early ideas were that this condition was some type of "brain damage." This idea was derived from the early studies of children who had suffered encephalitis in the encephalitis epidemic of 1917 and 1918. More recent studies of brain morphology involve modern and much more sophisticated measures. Hynd, Semrud-Clikeman, Lorys, Novey, and Elioplus (1990) produced magnetic resonance imaging findings, suggesting that children with ADD and normal plana temporal, but abnormal frontal lobes.

Giedd et al. (1994) demonstrated reduced volume in the rostrum and rostral body of the corpus callosum. This has been interpreted as being consistent with an alteration of functioning of the prefrontal and anterior cingulate cortices of the brain in addition to altered premotor function (Steere & Arnsten, 1995).

Pathophysiology of ADD has also been investigated using other imaging techniques including single photon emission computed tomography (SPECT) and positron emission tomography (PET) (Lou, Henriksen, Bruhn, Borner, & Nielsen, 1989; Zametkin et al., 1990). SPECT studies revealed focal cerebral hypofusion of striatum and hyperfusion in sensory and sensorimotor areas. The PET study by Zametkin et al. was of adults with ADD who had a child with ADD. Compared with normal adults, the adults with ADD had lower cerebral glucose metabolism in the promotor cortex and in the superior prefrontal cortex. These brain areas are involved in the control of motor activity and attention. The same authors used PET to study adolescents with ADD. The results were not as strong. Adolescent females with ADD did have reduced glucose metabolism globally compared with normal control females and males and compared with males with ADD (Cantwell, 1994b; Zametkin, 1993).

The results might be explained on the basis of the adults' having a "familial" and a "persistent" subtype of ADD. All adults in the Zametkin study continued to manifest the syndrome from childhood on and had a child with ADD. It may be that the adolescents did not all have a "familial" subtype and/or that their ADD will not persist into adult life.

There is general agreement that psychophysiological studies have not revealed global autonomic underactivity in children with ADD. However, a more specific pattern of underreactivity to stimulation has been suggested by studies showing more rapid heart rate deceleration and smaller orienting responses on galvanic skin response, greater slow-wave activities of the EEG, smaller amplitudes of response to stimulation, and more rapid habituation on average evoked responses to stimuli (Barkley, 1990).

Family genetic factors have been implicated as etiological in ADD for some 25 years. Heritability is estimated to be between .55 and .92. Concordance was 51% in monozygotic twins and 33% in dizygotic twins in one study (Goodman & Stevenson, 1989). Family aggregation studies have shown that the ADD syndrome and related problems do run in close family members (Biederman, Baldessarini, Wright, Knee, & Harmatz, 1989). Adoption studies support that this "running in families" is genetic rather than environmental (Barkley, 1990; Cantwell, 1975). At this point, no gene has been described or found, but this is an active area of research and is likely to bear fruit in the foreseeable future.

The positive response of ADD individuals to CNS stimulants and antidepressants logically suggested catecholamine abnormalities in ADD. There is a substantial body of literature reporting both animal and human studies that used blood, urine, and CSF, but results are inconsistent (Zametkin & Rapoport, 1986). Low dopamine and norepinephrine turnover is suggested by most studies. However, there is interaction between the serotonin and catecholamine systems and any "one drug–one neurotransmitter" hypothesis is too simplistic.

Psychosocial factors are not thought to play a primary etiological role. Various types of parent–child relationships and family dysfunction are found in families of children with ADD. Interaction conflicts with their mothers are more common in younger children with ADD than in older children with ADD. In the older adolescent age range, more noncompliant and negative verbalizations are reported in families of children with ADD than in families of normal children. These psychosocial factors are thought to be primarily related to development of oppositional defiant disorder and conduct disorder rather than to the core symptoms of ADD.

Some "environmental" etiological factors have been proposed. These include various pre- and perinatal abnormalities, toxins such as lead and various food additives, sugar intoxication, and orthomolecular theories of great need for vitamins and nutrients in children with ADD. None of these has received substantial empirical support (Arnold & Jensen, 1995; Barkley, 1990).

CORE CLINICAL CRITERIA

Although *DSM-III*, *DSM-III-R*, and *DSM-IV* differ on the exact core symptoms and how they are arranged, they are actually globally quite consistent. There is general agreement that the core symptoms consist of an inattention domain and a hyperactivity/impulsivity domain. *DSM-III* arranged these domains in three separate symptoms areas. *DSM-III-R* grouped them in one long symptom list and *DSM-IV* lists them as two core dimensions. There are nine symptoms of each dimension in *DSM-IV*. *DSM-IV* maintains the requirement of an early age of onset (before the age of 7 years), presence for 6 months or longer (to indicate chronicity), and presence in two or more settings (to indicate pervasiveness of symptoms). *DSM-IV* describes a combined subtype in which the individual has six or more symptoms out of nine from both the inattention dimension and the hyperactive/impulsive dimension. The predominantly inattentive subtype consists of six or more inattention symptoms and five or fewer hyperactive/impulsive symptoms. A predominantly hyperactive/impulsive type consists of six or more symptoms of the hyperactive/impulsive dimension and five or fewer of the inattention dimension. The symptoms must be more frequent and severe than those of children of comparable developmental level and must cause significant functional impairments. Across children the symptoms may vary in their frequency of occurrence, in their pervasiveness across settings, and in the degree of functional impairment in various areas. Also with the same child some settings may enhance or decrease symptom manifestation. For example, open classrooms may bring out more symptoms than classrooms that are more structured.

DEVELOPMENTAL PSYCHOPATHOLOGY

The core symptoms of ADD may change over time. Most of our knowledge base comes from studies of elementary school-age boys with ADD. There are fewer studies of younger children and adolescents and a growing body of literature on adults.

In the preschool age range, the most difficult differential diagnostic problem is with normally active, exuberant preschool children. Many parents of normal children describe their children as inattentive and hyperactive. The preschool child with true ADD, which persists over time, generally has such additional symptoms as temper tantrums, argumentative behavior, aggressive behavior (hitting others and taking others' possessions), and fearless behavior which leads to frequent accidental injury and noisy, boisterous behavior. Noncompliance is often a major problem with these youngsters as is sleep disturbance (Campbell, 1990). One follow-up study by Campbell (1990) showed that about one half of preschool children with a diagnosis of hyperactivity had a clear diagnosis of ADD by age 9. The children with more severe symptoms in preschool were likely to have the most persistent ADD over time.

The various *DSM* criteria have been based on the clinical picture in elementary school–age children. Cognitively effortful work is most difficult for these children. Thus, entering into the academic arena in the elementary school age range puts greater stress on the cognitive domain. In addition, their impulsivity, hyperactivity, and inattention often lead to difficulty in peer relationships, which first become manifest in the elementary school age range. Elementary school children also may begin to develop comorbid symptomatology such as noncompliant behavior.

The clinical presentation of ADD in adolescents has not been studied as systematically as in younger children (Barkley, 1990). Barkley suggests that not only do the symptom manifestations change with age, but that a lower number of symptoms should be considered as indicative of the diagnosis in the adolescent age range and possibly the adult age range. Adolescents are in junior high school or high school, where they no longer have one teacher in one class, but now have multiple teachers in multiple classes. In addition, adolescent demands for a greater degree of independence and development of both same-sex and opposite-sex peer relationships may present conflicts. The core symptoms may be manifest now as an internal sense of restlessness rather than gross motor activity. Their inattention and cognitive problems may lead to poorly organized approaches to school and work and poor follow-through on tasks. Failing to complete independent academic work is a hallmark in the adolescent age range, and a continuation of risky types of behaviors such as more frequent auto and bike accidents may also be manifestations (Weiss & Hechtman, 1994).

The study of the adult syndrome is a much more recent phenomenon. A variety of different symptoms in adults have been described by Wender (1994), Barkley (1995), Conners (1995), and Hallowell and Ratey (1994). The presence of disorganization continues to have an impact in the workplace, often requiring written lists of activities to be used as reminders. Poor concentration may continue to persist into adult life, leading to shifting activities, not finishing projects, and moving from one activity to another. Procrastination is present as is the presence of intermittent explosive outbursts, which may be related to comorbid mood symptomatology or may be a special type of labile mood described by Wender (1994).

COMORBIDITY

Comorbidity is a major problem in children, adolescents, and adults with the ADD syndrome. As many as two thirds of elementary school-age children with ADD who are referred for clinical evaluation have at least one other diagnosable psychiatric disorder (Arnold & Jensen, 1995; Cantwell, 1994b; Nottelmann & Jensen, 1995). The actual comorbid conditions and their prevalence rates may vary across different types of samples, depending on whether the sample is clinical or epidemiological and whether a clinical sample is pediatric or psychiatric. Conduct disorder and oppositional defiant disorder seem to be higher in psychiatric samples, learning disorders in pediatric samples. The major comorbid conditions include language and communication disorders, learning disorders, conduct and oppositional defiant disorder, anxiety disorders, mood disorders, and Tourette's syndrome or chronic tics (Cantwell, 1994b). A type of comorbidity described by Cantwell as "lack of social savoir-faire" is not a diagnosable condition in the *DSM* sense. However, it does describe a common problem that many ADD children, adolescents, and adults have. It is an inability to pick up on social cues, leading to difficulties in interpersonal relationships.

Comorbidity complicates the diagnostic process and can have an impact on natural history and prognosis and the management of children, adolescents, and adults with ADD. Assessment and treatment of the comorbid disorder is often equally as important as assessing and treating the ADD symptomatology. It may be that some of the comorbid conditions, such as ADD plus Tourette's syndrome or ADD plus conduct disorder, may identify subgroups of ADD children with different natural histories and possibly different underlying etiological factors and different responses to treatment. At present, the practicing clinician simply must carry a high index of suspicion for other types of disorders when assessing the child who has ADD. In particular, the internalizing problems such as anxiety and mood disorders may be underreported by parents and teachers, who are better able to see the externalizing behaviors.

DIFFERENTIAL DIAGNOSIS AND ASSESSMENT

It should be kept in mind that in the differential diagnosis of ADD in children there are conditions that in some cases may be comorbid and in other cases may mimic "true" ADD. A good example would be absence seizures, which may mimic the clinical presence of ADD in some cases and may be associated with a true ADD syndrome in others. The differential diagnosis must rule out the presence of other psychiatric disorders, developmental disorders, and medical and neurological disorders and determine whether these are comorbid or whether they are mimicking an ADD syndrome.

The diagnosis of ADD is a clinical diagnosis. It is made on the basis of a clinical picture that begins early in life, is persistent over time, is pervasive across different settings, and causes functional impairment at home, at school, or in leisure time activity. There is no laboratory test or set of tests that currently can be used to make a definitive diagnosis of ADD (Arnold & Jensen, 1995; Barkley, 1990). The clinician has a number of diagnostic tools, including parent and child interviews, observations of the parent and child, behavior rating scales, physical and neurological examinations, and cognitive testing. Laboratory studies, such as audiology and vision testing, may be useful in some cases but not others. Detailed speech and language evaluation may be appropriate in some cases. Developmental questionnaires and behavior rating scales for completion by the teacher and parents can be mailed out prior to the first visit. The initial parent visit should consist of a detailed developmental and symptomatic history and a detailed medical, neurological, family, and psychosocial history. The diagnostic process must occur in a developmental context. Symptoms are considered to be present and meaningful only if they are in excess of what woud be expected of a child of the same age and cognitive level.

The nature and content of the interview with the child vary, of course, with age and developmental levels. Nevertheless, the goal is the same: to obtain, both spontaneously and in response to direct questions, the patient's report of various types of psychiatric symptoms and their impact on the patient's life.

In the assessment process a variety of rating scales can be used to gather information from parents, teachers, significant others, and in some cases the patient. These can be generally divided into broad- and narrow-range scales. An example of a broad-range scale is the Child Behavior Checklist developed by Achenbach (1993). It contains items on a variety of dimensions, not just inattention and hyperactivity. It is useful as a broad-based screener. There is a parent and a teacher version.

More specific scales have been developed for ADD (Hinshaw, 1994), such as those developed by Conners (1994); the SNAP-IV, developed by Swanson (1995); and the Disruptive Behavior Disorder. Scale, developed by Pelham (1992). A diagnosis is not made on the basis of a score on one scale. Rather it is made when the clinician has collected all the available information and on that basis determines that ADD is present, determines whether there is or is not comorbidity, and determines what possibly important biological and psychosocial factors should be considered. Good measures of current intellectual functioning and current level of academic achievement are useful for every child. The need for further testing will then depend on the results of the clinical evaluation.

Specialized tests, such as the Continuous Performance Task (in its various permutations), the Wisconsin Cart-Sorting Test, the Matching Familiar Figures Test, and subtests of the WISC-R, should not be considered "diagnostic" of ADD (DuPaul, Anastopoulos, Shelton, Guevremont, & Metevia, 1992). Tests that measure cognitively effortful work, such as the Paired Associate Learning (PAL) Task, may be useful because they most approximate a laboratory measure of classroom learning. The PAL is likely to pick up "cognitive toxicity" caused by high dosages of medication, which may not be noticed simply by the use of behavior rating scales. However, the PAL is not diagnostic of ADD either. There is no specific diagnostic test for ADD (Cantwell & Swanson, 1992).

The core symptoms of ADD may occur in other psychiatric conditions and may be precipitated by medical and neurological conditions. In some cases a child, parent, or teacher may be unreliable as an informant. There may be negative findings in a brief, one-time interview with the child. All of these lead to pitfalls in the diagnostic process, but they can be overcome with the proper diagnostic approach. Such a diagnostic approach involves the following (Reiff, Benez, & Culbert, 1993):

1. A comprehensive interview with all parenting figures. This interview should pinpoint the child's symptoms so that the clinician can discern when, where, with whom, and with what intensity these symptoms occur. This should be complemented by a developmental, medical, school, and family social, medical, and mental health history.

2. A developmentally appropriate interview with the child to assess the child's view of the presence of signs and symptoms; the child's awareness of and explanation of any difficulties; and, most importantly, at least a screening for symptoms of other disorders—especially anxiety, depression, suicidal ideation, hallucinations, and unusual thinking.

3. An appropriate medical evaluation to determine general health status and to screen for sensory deficits, neurological problems, or other physical explanations for the observed difficulties.

4. Appropriate cognitive assessment of ability and achievement.

5. The use of both broad-spectrum and more narrowly ADD focused parent and teacher rating scales.

6. Appropriate adjunct assessments such as speech and language assessment, and evaluation of fine and gross motor function in selected cases (Braswell & Bloomquist, 1994).

NATURAL HISTORY

In the past it was believed that all children with ADD "outgrew their problem." This "outgrowing" was supposed to occur with puberty. We now know from prospective studies that this is not true. Cantwell (1985) has described three potential types of outcomes. One is described as a "developmental delay" outcome. This may occur in 30% of the subjects. With this outcome, sometimes early in young adult life the individual no longer manifests any functionally impairing ADD symptoms. The second outcome has been called the "continual display" outcome. This may occur in about 40% of child subjects. In this case, functionally impairing symptoms of ADD continue into adult life. In addition, these symptoms may be accompanied by a variety of different types of social and emotional difficulties. The last outcome, which may occur in as many as 30% of subjects, Cantwell describes as a "developmental decay" outcome. In these cases not only is there a continual display of core ADD symptoms, but there is the development of more serious psychopathology such as alcoholism, substance abuse, and antisocial personality disorder. One of the strongest predictors of this most negative outcome is the presence of comorbid conduct disorder with ADD in childhood.

Recent studies of adults with retrospectively diagnosed ADD suggest there may be people (particularly females) who had unrecognized ADD in childhood, who were not evaluated in childhood, and yet who seem to make a reasonable adjustment in adult life. They present with a wide range of comorbid adult disorders such as anxiety disorders and mood disorders (Wender, 1994), even though they have made a reasonable adjustment without treatment. A combination of psychosocial and medical interventions improves their functioning (Hallowell & Ratey, 1994; Wender, 1994). It is interesting that in most samples of those who present as adults with no childhood evaluation or treatment, a substantially greater number of females has been present.

MANAGEMENT

It is now recognized that management of the ADD syndrome requires a multiple-modality approach (American Academy of Child and Adolescent Psychiatry, 1991; Braswell, Bloomquist, & Pederson, 1991; Hechtman, 1993; Pelham, 1994; Swanson, 1992). A multiple-modality approach combines psychosocial interventions and medical interventions. The psychosocial interventions that have proven to be effective for children with ADD can be classified as those psychosocial interventions which focus on the family, the school, and the child. Among the family-focused interventions are education about what ADD is and what it is not. Support groups such as CHADD and ADDA are quite helpful in the psychoeducational process and are useful for other reasons such as providing group support and knowledge about working with school systems and about resources in the community. A number of books now available for parents, teachers, and the children themselves are useful adjuncts to treatment.

Parent management training is almost a sine qua non of psychosocial interventions with ADD. Training parents to use contingency management techniques and to cooperate with the school in a school–home daily report card and point/token response cost system is highly effective. Parent management training has been shown not only to reduce the childs' disruptive behavior in the home setting, but also to increase the parents' own self-confidence in their competence as parents and to decrease family stress. Both individual and group formats have been used for parents management training. Some clinicians such as Brown and Cantwell (1976) have used older siblings in additon to parents to serve as positive reinforcement and to make positive intercations. Assessment and treatment of parental psychopathology and more specific assessment and treatment of family dysfunction such as marital conflict are always indicated.

School-focused intervention should target academic performance. However, classroom behavior and peer relationships are also important. The most appropriate classroom environment is probably a structured classroom with the child placed in the front of the room, close to the teacher, where he or she may be less easily distracted and more able to focus. Children with ADD respond to predictable, well-organized schedules with rules that are known and clearly reinforced in the classroom setting. The use of contingency management and daily, teacher-completed report cards showing the child's progress in targeted areas of improvement are hallmarks of this type of intervention (Braswell & Bloomquist,

Annual Progress in Child Psychiatry and Development

1994). Incentives and tangible rewards, reprimands, and timeouts in the classroom setting can also be used in school as well as in the home.

School placement is a crucial issue. While many if not most children with ADD will remain in a regular classroom setting, some may need individual tutoring, some may need a resource program, some may need a self-contained special class (primarily for academic reasons), and others with complex problems may need a special school. The clinician can play a major role in assessing the need for specialized school intervention and in facilitating school placement.

The child-focused interventions include the use of individual psychotherapy to treat any depression, low self-esteem, anxiety, or other types of associated symptomatology. There should be a concerted effort to improve the child's impulse control, anger control, and social skills. Social skills-training programs focus on the child's entry into the social group, the development of conversational skills and problem-solving skills, as well as those factors noted above. Impaired social skills are an extremely important part of the negative aspect of children with ADD (Pelham & Bender, 1982). Problems caused by the "in your face" type of behavior associated with impulsivity and hyperactivity may be more easily treated than the lack of social savoir-faire described by Cantwell (1994b).

A number of summer treatment programs have been developed in which the child is in an intense school program for 8 weeks, 8 hours per day. The day involves not only academic work but behavioral management, social skills, and individual work with the child. There is then an attempt to carry over the school program into the regular school by the use of paraprofessionals in the regular classroom setting (Swanson, 1992).

The primary psychopharmacological agents used to treat ADD are the CNS stimulants (Cantwell, 1994a; Wilens & Biederman, 1992). The prototype drugs are dextroamphetamine, methylphenidate, and pemoline. There are a number of amphetamines including methamphetamine and dextroamphetamine, but dextroamphetamine probably enjoys the greatest use. Methylphenidate is probably used more than any of the other stimulants. At least 70% of children will have a positive response to one of the major stimulants on the first trial. If a clinician conducts a trial of dextroamphetamine, methylphenidate, and pemoline, the response rate to at least one of these is in the 85% to 90% range, depending on how response is defined (Elia, 1993).

While it is clear that the medications target classroom behavior, academic performance (Evans & Pelham, 1991), and productivity (Swanson, Cantwell, Lerner, & Hanna, 1991), there is also good evidence to show that ADD children with oppositional and conduct symptomatology and aggressive behavior also respond positively in these areas as well. Interactions between the child and peers, family, siblings, teachers, and significant others (such as scout masters and coaches) also improve. In addition, participation in leisure time activity, such as playing baseball, improves (Cantwell, 1994b). The main message is that stimulants are not "school time drugs." They should be used throughout the waking day and on the weekends as well. There is no way to pick the first stimulant to be tried because, essentially, they are all equally effective (Pelham et al., 1990). Some children respond better to one than they do to another, but response is idiosyncratic and cannot be predicted.

Side effect profiles may be better for one child with one drug than another, but in general, all stimulants share side effects of decreased appetite, insomnia, stomachache, headache, and irritability. Most side effects will dissipate with time and many can be managed with various types of manipulation (Cantwell, 1994b). Growth suppression appears to be dose-related, if it occurs at all. There does not seem to be strong evidence that adverse effects on the patient's ultimate height has been present in the long-term follow-up studies that have been done. However, there are individual children who do not seem to be able to adjust and adapt to the growth suppression. There is good evidence that the drugs do not lose their effect after puberty and that tolerance to the medication does not develop and lead to substance abuse (Greenhill & Setterberg, 1993). While there are some concerns about the use of stimulants in the ADD individuals who themselves have substance abuse in their past history or who have family members who are current substance abusers, this has not been a major problem.

The relationship of stimulant drugs to the development of tics is controversial. It is clear that a substantial number of children with ADD who are referred for clinical evaluation have motor or vocal tics or both. Some of these children experience worsening of their tics when stimulants are used. Recent data by Gadow, Sverd, Sprafkin, Noland, and Ezor (1995) suggest that a substantial majority of those children return to baseline, even when stimulants are continued. If this does not occur, adjunct treatment of the tics with medications such as haloperidol, pimozide, or clonidine is usually effective.

"Rebound" is a deterioration in behavior that follows the wearing off of short-acting stimulants (Johnston, Pelham, & Hoza, 1988). This rebound period may be one-half hour or more, and it is actually a worsening of behavior above baseline behavior. This occurs in a minority of children. Rebound can be managed by the use of longer-acting drugs which seem to have a smoother onset and offset.

Cantwell and Swanson (1992) have reported "cognitive toxicity" in a subgroup of patients at doses at which the behavioral effects of the medication are maximized. Thus, the maximum dosage the child receives for behavioral effects will have less than a maximal effect on cognitive functioning. In these cases the dose should be lowered.

The literature on stimulants consists of more than 100 studies of more than 4,500 elementary school-age children. There are several small studies of preschool children (approximately 130 subjects), a small number of studies of adolescents (approximately 113 subjects), and eight studies of adults (180 subjects). In general, the response rate is 70% or more in the elementary school age range and in the adolescent range. A more variable effect has been found in studies with preschool children and with adults (Cantwell, 1994b).

The use of nonstimulant medication to treat attention-deficit hyperactivity disorder has recently been reviewed by Cantwell (1994a). The medications that have been evaluated include the antidepressants, antianxiety agents (clonidine and guanfacine), neuroleptics, fenfluramine, lithium, and the anticonvulsants. The best studied of the nonstimulants are the heterocyclic antidepressants (Elia, 1991). Some studies suggest that approximately 70% of children with ADD will respond to desipramine at dosages up to 5 mg/kg per day with blood levels of 100 to 300 ng/mg per milliliter (Biederman et al., 1989; Plizska, 1987). All of the heterocyclics produce positive effects on hyperactivity, impulsivity, inattention, and most likely on anxiety and depressed mood. There is some question about whether there is a major effect on learning. The major side effects that are of concern are cardiovascular, especially the possible induction of arrhythmias. The report of the sudden death of several young children has led to a reconsideration of the use of the heterocyclics (Riddle et al., 1991).

Bupropion is an antidepressant that is not a serotonin reuptake blocker and is not a tricyclic. The side effect profile is very positive, and efficacy has been suggested in several studies published since 1986 in doses 5 to 6 mg/kg per day in three divided dosages.

The literature on serotonin reuptake blockers such as fluoxetine, sertraline, paroxetine, and fluvoxamine is limited, but it suggests that some individual children may get a positive response (Barrickman, Noyes, & Kuperman, 1991). Gammon and Brown (1993) reported on 32 subjects, aged 9 to 17 years, all with a diagnosis of ADD with multiple comorbid conditions. Mood disorders such as dysthymia were present in 78% of cases and major depressive disorder in 80% of cases. The addition of fluoxetine to the ongoing methylphenidate treatment led to a significant improvement in many measures in 30 of the 32 subjects.

Monoamine oxidase inhibitors have been shown in small studies to be effective in a substantial number of children, and in one study (Zametkin, Rapoport, & Murphy, 1986) their effect was equal to that of dextroamphetamine; however, multiple possible drug and diet reactions severely limit their use.

Clonidine and guanfacine are α_2-adrenergic agonists. The literature suggesting their efficacy alone in ADD is limited. In conjunction with stimulants, they may offer some adjunctive help in the treatment of associated aggressive hyperactive/hyperarousal behavior and they may benefit those children who have tics. The clonidine-methylphenidate combination has recently been associated with idiosyncratic episodes in a small number of cases; there have been three cases of sudden death. The exact role, if any, of the drugs in these deaths is unclear. Fenfluramine is a synthetic stimulant not shown to be useful in the usual case of ADD. Clinical data suggest a possible positive effect on ADD symptoms (Cantwell, 1994a) in those with mental retardation and pervasive developmental disorders.

The mood stabilizers, such as lithium, carbamazepine, and valproic acid, do not seem to have a positive effect on core ADD symptoms. Symptoms of episodic dyscontrol in some ADD individuals may be positively affected.

Early studies with neuroleptics suggested an effect on certain symptoms. Neuroleptics may be cognitively dulling, although the early studies at smaller doses did not show that. They are very rarely used today because of their negative side effect potential. However, haloperidol or pimozide plus stimulants may be a useful combination for those who have ADD plus Tourette's syndrome or tics.

It is now accepted that a multimodal approach to therapy that uses both psychosocial intervention and medication has the greatest chance of alleviating the multiple symptoms and domains of dysfunction with which ADD children present. Medical treatment and psychosocial treatment have complementary effects. Thus a wider range of symptoms may be treated than with either intervention alone. Psychosocial intervention may improve symptoms during the period of time that medication has worn off. The use of both interventions together may lead to lower medication dosage and a less complex psychosocial intervention program than with either treatment alone.

SUMMARY AND CONCLUSIONS

This review has attempted to highlight advances in ADD over the past 10 years. It does seem that advances have been made on all fronts. Neuroimaging and family genetic studies are providing enticing leads to possible underlying etiological factors. Treatment studies have added to the staple of treatment, which has remained psychostimulant medication. Various psychotherapeutic and psychosocial interventions play a major role in treatment. School-based interventions have become more common and are quite effective. More work needs to be done on long-term results of treatment in childhood. The syndrome of ADD remains a subject of intense research as one of our best-studied child psychiatric problems.

REFERENCES

Achenbach, T. M. (1993). *Empirically based taxonomy: How to use syndromes and profile types derived from the CBCL from 4 to 18, TRF, and WSR.* Burlington: University of Vermont Department of Psychiatry.

American Academy of Child and Adolescent Psychiatry. (1991). Practice parameters for the assessment and treatment of ADHD. *J. Am. Acad. Child Adolesc. Psychiatry, 30,* 1–3.

American Psychiatric Association. (1994). *Diagnostic and statistical manual of mental disorders* (pp. 63–65). Washington, DC: American Psychiatric Association.

Arnold, L. E., & Jensen, P. S. (1995). Attention deficit disorders. In H. Kaplan, B. Sadock, (Eds.). *Comprehensive textbook of psychiatry* (6th ed. pp. 2295–2310). Baltimore: Williams & Wilkins.

Barkley, R. A. (1990). *Attention deficit hyperactivity disorder: A handbook for diagnosis and treatment* (pp. 3–673). New York: Guilford Press.

Barkley, R. A. (1995). *Attention deficit disorder symptoms in adults.* Presented to the Bay State Psychiatric Hospital Symposium, Springfield, MA.

Barrickman, L., Noyes, R., & Kuperman, S. (1991). Treatment of ADHD with fluoxetine: A preliminary trial. *J. Am. Acad. Child Adolesc. Psychiatry, 30,* 762–767.

*Baumgaertel, A., Wolraich, M. L., & Dietrich, M. (1995). Comparison of diagnostic criteria for attention deficit disorders in a German elementary school sample. *J. Am. Acad. Child Adolesc. Psychiatry, 34,* 629–638.

Biederman, J., Baldessarini, R. J., Wright, V., Knee, D., & Harmatz, J. S. (1989). A double-blind placebo controlled study of desipramine in the treatment of ADD: I. Efficacy. *J. Am. Acad. Child Adolesc. Psychiatry, 28,* 777–784.

Braswell, L., & Bloomquist, M. (1994). *Cognitive behavior therapy of ADHD.* New York: Guilford Press.

Braswell, L., Bloomquist, M., & Pederson, S. (1991). *ADHD: A guide to understanding and helping children with attention deficit hyperactivity disorder in school settings.* Minneapolis: University of Minnesota Professional Development.

Brown, N. B., & Cantwell, D. P. (1976). Siblings as therapist: A behavioral approach. *Am. J. Psychiatry, 133,* 447–450.

Campbell, S. B. (1990). *Psychiatric disorder in preschool children.* New York: Guilford Publications.

Cantwell, D. P. (1975). The hyperactive child: Epidemiology, classification and diagnosis. In D. P. Cantwell, (Ed.). *The hyperactive child: Diagnosis, management, and current research,* New York: Spectrum Publications.

Cantwell, D. P. (1985). Hyperactive children have grown up. What have we learned about what happens to them? *Arch. Gen. Psychiatry, 42,* 1026–1028.

Cantwell, D. P. (1994a). *ADHD treatment with non-stimulants. Pediatric psychopharmacology.* Presented at Midyear Institute of the AACAP, February 1992. Washington, DC: AACAP Press.

Cantwell, D. P. (1994b). *Therapeutic management of attention deficit disorder: Participant workbook* (pp. 4–20), New York: SCP Communication.

Cantwell, D. P., Swanson, J. (1992). *Cognitive toxicity in ADHD children treated with stimulant medication.* Presented at the American Academy of Child and Adolescent Psychiatry Annual Meeting.

Conners, K. (1994). *Conners abbreviated symptom questionnaire.* North Tonawanda, NY: Multi Health Systems.

Conners, K. (1995). *Attention deficit disorder core criteria in adults.* Presented to Neuroscience Research Seminar, Lake Forest, IL.

DuPaul, G. J., Anastopoulos, A. D., Shelton, T. L., Guevremont, D. C., & Metevia, L. (1992). Multimethod assessment of attention-deficit hyperactivity disorder: The diagnostic utility of clinic-based tests. *J. Clin. Child Psychol., 21,* 194–402.

Elia, J. (1991). Stimulants and antidepressant pharmacokinetics in hyperactive children. *Psychopharmacol Bull., 27,* 411–415.

Elia, J. (1993). Drug treatment for hyperactive children. Therapeutic guidelines. *Drugs, 46,* 863–871.

Evans S. W., & Pelham W. E. (1991). Psychostimulant effects on academic and behavioral measures for ADHD junior high school students in a lecture format classroom. *J. Abnorm. Child Psychol., 19,* 537–552.

*Gadow, K. D., Sverd, J., Sprafkin, J., Noland, E. E., & Ezor, S. N. (1995), Efficacy of methylphenidate for attention deficit hyperactivity disorder in children with tic disorder. *Arch. Gen. Psychiatry, 52,* 444–455.

*Gammon, G. D., & Brown, T. E. (1993). Fluoxetine augmentation of methylphenidate for attention deficit and comorbid disorders. *J. Child Adolesc. Psychopharmacol., 3,* 1–10.

*Giedd, J. N., Castenalos, F. X., Korzuch, P., King, A. C., Hamburger, S. D., & Rapoport, J. L. (1994). Quantitative morphology of the corpus callosum in attention deficit hyperactivity disorder. *Am. J. Psychiatry, 151,* 665–669.

Goodman, R., & Stevenson, J. (1989). A twin study of hyperactivity: II. The aetiologic role of genes, family relationships, and perinatal adversity. *J. Child Psychol. Psychiatry, 30,* 691–709.

Greenhill, L. L., & Setterberg, S. (1993). Pharmacotherapy of disorders of adolescents. *Psychiatr. Clin. North Am., 16,* 793–814.

Hallowell, E., & Ratey, J. (1994). *Driven To distraction.* New York: Pantheon Books.

Hechtman, L. (1993). Aims and methodological problems in multimodal treatment studies. *Can. J. Psychiatry, 38,* 458–464.

Hinshaw, S. P. (1994). Behavior rating scales in the assessment of disruptive behavior disorders in childhood. In D. Shaffer & J. Richters, (Eds.), *Assessment in child psychopathology,* New York: Cambridge Press.

Hynd, G. W., Semrud-Clikeman, M., Lorys, A. R., Novey, E. S., & Elioplus, D. (1990). Brain morphology in developmental dyslexia and attention deficit disorder with hyperactivity. *Arch. Neurol.,* 919–926.

Johnston, C., Pelham, W. E., & Hoza, J. (1988). Psychostimulant rebound in attention deficit disordered boys. *J. Am. Acad. Child Adolesc. Psychiatry, 27,* 806–810.

Lou, H. C., Henriksen, L., Bruhn, P., Borner, H., & Nielsen, J. B. (1989). Striatal dysfunction in attention deficit and hyperkinetic disorder. *Arch. Neurol., 46,* 48–52

Nottelmann, E., & Jensen, P. (1995). Comorbidity of disorders in children and adolescents: Developmental perspectives. *Advances in clinical child psychology* (Vol. 17, pp. 109–155), New York: Plenum.

Pelham, W. E. (1992). Teacher ratings of *DSM-III-R* symptoms for the disruptive behavior disorders. *J. Am. Acad. Child Adolesc. Psychiatry, 31,* 210–218.

Pelham, W. E. (1994). *Attention deficit hyperactivity disorder: A clinician's guide.* New York: Plenum.

Pelham, W. E., & Bender, M. E. (1982). Peer relationships in hyperactive children: Description and treatment. In K. Gadow, & I. Bailer, (Eds.), *Advances in learning and behavioral disabilities* (pp. 365–436). Greenwich, CT: JAI Press.

*Pelham, W. E., Greenslade, K. E., Vodde-Hamilton, M. et al. (1990). Relative efficacy of long-acting stimulants on children with attention deficit-hyperactivity disorder: A comparison of standard methylphenidate, sustained released methylphenidate, sustained release dextroamphetamine, and pemoline. *Pediatrics, 86,* 226–237.

Plizska, S. R. (1987). Tricyclic antidepressants in the treatment of children with attention deficit disorder. *J. Am. Acad. Child Adolesc. Psychiatry, 26,* 127–132.

Reiff, M. I., Banez, G. A., & Culbert, T. P. (1993). Children who have attentional disorders: Diagnosis and evaluation. *Pediatr. Rev., 12,* 455–465.

Riddle, M. A., Nelson, J. C., Kleinman, C. S. et al. (1991). Sudden death in children receiving Norpramin™: A review of three reported cases and commentary. *J. Am. Acad. Child Adolesc. Psychiatry, 30,* 104–108.

Steere, G., & Arnsten, A. F. T. (1995). Corpus callosum morphology in ADHD. *Am. J. Psychiatry, 152,* 1105–1107.

*Swanson, J. M. (1992). *School-based assessment and interventions for ADD students.* Irvine, CA: KC Publications.

Swanson, J. M. (1995). *SNAP-IV scale.* Irvine, CA: University of California Child Development Center.

Swanson, J. M., Cantwell, D. P., Lerner, M., & Hanna, G. L. (1991). Effects of stimulant medication on learning in children with ADHD. *J. Learn. Disabil., 4,* 219–230, 255.

Weiss, G., & Hechtman, L. T. (1994). *Hyperactive children grown up* (2nd ed.). New York: Guilford Press.

Wender, P. (1994). *Attention deficit disorder in adults.* New York: Oxford Press.

Wilens, T., & Biederman, J. (1992). The stimulants. *Psychiatr. Clin. North Am., 15,* 191–222.

Wolraich, M. L., Hannah, J. N., Pinnock, T. Y., Baumgaertel, A., & Brown, J. (1996). Comparison of diagnostic criteria for attention-deficit hyperactivity disorder in a country-wide sample. *J. Am. Acad. Child Adolesc. Psychiatry, 35,* 319–324.

Zametkin, A. J. (1993). Brain metabolism in teenagers with attention deficit hyperactivity disorder. *Arch. Gen. Psychiatry, 50,* 333–340.

Zametkin, A. J., Nordahl, T. E., Gross, M. et al. (1990). Cerebral glucose metabolism in adults with hyperactivity of childhood onset. *N. Engl. J. Med., 323,* 1361–1366.

Zametkin, A. J., & Rapoport, J. L. (1986). The pathophysiology of attention deficit disorder with hyperactivity. In B. B. Lahey & A. E. Kasdin, (Eds.), *Advances in clinical child psychology* (Vol. 9). New York: Plenum.

Zametkin, A. J., Rapoport, J. L., & Murphy, D. L. (1986). Treatment of hyperactive children with monoamine oxidase inhibitors, I. Clinical efficacy. *Arch. Gen. Psychiatry, 42,* 962–966.

11

Pharmacotherapy of Attention-Deficit Hyperactivity Disorder Across the Life Cycle

Thomas J. Spencer, Joseph Biederman, and Timothy E. Wilens
Massachusetts General Hospital and Harvard Medical School

Margaret Harding, Deborah O'Donnell, and Susan Griffin
Massachusetts General Hospital

Objective: *To evaluate the scope of the available therapeutic armamentarium in attention-deficit hyperactivity disorder (ADHD).* **Method:** *The literature of medication trials in ADHD was systematically reviewed, with attention to issues of psychiatric comorbidity, age, gender, and ethnic background.* **Results:** *One hundred fifty-five controlled studies of 5,768 children, adolescents, and adults have documented the efficacy of stimulants in an estimated 70% of subjects. The literature clearly documents that stimulants not only improve abnormal behaviors of ADHD, but also self-esteem, cognition, and social and family function. However, response varied in different age groups and with certain comorbid conditions. In addition, there is an impressive body of literature documenting the efficacy of tricyclic antidepressants on ADHD in more than 1,000 subjects. Studies of alternative antidepressants, antipsychotics, antihypertensives, and other compounds were also reviewed.* **Conclusions:** *The available literature indicates the important role of psychopharmacological agents in the reduction of the core symptoms of ADHD and associated impairments. More research is needed on alternative pharmacological treatments and to further evaluate established therapeutics beyond school-age Caucasian boys. In addition, more research is needed on the efficacy of treatment for comorbid ADHD, use of combined medications, and the combination of medication and psychosocial treatment.*

Attention-deficit hyperactivity disorder (ADHD) is a heterogeneous disorder of unknown etiology. It is one of the major clinical and public health problems in the United States because of its associated morbidity and disability in children, adolescents, and perhaps in adults. Its impact on society is enormous in terms of the financial cost, the stress to families, the impact on academic and vocational activities, as well as the negative effects on self-esteem. Data from cross-sectional, retrospective, and follow-up studies indicate that children with ADHD are at risk for developing other psychiatric disorders in childhood, adolescence, and adulthood such as antisocial behaviors, alcoholism and substance abuse, as well as depressive and anxiety symptoms and disorders.

Reprinted with permission from *J. Am. Acad. Child Adolesc. Psychiatry*, 1996, Vol. 35(4), 409–432. Copyright © 1996 by the American Academy of Child and Adolescent Psychiatry.

Although its etiology remains unknown, data from family-genetic, twin, and adoption studies as well as segregation analysis suggest a genetic origin for some forms of this disorder (Biederman et al., 1990, 1992; Deutsch, Matthysse, Swanson, & Farkas 1990; Faraone & Biederman, 1994; Faraone et al., 1992; Goodman, 1989; Goodman & Stevenson, 1989a,b; Manshadi, Lippmann, O'Daniel, & Blackmon, 1983). However, other etiologies are also likely such as psychological adversity, perinatal insults, and perhaps other yet unknown biological causes (Biederman et al., 1994; Milberger, Biederman, Sprich-Buckminster, Faraone, & Krifcher-Lehman, 1993).

Even though follow-up studies show that ADHD persists into adulthood in 10% to 60% of childhood-onset cases (Gittelman, Mannuzza, Shenker, & Bonagura, 1985; Hechtman, 1992; Mannuzza et al., 1991, 1993; Weiss et al., 1985), little attention has been paid to the adult form of this disorder. Its high prevalence in childhood, combined with the follow-up results, suggests that approximately 2% of adults may suffer from ADHD. If so, this would make ADHD a relatively common adult disorder that may be underidentified in adult psychiatry clinics.

The nosology of ADHD has undergone a number of changes. The disorder was known as hyperkinetic reaction of childhood in *DSM-II*, and attention deficit disorder in *DSM-III*. It recently underwent yet another change with the introduction of *DSM-IV*. The disorder will continue to be known as attention-deficit/hyperactivity disorder. However, it is now possible for an individual to meet criteria for the disorder if they have symptoms of inattention and/or hyperactivity/impulsivity. A subtype is assigned depending on the symptoms endorsed (combined, predominantly hyperactive/impulsive, or predominantly inattentive). Additional criteria have been added requiring the presence of symptoms in two or more situations (e.g., at school and at home) to reduce the number of false-positive diagnoses.

While the stimulants are the most established treatment for this disorder, as many as 30% of affected individuals do not respond or may not tolerate such treatments (Wilens & Biederman, 1992). Over the last two decades, various alternative approaches have been proposed and evaluated. However, questions remain as to the effectiveness, tolerability, and safety of these alternative approaches. Another barrier to therapeutics is the increasing recognition that ADHD is a heterogeneous disorder with considerable comorbidity with conduct, mood, and anxiety disorders (Biederman, Newcorn, & Sprich, 1991) and tic disorders (Comings & Comings, 1988). It is not clear whether these groups respond preferentially to different psychotropics. Thus, a comprehensive review of the pharmacotherapeutics of ADHD requires evaluation of the body of knowledge on stimulant and alternative agents attending to issues of comorbidity.

To help understand these important issues, we systematically reviewed the literature addressing the pharmacotherapy of ADHD, attentive to issues of psychiatric comorbidity. We conducted a *Medline* search using specific search criteria. We limited our search to manuscripts published in the English language in peer-reviewed journals and those in which the methodology was at least minimally explicit (e.g., use of rating scales to document response). The current review includes and extends a previous, comprehensive review of stimulants by the authors (Wilens & Biederman, 1992). Based on the description in individual papers, we categorized the responses in controlled studies as (1) robust (>50% overall response); (2) moderate (30% to 50%); (3) poor (<30%); or (4) mixed (not categorizable). For open studies we used more restrictive response criteria: (1) robust (>70% overall response); (2) moderate (50% to 70%); (3) poor (<50%); or (4) mixed (not categorizable).

RESULTS

Stimulants

While stimulants produce a variety of neurochemical effects, it has been proposed that their ability to increase catecholamines (both dopamine and norepinephrine) in the synaptic cleft accounts for the clinical effects in ADHD (Zametkin & Rapoport, 1987). The available literature on stimulants clearly documents the efficacy and safety of stimulants in 155 controlled studies encompassing children, adolescents ($n = 5,608$), and adults ($n = 160$). One hundred forty (87%) of studies are of latency-age children (Table 1), with an average response of 70%. In contrast, a much more limited body of literature exists for other age groups. There are only five (3%) controlled studies of stimulants in preschool children encompassing only 144 children (Barkley, 1988; Barkley, Karlsson, Strzelecki, & Murphy, 1984; Conners, 1975; Mayes, Crites, Bixler, Humphrey, & Mattison, 1994; Schleifer et al., 1975). Those studies report a variable response with improvement noted in structured tasks as well as in mother–child interactions. Four of the five studies recorded a moderate ($n = 3$) to robust ($n = 1$) (Mayes et al., 1994) response to stimulants in preschool children and one a mixed response (Schleifer et al., 1975). A similarly limited body of literature is available on adolescents, with only seven studies (4%, $n = 122$ adolescents) (Brown & Sexson, 1988; Coons, Klorman, & Borgstedt, 1987; Evans & Pelham, 1991; Klorman, Coons, & Borgstedt, 1987; Lerer & Lerer, 1977; MacKay, Beck, & Taylor, 1973; Safer & Allen, 1975; Varley, 1983). In those studies, response was moderate to robust, with no abuse or tolerance noted. Six of the seven studies reported a robust response to stimulants in adolescents and one a moderate response. Six controlled studies (4%) assessed the efficacy of stimulants in adults with ADHD (Gualtieri, Ondrusek, & Finley, 1985; Mattes, Boswell, & Oliver, 1984; Spencer et al., 1995; Wender et al., 1981, 1985b; Wood, Reimherr, Wender, & Johnson, 1976). These studies report a variable response ranging from 25% to 78% with an average of 54%. The largest response was reported in a recent controlled study of methylphenidate in adult ADHD, using careful diagnostic methodology, childhood onset, and a robust dose (Spencer et al., 1995).

Of the stimulants studied, methylphenidate comprised 83% of all the studies ($n = 133$ studies, 4,033 patients), followed by amphetamine ($n = 22$ studies, 1,140 patients) and a much more limited body of literature on pemoline ($n = 6$ studies, 726 patients). The literature provides little evidence of differential response to the various stimulants.

Most of the studies included a crossover design. Most of the existing studies are very brief, of not more than a few weeks' duration at the most. Some studies were ultrashort, lasting only days. There is a dearth of evidence on long-term studies. Moreover, since most of the literature on the subject is limited to Caucasian males, there is very limited information about efficacy and safety of stimulants in females (Befera & Barkley, 1985; Pelham, Walker, Sturger, & Hoza, 1989) and minorities (Brown & Sexson, 1988).

The extant literature clearly documents that stimulants diminish behaviors prototypical of ADHD including motoric overactivity, impulsivity, and inattentiveness. In addition to improving core symptoms of ADHD, stimulants also improve associated behaviors, including on-task behavior, academic performance, and social function. These effects appear to be dose-dependent and cross-situational, including home, clinic, and school (Abikoff & Gittelman, 1985a; Barkley et al., 1984; Klein, 1987; Rapport & DuPaul, 1986; Swanson, Granger, & Kliewer, 1987; Tannock, Schachar, Carr, & Logan, 1989; Wilens & Biederman, 1992). In several studies, behaviors of the ADHD child became indistinguishable from those of their non-ADHD peers, including impulsivity, noncompliance, disruption, and overall hyperactivity (Whalen, 1989). In adults, occupational and marital dysfunction were noted to improve with stimulant treatment (Wender, Reimherr, Wood, & Ward, 1985a).

Observational studies also demonstrated stimulant-enhanced social skills in school and within families and with peers. Studies report improved maternal-child and sibling interactions (Barkley & Cunningham, 1979) and that families of stimulant-responsive children are more amenable to psychosocial interventions (Schachar, Hoppe, & Schell, 1987). Studies evaluating peer relationships in children with ADHD show that those treated with stimulants have increased abilities to perceive peer communications, self-perceptions, and situational cues. In addition, these children show improved modulation of the intensity of behavior, improved communication, and greater responsiveness with fewer negative interactions (Whalen, Henker, & Granger, 1990).

TABLE 1
Stimulants in Attention-Deficit Hyperactivity Disorder

	No. of Studies	Subject Information	Dose Range	Study Design/Duration	Response	Comments
Preschoolers	5	Total N = 144	MPH: 5–16 mg (0.3–1.0 mg/kg)	Controlled: n = 5 3–9 weeks	Mild to robust	Variability in response and side effects
Latency Age	140	Total N = 5403	Variable	Controlled: n = 140	70% of subjects	23–27% of children did not respond or could not tolerate stimulant treatment
Adolescents	7	Total N = 122	MPH: 10–60 mg (0.3–1.0 mg/kg)	Controlled: n = 4 Open: n = 3 3 weeks–2 years	*Controlled:* Moderate to robust *Open:* Response rates ranged from 60–100%	Stimulants are as effective in adolescents as in children Mild increased heart rate and blood pressure
Adults	9	Total N = 230	MPH: 38 mg (0.6 mg/kg) Pemoline: 65 mg (0.9 mg/kg) D-amphetamine 19 mg	Controlled: n = 6 Open: n = 3 2–6 weeks	*Controlled:* Mild to robust response to stimulants *Open:* Response to stimulants was 70%	Variable response 54% improved Relatively low doses used in some studies
Total Stimulants	161 Amphetamine: 22 MPH: 133 Pemoline: 6	Total N = 5899	Variable	Controlled studies; n = 155	Estimated overall response = 70%	Most common side effects: insomnia, diminished appetite, abdominal pain, irritability, headaches, weight loss

Note: An annotated version of the tables is available upon request. MPH = methylphenidate.

220

A multitude of studies documented stimulant-induced improvements in measures of vigilance, cognitive impulsivity, reaction time, short-term memory, and learning of verbal and nonverbal material in children with ADHD (Barkley, 1977; Klein, 1987; Rapport et al., 1988). Recent studies have shown consistent stimulant-associated improvements employing a simulated classroom paradigm (Barkley, 1991; DuPaul, Barkley, & McMurray, 1994). In addition, recent studies suggest that as with behavior, improvement in cognitive measures is also dose dependent (Douglas, Barr, Amin, O'Neill, & Britton, 1988; Klein, 1987; Kupietz, Winsberg, Richardson, Maitinsky, & Mendell, 1988; Pelham, Bender, Caddell, Booth, & Moorer, 1985; Rapport et al., 1987, 1989a,b; Tannock et al., 1989).

Tricyclic Antidepressants

Tricyclic antidepressants (TCAs) include secondary and tertiary amines with a wide range of receptor actions, efficacy, and side effects. Secondary amines are more selective (noradrenergic) with less side effects in sensitive populations such as juvenile and geriatric. There have been 29 studies of children, adolescents ($n = 1,016$), and adults ($n = 63$) evaluating the efficacy and safety of TCAs for ADHD (Table 2). Twenty-seven (93%) of the 29 studies reported either moderate ($n = 9$) or robust ($n = 18$) response rates to TCAs in ADHD. These studies were primarily of latency-age children (26/29 studies). Of the latency-age studies, 24 (92%) reported either moderate ($n = 8$) or robust ($n = 16$) response rates to TCAs. Four studies included preschool children (two controlled; two open) (Gross, 1973; Huessy & Wright, 1970; Krakowski, 1965; Watter & Dreyfuss, 1973). Two of the four studies recorded a robust respose to TCAs in preschool children and two moderate (Huessy & Wright, 1970; Watter & Dreyfuss, 1973). Eight studies (three controlled; five open) included adolescents, but only one was exclusively on adolescents (Gastfriend, Biederman, & Jellinek, 1985). Seven of the eight adolescent studies reported a robust response. Three of the studies that included adolescents specifically reported on age effects, and all three noted a robust response to TCAs in this age group (Biederman, Baldessarini, Wright, Knee, & Harmatz, 1989a; Gastfriend et al., 1985; Wilens, Biederman, Geist, Steingord, & Spencer, 1993). There have been two recent studies of TCAs in adults, one a retrospective review ($n = 37$) (Wilens, Biederman, Mick, & Spencer, 1995b) which reported a moderate response. The other adult study was controlled ($n = 26$) (Wilens et al., 1994) and reported a strong response to TCAs.

Of the 29 TCA studies, 12 evaluated imipramine (41%, 8 controlled, 4 open), 9 desipramine (31%, 6 controlled, 3 open), 3 amitriptyline (10%, 3 controlled), 4 nortriptyline (14%, 4 open), and 1 clomipramine (3%, 1 controlled). Imipramine was the TCA most studied in the 1970s. These studies used less stringent diagnostic criteria and a lower average daily dose (1.75 mg/kg). Ten of the 12 imipramine studies reporting a moderate (4/12) or a robust response (6/12). Two imipramine studies reported a poor response, one secondary to a high dropout rate (Quinn & Rapoport, 1975) and another from negative effects on motor performance in neuropsychological testing (Gualtieri & Evans, 1988). Desipramine has been studied more recently with more stringent methodology including improvements in diagnostic (Biederman et al., 1989a; Rapport, Carlson, Kelly, & Pataki, 1993) and testing (Rapport et al., 1993) methodology and higher average daily doses ($n = 9$ studies; 3.9 mg/kg) than those used with imipramine. Of nine studies of desipramine, all but two studies reported robust rates of improvement; the exceptions included a study by Garfinkel et al. (1983), which reported a moderate response, and a retrospective study of adults (Wilens et al., 1995b). Robust response was noted in investigations of amitriptyline ($n = 3/3$ studies) and nortriptyline ($n = 3/4$ studies). The one study of clomipramine reported moderate response; however, that study medicated only on weekdays (Garfinkel, Wender, Sloman, & O'Neill, 1983).

Sixty-two percent of TCA studies were controlled (2 single and 16 double-blind; $n = 18$ studies, 310 children, 26 adults), and of those 6 were of parallel design, 12 crossover. Responses in controlled

TABLE 2
Antidepressants in Attention-Deficit Hyperactivity Disorder

	No. of Studies	Dose Range (Children)	Subject Information	Study Design/ Duration	Response	Comparison to Stimulants	Comments (Side effects)
Tricyclics							
Imipramine	12	5–200 mg 1–3 mg/kg mean 1.75 mg/kg/day	Total N = 527 Age range: 3–32	Controlled: n = 8 Open: n = 4 2 weeks–2 years	*Controlled:* robust improvement; n = 5 moderate; n = 2 mixed; n = 1 *Open:* robust improvement; n = 1 moderate; n = 2 mixed; n = 1	Comparison to stimulants; n = 7 stimulant > IMI; n = 3 stimulant = IMI; n = 2 stimulant < IMI; n = 2	Most common side effects were anorexia, insomnia and dry mouth
Desipramine	9	25–100 mg 0.7–6.3 mg/kg mean 3.9 mg/kg/day	Total N = 196 Age range: 5–adult	Controlled: n = 6 Open: n = 3 2–52 weeks	*Controlled:* robust improvement; n = 5 moderate; n = 1 *Open:* robust improvement; n = 2 moderate; n = 1	Comparison to stimulants; n = 2 stimulant > DMI; n = 1 stimulant = DMI; n = 1	DMI well tolerated Side effects were mild and observed in initial stages of treatment Most common side effects were decreased appetite, dry mouth and dizziness
Amitriptyline	3	20–150 mg mean 1.6 mg/kg/day	Total: N = 92 Age range: 2–18	Controlled: n = 3 4 weeks–12 months	*Controlled:* robust improvement; n = 2 moderate; n = 1	Comparison to stimulants; n = 2 stimulant = AMI; n = 2 but more side effects with AMI	Side effects were minimal Most common side effect was drowsiness

Drug	No.	Dose	Total N / Age	Study type / Duration	Results	Comparison to stimulants	Side effects
Nortriptyline	4	10–75 mg; 0.4–4.5 mg/kg; mean 1.7 mg/kg/day	Total: $N = 252$; Age range: 2–20	Open: $n = 4$; 1–60 months	*Open:* robust improvement; $n = 3$; moderate; $n = 1$	Comparison to stimulants; $n = 1$; stimulant < NOR; $n = 1$	Nortriptyline well tolerated with minimal side effects. Most common side effects were irritability, lethargy and insomnia
Clomipramine	1	25–100 mg; mean 3.5 mg/kg/day (only on weekdays)	Total: $N = 12$; Age range: 5–11	Controlled: $n = 1$; 20 weeks	*Controlled:* 1 moderate; $n = 1$	Comparison to stimulants; $n = 1$; stimulant ≫ CLI; $n = 1$	Side effects were minimal
Total tricyclics	29	mean 2.2 mg/kg/day (not including nortriptyline)	$N = 1016$ children; $N = 63$ adults; Age range: 2–32	Controlled: $N = 18$; Open: $N = 11$; 2 weeks–2 years	*Controlled:* robust improvement; $n = 12$; moderate; $n = 5$; mixed; $n = 1$. *Open:* robust improvement; $n = 6$; moderate; $n = 4$; mixed; $n = 1$	Comparison to stimulants; $n = 13$; stimulant > TCA; $n = 5$; stimulant = TCA; $n = 5$; stimulant < TCA; $n = 3$	Common side effects: Anorexia, insomnia, dry mouth, dizziness, drowsiness, irritability, lethargy

(Continued)

TABLE 2 (*Continued*)

	No. of Studies	Dose Range	Subject Information	Study Design/ Duration	Response	Comments
Monoamine oxidase inhibitors						
Pargyline	4	30 mg	Age range: 6–43	Controlled: $n = 1$	*Controlled:* Robust improvement; $n = 1$ As good as dextroamphetamine by behavioral ratings and cognitive tests	Mild-moderate side effects
Clorgyline		12 mg	Total $N = 26$ children	Open: $n = 3$	*Open:* Moderate improvement; $n = 3$	
Tranylcypromine sulfate		10 mg	Total $N = 33$ adults			
Moclobemide		100–200 mg		4 weeks–15 months		
Deprenyl		30 mg				
SSRI's						
Fluoxetine	1	20–60 mg	$N = 19$ Age range: 7–15	Open: $n = 1$ 6 weeks	*Open:* Majority of subjects had at least moderate improvement	Common side effect was sedation, which diminished with medication adjustments. Medication was well tolerated
Other						
Bupropion	4	60–450 mg	Age range: 6–45 $n = 104$ children $n = 19$ adults	Controlled: $n = 2$ Open: $n = 2$ 6–8 weeks Open >8 weeks	*Controlled:* robust improvement; $n = 1$ moderate improvement; $n = 1$ *Open:* moderate improvement; $n = 2$	Minimal side effects (exception of children with comorbid tics)
Venlafaxine	2	50–150 mean 100 mg	$N = 34$ adults		*Open:* moderate improvement; $n = 2$	High rate of adverse effects. 11/34 could not tolerate drug

Total antidepressants

40

Children $N = 1165$
Adults: $N = 149$

Age range: 2–45

Controlled:
$n = 21$
Open: $n = 19$

2 weeks–2 years

Controlled:
robust improvement; $n = 14$
moderate; $n = 6$
mixed; $n = 1$

Open:
robust improvement; $n = 6$
moderate; $n = 12$
mixed; $n = 1$

Comparison to stimulants; $n = 14$
stimulant > TCA; $n = 5$
stimulant = TCA; $n = 6$
stimulant < TCA; $n = 3$

Side effects:
Anorexia, insomnia, dry mouth, dizziness, drowsiness, irritability, lethargy, nausea

Note: TCA = tricyclic antidepressant; SSRI = selective serotonin reuptake inhibitor.

studies were robust in 12, moderate in 5, and mixed in 1. Most of the studies (20/29, 69%) of TCAs were relatively brief, lasting weeks to several months, addressing short-term outcome only. Nine of 29 studies (31% extended up to 2 years. Outcomes in both short- and long-term studies were equally positive—primarily moderate or robust. Of the long-term studies, five reported robust responses, three moderate, and another mixed. Quinn et al. reported poor long-term outcome for imipramine (50% dropout rate); however, for those who continued to take imipramine, improvement was sustained for more than 1 year (Quinn & Rapoport, 1975). Recent studies of relatively higher doses of TCAs report sustained improvement (up to 1 year) with both desipramine (> 4 mg/kg) (Biederman, Gastfriend, & Jellinek, 1986; Gastfriend et al., 1985) and nortriptyline (Wilens et al., 1993) (2.0 mg/kg).

TCA studies were categorized as low dose (≤1 mg/kg/day), moderate dose (>1 mg/kg, <4 mg/kg), and high dose (≥4 mg/kg) for all TCAs except nortriptyline, which is as twice as potent. Studies of TCAs used doses that ranged widely from 5 up to 200 mg/day (0.4 to 6.3 mg/kg, average 2.2 mg/kg (imipramine, amitriptyline, desipramine, clomipramine); 10 to 75 mg/day, average 1.7 mg/kg for nortriptyline). In all, there were 6 studies of the low doses, 19 of moderate doses, and 6 of relatively higher doses. Response was equally positive in all the dose ranges (Table 2). Serum TCA levels have been examined in eight studies, six pediatric (Biederman et al., 1986, 1989a; Donnelly et al., 1986; Gastfriend et al., 1985; Rapport et al., 1993; Wilens et al., 1993) and two adult (Wilens et al., 1994, 1995b). These studies reported high interindividual variability with little relationship to response. In addition, there was no group association between dose and level, the exception being nortriptyline (Wilens et al., 1993). Two randomized trials have evaluated the effects of different doses of TCAs for ADHD. One reported a mixed response as measured by neuropsychological testing, at all doses (1, 2, and 3 mg/kg) with improvements in symptoms of ADHD but a negative dose-dependent decrement on motor performance (Gualtieri & Evans, 1988). The other study used low (1 mg/kg) and moderate doses (2 mg/kg) and found robust behavioral response at both doses but favoring the lowest (Werry, 1980).

Behavioral symptoms, as rated by clinicians, teachers, and parents, were most consistently responsive to TCAs. On the other hand, neuropsychological tests were variably responsive (Gualtieri & Evans, 1988; Quinn & Rapoport, 1975; Rapport et al., 1993; Werry, 1980). Thirteen (45%) of the 29 studies compared TCAs to stimulants on behavioral measures (Table 2). Five studies reported that stimulants were superior to TCAs (Garfinkel et al., 1983; Gittelman-Klein, 1974; Greenberg, Yellin, Spring, & Metcalf, 1975; Rapoport, Quinn, Bradbard, Riddle, & Brooks, 1974), five studies reported that stimulants were equal to TCAs (Gross, 1973; Huessy & Wright, 1970; Kupietz & Balka, 1976; Rapport et al., 1993; Yepes, Balka, Winsberg, & Bialer, 1977) and three studies reported that TCAs were superior to stimulants (Watter & Dreyfuss, 1973; Werry, 1980; Winsberg, Bialer, Kupietz, & Tobias, 1972).

Non-TCA Antidepressants

There have been 11 studies of non-TCA antidepressant treatment for ADHD in children, adolescents (6 studies; n = 149), and adults (5 studies; n = 86). Response was robust in 18% (2/11) and moderate in 82% (9/11). In latency-age children response was robust in one-third (n = 2/6) and moderate in two-thirds (4/6). In the latency plus adolescent studies, response was robust in one-half (1/2) (Barrickman et al., 1995) and moderate in one-half (1/2) (Barrickman et al., 1991). In adults, moderate responses were reported (5/5) (Adler, Resnick, Kunz, & Deuinsky, 1995; Reimherr, Hedges, Strong, & Wender, 1995; Wender & Reimherr, 1990; Wender, Wood, Reimherr, & Ward, 1983; Wood, Reimherr, & Wender, 1982). However, there were no studies of preschool children.

Medication studied included the monoamine oxidase inhibitors (MAOIs) (n = 4 studies, 1 controlled, 3 open), bupropion (n = 4 studies, 2 controlled, 2 open), fluoxetine (n = 1 study, open), and venlafaxine ($n = 2$ studies, open). All but one of the studies was of brief duration (4 to 12 weeks); the exception extended to 1 year (Wender & Reimherr, 1990). Studies of MAO-A (moclobemide, clorgyline) (Trott, Friese, Menzel, & Nissen, 1991; Zametkin, Rapoport, Murphy, Linnaila, & Ismond, 1985), MAO-B (pargyline and deprenyl) (Wender et al., 1983, 1985c; Wood et al., 1982), and mixed A and B (tranylcypromine sulfate) (Zametkin et al., 1985) inhibitors were examined in ADHD children ($n = 26$) and adults ($n = 33$). The one controlled MAOI study reported robust improvement ($n = 1/4$) and the others (open studies) reported moderate improvement (3/4).

Bupropion has been reported to be better than placebo in reducing ADHD symptoms in two controlled studies in children, including a four-center multisite study ($n = 72$) (Casat et al., 1987, 1989; Conners et al., in press), and in a comparison with methylphenidate ($n = 15$) (Barrickman et al., 1995). In addition, an open study of adults with ADHD ($n = 19$) (Wender & Reimherr, 1990) reported a moderate to marked response in 74% of subjects with minimal side effects. In that study, sustained improvement was noted up to 1 year with dosing for ADHD similar to that recommended for depression (Wender & Reimherr, 1990). Recently, two open studies of venlafaxine in ADHD adults with prominent mood symptoms reported moderate improvement; however, 11 of 34 adults could not tolerate adverse effects (Adler et al., 1995; Reimherr et al., 1995). A small ($n = 19$) open study (Barrickman, Noyer, Kuperman, Schumacher, & Verda, 1991) suggested that fluoxetine may be beneficial in the treatment of ADHD in children. However, this study did not have a denominator, making it difficult to assess the rate of response.

Antipsychotics

There have been 12 controlled studies including 242 children and young adolescents evaluating the efficacy and safety of antipsychotics for ADHD (Table 3). Much of this literature is dated and confounded by diagnostic uncertainty. Of 12 studies, 3 reported robust, 5 moderate, 1 mixed, and 3 poor rates of improvement. As reviewed by Klein (Gittelman, 1980), not more than 50% of ADHD subjects improve while being treated with antipsychotics. Studies only included children and adolescents from 4 to 14 years of age, with no studies of adults. Eighty-three percent ($n = 10/12$ studies) of the available studies evaluated phenothiazines; two evaluated haloperidol. Ten of the 12 studies were relatively brief, lasting 3 to 12 weeks. The two exceptions include one ultrashort (single dose) study reporting poor results (Sprague, Barnes, & Werry, 1970) and one study of up to 24 weeks reporting robust results (Alexandris & Lundell, 1968). There was no consistent pattern of response between parallel design ($n = 6/12$) and crossover design ($n = 6/12$) studies. Because of the paucity of information, little can be said about the relative efficacy of the various antipsychotics.

Dosage ranged widely from 15 up to 150 mg (0.25 to 1.75 mg/kg) for the phenothiazines and 0.025 to 0.05 mg/kg for haloperidol. Using a definition of a relatively high daily dose as greater than 90 mg (approximately 3 mg/kg) of chlorpromazine or its equivalent, the high-dose studies (33%, $n = 4/12$) reported either robust ($n = 2$) or moderate ($n = 2$) response. In contrast, of the low-dose studies (<90 mg; $n = 8/12$) there were an equal number of positive (robust, $n = 1$; moderate, $n = 3$) and negative (mixed, $n = 1$; poor, $n = 3$) results.

Nine of the 12 studies compared antipsychotics to stimulant treatments. In two thirds of the studies, stimulants were equal to ($n = 1$) or better than the antipsychotics ($n = 5/9$) in behavioral outcome. While there was no evidence of antipsychotic-associated impaired cognitive performance in these studies, there was no evidence of the cognitive enhancement obtained with the stimulants.

Other Drugs

Clonidine. Clonidine is an α_2-noradrenergic agonist. There have been four pediatric studies ($n = 2$ controlled, (Gunning, 1992; Hunt, Minderaa, & Cohen 1985), $n = 1$ open (Hunt, 1987), and $n = 1$

TABLE 3

Antipsychotics in Attention-Deficit Hyperactivity Disorder

	No. of Studies	Dose Range	Subject Information	Study Design/ Duration	Response	Comments
Phenothiazines						
Chlorpromazine	4	30–125 mg mean 96 mg	Total N = 77 Age range: 5–14	Controlled: n = 4 Parallel; n = 2 Crossover; n = 2 3–8 weeks	*Controlled:* robust improvement; n = 1 moderate; n = 2 mixed; n = 1 (sedation) *Comparison to stimulants; n = 3* stimulant > chlorpromazine; n = 2 stimulant ≥ chlorpromazine; n = 1	Side effects found with chlorpromazine in some studies Most common side effects were drowsiness and photosensitivity
Thioridazine	4	15–150 mg mean 107 mg 0.25–4.5 mg/kg	Total N = 81 Age range: 4–13	Controlled: n = 4 Parallel; n = 3 Crossover; n = 1 Single dose up to 24 weeks	*Controlled:* robust improvement; n = 1 moderate; n = 1 poor; n = 2 (single or low dose, diagnostic heterogeneity) *Comparison to stimulants; n = 3* stimulant > chlorpromazine; n = 2 stimulant ≥ chlorpromazine; n = 1	Side effects were minimal Most common side effects were insomnia, nasal congestion and tremors
Mesoridazine	1	30–100 mg mean 50 mg	n = 17 Age range: 7–14	Controlled: n = 1 Crossover; n = 1 4 weeks	*Controlled:* robust improvement; n = 1	No side effects reported
Perphenazine	1	8–16 mg	n = 30	Controlled: n = 1 Parallel: n = 1 7 weeks	*Controlled:* Poor improvement; n = 1	Side effects included drowsiness and dystonia

Haloperidol	2	0.025–0.05 mg/kg	Total $N = 56$ Age range: 4–12	Controlled: $n = 2$ Crossover: $n = 2$ 3 days–12 weeks	*Controlled:* moderate; $n = 2$ *Comparison to stimulants; $n = 2$* Mixed results: Lowest dose haloperidol = stimulant: $n = 2$ stimulant > moderate dose haloperidol: $n = 2$	High dose of haloperidol produced marked increases in side effects Most common side effects were drowsiness and dystonia
Total antipsychotics	12	low dose (<90 mg of chlorpromazine): $N = 8$ high dose: $N = 4$	Total $N = 242$ Age range: 4–14	Controlled: $n = 12$ Single dose up to 24 weeks	*Controlled:* robust improvement; $n = 3$ moderate; $n = 5$ mixed; $n = 1$ Poor; $n = 3$ *Comparison to stimulants; $n = 9$* stimulant > antipsychotic; $n = 5$ stimulant = antipsychotic; $n = 1$ stimulant < antipsychotic; $n = 1$ mixed $n = 2$	Common side effects: Drowsiness, dystonia, insomnia, nasal congestion, tremors, photosensitivity

TABLE 4

Antihypertensives, Mood-Stabilizers, and Antianxiety Drugs in Attention-Deficit Hyperactivity Disorder

	No. of Studies	Dose Range	Subject Information	Study Design/ Duration	Response	Comments
Antihypertensive drugs						
Clonidine	4	0.025–0.16 mg mean 0.2 mg/day mean 4.6 μg/kg	Total $N = 122$ Age range: 3–18	Controlled Crossover: $n = 1$ Parallel $n = 1$ Open $n = 2$ 8–10 weeks	*Controlled:* Robust improvement; $n = 1$ Moderate improvement; $n = 1$ *Open:* Robust improvement; $n = 1$ Moderate improvement; $n = 1$ *Comparison to stimulants*; $n = 3$ stimulant ≥ clonidine; $n = 3$	Clonidine was well tolerated, sedation was a common side effect
Propranolol	1	10–640 mg/day mean 528 mg/day	Total $N = 13$ Age range: 17–33	Open: $n = 1$ 8–9 weeks	Robust improvement 11/13 (85%) improved ADHD symptoms and temper tantrums improved	Medication well tolerated Most common side effect was mild drowsiness
Guanfacine	1	0.5–4 mg/day mean 3.2 mg/day	Total $N = 13$ Age range: 4–20	Open: $n = 1$ 4 weeks	Robust improvement over baseline	Medication well tolerated

Mood-stabilizing drugs

Lithium	1	900–1500 mg	$N = 9$ Age range: 6–16	Controlled: $n = 1$ 3 months	Majority of sample worsened or showed no improvements on lithium	Lithium is not helpful for hyperactive children who are unresponsive to stimulants

Antianxiety drugs

Meprobamate	1	*Meprobamate:* 800–1600 mg *Prochlorperazine:* 20–40 mg	Total $N = 77$ Meprobamate: $n = 24$ Prochlorperazine $n = 28$ Placebo: $n = 25$ Age range: 5–13	Controlled: $n = 1$ 11 weeks	Both meprobamate and prochlorperazine were not better than placebo	Side effects were mild Most common side effect was drowsiness
Hydroxyzine	1	150 mg	Total $N = 61$ Hydroxyzine: $n = 17$ Amphetamine: $n = 17$ Chlorpromazine: $n = 17$ Placebo: $n = 10$ Age range: 6–11	Controlled: $n = 1$ 8 weeks	Both amphetamine and chlorpromazine were better than placebo, hydroxyzine was not	Minimal side effects reported Most common side effects were appetite change, dizziness, and sleepiness

retrospective review (Steingard, Biederman, Spencer, Wilens, & Gonzalez, 1993)) reporting beneficial with effects of clonidine in the treatment of ADHD in children and adolescents ($n = 122$) with ADHD with daily doses of up to 4 to 5 μg/kg (average 0.2 mg/day). All studies reported positive behavioral response, with 50% to 70% of subjects having at least a moderate response. There was less effect on cognition.

Guanfacine. There is one open study ($n = 13$) of the more selective α_{2a}-agonist, guanfacine, in children and adolescents with ADHD. Beneficial effects on hyperactive behaviors and attentional abilities were reported (Hunt et al., 1995).

Propranolol. There has been a small open study ($n = 13$) of the antihypertensive propranolol for adults with ADHD and temper outbursts. This study reported beneficial effects (85% improved) on ADHD symptoms at very high doses (average 528 mg/day) over a period of 9 weeks (Mattes, 1986). Despite high doses, propranolol was very well tolerated.

Lithium. One report (Greenhill, Rieder, Wender, Buchsbaum, & Zhan, 1973) described a controlled, 3-month trial of lithium in the treatment of children ($n = 9$) with ADHD (Table 4). These authors found that ADHD children without comorbid affective disorders were unresponsive to lithium treatment.

Other compounds found to be ineffective in the treatment of ADHD include antianxiety drugs, meprobamate and hydroxyzine (Cytryn, Gilbert, & Eisenberg, 1960); a sympathomimetic amine, fenfluramine (Donnelly et al., 1989); dopamine agonists, amantadine and L-dopa (Gittelman-Klein, 1987); amino acid precursors, D, L-phenylalanine and L-tyrosine (Reimherr, Wender, Wood, & Ward, 1987); and caffeine (Firestone, Davey, Goodman, & Peters, 1978; Garfinkel, Webster, & Sloman, 1975, 1981; Gross, 1975; Harvey & Marsh, 1978; Schnackenberg, 1973) (Tables 4 and 5).

PSYCHIATRIC COMORBIDITY IN THE PHARMACOTHERAPY OF ADHD

ADHD plus Conduct Disorder and Aggression

The most studied comorbidity of ADHD is that with conduct disorder. There have been 17 controlled stimulant studies ($n = 647$) of aggressive ADHD children (Amery, Minichiello, & Brown, 1984; Barkley, McMurray, Edelbrock, & Robbins, 1989; Cunningham, Siegel, & Offord, 1991; Gadow, Nolan, Sverd, Sprafkin, & Paolicelli, 1990; Hinshaw et al., 1989, 1992; Klorman et al., 1988, 1989, 1994; Livingston, Dykman, & Ackerman, 1992; Murphy, Pelham, & Lang, 1992; Pelham et al., 1990; Pliszka, 1989; Taylor et al., 1987; Whalen et al., 1987; Winsberg et al., 1972, 1974) and adolescents (Kaplan, Busner, Kupietz, Wasserman, & Segal, 1990). These reports show robust improvement ($n = 14/15$ studies) in ADHD symptoms (behavioral, cognitive, attentional, and academic) in aggressive ADHD subjects. In addition, the stimulants suppressed physical and nonphysical aggression in these children ($n = 8/9$ studies) both at home and in school in a dose-dependent fashion. Doses used were from 0.3 mg/kg to 0.6 mg/kg of methylphenidate day. Responsive symptoms included verbal and physical aggression (Gadow et al., 1990; Hinshaw et al., 1989; Murphy et al., 1992), negative social interactions with peers in group settings (Whalen et al., 1987), and covert antisocial behavior (stealing, destroying property, but not cheating) (Hinshaw et al., 1992). There were mixed responses to retaliation to provocation (Hinshaw et al., 1989; Murphy et al., 1992), and little effect on social informational processing (Murphy et al., 1992) in these ADHD children. Preliminary studies of antidepressants for ADHD children with comorbid conduct disorder ($n = 4$ studies, $n = 137$ children) also indicate improvement of ADHD symptoms (Biederman, Baldessarini, Wright, Keenan, & Faraone, 1993b; Simeon et al., 1986; Wilens et al., 1993; Winsberg et al., 1972) ($n = 4/4$ studies) and aggressive symptoms ($n = 2/2$ studies) (Simeon, Ferguson, & Van Wyck Fleet, 1986; Winsberg et al., 1972).

TABLE 5

Other Pharmacotherapy in Attention-Deficit Hyperactivity Disorder

	No. of Studies	Dose Range	Subject Information	Study Design/ Duration	Response	Comments
Fenfluramine	1	2.0 mg/kg/d	$N = 20$	Controlled: $n = 1$ 6 week	No effect on behavior at low or high dosage	
Amino acids	7	*Carbidopa:* 10–350 mg	Total $N = 62$ Age range: 6–45	Controlled: $n = 3$ Open: $n = 4$ 2 weeks–3 months	*Controlled:* Some short-term benefits, not sustained over time *Open:* Some short-term benefits, not sustained over time	Amino acids not very helpful in the treatment of ADHD due to tolerance and side effects Most common side effects were nausea and fatigue
		L-Dopa: 10–1000 mg	*Carbidopa/ L-Dopa: n = 20*			
		D-Phenylalanine: 50–700 mg *L-Tyrosine:* 50–150 mg/kg/day	*D-Phenylalanine: n = 24* *L-Tyrosine: n = 12*			
Caffeine	12	30–500 mg 3–12 mg/kg	Total N: 169 Age range: 6–11	Controlled: $n = 1$ Open: $n = 1$ 5–13 weeks	*Controlled:* Only 3/11 studies reported caffeine better than placebo (one study, $n = 19$ in non-ADHD subjects) *Open:* Caffeine similar to MPH	Few side effects Most common side effect was insomnia
Amantadine	1	200 mg	Total $n = 9$ Age range: 10–13	Open: $n = 1$ 1 month	Stimulants > amantadine = placebo	Side effects were minimal One subject reported nausea on the first day of treatment

ADHD plus Depression and Anxiety

There have been 11 pediatric ($n = 584$) and 2 adult ($n = 55$) (Spencer et al., 1995; Wilens et al., 1995b) studies of ADHD with comorbid anxiety or depression (Table 6). Sixty-seven percent (6/9) of studies ($n = 260$ children and 23 adults; 6 controlled and 3 open) reported a lesser response to stimulants of ADHD symptoms (DuPaul et al., 1994; Pliszka, 1989; Swanson, Kinsbourne, Roberts, & Zucker, 1978; Tannock, Ickowicz, & Schachar, 1995; Taylor et al., 1987; Voelker, Lochar, & Gdowski, 1983). In contrast, all four TCA studies ($n = 134$ children and 32 adults; one controlled (Biederman et al., 1993b), one open (Cox, 1982), and two retrospective reviews (Wilens et al., 1993, 1995b)) reported an equal rate of response of ADHD symptoms in comorbid subjects. However, the effect of stimulants on the comorbid anxiety and depression symptoms was not assessed in any study. In the two TCA studies that examined the effect of medication on comorbid depressive symptoms, TCAs decreased symptoms of depression in children with ADHD (Biederman et al., 1993b; Garfinkel et al., 1983).

ADHD plus Tics

Open ($n = 72$) (Comings & Comings, 1984; Erenberg, Cruse, & Rothner 1985) and controlled studies ($n = 60$) (Gadow et al., 1992, 1995; Konkol, Fischer, & Newby, 1990; Sverd et al., 1989, 1992) have noted that methylphenidate treatment is highly effective for ADHD behaviors, aggression, and social skill deficits in children with TS or chronic tics (Table 6). While recent controlled studies report no exacerbation of tics ($n = 49$) (Gadow et al., 1995; Sverd et al., 1989, 1992), previous studies report tics worsening in 31% (95/306 patients, $n = 10$ studies) of comorbid ADHD/tic patients (Caine, Ludlow, Polinsky, & Ebert, 1984; Comings & Comings, 1988; Denckla, Bemporad, & Mackay, 1976; Erenberg, 1982; Erenberg et al., 1985; Golden, 1977, 1982; Konkol, Fischer, & Newby, 1990; Price, Leckman, Pauls, Cohen, & Kidd, 1986; Shapiro & Shapiro, 1981).

There have been eight studies ($n = 118$) of antidepressant treatment of children and adolescents with ADHD and tic disorders. Recent case reports and case series of the TCAs imipramine (Dillon, Salzman, & Schulsinger, 1985), nortriptyline (Spencer et al., 1993b), and desipramine (Hoge & Biederman, 1986; Riddle, Hardin, Cho, Woolston, & Leckman, 1988; Spencer et al., 1993a) have reported a high rate (82%; 42/51 of subjects) of improvement of ADHD symptoms with no change or improvement of the tic disorder over an extended follow-up period (Spencer et al., 1993a,b). In a controlled study ($n = 34$), Singer et al. (1994) reported that desipramine was significantly better than both clonidine and placebo in its ability to improve ADHD symptoms associated with the full Tourette's syndrome. In this study, desipramine was tic-neutral and clonidine also did not improve tics. In an open study ($n = 29$) of a (selective) MAO-B inhibitor, deprenyl improved ADHD symptoms in 90% of children with ADHD and tics and was generally well tolerated (Jankovic, 1993). Finally, a small case series described precipitation ($n = 2$) or exacerbation of tics ($n = 2$) in four children with comorbid ADHD treated with bupropion (Spencer, Biederman, Steingard, & Wilens, 1993c).

In a retrospective study ($n = 24$) and an open study ($n = 7$) of clonidine, Steingard et al. (Steingard et al., 1993) reported a high rate (96%) of response (moderate or greater) of ADHD symptoms in ADHD children and adolescents with comorbid tics. The authors also noted improvement in tic symptoms with clonidine. In the controlled study ($n = 34$) mentioned above, Singer et al. (1994) reported that clonidine was not better than placebo in its ability to improve ADHD symptoms associated with the full Tourette's syndrome. Finally, there is one open study ($n = 10$) of the more selective α_{2a}-agonist, guanfacine, reporting beneficial effects on phonic tics and neuropsychological measures of attention and impulsivity (the Continuous Performance Test) in children with ADHD and tics (Chappell, Schahill, Schultz, Riddle, & Leckman, 1994).

ADHD and Mental Retardation

As reviewed by Demb (1991), there is agreement among researchers that stimulants are effective for ADHD symptoms in mild to moderately retarded children (Table 6). There have been mixed findings in studies of children with more profound mental retardation (Aman, Marks, Turbott, Wilsher, & Merry, 1991; Demb, 1991) and those with pervasive developmental disorder not otherwise specified (Birmaher, Quintana, & Greenhill, 1988; Campbell et al., 1985; Strayhorn, Rapp, Donina, & Strain, 1988) along with concerns of increased stereotypics and constriction of attention. However, reports indicate that individual responses vary widely and that some children with moderate or profound mental retardation improve dramatically (Demb, 1991). The main predictor of response is reported to be the presence of clear ADHD symptoms (hyperactivity, impulsiveness, and inattention) as opposed to general behavioral disruption. Age, IQ, and other associated diagnoses were reported to be less predictive (Demb, 1991).

COMBINED PHARMACOTHERAPY

Little is known about combined pharmacotherapy in ADHD. Historically the first reports of combined pharmacotherapy in ADHD were of antipsychotics and stimulants. Despite the theoretical concern of contradictory dopaminergic mechanisms of action, there have been two controlled studies ($n = 181$) of combined neuroleptic and stimulant treatment of children with ADHD (Gittelman-Klein, Klein, Katz, Saraf, & Pollack, 1976; Weizman, Weitz, Szekely, Tyano, & Belmaker, 1984). In both studies, the combination was superior to stimulant medication alone, though only a trend in the larger study.

In one of the few studies of its kind, Rapport et al. (1993) evaluated the separate and combined effects of methylphenidate and desipramine in 16 hospitalized children. These investigators found that methylphenidate alone improved vigilance, both methylphenidate and desipramine alone produced positive affects on short-term memory and visual problem-solving, and their combination produced positive affects on learning of higher-order relationships. The authors speculated that performance on different cognitive measures may be modulated by separate neurotransmitter systems. Of note, the subjects in this study were children with ADHD and comorbid major depression (11/16), dysthymia (4/16), and anxiety (6/16). These investigators (Pataki, Carlson, Kelly, Rapport, & Biancaniello, 1993) also reported that, although this combined pharmacotherapy was associated with more side effects than monotherapy, there was no evidence that the combined use of both drugs was associated with unique or serious side effects. Finally, there is a report indicating that β-blockers ($n = 3$) may be helpful in combination with the stimulants (Ratey, Greenberg, & Lindem, 1991).

There are several single reports of the use of multiple agents in the treatment of concurrent disorders with ADHD. There is one open report of the successful use of fluoxetine with stimulants in the management of concurrent depressive disorders ($n = 32$) (Gammon & Brown, 1993). There are open reports of the successful use of clonidine with stimulants for conduct disorder (Conners, unpublished) and sleep disorders (Brown & Gammon, 1992; Prince, Wilens, Spenier, Wozniak, & Biederman, 1994) in children with ADHD. The combined use of other agents with anti-ADHD drugs (stimulants or TCAs) such as benzodiazepines for anxiety or lithium carbonate or carbamazepine for mania has not been systematically evaluated.

DISCUSSION

Although little doubt remains regarding the efficacy of stimulants in the treatment of ADHD, this extensive literature has largely documented the short-term efficacy of methylphenidate treatment in latency-age Caucasian boys (Figs. 1 and 2). A much more limited body of literature exists for

TABLE 6
Pharmacotherapy of Comorbidity in Attention-Deficit Hyperactivity Disorder

No. of Studies	Duration	Subject Information	Study Design	Comorbidity	Response of ADHD Symptoms	Response of Comorbid Symptoms
ADHD + Conduct Disorder/Aggressive Behavior						
Stimulant $n = 17$ studies	**Stimulant** single dose to 6 weeks	**Stimulant** $n = 647$ all latency; ($N = 9$) adolescent also	**Stimulant** 17 controlled crossover studies (15 methylphenidate, 4 D-amphetamine, 1 pemoline)	ADHD + aggression	**Stimulant:** 14/15 studies reported improvement of ADHD symptoms 1/15 mixed response	**Stimulant** 8/9 stimulant studies reported improvement of aggressive symptoms
Antidepressant $n = 4$ studies	**Antidepressant** 6 weeks up to 1 year	**Antidepressant** $n = 137$ latency + adolescent	**Antidepressant** 2 controlled (imipramine, desipramine); 2 open (bupropion, nortriptyline)		**Antidepressant:** 4/4 studies reported improvement of ADHD symptoms	**Antidepressant** 2/2 studies reported improvement of aggressive symptoms
ADHD + Anxiety/Depression						
Stimulant $n = 9$ studies **TCAs** $n = 4$ studies	4 weeks up to 1 year	**Stimulant** 450 children; 23 adults; **TCAs** 134 children; 32 adults	**Stimulant** $n = 6$ controlled $n = 3$ open **TCAs** $n = 1$ controlled $n = 3$ open	**Stimulant** Depression; $n = 2$ Anxiety; $n = 7$ (Both; $n = 2$) **TCAs** Depression; $n = 4$ Anxiety; $n = 3$ (Both; $n = 3$)	**Stimulant** Equal response; $n = 3$ Less response; $n = 6$ **TCAs** Equal response; $n = 4$ Less response; $n = 0$	**Stimulant** Effect of on comorbid anxiety and depression not assessed **TCAs** In 2 studies, decreased comorbid depression

ADHD + Tics/Tourette's

Number of studies	Duration	Number of subjects	Study design	ADHD + tics/Tourette's	ADHD symptoms	Tics/Tourette's
Stimulant n = 13 studies of tics; n = 6 studies of ADHD	Weeks up to 1 year	**Stimulant** n = 355 subjects; studies of tics, n = 132 subjects; studies of ADHD	**Stimulant** 9 open studies; 5 controlled studies		**Stimulant** In two open and four controlled studies of ADHD/tic subjects, ADHD symptoms improved dramatically with stimulants	**Stimulant** Tics worsened in 27% (95/355) of ADHD/tic subjects treated with stimulants. In the five controlled studies, 11% (7/66) subjects had worsening tics
TCAs n = 6 studies		**TCAs** n = 92 subjects	**TCAs** 5 open studies 1 controlled study		**TCAs** In 82% (42/51), ADHD symptoms improved with TCAs in open studies; improvement in the one controlled study	**TCAs** No exacerbation of tic symptoms
MAOIs n = 1 study		**MAOIs** n = 29 subjects	**MAOIs** open		**MAOIs** Improvement of 90% of the one open study	**MAOIs** No exacerbation of tic symptoms
Clonidine n = 3 studies		**Clonidine** n = 65 subjects	**Clonidine** 2 open studies 1 controlled		**Clonidine** In 96% (23/24), ADHD symptoms improved with TCAs in open studies; improvement in the one controlled study	**Clonidine** In 75% (18/24), tic symptoms improved with TCAs in open studies; no improvement in the one controlled study

ADHD + Mental Retardation

Number of studies	Duration	Number of subjects	Study design	ADHD + Mental Retardation	Response	
Stimulant n = 12 studies	3 weeks to 29 months	**Stimulant** n = 343	**Stimulant** 10 controlled 2 open	1 severe MR 9 mild-moderate 2 mild-severe	**Stimulant** Response moderate (6) to robust (3) in 9/12. Response moderate to robust in 7/10 in controlled studies. Response moderate to robust in 9/11 with mild-moderate MR. 1/3 studies of severe retardation found moderate response	**Stimulant** Not assessed

Note: TCA = tricyclic antidepressant; MAOI = monoamine oxidase inhibitor.

237

A. Medication Type

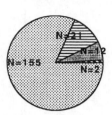

☒ Stimulants

☰ Antidepressants

▦ Neuroleptics

◨ Clonidine

N=6,472 Subjects

B. Age of Subjects

☒ Latency

☰ Adolescents

▦ Adults

◨ Preschoolers

N=6,472 Subjects

C. Studies of Stimulants

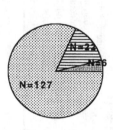

☒ Methylphenidate

☰ D-Amphetamine

▦ Pemoline

N=5,768 Subjects

D. Studies of Antidepressants

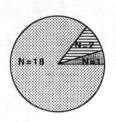

☒ Tricyclics

☰ Bupropion

▦ MAOI's

N=487 Subjects

Figure 1. Controlled studies in attention-deficit hyperactivity disorder (all ages). MAOI = monoamine oxidase inhibitor.

A. Duration

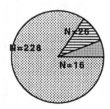

☒ Short < 2 month

☰ Medium ≤ 1 year

▦ Long > 1 year

B. Gender

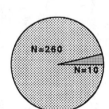

☒ Boys only

▦ Gender comparison

C. Ethnicity

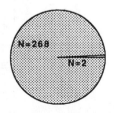

☒ Caucasian

▦ Non-Caucasian

N= > 7,500 Subjects

Figure 2. Medication studies in attention-deficit hyperactivity disorder (open and controlled).

stimulants at other ages, for females, and for ethnic minorities. Despite small numbers, the few studies of stimulants in adolescents reported rates of response highly consistent with those seen in latency-age children. In contrast, the few studies on preschool children appear to indicate that young children respond less well to stimulant therapy, suggesting that preschool children with ADHD may be more treatment refractory. On the other hand, studies of stimulants in adults have reported conflicting results, with some studies reporting good and others poor responses. However, a recent study in adult ADHD (Spencer et al., 1995), using robust daily doses (1 mg/kg per day) and careful diagnostic methodology (childhood onset, persistent symptomatology, and full *DSM-III-R* criteria), has reported a response of 78%, consistent with that of younger ADHD patients.

In latency-age children, the literature clearly documents that treatment with stimulants not only improves abnormal behaviors of ADHD but also self-esteem and cognitive, social, and family function (Abikoff & Gittelman, 1985b; Barkley et al., 1984; Klein, 1987; Rapport & DuPaul, 1986; Swanson et al., 1987; Tannock et al., 1989; Wilens & Biederman, 1992). These findings support the importance of treating children with ADHD beyond school hours to include evenings, weekends, and vacations. Treatment with stimulants also improves a wide variety of cognitive abilities (Barkely, 1977; Klein, 1987; Rapport et al., 1988), increases school-based productivity (Famularo & Fenton, 1987), and improves performance in academic testing (Abikoff et al. personal communication). However, despite these beneficial cognitive effects, it is important to be aware that children with ADHD commonly manifest additional learning disabilities that are not responsive to pharmacotherapy (Bergman, Winters, & Cornblatt, 1991; Faraone et al., 1993) but may respond to educational remediation.

The relationship between dose and response remains a source of active controversy. An influential early study (Sprague & Sleator, 1977) reported that higher stimulant doses were required to ameliorate behavior but that these higher doses degraded performance on cognitive tasks. Yet more recent studies challenged this notion by failing to reveal evidence of cognitive impairment on standard (0.3 to 2.0 mg/kg per day) doses of stimulants. Moreover, recent studies indicate that both behavior and cognitive performance improve with stimulant treatment in a dose-dependent fashion (Douglas et al., 1988; Klein, 1987; Kupietz et al., 1988; Pelham et al., 1985; Rapport et al., 1987, 1989a,b; Tannock et al., 1989). Elia et al. reported a very robust response (96%) to either methylphenidate or dextroamphetamine using high doses of medication. However, a large number of responders had adverse effects (Borcherding, Keysor, Rapoport, Elia, & Amass, 1990; Elia, Borcherding, Rapoport, & Keysor, 1991). In addition, earlier concerns that stimulants were associated with constriction of attention or "overfocusing" have been recently refuted (Douglas, Barr, Desilets, & Sherman, 1995; Solanto & Wender, 1989). Also, there is no evidence that improved behavior comes at the cost of "zombification," as studies have shown increased prosocial behavior on stimulant medication (Gittelman, 1980; Whalen et al., 1990). Despite beneficial effects on social skills, some ADHD-associated interpersonal difficulties could represent additional brain-based abnormal social behavior, akin to learning disabilities (Weintraub, Mesulam, & Kramer, 1981), that are not drug sensitive but may require psychosocial treatment strategies.

Other areas of controversy and concern about stimulant use include growth suppression (Mattes & Gittelman, 1983; Safer, Allen, & Barr, 1972), the development of tics (Lowe, Cohen, & Detlor, 1982), drug abuse (Jaffe, 1991), use in adolescents (Evans & Pelham, 1991), and rebound (Johnston, Pelham, Hoza, & Sturges, 1988). Although stimulants routinely produce anorexia and weight loss, their effect on growth in height is less certain. While initial reports suggested that there was a persistent stimulant-associated decrease in growth in height in children (Mattes & Gittelman, 1983; Safer et al., 1972), other reports have failed to substantiate this claim (Gross, 1976; Satterfield, Cantwell, Schell, & Blaschke, 1979). Ultimate height appears to be unaffected if treatment is discontinued in adolescence (Gittelman & Mannuzza, 1988); however, there are no studies of growth in children treated continually from childhood through adolescence and young adulthood. Moreover, the literature on stimulant-associated growth deficits did not examine the possibility that growth deficits may represent maturational delays related to ADHD itself (i.e., dysmaturity) and not its treatment. In fact, preliminary work from our group supports this dysmaturity hypothesis (Spencer et al., unpublished data). This state of affairs does not support the common practice of drug holidays in children without evidence of growth deficits. However, until more is known, it seems prudent that children suspected of stimulant-associated growth deficits be provided with drug holidays or alternative treatment. This recommendation should be carefully weighed against the risk for exacerbation of symptoms due to drug discontinuation.

Early reports indicated that children with a personal or family history of tic disorders were at greater risk for developing a tic disorder when exposed to stimulants (Lowe et al., 1982). However, recent work has increasingly challenged this view (Comings & Comings, 1988; Gadow et al., 1992, 1995). For example, in a recent short-term, controlled study of children with ADHD and tics ($n = 34$) using multiple informants and direct observation, Gadow et al. (1995) reported that methylphenidate effectively suppressed ADHD symptoms, with only a weak effect on the frequency of tics. Although this work is reassuring, clearly more information is needed in larger numbers of subjects over a longer period of time to obtain closure on this issue. Until more is known, it seems prudent to weigh risks and benefits in individual cases with appropriate discussion with the child and family about the benefits and pitfalls of the use of stimulants in children with ADHD and tics. Similar uncertainties remain about the abuse potential of stimulants in children with ADHD. Despite the concern that ADHD may increase the risk of abuse in adolescents and young adults (or their associates), there are no scientific data confirming the abuse of prescribed stimulants by ADHD children who are receiving appropriate diagnosis and careful follow-up. Moreover, recent work has shown that the most commonly abused substance in adolescents and adults with ADHD is marijuana, not stimulants (Biederman et al., 1995b). Despite their clinical importance, issues of interdose rebound have not been adequately examined in the literature. Poststimulant worsening of symptoms may be particularly taxing in the evening, when family life takes place. Treatment options include the use of long-acting preparations of the stimulants or alternative medications such as antidepressants.

After the stimulants the most extensive literature on the pharmacotherapy of ADHD is on the TCAs. We identified 29 studies of TCAs involving more than 1,000 children, adolescents, and adults with ADHD. These studies showed that various TCAs are effective in the treatment of symptoms of ADHD at different doses with an unclear relationship to serum levels. Advantages of TCAs over stimulants include a longer duration of action, the feasibility of once-daily dosing without symptom rebound or insomnia, greater flexibility in dosage, the readily available option of monitoring plasma drug levels (Preskorn, Weller, Weller, & Glotzbach, 1983), and minimal risk of abuse or dependence (Gittelman, 1980; Rapoport & Mikkelsen, 1978). Although the early literature suggested that the beneficial effects of TCAs in ADHD were short-lived, more recent studies have challenged this view. Recent studies have shown that improvement could be maintained over time using doses of 3 to 5 mg/kg per day (Biederman et al., 1986, 1989a; Gastfriend et al., 1985; Wilens et al., 1993). Thus, it could be that short-lived effects reported in previous studies could have been due to low doses (<3 mg/kg) without appropriate adjustment in dose over time. Although the literature is limited and inconclusive, studies of response to TCAs reported less consistent effect on cognition than on behavior compared with the stimulants. More work is needed to define better the cognitive effects of both TCAs and stimulants in children with ADHD.

Despite an extensive body of literature documenting relatively benign and predictable TCA-associated cardiac effects (Biederman et al., 1993a), four cases of sudden death in desipramine-treated children identified in postmarketing surveillance (*Medical Letter*, 1990) have increased fears of cardiac toxicity of TCAs in children (Biederman et al., 1989b; Preskorn et al., 1983; Winsberg, Goldstein, & Yepes, 1975). A recent report estimated that the magnitude of desipramine-associated risk of sudden death in children may not be much larger than the baseline risk of sudden death in this age group (Biederman et al., 1995a). Thus, until more is known, TCAs should be used as second-line treatment for ADHD and only after carefully weighing the risks and benefits of treating or not treating an affected child.

In addition to the TCAs, there is a small number of publications suggesting that other antidepressants with predominately noradrenergic or a dopaminergic mechanism of activity such as bupropion and MAOIs may also be effective in the treatment of ADHD. Although bupropion has been found helpful in ADHD, it has been associated with a somewhat greater risk of seizures than other antidepressants. However, this risk has been linked to high doses, a previous history of seizures, and eating disorders. Thus, by avoiding these risk factors, and by dividing the daily dose, the risk of seizures may be comparable with that accompanying other antidepressants. The literature on MAOIs is limited, making evaluation of the usefulness of these compounds in ADHD uncertain. In addition, dietetic restrictions and potential drug–drug interactions leading to hypertensive crisis and the serotonergic syndrome make these compounds less than ideal therapies for ADHD. Nonetheless, the MAOIs may be important to consider in individuals with treatment-refractory ADHD. The literature on selective serotonin reuptake inhibitors is limited to a single positive small open study without a denominator. Although more work is needed to evaluate the role, if any, of selective serotonin reuptake inhibitors in the treatment of ADHD, there is little clinical or scientific evidence implicating serotonergic systems in the pathophysiology of ADHD.

Besides stimulants and antidepressants, the antipsychotics and clonidine have also been evaluated in the treatment of ADHD. Although early reports documented some efficacy for antipsychotic drugs in the pharmacotherapy of the behavioral symptoms of ADHD (Table 3), the risk for neuroleptic-associated tardive dyskinesia and neuroleptic malignant syndrome make their use in this disorder less desirable. Thus, antipsychotics should be reserved as a last resort in patients with treatment-refractory ADHD. Although limited, there is a small body of literature on clonidine documenting that this compound is helpful for the control of behavioral symptoms of ADHD, particularly disinhibition and aggression. However, clonidine is short-acting and highly sedating, with unclear cognitive effects. Recently guanfacine, another antihypertensive with clonidine-like α-adrenergic properties, has been advanced as an alternative to clonidine in the treatment of ADHD. More work is needed to evaluate the role of clonidine and guanfacine in ADHD. Both are considered third-line treatments for this disorder.

Recent work has documented an increasingly expanding range of comorbid disorders with ADHD beyond oppositional defiant, conduct, and tic disorders, showing high levels of depression, bipolarity, and anxiety (Biederman et al., 1991; Wozniak et al., 1995). However, uncertainty remains as to whether the presence of a comorbid disorder has an impact on the treatment of ADHD and whether agents used to treat ADHD improve or worsen the comorbid symptoms. Several reports indicate that stimulant treatment of children with ADHD and comorbid aggression or conduct disorder helps both the ADHD and the aggressive/conduct symptoms. Although these findings are of great clinical significance, they do not support the use of stimulants to treat aggression outside ADHD. Moreover, the literature on the topic did not fully distinguish between impulsive and predatory aggression, making the role of stimulants for predatory antisocial aggression even more uncertain. Until more is known, clinicians should be discouraged from treating non-ADHD predatory delinquents with stimulants. Much less is known about the impact of pharmacotherapy in children with ADHD and comorbid anxiety or mood disorders. The emerging literature suggests that, with regard to their ADHD symptoms, anxious ADHD children respond more poorly to stimulants than do nonanxious ADHD children (Table 6). In addition, stimulants are thought to be anxiogenic, suggesting that caution be used in the treatment of individuals with ADHD and comorbid anxiety disorders. Nothing is known about the effect of stimulants on ADHD and comorbid mood disorders. Although stimulants may be depressogenic, it is possible that demoralization and failure due to ADHD may improve with stimulants by improving performance in the affected ADHD patient. Also, caution should be exercised in distinguishing stimulant-induced depressive symptoms from emerging depression in children with ADHD. This important clinical issue requires further clinical research. Despite increasing recognition of the co-occurrence of ADHD and bipolarity (Wozniak et al., 1995), nothing is known about the pharmacotherapy of the combined condition. Considering the potential for activation of individuals with ADHD and mania, caution should be used in treating ADHD and mania with stimulants and antidepressants. Since mania can produce severe cognitive and behavioral symptoms, it is crucial to first stabilize the mood disorder with mood stabilizers. As mentioned earlier, recent literature has challenged the absolute contraindication of stimulants with ADHD and tics. For children with ADHD and tics with documented exacerbation of tics by stimulants, alternative agents should be explored. On the other hand, many children with this comorbidity respond to stimulants without worsening of tics. Although limited, the literature on mental retardation is clear: it suggests that mentally retarded individuals suffering from ADHD, at least in the mild to moderate range, can benefit from the same pharmacotherapeutic interventions found effective for nonretarded ADHD individuals. Considering the extraordinary importance of augmenting functional abilities of mentally retarded individuals, clinicians should be proactive in identifying and treating ADHD in developmentally disordered individuals.

Although in clinical practice many ADHD patients receive multiple treatments, the literature on combined pharmacotherapy is very sparse, not permitting the development of clear therapeutic guidelines. In contrast to polypharmacy, rational combined pharmacological approaches can be used for the treatment of comorbid ADHD, as augmentation strategies for patients with insufficient response to a single agent and for the management of treatment-emergent adverse effects. Examples of the rational use of combined treatment include the use of an antidepressant plus a stimulant for ADHD and comorbid depression, the use of clonidine to ameliorate stimulant-induced insomnia, and the use of lithium plus an anti-ADHD agent to treat ADHD comorbid with bipolar disorder (Wilens, Spencer, Biederman, Wozniak, & Connor, 1995a).

Summary

There is a substantial body of literature documenting the efficacy of multiple unrelated pharmacological agents in ADHD individuals throughout the life cycle. The literature documents that pharmacological treatment leads to improvement not only on core behavioral symptoms but also on associated impairments including cognition, social skills, and family function. The armamentarium of anti-ADHD compounds includes not only the stimulants, but also several antidepressants, antipsychotics, and clonidine. Effective pharmacological treatments for ADHD seem to share noradrenergic and dopaminergic mechanisms of action. While studies include a wide variety of medications, by far the greatest proportion of existing studies are on stimulant drugs in general and methylphenidate in particular. In addition, there is a large body of literature documenting the efficacy of TCAs on ADHD. While clonidine provides a distinct alternative, to date there is a paucity of data. The efficacy of neuroleptics is less robust and includes the risk of tardive dyskinesia. Despite great progress over the last three decades, little is known about the treatment of ADHD in preschool children, adolescents, adults, females, and minorities. Although there is increasing recognition that ADHD is a heterogeneous disorder with considerable and varied comorbidity, increased attention to comorbidity in ADHD has not been matched by therapeutic advances. There are limited data on the differential response of medications in comorbid ADHD, on the effects of combined pharmacotherapy, and on combined pharmacotherapy and psychotherapy. It is hoped that ongoing and future research will fill these gaps.

REFERENCES

Abikoff, H., & Gittelman, R. (1985a). Hyperactive children treated with stimulants. *Arch. Gen. Psychiatry, 42*, 953–961.

Abikoff, H., & Gittelman, R., (1985b). The normalizing effects of methylphenidate on the classroom behavior of ADDH children. *J. Abnorm. Child Psychol., 13*, 33–44.

Adler, L., Resnick, S., Kunz, M., & Devinsky, O. (1995). *Open-label trial of venlafaxine in attention deficit disorder*. Presented at the New Clinical Drug Evaluation Unit Program, Orlando, FL.

Alexandris, A., & Lundell, F. W. (1968). Effect of thioridazine, amphetamine and placebo on the hyperkinetic syndrome and cognitive area in mentally deficient children. *Can. Med. Assoc. J., 98*, 92–96.

Aman, M. G., Marks, R. E., Turbott, S. H., Wilsher, C. P., & Merry, S. N. (1991). Clinical effects of methylphenidate and thioridazine in intellectually subaverage children. *J. Am. Acad. Child Adolesc. Psychiatry, 30*, 246–256.

Amery, B., Minichiello, M., & Brown, G. (1984). Aggression in hyperactive boys: Response to D-amphetamine. *J. Am. Acad. Child Psychiatry, 23*, 291–294.

Barkley, R. A. (1977). A review of stimulant drug research with hyperactive children. *J. Child Psychol. Psychiatry, 18*, 137–165.

Barkley, R. A. (1988). The effects of methylphenidate on the interactions of preschool ADHD children with their mothers. *J. Am. Acad. Child Adolesc. Psychiatry, 27*, 336–341.

Barkley, R. A. (1991). The ecological validity of laboratory and analogue assessment methods of ADHD symptoms. *J. Abnorm. Child Psychol., 19*, 149–178.

Barkley, R. A., & Cunningham, C. (1979). The effects of methylphenidate on the mother–child interactions of hyperactive children. *Arch. Gen. Psychiatry, 36*, 201–208.

Barkley, R. A., Karlsson, J., Strzelecki, E., & Murphy, J. V. (1984). Effects of age and Ritalin dosage on mother–child interactions of hyperactive children. *J. Consult. Clin. Psychol., 52*, 750–758.

Barkley, R. A., McMurray, M. B., Edelbrock, C. S., & Robbins, K. (1989). The response of aggressive and nonaggressive ADHD children to two doses of methylphenidate. *J. Am. Acad. Child Adolesc. Psychiatry, 28*, 873–881.

Barrickman, L., Noyes, R., Kuperman, S., Schumacher, E., & Verda, M. (1991). Treatment of ADHD with fluoxetine: A preliminary trial. *J. Am. Acad. Child Adolesc. Psychiatry, 30*, 762–767.

Barrickman, L., Perry, P., Allen, A. et al. (1995). Bupropion versus methylphenidate in the treatment of attention-deficit hyperactivity disorder. *J. Am. Acad. Child Adolesc. Psychiatry, 34*, 649–657.

Befera, M., & Barkley, R. A. (1985). Hyperactive and normal girls and boys: Mother–child interactions, parent psychiatric status, and child psychopathology. *J. Child Psychol. Psychiatry, 26*, 439–452.

Bergman, A., Winters, L., & Cornblatt, B. (1991). Methylphenidate: Effects on sustained attention. In L. Greenhill & B. Osman (Eds.), *Ritalin: Theory and patient management* (pp. 223–231). New York: Mary Ann Liebert.

Biederman, J., Baldessarini, R., Goldblatt, A., Lapey, K., Doyle, A., & Hesslein, P. (1993a). A naturalistic study of 24-hour electrocadiographic recordings and echocardiographic findings in children and adolescents treated with desipramine. *J. Am. Acad. Child Adolesc. Psychiatry, 32*, 805–813.

Biederman, J., Baldessarini, R. J., Wright, V., Keenan, K., & Faraone, S. (1993b). A double-blind placebo controlled study of desipramine in the treatment of attention deficit disorder: III. Lack of impact of comorbidity and family history factors on clinical response. *J. Am. Acad. Child Adolesc. Psychiatry, 32*, 199–204.

Biederman, J., Baldessarini, R., Wright, V., Knee, D., & Harmatz, J. (1989a). A double-blind placebo controlled study of desipramine in the treatment of attention deficit disorder: I. Efficacy. *J. Am. Acad. Child Adolesc. Psychiatry, 28*, 777–784.

Biederman, J., Baldessarini, R., Wright, V., Knee, D., Harmatz, J., & Goldblatt, A. (1989b). A double-blind placebo controlled study of desipramine in the treatment of attention deficit disorder: II. Serum drug levels and cardiovascular findings. *J. Am. Acad. Child Adolesc. Psychiatry, 28*, 903–911.

Biederman, J., Faraone, S. V., Keenan, K. et al. (1992). Further evidence for family-genetic risk factors in attention deficit hyperactivity disorder (ADHD): Patterns of comorbidity in probands and relatives in psychiatrically and pediatrically referred samples. *Arch. Gen. Psychiatry, 49*, 728–738.

Biederman, J., Faraone, S. V., Keenan, K., Knee, D., & Tsuang, M. T. (1990). Family-genetic and psychosocial risk factors in *DSM-III* attention deficit disorder. *J. Am. Acad. Child Adolesc. Psychiatry, 29*, 526–533.

Biederman, J., Gastfriend, D. R., & Jellinek, M. S. (1986). Desipramine in the treatment of children with attention deficit disorder. *J. Clin. Psychopharmacol., 6*, 359–363.

Biederman, J., Milberger, S., Faraone, S. et al. (1994). Family environmental risk factors for attention deficit hyperactivity disorder: A test of Rutter's indicators of adversity. *Scientific Proceedings of the Annual Meeting of the American Academy of Child and Adolescent Psychiatry*, New York.

Biederman, J., Newcorn, J., & Sprich, S. (1991). Comorbidity of attention deficit hyperactivity disorder with conduct, depressive, anxiety, and other disorders. *Am. J. Psychiatry, 148*, 564–577.

Biederman, J., Thisted, R., Greenhill, L., & Ryan, N. (1995a). Estimation of the association between desipramine and the risk for sudden death in 5- to 14-year-old children. *J. Clin. Psychiatry, 56*, 87–93.

Biederman, J., Wilens, T., Mick, E., Milberger, S., Faraone, S., & Spencer, T. (1995b). Psychoactive substance use disorder in adults with attention deficit hyperactivity disorder. *Am. J. Psychiatry, 152*, 1652–1658.

Birmaher, B., Quintana, H., & Greenhill, L. (1988). Methylphenidate treatment of hyperactive autistic children. *J. Am. Acad. Child Adolesc. Psychiatry, 27*, 248–251.

Borcherding, B. G., Keysor, C. S., Rapoport, J. L., Elia, J., & Amass, J. (1990). Motor/vocal tics and compulsive behaviors on stimulant drugs: Is there a common vulnerability? *Psychiatry Res., 33*, 83–94.

Brown, T. E., & Gammon, G. D. (1992). *ADHD-associated difficulties falling asleep and awakening: Clonidine and methylphenidate treatments.* Presented at the American Academy of Child and Adolescent Psychiatry, Washington, DC.

Brown, R. T., & Sexson, S. B. (1988). A controlled trial of methylphenidate in black adolescents. *Clin. Pediatr. (Phila), 27*, 74–81.

Caine, E., Ludlow, C., Polinsky, R., & Ebert, M. (1984). Provocative drug testing in Tourette's syndrome: D- and L-amphetamine and haloperidol. *J. Am. Acad. Child Psychiatry, 23*, 147–152.

Campbell, M., Green, W. H., & Deutsch, S. I. (1985). *Child and Adolescent Psychopharmacology.* Beverly Hills, CA: Sage Publications.

Casat, C. D., Pleasants, D. Z., Schroeder, D. H., & Parler, D. W. (1989). Bupropion in children with attention deficit disorder. *Psychopharmacol. Bull., 25*, 198–201.

Casat, C. D., Pleasants, D. Z., & Van Wyck Fleet, J. (1987). A double-blind trial of bupropion in children with attention deficit disorder. *Psychopharmacol. Bull., 23*, 120–122.

Chappell, P., Scahill, L., Schultz, R., Riddle, M., & Leckman, J. (1994). Guanfacine treatment of children with ADHD and tics: Preliminary clinical experience (abstract). *Proceedings of the NCDEU 34th Annual Meeting*, p. 29.

Comings, D. E., & Comings, B. G. (1984). Tourette's syndrome and attention deficit disorder with hyperactivity: Are they genetically related? *J. Am. Acad. Child Psychiatry, 23*, 138–146.

Comings, D. E., & Comings, B. G. (1988). Tourette's syndrome and attention deficit disorder. In D. J. Cohen, R. D. Bruun, & J. F. Leckman (Eds.), *Tourette's syndrome and tic disorders: Clinical understanding and treatment* (pp. 119–136). New York: Wiley.

Conners, C. K. (1975). Controlled trial of methylphenidate in preschool children with minimal brain dysfunction. *Int. J. Ment. Health, 4*, 61–74.

Conners, C., Casat, C., Gualtieri, C. et al. (in press). Bupropion hydrochloride in attention deficit disorder with hyperactivity. *J. Am. Acad. Child Adolesc. Psychiatry.*

Coons, H. W., Klorman, R., & Borgstedt, A. D. (1987). Effects of methylphenidate on adolescents with a childhood history of attention deficit disorder: II. Information processing. *J. Am. Acad. Child Adolesc. Psychiatry, 26*, 368–374.

Cox, W. (1982). An indication for the use of imipramine in attention deficit disorder. *Am. J. Psychiatry, 139,* 1059–1060.

Cunningham, C., Siegel, L., & Offord, D. (1991). A dose-response analysis of the effects of methylphenidate on the peer interactions and simulated classroom performance of ADD children with and without conduct problems. *J. Child Psychol. Psychiatry, 32,* 439–452.

Cytryn, L., Gilbert, A., & Eisenberg, L. (1960). The effectiveness of tranquilizing drugs plus supportive psychotherapy in treating behavior disorders of children: A double-blind study of eighty outpatients. *Am. J. Orthopsychiatry, 30,* 113–129.

Demb, H. (1991). Use of Ritalin in the treatment of children with mental retardation. In L. Greenhill & B. Osman (Eds.), *Ritalin: Theory and patient management* (pp. 155–170). New York: Mary Ann Liebert.

Denckla, M. B., Bemporad, J. R., & MacKay, M. C. (1976). Tics following methylphenidate administration: A report of 20 cases. *JAMA, 235,* 1349–1351.

Deutsch, C. K., Matthysse, S., Swanson, J. M., & Farkas, L. G. (1990). Genetic latent structure analysis of dysmorphology in attention deficit disorder. *J. Am. Acad. Child Adolesc. Psychiatry, 29,* 189–194.

Dillon, D. C., Salzman, I. J., & Schulsinger, D. A. (1985). The use of imipramine in Tourette's syndrome and attention deficit disorder: Case report. *J. Clin. Psychiatry, 46,* 348–349.

Donnelly, M., Rapoport, J. L., Potter, W. Z., Oliver, J., Keysor, C. S., & Murphy, D. L. (1989). Fenfluramine and dextroamphetamine treatment of childhood hyperactivity. *Arch. Gen. Psychiatry, 46,* 205–212.

Donnelly, M., Zametkin, A. J., Rapoport, J. L. et al. (1986). Treatment of childhood hyperactivity with desipramine: Plasma drug concentration, cardiovascular effects, plasma and urinary catecholamine levels, and clinical response. *Clin. Pharmacol. Ther., 39,* 72–81.

Douglas, V., Barr, R., Amin, K., O'Neill, M., & Britton, B. (1988). Dosage effects and individual responsivity to methylphenidate in attention deficit disorder. *J. Child Psychol. Psychiatry, 29,* 453–475.

Douglas, V., Barr, R., Desilets, J., & Sherman, E. (1995). Do high doses of stimulants impair flexible thinking in ADHD? *J. Am. Acad. Child Adolesc. Psychiatry, 34,* 877–885.

DuPaul, G., Barkley, R., & McMurray, M. (1994). Response of children with ADHD to methylphenidate: Interaction with internalizing symptoms. *J. Am. Acad. Child Adolesc. Psychiatry, 33,* 894–903.

Elia, J., Borcherding, B. G., Rapoport, J. L., & Keysor, C. S. (1991). Methylphenidate and dextroamphetamine treatments of hyperactivity: Are there true nonresponders? *Psychiatry Res., 36,* 141–155.

Erenberg, G. (1982). Stimulant medication in Tourette's syndrome (letter). *JAMA, 248,* 1062.

Erenberg, G., Cruse, R. P., & Rothner, A. D. (1985). Gilles de la Tourette's syndrome: Effects of stimulant drugs. *Neurology, 35,* 1346–1348.

Evans, S. W., & Pelham, W. E. (1991). Psychostimulant effects on academic and behavioral measures for ADHD junior high school students in a lecture format classroom. *J. Abnorm. Child Psychol., 19,* 537–552.

Famularo, R., & Fenton, T. (1987). The effect of methylphenidate on school grades in children with attention deficit disorder without hyperactivity: A preliminary report. *J. Clin. Psychiatry, 48,* 112–114.

Faraone, S., & Biederman, J. (1994). Is attention deficit hyperactivity disorder familial? *Harv. Rev. Psychiatry, 1,* 271–287.

Faraone, S., Biederman, J., Chen, W. J. et al. (1992). Segregation analysis of attention deficit hyperactivity disorder: Evidence for single gene transmission. *Psychiatry Genet., 2,* 257–275.

Faraone, S. V., Biederman, J., Krifcher Lehman, B. et al. (1993). Intellectual performance and school failure in children with attention deficit hyperactivity disorder and in their siblings. *J. Abnorm. Psychol., 102,* 616–623.

Firestone, P., Davey, J., Goodman, J. T., & Peters, S. (1978). The effects of caffeine and methylphenidate on hyperactive children. *J. Am. Acad. Child Psychiatry, 17,* 445–456.

Gadow, K., Nolan, E., & Sverd, J. (1992). Methylphenidate in hyperactive boys with comorbid tic disorder, II. Short-term behavioral effects in school settings. *J. Am. Acad. Child Adolesc. Psychiatry, 31,* 462–471.

Gadow, K. D., Nolan, E. E., Sverd, J., Sprafkin, J., & Paolicelli, L. (1990). Methylphenidate in agressive-hyperactive boys: I. Effects on peer aggression in public school settings. *J. Am. Acad. Child Adolesc. Psychiatry, 29,* 710–718.

Gadow, K., Sverd, J., Sprafkin, J., Nolan, E., & Ezor, S. (1995). Efficacy of methylphenidate for ADHD in children with tic disorder. *Arch. Gen. Psychiatry, 52*, 444–455.

Gammon, G. D., & Brown, T. E. (1993). Fluoxetine and methylphenidate in combination for treatment of attention deficit disorder and comorbid depressive disorder. *J. Child Adolesc. Psychopharmacol., 3*, 1–10.

Garfinkel, B. D., Webster, C. D., & Sloman, L. (1975). Methylphenidate and caffeine in the treatment of children with minimal brain dysfunction. *Am. J. Psychiatry, 132*, 723–728.

Garfinkel, B. D., Webster, C. D., & Sloman, L. (1981). Responses to methylphenidate and varied doses of caffeine in children with attention deficit disorder. *Am. J. Psychiatry, 26*, 395–401.

Garfinkel, B. D., Wender, P. H., Sloman, L., & O'Neill, I. (1983). Tricyclic antidepressant and methylphenidate treatment of attention deficit disorder in children. *J. Am. Acad. Child Psychiatry, 22*, 343–348.

Gastfriend, D. R., Biederman, J., & Jellinek, M. S. (1985). Desipramine in the treatment of attention deficit disorder in adolescents. *Psychopharmacol. Bull., 21*, 144–145.

Gittelman, R. (1980). Childhood disorders. In D. Klein, F. Quitkin, A. Rifkin, & R. Gittelman (Eds.), *Drug treatment of adult and child psychiatric disorders* (pp. 576–756). Baltimore: Williams & Wilkins.

Gittelman, R., & Mannuzza, S. (1988). Hyperactive boys almost grown up: III. Methylphenidate effects on ultimate height. *Arch. Gen. Psychiatry, 45*, 1131–1134.

Gittelman, R., Mannuzza, S., Shenker, R., & Bonagura, N. (1985). Hyperactive boys almost grown up: I. Psychiatric status. *Arch. Gen. Psychiatry, 42*, 937–947.

Gittelman-Klein, R. (1974). Pilot clinical trial of imipramine in hyperkinetic children. In C. Conners (Ed.), *Clinical use of stimulant drugs in children* (pp. 192–201). The Hague: Excerpta Medica.

Gittelman-Klein, R. (1987). Pharmacotherapy of childhood hyperactivity: An update. In H. Y. Meltzer (Ed.), *Psychopharmacology: The third generation of progress* (pp. 1215–1224). New York: Raven Press.

Gittelman-Klein, R., Klein, D. F., Katz, S., Saraf, K., & Pollack, E. (1976). Comparative effects of methylphenidate and thioridazine in hyperkinetic children. *Arch. Gen. Psychiatry, 33*, 1217–1231.

Golden, G. (1977). The effect of central nervous system stimulants on Tourette syndrome. *Ann. Neurol., 2*, 69–70.

Golden, G. (1982). Stimulant medication in Tourette's syndrome (letter). *JAMA, 248*, 1063.

Goodman, R. (1989). Genetic factors in hyperactivity account for about half of the explainable variance. *Br. Med. J., 298*, 1407–1408.

Goodman, R., & Stevenson, J. (1989a). A twin study of hyperactivity: I. An examination of hyperactivity scores and categories derived from Rutter teacher and parent questionnaires. *J. Child Psychol. Psychiatry, 30*, 671–689.

Goodman, R., & Stevenson, J. (1989b). A twin study of hyperactivity: II. The aetiological role of genes, family relationships and perinatal adversity. *J. Child Psychol. Psychiatry, 30*, 691–709.

Greenberg, L., Yellin, A., Spring, C., & Metcalf, M. (1975). Clinical effects of imipramine and methylphenidate in hyperactive children. *Int. J. Ment. Health, 4*, 144–156.

Greenhill, L. L., Rieder, R. O., Wender, P. H., Buchsbaum, M., & Zhan, T. P. (1973). Lithium carbonate in the treatment of hyperactive children. *Arch. Gen. psychiatry, 28*, 636–640.

Gross, M. (1973). Imipramine in the treatment of minimal brain dysfunction in children. *Psychosomatics, 14*, 283–285.

Gross, M. D. (1975). Caffeine in the treatment of children with minimal brain dysfunction or hyperkinetic syndrome. *Psychosomatics, 16*, 26–27.

Gross, M. (1976). Growth of hyperkinetic children taking methylphenidate, dextroamphetamine, or imipramine/desipramine, *J. Pediatr. 58*, 423–431.

Gualtieri, C. T., & Evans, R. W. (1988). Motor-performance in hyperactive children treated with imipramine. *Percept. Mot. Skills, 66*, 763–769.

Gualtieri, C. T., Ondrusek, M. G., & Finley, C. (1985). Attention deficit disorders in adults. *Clin. Neuropharmacol., 8*, 343–356.

Gunning, B. (1992). *A controlled trial of clonidine in hyperkinetic children*. Thesis, Department of Child and Adolescent Psychiatry, Academic Hospital Rotterdam, Sophia Children's Hospital Rotterdam, the Netherlands.

Harvey, D. H. P., & Marsh, R. W. (1978). The effects of decaffeinated coffee versus whole coffee on hyperactive children. *Dev. Med. Child Neurol., 20,* 81–86.

Hechtman, L. (1992). Long-term outcome in attention-deficit hyperactivity disorder. *Psychiatr. Clin. North Am., 1,* 553–565.

Hinshaw, S., Buhrmester, D., & Heller, T. (1989). Anger control in response to verbal provocation: Effects of stimulant medication for boys with ADHD. *J. Abnorm. Child Psychol., 17,* 393–407.

Hinshaw. S. P., Heller, T., & McHale, J. P. (1992). Covert antisocial behavior in boys with attention-deficit hyperactivity disorder: External validation and effects of methylphenidate. *J. Consult. Clin. Psychol., 60,* 274–281.

Hoge, S. K., & Biederman, J. (1986). A case of Tourette's syndrome with symptoms of attention deficit disorder treated with desipramine. *J. Clin. Psychiatry, 47,* 478–479.

Huessy, H., & Wright, A. (1970). The use of imipramine in children's behavior disorders. *Acta Paedopsychiatr., 37,* 194–199.

Hunt, R. D. (1987). Treatment effects of oral and transdermal clonidine in relation to methylphenidate: An open pilot study in ADDH. *Psychopharmacol. Bull., 23,* 111–114.

Hunt, R. D., Arnsten, A. F. T., & Asbell, M. D. (1995). An open trial of guanfacine in the treatment of attention-deficit hyperactivity disorder. *J. Am. Acad. Child Adolesc. Psychiatry, 34,* 50–54.

Hunt, R. D., Minderaa, R. B., & Cohen, D. J. (1985). Clonidine benefits children with attention deficit disorder and hyperactivity: Report of a double-blind placebo-crossover therapeutic trial. *J. Am. Acad. Child Psychiatry,* 617–629.

Jaffe, S. (1991). Intranasal abuse of prescribed methylphenidate by an alcohol and drug abusing adolescent with ADHD. *J. Am. Acad. Child Adolesc. Psychiatry, 30,* 773–775.

Jankovic, J. (1993). Deprenyl in attention deficit associated with Tourette's syndrome. *Arch. Neurol., 50,* 286–288.

Johnston. C., Pelham, W. E., Hoza, J., & Sturges, J. (1988). Psychostimulant rebound in attention deficit disordered boys. *J. Am. Acad. Child Adolesc. Psychiatry, 27,* 806–810.

Kaplan, S. L., Busner, J., Kupietz, S., Wasserman, E., & Segal, B. (1990). Effects of methylphenidate on adolescents with aggressive conduct disorder and ADDH: A preliminary report. *J. Am. Acad. Child Adolesc. Psychiatry, 29,* 719–723.

Klein, R. G. (1987). Pharmacotherapy of childhood hyperactivity: An update. In H. Y. Meltzer (Ed.), *Psychopharmacology: The third generation of progress* (pp. 1215–1225). New York: Raven Press.

Klorman, R., Brumaghim, J., Fitzpatrick, P., Borgstedt, A., & Strauss, J. (1994). Clinical and cognitive effects of methylphenidate on children with attention deficit disorder as a function of aggression/oppositionality and age. *J. Abnorm. Psychol., 103,* 206–221.

Klorman, R., Brumaghim, J. T., Salzman, L. F. et al. (1988). Effects of methyl-phenidate on attention-deficit hyperactivity disorder with and without aggressive/noncompliant features. *J. Abnorm. Psychol., 97,* 413–422.

Klorman, R., Brumaghim, J. T., Salzman, L. F. et al. (1989). Comparative effects of methylphenidate on attention-deficit hyperactivity disorder with and without aggressive/noncompliant features. *Psychopharmacol. Bull., 25,* 109–113.

Klorman, R., Coons, H. W., & Borgstedt, A. D. (1987). Effects of methylphenidate on adolescents with a childhood history of attention deficit disorder: I. Clinical findings. *J. Am. Acad. Child Adolesc. Psychiatry, 26,* 363–367.

Konkol, R., Fischer, M., & Newby, R. (1990). Double-blind, placebo-controlled stimulant trial in children with Tourette's syndrome and ADHD (abstract). *Ann. Neurol., 28,* 424.

Krakowski, A. J. (1965). Amitriptyline in treatment of hyperkinetic children: A double-blind study. *Psychosomatics, 6,* 355–360.

Kupietz, S. S., & Balka, E. B. (1976). Alterations in the vigilance performance of children receiving amitriptyline and methylphenidate pharmacotherapy. *Psychopharmacology, 50,* 29–33.

Kupietz, S. S., Winsberg, B. G., Richardson, E., Maitinsky, S., & Mendell, N. (1988). Effects of methylphenidate dosage in hyperactive reading-disabled children: I. Behavior and cognitive performance effects. *J. Am. Acad. Child Adolesc. Psychiatry, 27*, 70–77.

Lerer, R. J., & Lerer, M. P. (1977). Responses of adolescents with minimal brain dysfunction to methylphenidate. *J. Learn. Disabil., 10*, 223–228.

Livingston, R., Dykman, R., & Ackerman, P. (1992). Psychiatric comorbidity and response to two doses of methylphenidate in children with attention deficit disorder. *J. Child Adolesc. Psychopharmacol., 2*, 115–122.

Lowe, T. L., Cohen, D. J., & Detlor, J. (1982). Stimulant medications precipitate Tourette's syndrome. *JAMA, 247*, 1168–1169.

MacKay, M. C., Beck, L., & Taylor, R. (1973). Methylphenidate for adolescents with minimal brain dysfunction. *NY State J. Med., 73*, 550–554.

Mannuzza, S., Gittelman-Klein, R., Bonagura, N., Malloy, P., Giampino, T. L., & Addalli, K. A. (1991). Hyperactive boys almost grown up: V. Replication of psychiatric status. *Arch. Gen. Psychiatry, 48*, 77–83.

Mannuzza, S., Klein, R. G., Bessler, A., Malloy, P., & LaPadula, M. (1993). Adult outcome of hyperactive boys: Educational achievement, occupational rank and psychiatric status. *Arch. Gen. Psychiatry, 50*, 565–576.

Manshadi, M., Lippmann, S., O'Daniel, R. G., & Blackman, A. (1983). Alcohol abuse and attention deficit disorder. *J. Clin. Psychiatry, 44*, 379–380.

Mattes, J. A. (1986). Propranolol for adults with temper outbursts and residual attention deficit disorder. *J. Clin. Psychopharmacol., 6*, 299–302.

Mattes, J. A., Boswell, L., & Oliver, H. (1984). Methylphenidate effects on symptoms of attention deficit disorder in adults. *Arch. Gen. Psychiatry, 41*, 1059–1063.

Mattes, J. A., & Gittelman, R. (1983). Growth of hyperactive children on maintenance regimen of methylphenidate. *Arch. Gen. Psychiatry, 40*, 317–321.

Mayes, S., Crites, D., Bixler, E., Humphrey, F., & Mattison, R. (1994). Methylphenidate and ADHD: Influence of age, IQ and neurodevelopmental status. *Dev. Med. Child Neurol., 36*, 1099–1107.

Medical Letter (1990). *32*, 37–40.

Milberger, S., Biederman, J., Sprich-Buckminster, S., Faraone, S., & Krifcher-Lehman, B. (1993). Are perinatal complications relevant to the manifestation of attention-deficit hyperactivity disorder? *Scientific Proceedings of the Annual Meeting of the American Academy of Child and Adolescent Psychiatry*, San Antonio, TX.

Murphy, D., Pelham, W., & Lang, A. (1992). Aggression in boys with ADHD: Methylphenidate effects on naturalistically observed aggression, response to provocation, and social information processing. *J. Abnorm. Child Psychol., 20*, 451–466.

Pataki, C., Carlson, G., Kelly, K., Rapport, M., & Biancaniello, T. (1993). Side effects of methylphenidate and desipramine alone and in combination in children. *Am. J. Psychiatry, 32*, 1065–1072.

Pelham, W. E., Bender, M. E., Caddell, J., Booth, S., & Moorer, S. H. (1985). Methylphenidate and children with attention deficit disorder. *Arch. Gen. Psychiatry, 42*, 948–952.

Pelham, W., Greenslade, K., Vodde-Hamilton, M. et. al. (1990). Relative efficacy of long-acting stimulants on children with attention deficit-hyperactivity disorder: A comparison of standard methylphenidate, sustained-release methylphenidate, sustained-release dextroamphetamine, and pemoline. *Pediatrics, 86*, 226–237.

Pelham, W. E., Walker, J. L., Sturges, J., & Hoza, J. (1989). Comparative effects of methylphenidate on ADD girls and boys. *J. Am. Acad. Child Adolesc. Psychiatry, 28*, 773–776.

Pliszka, S. R. (1989). Effect of anxiety on cognition, behavior, and stimulant response in ADHD. *J. Am. Acad. Child Adolesc. Psychiatry, 28*, 882–887.

Preskorn, S. H., Weller, E. B., Weller, R. A., & Glotzbach, E. (1983). Plasma levels of imipramine and adverse effects in children. *Am. J. Psychiatry, 140*, 1332–1335.

Price, A. R., Leckman, J. F., Pauls, D. L., Cohen, D. J., & Kidd, K. K. (1986). Gilles de la Tourette's syndrome: Tics and central nervous system stimulants in twins and nontwins. *Neurology, 36*, 232–237.

Prince, J., Wilens, T., Spencer, T., Wozniak, J., & Biederman, J. (1994). Clonidine for ADHD related sleep disturbances. *Scientific Proceedings of the 41st Annual Meeting of the American Academy of Child and Adolescent Psychiatry*, New York.

Quinn, P. O., & Rapoport, J. L. (1975). One-year follow-up of hyperactive boys treated with imipramine or methylphenidate. *Am. J. Psychiatry, 132*, 241–245.

Rapoport, J., & Mikkelsen, E. (1978). Antidepressants. In J. Werry (Ed.), *Pediatric psychopharmacology* (pp. 208–233). New York: Brunner/Mazel.

Rapoport, J. L., Quinn, P., Bradbard. G., Riddle, D., & Brooks, E. (1974). Imipramine and methylphenidate treatment of hyperactive boys: A double-blind comparison. *Arch. Gen. Psychiatry, 30*, 789–793.

Rapport, M. D., Carlson, G. A., Kelly, K. L., & Pataki, C. (1993). Methylphenidate and desipramine in hospitalized children: I. Separate and combined effects on cognitive function. *J. Am. Acad. Child Adolesc. Psychiatry, 32*, 333–342.

Rapport, M. D., & DuPaul, G. J. (1986). Hyperactivity and methylphenidate: Rate-dependent effects on attention. *Int. Clin. Psychopharmacol., 1*, 45–52.

Rapport, M. D., DuPaul, G. J., & Kelly, K. L. (1989a). Attention deficit hyperactivity disorder and methylphenidate: The relationship between gross body weight and drug response in children. *Psychopharmacol. Bull., 25*, 285–290.

Rapport, M. D., Jones, J. T., DuPaul, G. J. et al. (1987). Attention deficit disorder and methylphenidate: Group and single-subject analyses of dose effects on attention in clinic and classroom settings. *J. Clin. Child Psychol., 16*, 329–338.

Rapport, M. D., Quinn, S. O., DuPaul, G. J., Quinn, E. P., & Kelly, K. L. (1989b). Attention deficit disorder with hyperactivity and methylphenidate: The effects of dose and mastery level on children's learning performance. *J. Abnorm. Child Psychol., 17*, 669–689.

Rapport, M. D., Stoner, G., DuPaul, G. J., Kelly, K. L., Tucker, S. B., & Shroeler, T. (1988). Attention deficit disorder and methylphenidate: A multilevel analysis of dose-response effects on children's impulsivity across settings. *J. Am. Acad. Child Adolesc. Psychiatry, 27*, 60–69.

Ratey, J., Greenberg, M., & Lindem, K. (1991). Combination of treatments for attention deficit disorders in adults. *J. Nerv. Ment. Dis., 176*, 699–701.

Reimherr, F., Hedges, D., Strong, R., & Wender, P. (1995). *An open-trial of venlafaxine in adult patients with attention deficit hyperactivity disorder*. Presented at the New Clinical Drug Evaluation Unit Program, Orlando, FL.

Reimherr, F. W., Wender, P. H., Wood, D. R., & Ward, M. (1987). An open trial of L-tyrosine in the treatment of attention deficit disorder, residual type. *Am. J. Psychiatry, 144*, 1071–1073.

Riddle, M. A., Hardin, M. T., Cho, S. C., Woolston, J. L., & Leckman, J. F. (1988). Desipramine treatment of boys with attention-deficit hyperactivity disorder and tics: preliminary clinical experience. *J. Am. Acad. Child Adolesc. Psychiatry, 27*, 811–814.

Safer, D. J., & Allen, R. P. (1975). Stimulant drug treatment of hyperactive adolescents. *Dis. Nerv. Syst., 36*, 454–457.

Safer, D. J., Allen, R. P., & Barr, E. (1972). Depression of growth in hyperactive children on stimulant drugs. *N. Engl. J. Med., 287*, 217–220.

Satterfield, J. H., Cantwell, D. P., Schell, A., & Blaschke, T. (1979). Growth of hyperactive children treated with methylphenidate. *Arch. Gen. Psychiatry, 36*, 212–217.

Schachar, R., Hoppe, C., & Schell, A. (1987). Changes in family function and relationships in children who respond to methylphenidate. *J. Am. Acad. Child Adolesc. Psychiatry, 26*, 728–732.

Schleifer, N., Weiss, G., Cohen, N., Elman, M., Cvejic, H., & Kruger, E. (1975). Hyperactivity in preschoolers and the effect of methylphenidate. *Am. J. Orthopsychiatry, 45*, 38–50.

Schnackenberg, R. C. (1973). Caffeine as a substitute for schedule II stimulants in hyperkinetic children. *Am. J. Psychiatry, 130*, 796–798.

Shapiro, A. K., & Shapiro, E. (1981). Do stimulants provoke, cause, or exacerbate tics and Tourette syndrome? *Compr. Psychiatry, 22*, 265–273.

Simeon, J. G., Ferguson, H. B., & Van Wyck Fleet, J. (1986). Bupropion effects in attention deficit and conduct disorders. *Can. J. Psychiatry, 31*, 581–585.

Singer, S., Brown, J., Quaskey, S., Rosenberg, L., Mellits, E., & Denckla, M. (1994). The treatment of attention-deficit hyperactivity disorder in Tourette's syndrome: A double-blind placebo-controlled study with clonidine and desipramine. *Pediatrics, 95*, 74–81.

Solanto, M. V., & Wender, E. H. (1989). Does methylphenidate constrict cognitive functioning? *J. Am. Acad. Child Adolesc. Psychiatry, 28*, 897–902.

Spencer, T., Biederman, J., Kerman, K., Steingard, R., & Wilens, T. (1993a). Desipramine in the treatment of children with tic disorder or Tourette's syndrome and attention deficit hyperactivity disorder. *J. Am. Acad. Child Adolesc. Psychiatry, 32*, 354–360.

Spencer, T., Biederman, J., Wilens, T., Steingard, R., & Geist, D. (1993b). Nortriptyline in the treatment of children with attention deficit hyperactivity disorder and tic disorder or Tourette's syndrome. *J. Am. Acad. Child Adolesc. Psychiatry, 32*, 205–210.

Spencer, T. J., Biederman, J., Steingard, R., & Wilens, T. (1993c). Bupropion exacerbates tics in children with attention deficit hyperactivity disorder and Tourette's disorder. *J. Am. Acad. Child Adolesc. Psychiatry, 32*, 211–214.

Spencer, T., Wilens, T. E., Biederman, J. Faraone, S. V., Ablon, S., & Lapey, K. (1995). A double blind comparison of methylphenidate and placebo in adults with attention deficit hyperactivity disorder. *Arch. Gen. Psychiatry, 52*, 434–443.

Sprague, R. L., Barnes, K. R., & Werry, J. S. (1970). Methylphenidate and thioridazine: Learning, reaction time, activity, and classroom behavior in disturbed children. *Am. J. Orthopsychiatry, 40*, 615–628.

Sprague, R. L., & Sleator, E. K. (1977). Methylphenidate in hyperkinetic children: Differences in dose effects on learning and social behavior. *Science, 198*, 1274–1276.

Steingard, R., Biederman, J., Spencer, T., Wilens, T., & Gonzalez, A. (1993). Comparison of clonidine response in the treatment of attention deficit hyperactivity disorder with and without comorbid tic disorders. *J. Am. Acad. Child Adolesc. Psychiatry, 32*, 350–353.

Strayhorn, J., Rapp, N., Donina, W., & Strain, P. (1988). Randomized trial of methylphenidate for an autistic child. *J. Am. Acad. Child Adolesc. Psychiatry, 27*, 244–247.

Sverd, J., Gadow, K., Nolan, E., Sprafkin, J., & Ezor, S. (1992). Methylphenidate in hyperactive boys with comorbid tic disorder: I. Clinical evaluations. *Adv. Neurol., 58*, 271–282.

Sverd, J., Gadow, K. D., & Paolicelli, L. M. (1989). Methylphenidate treatment of attention-deficit hyperactivity disorder in boys with Tourette's syndrome. *J. Am. Acad. Child Adolesc. Psychiatry, 28*, 574–579.

Swanson, J. M., Granger, D., & Kliewer, W. (1987). Natural social behaviors in hyperactive children: Dose effects of methylphenidate. *J. Consult. Clin. Psychol., 55*, 187–193.

Swanson, J., Kinsbourne, M., Roberts, W., & Zucker, K. (1978). Time-response analysis of the effect of stimulant medication on the learning ability of children referred for hyperactivity. *Pediatrics, 61*, 21–24.

Tannock, R., Ickowicz, A., & Schachar, R. (1995). Differential effects of methylphenidate on working memory in ADHD children with and without comorbid anxiety. *J. Am. Acad. Child Adolesc. Psychiatry, 34*, 886–896.

Tannock, R., Schachar, R. J., Carr, R. P., & Logan, G. D. (1989). Dose-response effects of on academic performance and overt behavior in hyperactive children. *Pediatrics, 84*, 648–657.

Taylor, E., Schachar, R., Thorley, G., Wieselberg, H. M., Everitt, B., & Rutter, M. (1987). Which boys respond to stimulant medication? A controlled trial of methylphenidate in boys with disruptive behaviour. *Psychol. Med., 17*, 121–143.

Trott, G. E., Friese, H. J., Menzel, M., & Nissen, G. (1991). Use of moclobemide in children with attention deficit hyperactivity disorder (Wirksamkeit und vertraglichkeit des selektiven MAO-A-Inhibitors moclobemid bei kindern mit hyperkinetischem syndrom) (both English and German versions). *Jugendpsychiat., 19*, 248–253.

Varley, C. K. (1983). Effects of methylphenidate in adolescents with attention deficit disorder. *J. Am. Acad. Child Psychiatry, 22*, 351–354.

Voelker, S. L., Lachar, D., & Gdowski, L. L. (1983). The personality inventory for children and response to methylphenidate: Preliminary evidence for predictive validity. *J. Pediatr. Psychol., 8*, 161–169.

Watter, N., & Dreyfuss, F. E. (1973). Modifications of hyperkinetic behavior by nortriptyline. *Va. Med. Monthly, 100*, 123–126.

Weintraub, S., Mesulam, M. M., & Kramer, L. (1981). Disturbances in prosody. *Acta. Neurol., 38*, 742–744.

Weiss, G., Hechtman, L., Milroy, T., & Perlman, T. (1985). Psychiatric status of hyperactives as adults: A controlled prospective 15-year follow-up of 63 hyperactive children. *J. Am. Acad. Child Psychiatry, 24*, 211–220.

Weizman, A., Weitz, R., Szekely, G., Tyano, S., & Belmaker, R. (1984). Combination of neuroleptic and stimulant treatment in ADHD. *J. Am. Acad. Child Psychiatry, 23*, 295–298.

Wender, P. H., & Reimherr, F. W. (1990). Bupropion treatment of attention-deficit hyperactivity disorder in adults. *Am. J. Psychiatry, 147*, 1018–1920.

Wender, P. H., Reimherr, F. W., & Wood, D. R. (1981). Attention deficit disorder ("minimal brain dysfunction") in adults. A replication study of diagnosis and drug treatment. *Arch. Gen. Psychiatry, 38*, 449–456.

Wender, P., Reimherr, F., Wood, D., & Ward, M. (1985a). A controlled study of methylphenidate in the treatment of attention deficit disorder, residual type, in adults. *Am. J. Psychiatry, 142*, 547–552.

Wender, P. H., Reimherr, F. W., Wood, D., & Ward, M. (1985b). A controlled study of methylphenidate in the treatment of attention deficit disorder, residual type, in adults. *Am. J. Psychiatry, 142*, 547–552.

Wender, P. H., Wood, D. R., & Reimherr, F. W (1985c). Pharmacological treatment of attention deficit disorder, residual type (ADD, RT, "minimal brain dysfunction," "hyperactivity") in adults. *Psychopharmacol. Bull., 21*, 222–230.

Wender, P. H., Wood, D. R., Reimherr, F. W., & Ward, M. (1983). An open trial of pargyline in the treatment of attention deficit disorder, residual type. *Psychiatry, Res., 9*, 329–36.

Werry. J. (1980). Imipramine and methylphenidate in hyperactive children. *J. Child Psychol. Psychiatry, 21*, 27–35.

Whalen, C. (1989). Does stimulant medication improve the peer status of hyperactive children: *J. Consult. Clin. Psychol., 57*, 545–549.

Whalen, C., Henker, B., & Granger, D. (1990). Social judgement processes in hyperactive boys: Effects of methylphenidate and comparisons with normal peers. *J. Abnorm. Child Psychol., 18*, 297–316.

Whalen, C., Henker, B., Swanson, J., Granger, D., Kliewer, W., & Spencer, J. (1987). Natural social behaviors in hyperactive children: Dose effects of methylphenidate. *J. Consult. Clin. Psychol., 55*, 187–193.

Wilens, T. E., & Biederman, J. (1992). The stimulants. *Psychiatr. Clin. North Am., 15*, 191–222.

Wilens, T. E., Biederman, J., Geist, D. E., Steingard, R., & Spencer, T. (1993). Nortriptyline in the treatment of attention deficit hyperactivity disorder: A chart review of 58 cases. *J. Am. Acad. Child Adolesc. Psychiatry, 32*, 343–349.

Wilens, T. E., Biederman, J. B., Mick, E., & Spencer, T. (1995b). A systematic assessment of tricyclic antidepressants in the treatment of adult attention-deficit hyperactivity disorder. *J. Nerv. Ment. Dis., 183*, 48–50.

Wilens, T., Prince, J., Spencer, T. et al. (1994). Double-blind comparison of desipramine and placebo in adults with attention deficit hyperactivity disorder: Preliminary results. *Scientific Proceedings of the 41st Annual Meeting of the American Academy of Child and Adolescent Psychiatry*, New York.

Wilens, T., Spencer, T., Biederman, J., Wozniak, J., & Connor, D. (1995a). Combined pharmacotherapy: An emerging trend in pediatric psychopharmacology. *J. Am. Acad. Child Adolesc. Psychiatry, 34*, 110–112.

Winsberg, B. G., Bialer, I., Kupietz, S., & Tobias, J. (1972). Effects of imipramine and dextroamphetamine on behavior of neuropsychiatrically impaired children. *Am. J. Psychiatry, 128*, 1425–1431.

Winsberg, B. G., Goldstein, S., & Yepes, L. E. (1975). Imipramine and electrocardiographic abnormalities in hyperactive children. *Am. J. Psychiatry, 132*, 542–547.

Winsberg, B. G., Press, M., Bialer, I., & Kupietz, S. (1974). Dextroamphetamine and methylphenidate in the treatment of hyperactive/aggressive children. *Pediatrics, 53*, 236–241.

Wood, D., Reimherr, F., & Wender, P. (1982). *The use of L-deprenyl in the treatment of attention deficit disorder, residual type.* Presented at the American College of Neuropsychopharmacology, San Juan, PR.

Wood, D. R., Reimherr, F. W., Wender, P. H., & Johnson, G. E. (1976). Diagnosis and treatment of minimal brain dysfunction in adults: A preliminary report. *Arch. Gen. Psychiatry, 33*, 1453–1460.

Wozniak, J., Biederman, J., Kiely, K. et al. (1995). Mania-like symptoms suggestive of childhood onset bipolar disorder in clinically referred children. *J. Am. Acad. Child Adolesc. Psychiatry, 34*, 867–876.

Yepes, L. E., Balka, F. B., Winsberg, B. G., & Bialer, I. (1977). Amitriptyline and methylphenidate treatment of behaviorally disordered children. *J. Child Psychol. Psychiatry, 18*, 39–52.

Zametkin, A. J., & Rapoport, J. L., (1987). Neurobiology of attention deficit disorder with hyperactivity: Where have we come in 50 years? *J. Am. Acad. Child Adolesc. Psychiatry, 26*, 676–686.

Zametkin, A., Rapoport, J. L., Murphy, D. L., Linnoila, M., & Ismond, D. (1985). Treatment of hyperactive children with monoamine oxidase inhibitors: I. Clinical efficacy. *Arch. Gen. Psychiatry, 42*, 962–966.

12

Growth Deficits in ADHD Children Revisited: Evidence for Disorder-Associated Growth Delays?

Thomas J. Spencer, Joseph Biederman, Margaret Harding, Deborah O'Donnell, Stephen V. Faraone, and Timothy E. Wilens
Massachusetts General Hospital and Harvard Medical School

Objective: *To reevaluate the hypothesis that stimulants cause growth deficits in children with attention-deficit hyperactivity disorder (ADHD).* **Method:** *Growth deficits in height and weight were examined in 124 children and adolescents with ADHD and 109 controls, using appropriate correction by age and parental height measures and attending to issues of pubertal stage, treatment, and psychiatric comorbidity.* **Results:** *Small but significant differences in height were identified between ADHD children and controls. However, height deficits were evident in early but not late adolescent ADHD children and were unrelated to use of psychotropic medications. There was no evidence of weight deficits in ADHD children relative to controls, and no relationship between measures of malnutrition and short stature was identified.* **Conclusions:** *ADHD may be associated with temporary deficits in growth in height through mid-adolescence that may normalize by late adolescence. This effect appears to be mediated by ADHD and not its treatment.*

Since the publication of reports by Safer et al. in the early 1970s, the issue of stimulant-associated growth deficits in children with attention-deficit hyperactivity disorder (ADHD) has remained an unresolved area of clinical and scientific debate. The studies by Safer et al. (Safer & Allen, 1973; Safer, Allen, & Barr 1972, 1975) indicated that long-term stimulant treatment in children with ADHD was associated with statistically significant suppression of growth in weight and height (3 cm over 3 years). These initial reports were followed by several similar findings. Loney, Whally, Ponto, and Adney (1981) reported statistically significant stimulant-associated height and weight growth deficits over a 5-year follow-up period in ADHD children and adolescents. Mattes and Gittelman (1983) found a progressive, stimulant-associated deterioration in growth in height (3.3 cm over a 4-year follow-up period) despite frequent summer discontinuation of medication. Similarly, Spencer, Blederman, Wright, and Danon (1992) reported modest methylphenidate-associated growth deficits in weight and height (1.5 cm) in ADHD children treated for more than 1 year.

Reprinted with permission from *J. Am. Acad. Child Adolesc. Psychiatry*, 1996, Vol. 35(11), 1460–1469. Copyright © 1996 by the American Academy of Child and Adolescent Psychiatry.
Preparation of this article was supported by NIMH grant K20 MH01169-01 (Dr. Spencer).

Although these studies showed stastically significant associations between stimulant treatment and growth deficits in ADHD children, uncertainties remain as to their clinical significance and permanence. Statistical significance is not synonymous with clinical significance, and whether growth deficits in ADHD children are temporary or permanent has very different clinical implications. Even if small, permanent deficits in growth in height in ADHD children could raise grave concerns for children, parents, and clinicians, considering the social value of height in our culture. If, on the other hand, growth deficits are temporary, that would reassure affected children and families.

Gittelman and Mannuzza (1988) found that early differences in height prior to puberty in stimulant-treated ADHD children did not compromise ultimate adult height at follow-up into late adolescence and young adulthood. This study suggested that the catchup growth observed in this sample could have been due to drug discontinuation, since children had stimulant treatment discontinued in early adolescence. However, another study by Satterfield Cantwell, Schell, and Blaschke (1979) reported that initial height deficits observed in ADHD children after 1 year of stimulant treatment dissipated by the second year of treatment despite persistent weight deficits and uninterrupted treatment. These findings raised the possibility that height deficits in ADHD children may be temporary developmental deviations, not complications of stimulant treatment. The testing of such a hypothesis requires examining growth in younger and older ADHD children. Since most studies of growth deficits in ADHD children have evaluated samples of prepubertal children, there is a need to reevaluate growth deficits in ADHD children, attending to these developmental issues.

However, studies of growth deficits in children of different ages raise complex methodological issues. Since height does not vary linearly with age, the wider the age range of the sample being studied the more vulnerable are direct comparisons of averaged height measurements to produce spurious results (Chinchilli McEnery, & Chan, 1990). Similar problems emerge when using percentiles from standardized growth charts. This approach is not free of distortions because the averaging of percentiles overemphasizes small differences near the mean at the expense of similar differences at the extremes. For instance, a five percentile difference in 11-year-old boys equates to a 0.83-cm height difference between the 53rd percentile and 48th percentiles, but the same percentile difference yields a 5.2-cm difference between the 6th percentile and the 1st percentile. One method of dealing with these issues is to use Z scores for analysis of height parameters. This method corrects for age, avoids mathematical distortions, and is sensitive to height changes at all levels of height. Although the use of Z scores to standardize height data is universally accepted as the most valid method for assessing height variability in pediatric samples (Chinchilli et al., 1990), it has never before been used in assessing height deficits in ADHD research.

Height deficits in ADHD children could be related to parental stature and not to ADHD or its treatment. Although genetic influences are known to be important contributors to height (Tanner, 1986), the effect of parental height has not been examined in previous studies of ADHD-associated growth deficits. Another important factor in assessing height in ADHD children is pubertal development. Although the timing of the adolescent growth spurt does not closely correspond to the stage of sexual maturity, pubertal stages may provide an additional index of maturity that may be informative when evaluating adolescent growth delays. Thus, a comprehensive evaluation of height deficits in ADHD children requires the assessment of the contribution of parental height to the child's height as well as pubertal staging.

Another important factor in evaluating growth deficits associated with ADHD is the known clinical and possible etiological heterogeneity of the disorder. ADHD shows a high level of comorbidity with conduct, mood, and anxiety disorders. Since these comorbid disorders might also affect growth (Biederman, Newcorn, & Sprich, 1991; Kutcher et al., 1991; Pine, Cohen, & Brook 1995; Puig-Antich et al., 1981; Uhde, 1994), it remains to be determined whether growth deficits in ADHD children are due to co-occurring disorders. Since familial ADHD may be a more biological subtype (Faraone & Biederman, 1994), it may have a larger impact on growth and maturation in ADHD than other forms of the disorder. Thus, a reassessment of growth deficits in ADHD children requires attention to issues of comorbidity and familiality.

The purpose of this report is the systematic reevaluation of growth deficits and ADHD, with attention to issues of dysmaturity, therapeutics, comorbidity, and familiality, using developmentally sensitive methodology. Based on the literature, we expected to find growth deficits in height and weight in ADHD children compared with controls. To account for these growth deficits, we examined the following competing hypotheses: (1) if deficits in height are due to deficits in weight, then we would expect to find an association between the two; (2) if growth deficits are due to pharmacological treatment, then they should be more marked in children who were pharmacologically treated; (3) if growth deficits are due to comorbid psychopathology, then these deficits will be more marked in subjects with comorbid disorders; (4) if growth deficits are limited to a genetic subtype of ADHD, then they should be limited to familial cases; and (5) if growth deficits are due to developmental "dysmaturity," then growth deficits will be observable during early but not late puberty.

METHOD

As reported earlier, this was the 4-year follow-up of an ongoing longitudinal study of ADHD children (Biederman et al., 1996). The sample consisted of 245 children (132 ADHD and 113 normal controls) representing 94.6% of the 140 ADHD children and 94% of the 120 normal controls seen at baseline (Biederman et al., 1996). Of these 245 children, we had growth measures on 95% ($n = 233$; 124 ADHD and 109 normal controls). There were no significant differences between subjects successfully followed up and those lost to follow-up on each of the measures used in this study (all p values $> .05$). Children were chosen from psychiatric and nonpsychiatric settings (Biederman et al., 1992). Within each setting, ADHD-diagnosed children and non-ADHD normal controls were included.

Eligible subjects were Caucasian, non-Hispanic, male children and adolescents, 6 to 17 years of age, with an IQ greater than 80. We excluded adopted and stepchildren, children with major sensorimotor handicaps (paralysis, deafness, blindness), and children or parents with mental retardation or very severe and unstable psychopathology (Psychosis, autism, suicidality). Also, subjects from the lowest socioeconomic class were excluded to avoid the confounds of extreme social adversity (Hollingshead, 1975).

Diagnostic Assessments

All diagnostic assessments were made using *DSM-III-R*-based structured interviews. Subjects were evaluated by raters who were blind to their clinical status and ascertainment site. ADHD and control children were assessed at baseline and reassessed at 1- and 4-year follow-up with identical assessment methodology. All follow-up assessments were made blind to prior assessments of the same subjects.

Psychiatric assessments of children were made using the Schedule for Affective Disorders and Schizophrenia for School-Age Children-Epidemiologic version (Orvaschel, 1985) and were based on independent interviews with the mothers and direct interviews of probands and siblings, except for children younger than 12 years, who were not directly interviewed. Diagnoses were considered positive if, based on the interview results, *DSM-III-R* criteria were unequivocally met. For every diagnosis, information was gathered regarding the associated level of impairment (mild, moderate, or severe), ages at onset and offset of symptoms, number of episodes, and treatment history. We computed κ coefficients of agreement by having three experienced, board-certified child and adult psychiatrists diagnose subjects from audiotaped interviews made by the assessment staff. Based on 173 interviews, the median κ was .86.

A sign-off committee of board-certified child and adult psychiatrists chaired by the Program Director (J.B.) resolved all diagnostic uncertainties. As suggested by others (Gershon et al., 1982; Weissman et al., 1984), we diagnosed major depression only if the depressive episode was associated with marked impairment. Since the anxiety disorders comprise many syndromes with a wide range of severity, we used two or more anxiety disorders to indicate the presence of a clinically meaningful anxiety syndrome and refer to this as "multiple anxiety disorders" as we have elsewhere (Biederman et al., 1990).

Assessments of Growth and Pubertal Development

Growth measures were obtained only at the 4-year follow-up assessment. All probands and relatives were weighed and measured using the same scale. Measurements were obtained with the subjects lightly clothed but without shoes. We used a Physician's Beam Scale (Detecto, Webb City, MO), which is a high-calibration scale with a height rod for precise measurement of height. Subjects were erect, with height examined at the vertex. Growth measurements were plotted on National Center for Health Statistics growth tables (Hamill, Drizd, Johnson, Reed, & Roche, 1979). These growth charts are sex-specific and standardized. Thus, they permit comparisons of growth deficit findings to normal population data (Hamill et al., 1979).

To assess pubertal staging, children of age 12 to 18 years were asked questions about pubertal development. Questions included presence or absence of a full beard, axillary hair, and pubertal hair as well as the age attainment of each stage. Based on these questions estimates of Tanner stages were developed as follows: attainment of pubertal hair, Tanner stage 2 to 3; attainment of axillary hair, Tanner stage 3 to 4; attainment of facial hair, Tanner stage 4 to 5.

Based on growth measurements, the following height and weight indices were made: (1) Absolute height was the uncorrected height in centimeters. (2) Age-corrected height (Abitbol, Foreman, Strife, & McEnery, 1989; Chinchilli et al., 1990) values were converted to a height "Z score," defined as the difference of an individual height from the mean height, for children of the same age and sex, divided by the standard deviation of height for that subgroup. Height Z scores were calculated in four steps. First, the mean height, for the age of the child, was obtained from the growth table as the height at the 50th percentile for that age group; second, the difference between the child's actual height and the mean height for children of the same age and sex was calculated; third, the standard deviation of height for age was calculated as the height difference between the 90th and 10th cumulative frequency percentiles at the child's age on the growth table, divided by a constant (2.56); finally, the difference between the child's actual height and the mean height was then divided by the standard deviation of height for that age. (3) We calculated parent- and age-corrected height. First we calculated height Z scores for parents, using the methodology described above. We then examined the relationship of the child's height to the parents' height by regression analysis in the controls. The estimated regression equation was used to determine the child's predicted height from the parents' heights. The difference between the child's actual height (Z score) and the child's predicted height based on parental height (Z score) was defined as the parent- and age-corrected height. (4) Absolute weight was the uncorrected weight in kilograms. (5) Age- and height-corrected weight index (Polito, Oporto, Totino, La Manna, & Toro, 1986; Spencer et al., 1992) was computed by examining the "weight as percentage of expected (or standard) weight for height" consistent with studies of malnutrition in Third World countries (Anderson, 1979; McLaren & Read, 1975; Waterlow, 1972, 1973, 1974). The expected weight for height was derived from standard growth tables (Hamill, Drizd, Johnson, Reed, & Roche, 1979). The 50th percentile curve in the height growth chart was compared to the child's height. The height-age is the age at which the child's height is the same as the value on the 50th percentile curve on the height growth chart. The expected weight for height is the 50th percentile weight on the weight growth chart for the height age just derived. Studies have suggested that if malnutrition were to affect height growth, this would not be manifested until the malnutrition is severe, as expressed in a ratio of weight to height-corrected expected weight of less than 85% (grade 1 malnutrition) (Anderson, 1979; Waterlow, 1972). In contrast, a weight index of 115% would be overweight and 120% obese.

Data Analysis

Categorical data were analyzed by χ^2 analysis of Fisher's Exact Test. Parametric testing of continuous data were analyzed by one-way analysis of variance, nonparametric data by the rank-sum test. Binary and ordinal dependent variables were analyzed using standard and ordinal logistic regressions. Survival analysis was performed by the Kaplan-Meier method. Associations between continuous variables were examined using the Pearson Correlation Coefficient. All analyses were two-tailed, and statistical significance was defined at the 5% level.

RESULTS

The control sample was slightly older and had a somewhat higher socioeconomic status (SES) than the ADHD sample (Table 1). Therefore, all comparisons were statistically corrected for age and SES. There were no statistically significant differences between the ADHD and control samples in the percentage of intact families. As shown in Table 1, there were no differences between ADHD and control probands in the age of onset of estimated Tanner stages. Although a greater proportion of ADHD probands than controls were at the lower Tanner stages ($p = .006$), this was accounted for by differences in age between ADHD and control children ($p < .001$).

Table 1 shows that 89% of ADHD children had received pharmacological treatment at some time in their lives ($n = 110$), and 70% in the previous 2 years ($n = 83$). Stimulant doses were converted to methylphenidate equivalents (twice the dextroamphetamine dose; one half of the pemoline dose). Over the preceding 2 years, 45% ($n = 53$) had been treated with stimulants at an average daily dose of methylphenidate (or its equivalent) of 38 ± 24 mg/day (5 to 120) and of those, 71% had been treated continuously.

TABLE 1
Demographics of ADHD Probands, Normal Controls, and Their Parents

	ADHD ($n = 124$)		Controls ($n = 109$)		Significance (p)
Age, yr: mean (*SD*)					
Children	14.5*	(3.0)	15.5	(3.7)	.03
Parents	40.7*	(6.2)	41.9	(5.7)	.03
SES: mean (*SD*)	1.9**	(1.0)	1.50	(0.7)	.005
Estimated Tanner stages: age of					
onset, yr: mean (*SD*)					
Stage 2–3	11.9	(0.9)	12	(1.2)	NS
Stage 3–4	13.1	(1.4)	13.3	(1.1)	NS
Stage 4–5	15.5	(1.2)	15.4	(1.1)	NS
Pharmacotherapy: No. (%)					
Lifetime history	110	(89)	NA		NA
Last 2 yr (any medication)	83	(70)	NA		NA
Last 2 yr (stimulant)	53	(45)	NA		NA

Note: ADHD = attention-deficit hyperactivity disorder; SES = socioeconomic status; NS = not significant: NA = not applicable.
* $p < .05$; ** $p < .01$ (ADHD vs. controls).

Growth in Height

Although on an average, ADHD children were 3 cm shorter than controls, this difference failed to reach statistical significance (Table 2). However, when heights were converted to age-specific Z scores, the difference in height between ADHD children and controls was found to be statistically significant (0.21 versus 0.47; $p = .03$). Similar results were obtained after correcting by parental height (-0.24 versus 0.01; $p = .03$). These findings were accounted for by shorter stature in the adolescent ADHD group but not in the postadolescent group. In contrast, there were no meaningful differences in height between parents of ADHD and control children. Children's heights were highly correlated with parental heights (r values $= .28$ to $.38$; p values $<.001$) in both ADHD and control children, with the exception of ADHD children's and mothers' heights, which were only modestly correlated ($r = .17$; $p = .03$). Findings in ADHD and control probands were further examined for extremes of stature defined as being at least two standard deviations below the mean for controls. This analysis revealed that there were more ADHD probands who were very short compared with controls (12/124 versus 1/109, $\chi^2 = 7.6$, $p = 08$; 12/118 versus 2/105, $\chi^2 = 5.7$, $p = .02$; for ADHD and controls, age-corrected and age- and parent-corrected heights, respectively).

Growth in Weight

Although on average, ADHD children weighted 4 kg less than controls, this difference failed to reach statistical significance (58 ± 17 versus 62 ± 19 kg; $F = 2$, $p =$ not significant [NS]). Even after correcting for height and age, both ADHD probands and controls were found to have more than adequate body mass (age- and height-corrected weight indices: 109 ± 15 versus 111 ± 19; $F = 0.5$, $p = $ NS; ADHD and controls, respectively; as described earlier under "Method," an index of 100 indicates that a subject's weight is the average expected weight for height and age; an index greater than 100 indicates greater than the average expected weight). No significant effect of age or pubertal stage on the age- and height-corrected weight index could be identified.

Impact of Psychopharmacological Treatment on Growth

No meaningful differences in height measures were detected between psychopharmacologically treated (either lifetime or currently) and untreated ADHD subjects (Table 3). No associations were found between height measures with either dose or duration of stimulant treatment. Although ADHD probands with a lifetime history of psychopharmacological treatment had a lower absolute weight than those without such a history, these subjects were not thin. When weight was corrected for age and height, treated ADHD probands were found to have more than adequate body mass (age- and height-corrected weight index $= 108$). No meaningful effects of recent stimulant treatment on weight were detected when weight was corrected for age and height (Table 3).

Associations between Height and Weight

There was no meaningful association between weight and height (r values $= -.15$ to $.11$; NS). Using the 85% cutoff for severe malnutrition, there was only one ADHD child and two controls who had an abnormal age- and height-corrected weight index. Despite being "malnourished," all three children were of average height. In addition, analysis of the weights of children who were very short as defined above (two standard deviations below the mean of controls) failed to reveal that these children had an abnormal age- and height-corrected weight index (<85); all had more than adequate body mass (average weight indices >110).

TABLE 2
Height in Children and Parents

Height	ADHD (n = 124)						Controls (n = 109)					
	Height (cm)		Age-Corrected Height (Z Score)		Parent- & Age-Corrected Height (Z Score)		Height (cm)		Age-Corrected Height (Z Score)		Parent- & Age-Corrected Height (Z Score)	
	Mean	SD	Mean	SD	Mean	SD	Mean	SD	Mean	SD	Mean	SD
All probands	166	15	0.21*	1.1	−0.24*	1.1	169	15	0.47	0.86	0.01	0.74
Children (<12 yr)	146	6	0.35	0.8	−0.14	0.8	147	7	0.53	0.9	0.06	0.8
Adolescent (12–18 yr)	167*	13	0.15*	1.1	−0.24*	1.1	174	10	0.47	0.8	0.01	0.7
Young Adults (>18 yr)	180	8	0.42	1.1	−0.03	0.8	179	6	0.42	0.9	−0.02	0.7
Mothers	165	7	0.18	1.3	NA		164	6	0.09	1.1	NA	
Fathers	179	7	0.30	1.0	NA		179	7	0.32	1.0	NA	

Note: ADHD (child n = 17, adolescent n = 82, young adult n = 25; control (child n = 25, adolescent n = 46, young adult n = 38). ADHD = attention-deficit hyperactivity disorder; NA = not applicable.

* $p < .05$; (ADHD vs. controls; statistical analysis controlled for age and socioeconomic status by logistic regression).

TABLE 3
Growth in ADHD Probands Stratified by Psychopharmacological Treatment History

Growth Variable	Lifetime History (Any Medication)				Last 2 Years (Any Medication)				Last 2 Years (Stimulant)			
	Yes (n = 110)		No (n = 13)		Yes (n = 83)		No (n = 36)		Yes (n = 53)		No (n = 66)	
	Mean	SD	Mean	SD	Mean	SD	Mean	SD	Mean	SD	Mean	SD
Height												
Absolute (cm)	165	14	173	15	163	14	170	14	160	14	169	13
Age-corrected (Z score)	0.15	1.1	0.64	0.96	0.14	1.0	0.37	1.2	0.23	0.96	0.17	1.2
Parent- and age-corrected (Z score)	−0.29	1.0	0.18	1.0	−0.35	1.0	0.00	1.1	−0.25	0.83	−0.23	1.2
Weight												
Absolute (kg)	57**	16	72	26	56	16	64	19	54	16	62	17
Age- and height-corrected weight index	108	15	115	18	109	15	109	14	110	15	108	15

** $p < .01$.

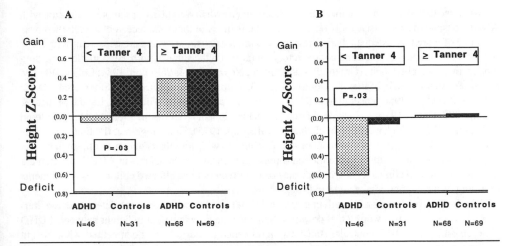

Figure 1. Height of probands by maturational stage: age-corrected height (A); parent- and age-corrected height (B). ADHD = attention-deficit hyperactivity disorder.

Impact of Comorbidity and Familiality on Growth

With one exception, height and maturational findings were not affected by comorbidity with major depression, anxiety, or conduct disorder or family history of ADHD; the exception was that ADHD children with a history of major depression were shorter than ADHD children without depression as measured by age-corrected height (0.38 versus −0.01; $p = .05$).

Impact of Development on Growth

Examination of developmental data revealed differences in age-corrected heights between ADHD probands and controls in early pubertal ADHD children (Tanner 2 to 3 or lower) but not in late pubertal ADHD children (Tanner 3 to 4 and above; $p = .03$) (Fig. 1A). Similarly, there were meaningful differences in age- and parent-corrected heights between ADHD probands and controls in early pubertal ADHD children (Tanner 2 to 3 or lower) but not in late pubertal ADHD children (Tanner 3 to 4 and above; $p = .03$) (Fig. 1B). Although a significantly greater proportion of early pubertal children (Tanner 2 to 3 or lower) had been medicated over the previous 2 years (85% versus 61%; $p = .005$), mostly with stimulants (62% versus 34%; $p = .005$), these differences in height were not accounted for by medication status. Neither recent nor past history of medication use nor the use of stimulants significantly affected height measures in either early or late pubertal ADHD children.

DISCUSSION

In a comprehensive reevaluation of growth deficits in a large sample of referred children and adolescents with ADHD, we found modest height deficits in ADHD patients compared with controls. However, these height deficits were evident only in early adolescence and were unrelated to weight deficits or stimulant treatment. In contrast, we found no evidence of delayed pubertal development, weight deficits, or relationship between measures of malnutrition and short stature. These findings are most consistent with the hypothesis that ADHD may be associated with a delayed tempo of growth in height and not with arrested growth.

We failed to find evidence for meaningful effects on growth in weight in our sample of children with ADHD, despite the aggressive daily doses of stimulants many of them had received. In fact, there was evidence of more than adequate body mass in our sample. Thus, our results are consistent with some but not all of the rather mixed and contradictory literature on the subject, with some studies reporting modest mean weight deficits (Greenhill, Puig-Antich, Novacenko, & Solomon, 1984; Loney, Whaley, Ponto, & Adney, 1981; Mattes & Gittelman, 1983; Quinn & Rapoport, 1975; Safer et al., 1972; Satterfield et al., 1979; Spencer et al., 1992) and others reporting none (Gittelman, Landa, Mattes, & Klein, 1988; Gross, 1976; Kalachnik, Sprague, Sleator, Cohen, & Ullmann, 1982; McNutt, Boilequ, & Cohen, 1977; Millichap, 1978; Millichap & Millichap, 1975). Taken together, the findings of this and other studies suggest that treatment of ADHD children with stimulants may result in small effects in growth in weight in some children. Even if present, modest weight deficits in ADHD children are generally of limited clinical concern since they can be offset in most affected children by adjustments in timing of medication intake and food supplementation.

Our findings on deficits in growth in height in ADHD children are largely consistent with the literature. However, it is noteworthy that despite a 3-cm average growth deficit in height between ADHD children and non-ADHD controls, statistical significance could only be documented when height findings were converted to Z scores to correct for age and not when absolute heights were compared. Moreover, statistical significance in height between ADHD children and non-ADHD controls could also be documented when height findings were corrected by parental height. This was the case despite the absence of meaningful differences in height between parents of ADHD children and parents of control children and despite significant associations between children's and their parents' heights.

Although the use of Z scores to assess height deficits is universally accepted as the most valid method for assessing height variability in pediatric samples (Chinchilli et al. 1990), it has not been previously used in studies of growth deficits in children with ADHD. Instead, previous ADHD growth studies have used more than eight different methods of assessing growth, including direct comparisons of averaged absolute height or percentiles from standardized growth charts (Spencer et al., 1992), methods subject to artifactual distortion and low sensitivity (Chinchilli et al., 1990). Sensitivity is a critical issue in evaluating growth deficits because mean height deficits in our study as well as in previous studies have been generally small. Thus, some methods of assessing growth would have low power to find differences should they exist (type II error). The greater sensitivity of Z scores was evident in our sample: the effect size (mean difference/standard deviation) for absolute height was 20%, whereas it was 28% for Z scores (Table 2). Since Z scores are more sensitive and less vulnerable to distortions in a sample with a wide range of ages such as ours, they may more accurately reflect ADHD-associated height deficits than absolute height.

Although for the most part height deficits were small, 10% of our ADHD children (versus 1% of the controls) were more than two standard deviations (i.e., approximately 14 cm in 15-year-old males) below that of the average height of the non-ADHD controls. This finding indicates that a small minority of ADHD children may have marked delays in growth in height. Since it is not known whether this subgroup of ADHD children will outgrow these deficits or whether they may be at high risk for short stature, it may be prudent to be vigilant and consider appropriate clinical evaluation for such children.

As implied by average Z scores greater than 0, both controls and ADHD probands were slightly taller than the population norms. This finding is consistent with a cohort effects in which each generation tends to be taller than its predecessor (Goldstein, 1978). If confirmed, this would cast doubt on the informativeness of results from studies based solely on comparisons of heights in treated ADHD children to population norms.

A key finding in our study was that height deficits were evident in younger but not in older ADHD children. Similar developmental variability in height deficits has been reported by other investigators. Gross (1976) failed to identify height deficits in adolescents despite earlier decreases in height percentiles. Gittelman et al. and Hechtman et al. showed that ultimate height in grownup ADHD children was not compromised despite preadolescent height deficits (Gittelman and Mannuzza, 1988; Hechtman, Weiss, & Perlman, 1984). Taken together, these findings raise the possibility that ADHD may be associated with a delayed tempo of growth in height and not with permanent stunting of growth.

Support for this intriguing hypothesis can be derived from our failing to find an association between height deficits and stimulant treatment. Despite comprehensive efforts to examine the impact on growth in height of various drug classes (stimulant or other), various dose regimens (robust or mild), and duration of treatment, we were unable to identify meaningful associations between height deficits and treatment variables in our sample.

These results are consistent with some of the mixed literature on the subject; of the six previous studies that compared height deficits in treated and untreated ADHD children, three studies (Safer, 1973; Safer et al., 1972, 1975) reported stimulant-associated height deficits in ADHD children and three did not (Kalachnik et al., 1982; McNutt et al., 1977; Quinn and Rapoport, 1975). Moreover, those studies that reported stimulant-associated height deficits evaluated preadolescent samples and could not fully assess normalization of height over time. Similarly, although three out of four studies that evaluated the impact of drug holidays in ADHD children found that continued stimulant treatment was associated with height suppression and that rebound growth occurred during drug holidays (Gittelman et al., 1988; Safer & Allen, 1973; Safer et al., 1975; Satterfeld et al., 1979), it remains unclear whether increased growth in height during drug holidays reflects spontaneous normalization of growth in height over time (Dickinson et al., 1979; Gross, 1976; Satterfield et al., 1979).

Also consistent with this hypothesis is our finding of no association between weight loss and height deficits. Although an early report linked stimulant-associated weight loss with height loss (Safer et al., 1972), more recent reports have failed to replicate this finding (Dickinson et al., 1979; Gittelman et al., 1988; Safer & Allen, 1973; Satterfield et al., 1979; Spencer et al., 1992). These findings add to the growing consensus that stimulant-associated weight deficits are not implicated in ADHD-associated height deficits and support the hypothesis that developmental growth in height deficits may be operant in ADHD.

The hypothesis that ADHD may be associated with delays in growth in height is consistent with a dysmaturity hypothesis of ADHD that proposes that the pathological manifestations of ADHD in some children may represent developmental lags that will be eventually outgrown (Cantwell, 1985). Consistent with this hypothesis is the commonly observed decline in some children of core behavioral symptoms of the disorder over time, predominantly those of motoric hyperactivity. Thus, it is possible that developmental delays in some ADHD children include not only the core behavioral and cognitive signs and symptoms of the disorder but perhaps physical growth as well. If confirmed, these findings would suggest that previously reported stimulant-associated height deficits in ADHD children may be temporary pre- and early pubertal manifestations of ADHD itself and not complications of its treatment.

Clinically, these findings do not support the common practice of drug holidays in children without evidence of growth deficits. However, until more is known, it seems prudent to provide drug holidays or alternative treatment for children in whom stimulant-associated growth deficits are suspected. This recommendation should be carefully weighed against the risk of exacerbation of symptoms due to drug discontinuation.

In our sample, the largest effects on growth in height in ADHD children were observed in those with comorbid major depression. This is a novel finding not previously reported in ADHD research. An association has been previously reported between childhood anxiety disorders and later short stature (Pine et al., 1995). Considering the frequent comorbidity between anxiety and depressive disorders, similar findings could also be observed in depressed children. However, in our study comorbidity with anxiety disorders was not associated with reductions in growth in height. While the clinical significance of these preliminary findings remains uncertain, they highlight the importance of taking into account comorbidity with depression and anxiety in future studies examining growth in ADHD children.

The apparent slower tempo of growth in height observed in our sample was not associated with pubertal development. The ages of onset of Tanner stages were equivalent between the groups (Table 1) and consistent with the published age of onset of Tanner stages in the general population (12 years for initial public hair; approximately 13 years 5 for axillary hair and approximately 14.5 years for beard) (Marshall & Tanner, 1986; Tanner & Davies, 1985). A similar dissociation between Tanner stages and timing of pubertal growth in height has been well documented in males in the general population (Marshall & Tanner, 1986). Although the reasons for the observed dissociation between growth in height and pubertal development remain unknown and require further study, our findings suggest that height delays in ADHD children are not accounted for by pubertal delays.

The findings reported here should be evaluated against the methodological limitations. It would have been optimal to have the same individual perform all the measurements; however, this was not practical given the number of subjects involved. As this study was naturalistic and cross-sectional, there were chance differences in age and SES. Although growth measures were not found to be significantly correlated with age or SES, all analyses corrected by age and SES. Pubertal stages were based on probands' self-report and not on direct physical examination. However, studies have shown that self-assessed pubertal stages may be highly concordant with physican-assessed pubertal staging (Duke, Litt, & Grass 1980). Since growth parameters were assessed at the follow-up assessment only, our cross-sectional findings permit only weak developmental inferences. However, we could compare growth parameters in younger and older subjects, permitting the generation of initial developmental hypotheses to be tested in future longitudinal studies.

Despite these limitations, our findings confirm previous reports showing small but statistically significant deficits in growth in height in ADHD children in general and in those with comorbid major depression in particular compared with non-ADHD healthy children. In addition, our findings also show that height deficits in ADHD children may not be associated with delayed pubertal development and may normalize in late adolescence regardless of medication use. These findings are consistent with the hypothesis that ADHD may be associated with a temporary delay in the tempo of growth in height. If confirmed, these findings can be reassuring to patients and families and could provide new insights into the pathophysiology of ADHD.

REFERENCES

Abitbol, C., Foreman, J. W., Strife, C. F., & McEnery, P. T. (1989). Quantification of growth deficits in children with renal diseases. *Semin Nephrol*, *9*, 31–36.

Anderson, M. A. (1979). Comparison of anthropometric measures of nutritional status in preschool children in five developing countries. *Am. J. Clin. Nutr.*, *32*, 2339–2345.

Biederman, J., Faraone, S. V., Keenan, K. et al. (1992). Further evidence for family-genetic risk factors in attention deficit hyperactivity disorder (ADHD): Patterns of comorbidity in probands and relatives in psychiatrically and pediatrically referred samples. *Arch. Gen. Psychiatry*, *49*, 728–738.

Biederman, J., Faraone, S., Milberger, S. et al. (1996). A prospective four-year follow-up study of attention deficit hyperactivity and related disorders. *Arch. Gen. Psychiatry*, *53*, 437–446.

Biederman, J., Newcorn, J., & Sprich, S. (1991). Comorbidity of attention deficit hyperactivity disorder with conduct, depressive, anxiety, and other disorders. *Am. J. Psychiatry*, *148*, 564–577.

Biederman, J., Rosenbaum, J. F., Hirshfeld, D. R. et al. (1990). Psychiatric correlates of behavioral inhibition in young children of parents with and without psychiatric disorders. *Arch. Gen. Psychiatry*, *47*, 21–26.

Cantwell, D. P. (1985). Hyperactive children have grown up: What have we learned about what happens to them? *Arch. Gen. Psychiatry*, *42*, 1026–1028.

Chinchilli, V. M., McEnery, P. T., & Chan, J. C. M. (1990). Statistical methods and determination of sample size in the growth failure in children with renal diseases study. *J. Pediatr*, *116*, S32–S36.

Dickinson, L. C., Lee, J., Ringdahl, I. C., Schedewie, H. K., Kilgore, B. S., & Elders, M. J. (1979). Impaired growth in hyperkinetic children receiving pemoline. *Pediatrics*, *94*, 538–541.

Duke, P., Litt, I., & Gross, R. (1980). Adolescents' self-assessment of sexual maturation. *Pediatrics*, *66*, 918–920.

Faraone, S., & Biederman, J. (1994). Genetics of attention-deficit hyperactivity disorder. *Child Adolesc. Psychiatr. Clin. North. Am.*, *3*, 285–302.

Gershon, E. S., Hamovit, J., Guroff, J. J. et al. (1982). A family study of schizoaffective, bipolar I, bipolar II, unipolar and normal control probands. *Arch. Gen. Psychiatry*, *39*, 1157–1167.

Gittelman, R., Landa, B., Mattes, J., & Klein, D. (1988). Methylphenidate and growth in hyperactive children: A controlled withdrawal study. *Arch. Gen. Psychiatry*, *45*, 1127–1130.

Gittelman, R., & Mannuzza, S. (1988). Hyperactive boys almost grown up III: Methylphenidate effects on ultimate height. *Arch. Gen. Psychiatry*, *45*, 1131–1134.

Goldstein, H. (1978). Sampling for growth studies. In F. Falkner & J. Tanner (Eds.), *Human Growth* (pp. 183–208). New York: Plenum Press.

Greenhill, L. L., Puig-Antich, J., Novacenko, M. A., & Solomon, M. (1984). Prolactin, growth hormone and growth responses in boys with attention deficit disorder and hyperactivity treated with methylphenidate. *J. Am. Acad. Child Psychiatry 23*, 58–67.

Gross, M. (1976). Growth of hyperkinetic children taking methylphenidate, dextroamphetamine, or imipramine/desipramine. *J. Pediatr*, *58*, 423–431.

Hamill, P. V. V., Drizd, T. A., Johnson, C. L., Reed, R., & Roche, A. (1979). Physical growth: National Center for Health Statistics percentiles. *Am. J. Clin. Nutr.*, *32*, 607–629.

Hechtman, L., Weiss, G., & Perlman, T. (1984). Young adult outcome of hyperactive children who received long-term stimulant treatment. *J. Am. Acad. Child Psychiatry*, *23*, 261–269.

Hollingshead, A. B. (1975). *Four factor index of social status*. New Haven, CT: Yale University Department of Sociology.

Kalachnik, J. E., Sprague, R. L., Sleator E. K., Cohen M. N., & Ullmann, R. K. (1982). Effect of methylphenidate hydrochloride on stature of hyperactive children. *Dev. Med. Child Neurol.*, *70*, 987–992.

Kutcher, S., Malkin, D., Silverberg, J. et al. (1991). Nocturnal cortisol, thyroid stimulating hormone, and growth hormone secretory profiles in depressed adolescents. *J. Am. Acad. Child Adolesc. Psychiatry*, *30*, 407–414.

Loney, J., Whaley, K. M. A., Ponto, L. B., & Adney, K. (1981). Predictors of adolescent height and weight in hyperkinetic boys treated with methylphenidate (proceedings). *Psychopharmacol Bull.*, *17*, 132–4.

Marshall, W., & Tanner, J. (1986). Puberty. In F. Falkner & J. Tanner (Eds.), *Human growth: A comprehensive treatise* (2nd ed., pp. 171–209). New York: Plenum.

Mattes, J. A., & Gittelman, R. (1983). Growth of hyperactive children on maintenance regimen of methylphenidate. *Arch. Gen. Psychiatry*, *40*, 317–321.

McLaren, D. S, & Read, W. W. C. (1975). Weight/length classification of nutritional status. *Lancet*, *2*, 219–221.

McNutt, B. A., Boileau, R. A., & Cohen M. N. (1977). The effects of long-term stimulant medication on the growth and body composition of hyperactive children. *Psychopharmacol Bull.*, *13*, 36–38.

Millichap, J. G. (1978). Dr. Gross's findings supported (letter). *Pediatrics*, *61*, 146–147.

Millichap, J. G., & Millichap, M. (1975). Growth of hyperactive children. *N. Engl. J. Med. 292*, 1300.

Orvaschel, H. (1985), Psychiatric interviews suitable for use in research with children and adolescents. *Psychopharmacol Bull.*, *21*, 737–745.

Pine, D., Cohen, P., & Brook, J. (1995). *Youth emotional problems as predictors of early adulthood stature*. Presented at 42nd Annual Meeting of American Academy of Child and Adolescent Psychiatry, New Orleans.

Polito, C., Oporto, M. R., Totino, S. F., La Manna, A., & Di Toro, R. (1986). Normal growth of nephrotic children during long-term alternate-day prednisone therapy. *Acta. Paediatr. Scand. 75*, 245–250.

Puig-Antich, J. Tabrizi, M. A., Davies, M. et al. (1981). Prepubertal endogenous major depressives hyposecrete growth hormone in response to insulin-induced hypoglycemia. *Biol. Psychiatry, 16*, 801–818.

Quinn, P. O., & Rapoport, J. L. (1975). One-year follow-up of hyperactive boys treated with imipramine or methylphenidate. *Am. J. Psychiatry, 132*, 241–245.

Safer, D., & Allen, R. (1973). Factors influencing the suppressant effects of two stimulant drugs on the growth of hyperactive children. *J. Pediatr., 51*, 660–667.

Safer, D., Allen, R., & Barr, E. (1975). Growth rebound after termination of stimulant drugs. *J. Pediatr., 86*, 113–116.

Safer, D. J. (1973). A familial factor in minimal brain dysfunction. *Behav. Genet, 3*, 175–186.

Safer, D. J., Allen, R. P., & Barr, E. (1972). Depression of growth in hyperactive children on stimulant drugs. *N. Engl. J. Med., 287*, 217–20.

Satterfield, J. H., Cantwell, D. P., Schell, A., & Blaschke, T. (1979). Growth of hyperactive children treated with methylphenidate. *Arch. Gen. Psychiatry, 36*, 212–217.

Spencer, T., Biederman, J., Wright, V., & Danon M. (1992). Growth deficits in children treated with desipramine: a controlled study. *J. Am. Acad. Child Adolesc Psychiatry, 31*, 235–423.

Tanner, J. (1986). Use and abuse of growth standards. In F. Falkner & J. Tanner (Eds.), *Human growth: a comprehensive treatise* (pp. 95–109). New York: Plenum.

Tanner, J., & Davies, P. (1985). Clinical longitudinal standards for height and height velocity for North American children. *J. Pediatr., 107*, 317–329.

Uhde, T. (1994). Anxiety and growth disturbance: Is there a connection? A review of biological studies in social phobia. *J. Clin. Psychiatry, 55*, 17–27.

Waterlow, J. C. (1972). Classification and definition of protein-calorie malnutrition. *Br. Med. J., 3*, 566–569.

Waterlow, J. C. (1973). Note on the assessment and classification of protein-energy malnutrition in children. *Lancet, 2*, 87–89.

Waterlow, J. C. (1974). Some aspects of childhood malnutrition as a public health problem. *Br. Med. J., 4*, 88–90.

Weissman, M. M., Gershon, E. S., Kidd, K. K. et al. (1984), Psychiatric disorders in the relatives of probands with affective disorders. *Arch. Gen. Psychiatry, 41*, 13–21.

PART III: CLINICAL ISSUES

13

Developmental Pathways in Depression: Multiple Meanings, Antecedents, and Endpoints

Richard Harrington, Michael Rutter, and Eric Fombonne

MRC Child Psychiatry Unit, London

This article presents an overview of work conducted at the Institute of Psychiatry over the past 30 years on childhood depression. The work began with the basic question of definition and measurement. Epidemiological studies showed that depressive symptoms were quite common in children and were a good, if nonspecific, indicator of psychological disturbance. Further work in both epidemiological and clinical samples provided some evidence for the validity of a depressive syndrome. However, this work also showed that these depressive syndromes represented a heterogeneous group of phenomena. The validity of major depressive disorder in children was therefore tested further in longitudinal and family-genetic studies. These studies supported the validity of the concept but confirmed that there was heterogeneity in respect to both developmental stage at the time of onset and comorbidity with conduct disorder. We concluded that there are probably several different kinds of depressive syndromes in children. Some are strongly linked with depressive disorders in adulthood, but others are probably better conceptualized as part of another psychopathological problem altogether.

Over the past 15 years the use of symptom-oriented personal interviews with children has led to widespread recognition that disorders resembling adult depression can occur in children. Indeed, the prevailing psychiatric classifications give the impression that depressive disorder in young people is a neat, defined syndrome with core symptoms that are the same across the agespan. Thus, in the *Diagnostic and Statistical Manual of the Mental Disorders* (American Psychiatric Association, 1994) the essential criteria for major depression are similar for prepubertal children, adolescents, and adults. The hypothesis that depressive disorders in young people are isomorphic with depression in adulthood is supported by the consistent finding from longitudinal studies that depressed young people have an increased risk of depressive conditions in adulthood. We found that in comparison with a nondepressed child psychiatric control group, children who had been depressed had a greatly increased risk of major depression and suicidality when followed up 18 years later (Harrington et al., 1994; Harrington, Fudge,

Reprinted with permission from *Development and Psychopathology*, 1996, Vol. 8, 601–616. Copyright © 1996 by the Cambridge University Press.

The work described in this article has been supported by various bodies, including the Department of Health, the Medical Research Council, and the MacArthur Foundation Network on Risk and Protective Factors in the Major Mental Disorders.

Rutter, Pickles, & Hill, 1990). The fact that further follow-up studies of different samples showed the same basic pattern (Rao et al., 1995; Rao, Weissman, Martin, & Hammond, 1993) would seem to end the matter.

However, in spite of this apparently clearcut pattern of direct, predictable continuity from childhood into adult life, research findings also indicate a more complex picture in which continuities are often indirect and the outcomes diverse. Thus, *looking backwards*, it is clear that depressive disorders in adulthood can be preceded by a wide range of childhood psychopathology (Zeitlin, 1986) and that only a minority of depressed adults showed depressive syndromes as children (Smith & Weissman, 1992). Similarly, it seems that the children of depressed parents are at risk of a wide range of psychiatric disorders, not just depression (Weissman et al., 1987). Then there are the findings that *looking forwards* it is not only depression that predicts subsequent affective disorders but other symptoms as well. For instance, childhood conduct disorder has been shown to predict depressive symptomatology in adulthood (Rutter, 1991; Rutter, Harrington, Quinton, & Pickles, 1994). Moreover, depression in adolescents predicts not only subsequent depression but many other problems too, including impaired social relationships and negative life experiences (Garber, Kriss, Koch, & Lindholm, 1988; Kandel & Davies, 1986).

This diversity of nonspecific connections in which supposedly distinct syndromes have a similar outcome and in which the same problem has diverse outcomes raises fundamental questions about the validity of the concept of depressive disorder in young people. Should we abandon the whole concept altogether and move back to the situation that applied 30 years ago in which there was a nondifferentiated global concept of childhood emotional disorder? If not, in what circumstances is it sensible to regard children as suffering from the same kinds of depressive conditions as adults?

In this article we present an overview of a series of studies conducted at the Institute of Psychiatry in London over the past 30 years (The Institute of Psychiatry Studies of Child and Adolescent Depression) that provide data on the nature of childhood depression and the mechanisms involved in its persistence and desistance over time. The article has four parts. In the first part, we begin by charting the phenomenon of depression using data both from epidemiological studies of the general population and from studies of clinical groups. The findings showed that symptoms of misery could and did occur in children and that they were a good, if nonspecific, indicator of psychological disturbance. Moreover, clinical studies showed that depressive symptoms tended to cluster together into distinct syndromes.

It was also clear, however, that these depressive syndromes represented a heterogeneous group of phenomena ranging from nonspecific clusters of symptoms that were usually part of another psychopathological problem through to what appeared to be distinctive depressive disorders. It was therefore necessary to conduct more stringent tests of validity. In the second part of this article, we show how this was achieved through longitudinal and family-genetic research strategies. Childhood depression was associated with a greatly increased risk of depressive disorders in adulthood and with an increased familial loading for depression.

Having established that depressive disorders in young people did have longitudinal and familial linkages with depressive conditions in adult life, the next step was to determine whether these linkages could be used to investigate the heterogeneity of depression that had been found in the epidemiological studies. In the third part of this article, we demonstrate how leads from the epidemiological studies were used to identify the groups at highest risk of major depression in adulthood. Results showed that there was some heterogeneity related to both age at onset and comorbidity with conduct disorder. Apparently identical childhood depressive conditions can have different outcomes (multifinality), and there may be different childhood precursors of the same adult outcome (equifinality). In the fourth part, we make some suggestions for future research.

DEPRESSIVE PHENOMENA

The story necessarily begins with a charting of the phenomena of depression using both general population epidemiological samples and clinical groups. At the time we started our studies 30 years ago, there was considerable skepticism about the notion that depressive disorders could occur in young people, and adequate standardized measures specifically focused on depressive features in childhood and adolescence were not available. Both questionnaire and interview measures to tap a wide range of psychopathology were devised and shown to be reliable and valid (Rutter, Tizard, & Whitmore, 1970). Findings from both types of measures showed that symptoms of misery in young people were frequently reported by teachers, parents, and the children themselves. Thus, on both parent and teacher questionnaires, about 1 in 10 ten-year-olds were reported as showing misery. Most strikingly, the item "often appears miserable, unhappy, tearful, or distressed," as reported by teachers or parents for both boys and girls, was a good discriminator of overall psychopathology. Thus, 60% of girls with psychiatric disorder (as assessed on the basis of detailed interviews with parents and children) showed misery on the parental account, as contrasted with 11% of those without disorder; the comparable figures on the teacher scale were 28% and 7%. For boys, the contrasts were 38% versus 10% and 20% versus 9% on the parent and teacher scales, respectively.

It was also evident, however, that misery was associated with a wide range of psychopathology including conduct disorders and reading retardation, as well as emotional disturbance (Rutter et al., 1970). Thus, some 30% to 40% of 10-year-old children with any of these diagnoses exhibited depressive phenomena (see Table 1). It seemed that, whatever else it was, depressive mood constituted a good, but nonspecific, indicator of psychological disturbance. It could be argued, of course, that this nonspecificity was an artifact of the crude tools of measurement available at the time. That was not the case, however, as is shown by similar findings from all more recent studies (Harrington, 1993).

To address the need to develop much more detailed standardized parent and child interviews for assessing the range of psychopathological phenomena considered relevant for modern psychiatric diagnoses, the Child and Adolescent Psychiatric Assessment (CAPA) was devised and shown to have good reliability (Angold & Costello, 1995; Angold, Prendergast, Cox, Rutter, & Harrington, 1995). This assessment was used in the Virginia Twin Study of Adolescent Behavioral Development (VTSABD), an epidemiological study of some 1400 twin pairs aged 8 to 16 years (Eaves et al., 1996; Hewitt et al., 1996; Simonoff et al., 1996). As in the Isle of Wight study some 30 years earlier, depressive symptomatology was quite strongly associated with conduct and oppositional disorders, as well as anxiety and depressive disorders. This was true for both questionnaire and interview measures.

The early epidemiological studies on the Isle of Wight also brought out two other crucial features that continue to present conceptual and methodological difficulties. First, there was low agreement

TABLE 1
Psychiatric Ratings (%) from Interviews with 10-Year-Olds (Rutter et al., 1970)

		Disorder		
	Controls	Emotional	Conduct	Mixed
Preoccupation with depressive topics	9	42	26	43
Depressed mood	13	38	35	43
Lack of smiling	17	44	38	32
Poor emotional responsiveness	15	31	31	36

TABLE 2
Psychiatric Ratings (%) from Interviews with
Adolescents in the General Population
(Rutter et al., 1976)

	Boys (N = 96)	Girls (N = 88)
Items reported by adolescent		
Misery	42	48
Self-depreciation	20	23
Suicidal ideas	7	8
Ideas of reference	28	31
Items observed by psychiatrist		
Anxiety	20	28
Sadness/misery	13	15

between parents and children in their reports on depressive symptomatology shown by young people. At first, it was considered that this might represent weak measures but, once more, the VTSABD findings (Hewitt et al., 1996; Simonoff et al., 1996), as well as those of other modern studies, have shown the same. Second, when interviewed in standardized fashion, adolescent girls reported substantially higher levels of misery and suicidal ideation than noted by their parents. What was not clear, however, was whether this disparity arose because parents were failing to appreciate serious mood disturbances in their children or, rather, because young people were overreacting to, or misperceiving, normal variations in mood, perhaps because they were less accustomed than adults to the negative cognitions associated with depressive feelings. That the latter might be part of the story was suggested by the disparity between depression as *reported* by adolescents and as *observed* by psychiatrists (Rutter, Graham, Chadwick, & Yule, 1976). Only about 1 in 7 adolescents *showed* sadness at a psychiatric interview but some 2 out of 5 *reported* this feeling in the same interview (see Table 2). The query regarding the relative validity of parent and child reports, however, remains unanswered. Evidence on predictive validity to later episodes of major depressive disorder, with accompanying social impairment, is likely to be most informative on this issue. It should be added that the parent–child difference in level of depressive phenomena does not apply in the same way to referred patient groups (Harrington, 1993); this is likely to be a consequence of the fact that parents initiate most child psychiatric referrals.

Depression as a Syndrome and as a Mood Feature

After establishing the importance of depression as a nonspecific indicator of psychopathology, the next step was to determine whether it also indexed a meaningfully distinctive syndrome, or diagnostic category, as well. Pearce (1974, 1978) used Maudsley Hospital item-sheet data (symptom codings made routinely at the time of initial clinical assessment) to examine this issue. He found a significant tendency for depression-related symptomatology to cluster together, and an operationally defined depression cluster occurred in some 12% of all child and adolescent referrals. It became more frequent and also showed an increasing female preponderance across the transition from childhood to adolescence.

The next question concerned the connections between depression as a mood feature and depression as a diagnostic category. This issue needed to be tackled initially by determining whether the epidemiological findings and adult outcome differed between the two. Zeitlin (1986) applied the latter criterion in his study of patients who had attended the Maudsley Hospital as both children and adults. The findings were illuminating in several aspects. First, there was strong continuity between an operationally defined depressive syndrome in childhood and a similarly defined syndrome in adult life; 84% of the individuals with the childhood syndrome showed the same syndrome in adult life compared with 44% of those without the depressive constellation in childhood. Second, there was similarly strong continuity at the symptom level but, in both age periods, the symptom of depression was associated with a wide range of other psychopathology. Third, there was no support for the concept of "masked" depression in childhood (a popular concept in the 1970s and early 1980s); there was no continuity to adult depression for constellations of depression-related symptomatology in the absence of the symptom of depression. Fourth, the *majority* of cases of depressive disorder in adult life had *not* been preceded by depressive syndromes in childhood. In other words, major depressive disorders frequently had their first onset in adult life; this was particularly so far affective psychoses.

These results confirmed the earlier findings on depressive mood as a nonspecific indicator of psychopathology and began to provide validation of the childhood category of depressive disorder that derived from Pearce's research. However, the results additionally indicated that depression as a mood feature also showed substantial continuity over time and might, therefore, represent a meaningful dimension—perhaps as a personality feature associated with mental disorder.

Age and sex trends provided another way of examining connections between the diagnostic category and the mood feature. The Isle of Wight data suggested a major increase in the rate of depressive disorder over the years between 10 and 15 years of age—3 cases out of about 2000 children in the general population at age 10, but 9 cases of "pure" depressive disorder and 26 cases of mixed affective disorder in the same cohort some 4 years later. The findings were suggestive but were severely limited by measurement constraints.

Accordingly, the next step was to turn again to Maudsley Hospital item-sheet data. Angold and Rutter (1992) examined age and sex trends in 3519 8- to 16-year-old psychiatric patients. Figure 1 shows the findings for girls using the same operationalized symptom constellation as that employed by Pearce (1974) and Zeitlin (1986). There was no substantial rise over the years of early adolescence in girls who had yet to reach puberty or in those who were postpubertal. There was a marked rise,

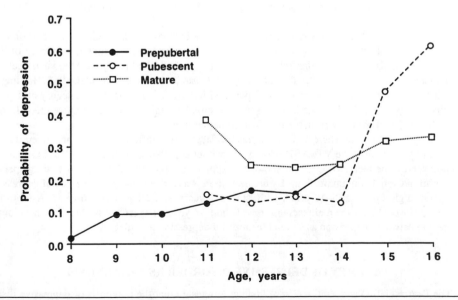

Figure 1. Effect of age on syndromic depression in girls attending the Maudsley hospital, by pubertal status (Angold & Rutter, 1992).

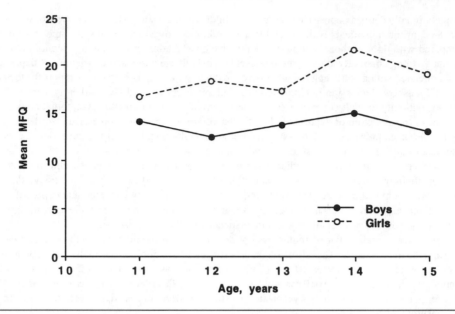

Figure 2. Mean MFQ self-report score by age and sex in a London secondary school sample (Harrington et. al., 1996a).

most evident at age 14, in those who were pubescent (i.e., still passing through puberty). Multivariate analyses indicated that age had a greater effect than puberty, but the difference in curves according to stage of puberty indicates that caution should be exercised in taking that finding at face value. The age trend findings in boys were inconsistent and much less striking; overall, girls showed the main increase in depressive syndromes.

The question that followed was whether the same age and sex trends applied to depression considered as a mood feature. To answer that question, we undertook a questionnaire survey of 724 11- to 15-year-olds in three London schools (Harrington et al., 1996a) using the Mood and Feelings Questionnaire (Angold, Costello et al., 1995; Angold, Costello, Pickles, & Winder, 1987; Harrington & Shariff, 1992). The trends were trivial compared with those for the diagnostic category of depressive disorder (see Fig. 2). The implication is that questionnaire measures of depressive mood have a somewhat different meaning from the diagnosis of depression.

The important limitation here, however, is that the data apply to different populations. Accordingly, we need to turn again to the VTSABD findings (Hewitt et al., 1996; Simonoff et al., 1996). As in the London survey, the mean MFQ scores showed no appreciable rise over the 8- to 16-year age period (Simonoff, personal communication). By contrast, there was a rise with age in the rate of depressive disorders; in girls 0.6% at 8–10 years, 1.0% at 11–13 years, and 3.1% at 14–16 years. As with the Maudsley Hospital data, the main increase was at about 14 years of age. Clearly, there is a meaningful distinction between depression as a mood feature and depression as a diagnosis.

VALIDITY OF DEPRESSIVE DISORDER AS A DIAGNOSIS

The Pearce (1974) and Zeitlin (1986) findings suggested that the diagnosis of depressive disorder in childhood had some discriminative validity, but it was necessary to undertake more rigorous

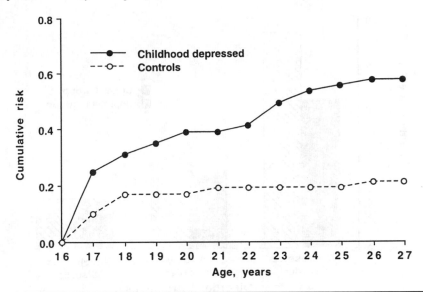

Figure 3. Cumulative risk of depressive disorder in adult life in childhood depressed cases and controls ($n = 52$ pairs) (Harrington et al., 1990).

testing of validity. We did that through the use of a follow-up into adult life combined with a family study.

Temporal Continuities

Our previous research had consistently shown that depressive conditions in young people often occurred in conjunction with other problems (Pearce, 1974; Rutter et al., 1970; Zeitlin, 1986), so in designing the follow-up it was first necessary to devise a set of outcome measures capable of measuring a wide range of relevant outcomes. We accomplished this in a series of pilot studies (Harrington et al., 1988; Hill, Harrington, Fudge, Rutter, & Pickles, 1989, 1995).

These measures were then used in a follow-up of the 80 Maudsley Hospital depressed cases who had been studied by Pearce (1974, 1978), together with a closely matched control group of 80 nondepressed child psychiatric cases (Harrington et al., 1990). Subjects were a mean age of 13 years at the time of their initial clinic attendance, and were reexamined at a mean age of 31 years, with outcome data on 82% of the total sample. Figure 3 shows the risk of an episode of major or minor depression in adult life, analyzed using a proportional hazards model. The childhood depressed group had a much greater risk for a depressive disorder in adulthood than the controls. No other disorder was increased, suggesting that the risk was specific to depression.

Family-Genetic Associations

The course of a disorder may be affected by many extraneous factors. It was therefore necessary to study other kinds of correlates that were, at least to some extent, independent of the disorder itself. Family-genetic findings represent one such correlate, and we therefore conducted a family-interview study on the first-degree relatives (FDRs) of the depressed children and nondepressed child psychiatric controls who were described in the previous section (Harrington et al., 1993). Efforts were made to

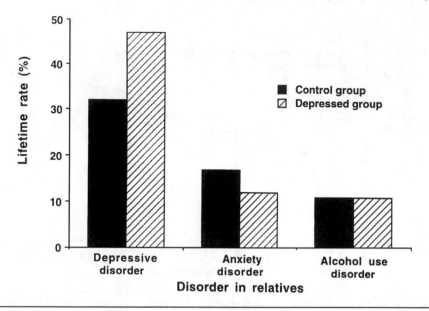

Figure 4. Lifetime risk of disorder among first degree relatives of depressed children and nondepressed child psychiatric controls (Harrington et al., 1993).

obtain interviews with all available FDRs, and the prevalence of lifetime psychiatric disorders was assessed with the methodologies used in the follow-up.

In line with the follow-up findings, the FDRs of depressed children had significantly higher rates of depressive disorder than the relatives of the controls, with an odds ratio of nearly 2. Once again, it was necessary to establish whether the risk was specific for depression, or whether it included other psychiatric problems as well. The only psychiatric disorder that was increased in relatives of the depressed probands was depression (see Fig. 4).

Of course, depressive disorders are common in the general population and often arise for reasons unassociated with factors leading to familial aggregation. Such cases necessarily add "noise" to familial data. A partial way around this difficulty was afforded by a focus on the proportion of individuals having at least two affected relatives. This proportion was significantly higher in the depressed group than in controls (37% vs. 18%), with an odds ratio of more than 2.5 (Harrington et al., 1993). The finding that the excess familial loading was restricted to a minority subgroup implied the possibility of some heterogeneity within the broad construct of childhood depression.

HETEROGENEITY IN DEPRESSIVE DISORDERS

The question, therefore, arose as to whether there were subgroups that had particularly strong continuities with adult depressive conditions. This was a crucial question because research on other aspects of the validity of childhood depression, such as its neurobiology and its response to antidepressants, had produced equivocal results (Harrington, 1994). An important possible explanation for the apparent failure of these studies was that juvenile depressive disorders were highly heterogeneous.

TABLE 3
Cumulative Probability (%) of Depression in Adulthood (Harrington et al., 1990)

	Chart Diagnosis in Childhood		
	Group 1	Group 2	Group 3
Adult Outcome	No Depression or Minor Depression ($N = 75$)	Major Depression ($N = 27$)	Major Depression and Clinical Diagnosis ($N = 18$)
Any affective disorder	29[a]	70	61
Major depression	4[a]	26	50[b]

[a]Group 1 versus Group 3; $p < .01$.
[b]Group 2 versus Group 3; $p = .06$.

Patterns of Depressive Symptoms

Earlier studies had suggested several potential markers of heterogeneity. First, the follow-back findings (Zeitlin, 1986) had shown that continuities were stronger when there was particularly obvious depressive symptomatology. Indeed, only a minority of the depressed probands in our follow-up study were given a clinical diagnosis of depression by the examining psychiatrist, probably because their presentation differed from the typical picture of adult depressive disorders (Harrington et al., Pearce, 1974).

To examine the influence that the clinical picture had on the risk of adult depression, the charts of the depressed and control children were rated by a psychiatrist who had not been involved in the follow-up, and the sample was reclassified into three groups: (a) those with either no chart Research Diagnostic Criteria (RDC; Spitzer, Endicott, & Robins, 1978) for an affective diagnosis or a diagnosis of minor depression; (b) those with an RDC chart diagnosis of major depression but without a clinical diagnosis of depression; and (c) those with both a chart diagnosis of major depression *and* a clinical diagnosis of depressive disorder by the psychiatrist who had examined them at the time of the index episode.

Table 3 shows the cumulative probability of depressive disorder in adulthood for these groups. The more closely the clinical picture in childhood resembled adult depression, the greater the risk of an episode of major depression in adulthood. Of those with the best evidence of a major depressive disorder in childhood, half developed a similar major disorder in adult life compared with only 1 in 25 of those without a major depressive disorder in childhood. The clinical picture in childhood seemed to have an important influence on the adult outcome. However, there was a quite different picture for minor depressive disorders in adult life. These were very common (29%) in individuals who had *not* had, as well as those who had had a major depressive disorder in childhood.

Multifinality of Outcomes: The Example of Depression and Conduct Disorder

The second possible indicator of heterogeneity in depressive disorder was the presence of conduct disorder. When we started our studies 30 years ago, it was widely believed that depressive disorders in children were expressed through "equivalents," and that symptoms such as behavioral problems were often expressions of an underlying "masked" depression. However, our research in both epidemiological and clinical samples had produced evidence that depressive disorders had a different meaning when they occurred in conjunction with conduct disorder. For example, Angold and Rutter (1992) found that the gender and age effects that were common to all other depression groups were absent in mixed disorders of conduct and emotions. The *only* form of depressive disorder that did not increase during adolescence and that was not more common in girls was depressive conduct disorder.

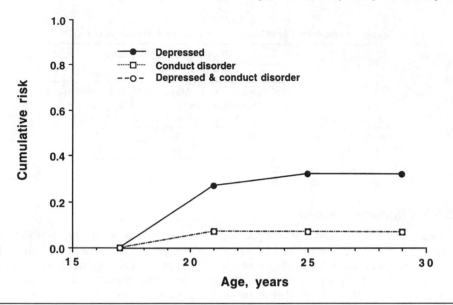

Figure 5. Cumulative risk of major depressive disorder in adult life in children with depression only, children with conduct disorder only and children with both depression and conduct disorder (Harrington et al., 1991).

The question, therefore, arose as to whether this comorbid group resembled children with "pure" depression in its adult outcome, or whether its outcome was similar to that of children with "pure" conduct disorder. To tackle this question, the depressed probands from the follow-up study were divided into two groups: those without conduct problems and those with conduct disorder (three or more conduct symptoms) (Harrington, Fudge, Rutter, Pickles, & Hill, 1991). These two depressed groups were compared with a third group of children with conduct disorders who were obtained from the control sample, described earlier.

The results showed that childhood conduct disorder was associated with a much increased risk of adult criminality (assessed from official crime records). There was no increased risk of criminality associated with childhood depression, either on its own or in combination with conduct disturbance (Harrington et al., 1991). As with the adult depressive outcome, not only was the raised risk very marked, but also it was syndrome-specific.

Figure 5 deals with the risk of adult depression in the same way. The overlap group that showed both conduct disturbance and depression in childhood had no increase in risk for adult depression, compared with those without depression in childhood. The finding was all the more noteworthy because this overlap group was more severely disturbed than the pure depressed group in many respects (Harrington et al., 1991).

These findings were clear-cut in showing the distinctiveness of the long-term course of depressive and conduct disorders. We could reject the idea that they represented different manifestations of the same underlying psychopathology. Major depression in childhood was associated with a much increased risk of major depression in adult life, but no increase in the risk of adult criminality. Conversely, adult criminality was predicted by conduct disorder in childhood but not by depressive conditions early in life. The main interest with respect to the issues considered in this section lies in the

TABLE 4

Adult Depression in Subjects with Pervasive Social Dysfunction
in Adulthood, by Antisocial Personality Disorder (Follow-up of
Child Psychiatric Clinic Attenders; Rutter et al., 1994)

| | Antisocial Personality Disorder | | |
	Absent	Present	χ^2
Adult minor depression	18 (5)	23 (4)	0.2
Adult major depression	46 (13)	6 (1)	8.1**

Note: Values are percentages with mean number of cases (*n*) in parentheses.
**p < .01

adult outcome of the comorbid depression plus conduct disorder group. The rate of adult depressive disorder in this group was much the same as that in the group *without* depressive disorder in childhood. This finding seemed more compatible with the hypothesis that the depressive problems in childhood for this comorbid group were in some sense secondary to the conduct disorder. Once again the concept of masked depression was not supported.

These analyses dealt with the adult outcome for conduct disturbance solely in terms of criminality and with the adult outcome for depression in terms of major depression only. The next issue was whether the outcomes were as distinctive when broader aspects of social functioning were included and when the outcome was minor rather than major depression. We found that people who had shown conduct disorder as children usually had a much more pervasive form of social dysfunction in adult life than those who had shown other forms of psychiatric disturbance (Rutter et al., 1994). This pervasive dysfunction was characterized by a poor employment history and difficulties keeping friends. In many instances this dysfunction took the form of antisocial personality disorder.

Table 4 focuses on all the subjects who had pervasive social dysfunction at follow-up and subdivides them according to whether or not they had antisocial personality disorder. The top line shows that both groups had a similar rate of minor depression in adult life. Minor depression is clearly associated with a range of problems in adulthood, including antisocial personality disorder. However, as the bottom line of the table shows, major depression in adulthood was very uncommon in the antisocial group. Major depression constitutes a much more specific form of psychopathology with a high degree of consistency over time.

These findings point to the need to separate minor and major affective disorders, but also they suggest that conduct disorder may play a role as a risk factor for the former, although clearly it does not for the latter. The data from this follow-up of a clinic sample, however, were less decisive in differentiating between a risk based on comorbidity between emotional and conduct disturbance already established in childhood and a risk process by which conduct problems in childhood predisposed to the *later* onset of minor depression. To make this differentiation, we turned to the data set provided by the British National Child Development Study, a longitudinal study from birth to adulthood of some 17,000 children born in a particular week in 1978 (Rutter, 1991). Emotional and conduct disturbance in childhood was assessed using the parent and teacher questionnaires developed for the Isle of Wight studies (Rutter et al., 1970), and emotional disturbance in adult life by the Malaise Inventory (which largely taps minor depressive symptomatology but includes some anxiety and somatic items), which was developed for the same studies. Not surprisingly, emotional difficulties in childhood were associated with a two- to three-fold increase in emotional disturbance at age 23 years. But the same size of increased risk for minor depression in adult life applied to conduct disturbance in childhood, even after controlling for the presence of emotional symptoms in childhood. Thus, as

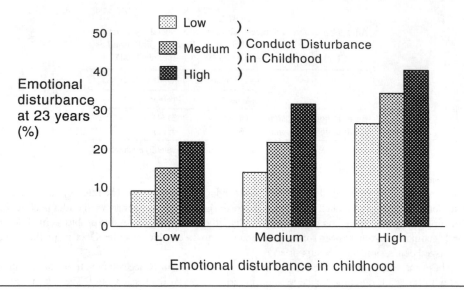

Figure 6. Emotional/conduct disturbance in childhood and probability of a high Malaise score in females at 23 years (Rutter, 1991).

shown in Fig. 6, within the group with little or no evidence of emotional difficulties in childhood, high conduct disturbance was associated with a three-fold increase in the risk of a high score on the Malaise Inventory—from 3% to 10%. It may be concluded that there is meaningful continuity between conduct problems in childhood and minor depressive symptomatology in early adult life. Taken with the clinic follow-up study findings, the evidence points to a route via personality difficulties and social malfunction.

To take this issue one stage further, a 20-year follow-up study was undertaken of children first studied at the age of 10 years using the same Isle of Wight questionnaires, but this time using a general population sample in inner London (Champion, Goodall, & Rutter, 1995). As shown in Fig. 7, conduct problems at age 10 years were associated with a doubling of the risk of severely negative life events and experiences nearly two decades later. As these events and experiences were chosen to represent those shown in earlier studies (Brown & Harris, 1978) to precipitate depressive disorders in adults, it is likely that they played a role in the route from conduct difficulties in childhood to minor depression in adult life.

Equifinality of Outcomes: The Example of Suicidal Behavior

The findings in respect to depression and conduct disorder emphasized the distinctiveness of the outcomes of these disorders. They also showed how an apparently similar phenotype (childhood depressive disorder) could have a different outcome depending on the context in which it occurred. However, to understand better the heterogeneity of childhood affective disturbance, we also needed to pose the question the other way around. Were there instances in which different pathways led to the same endpoint (equifinality)?

This question was tackled using the data on suicidal behavior in the follow-up (Harrington et al., 1994). Two risk factors in childhood (depression and conduct disorder) were identified for a suicidal attempt in adult life (Table 5), but the strongest risk factor was depressive disorder in adulthood.

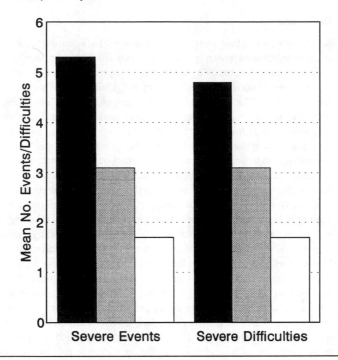

Figure 7. Severe events and difficulties in early adult life and type of disturbance at 10 years, in females (Champion et al., 1995). Black bars conduct/mixed; shaded bars emotional disturbance; white bars no disturbance.

It seemed, then, that depression in childhood was associated with an attempt in adulthood largely because it predicted subsequent depressive disorder. However, logistic regression analyses showed that conduct disorder had an independent "direct" effect on the risk of an episode of self-harm in adult life (Harrington et al., 1994) that did not depend on subsequent depressive disorder. These findings suggest that there are different pathways to a suicidal attempt in adulthood, one through depression and the other through conduct disorder. They also highlight the fact that the pathways from childhood psychopathology to adult outcomes depend crucially on what happens later in life.

TABLE 5
Predictors of a Suicidal Attempt in Adulthood (Harrington et al., 1994)

		Childhood Status			
		Control Adult Attempt (*N*)		Depressed Adult Attempt (*N*)	
		No	Yes	No	Yes
No major depression in adult life					
Conduct disorder	No	45	3	26	5
	Yes	11	4	12	1
Major depression in adult life					
Conduct disorder	No	3	0	3	12
	Yes	0	1	0	1

Developmental Differences

The final issue concerned whether there were differences between depressive conditions that start in preadolescence and those apparently identical conditions that start during or after puberty. For the past 20 years or so it has become customary to regard prepubertal depressive disorders as essentially the same kind of condition as adolescent and adult forms of the condition. However, findings from studies such as the Maudsley Item Sheet research (Angold & Rutter, 1992; Pearce, 1974) have consistently pointed to important differences between prepubertal and later onset varieties of depressive disorder, of which perhaps the most robust has been the absence of a female preponderance in prepubertal depression. The question, therefore, arose as to whether prepubertal onset depressive disorders differed from later onset depressive conditions in respect of outcome, family history, or both.

To explore this issue, we divided the probands in the follow-up study according to whether the onset of depression was pre- or postpubertal (including those who were pubescent). Prepubertal and postpubertal depressed cases differed in their outcomes. Continuity to major depression in adulthood was significantly lower in prepubertal probands than in postpubertal cases (Harrington et al., 1990). Once again, it was necessary to test the validity of the longitudinal findings with data from the family study. Compared with controls, both those with a prepubertal and those with a postpubertal onset of major depressive disorder showed an increased familial loading for depressive disorders in first- and second-degree relatives. However, there were important differences in pattern according to the age of onset (Harrington et al., 1996b). Criminality, alcohol abuse, and intrafamilial discord were all significantly more common in the families of prepubertal depressed cases as compared with postpubertal depressed cases. Also, the relatives with depression were more likely to have a depressive disorder that was comorbid with criminality. These differences were found even when the effects of potential confounding variables, such as conduct disorder, year of birth, type of depression, and gender were controlled in proportional hazards analyses.

DISCUSSION

Conclusions

Since the Institute of Psychiatry studies started 30 years ago, great progress has been made in the definition and measurement of depressive disorder in children and adolescents. As a result, there is now much greater consistency in the findings from epidemiological studies, which tend to show that age and sex trends for depressive disorder differ from those for other psychological symptoms. Other findings, too, support the nosological validity of the concept of depressive disorder among the young. Children with severe depressive disorders have an increased risk of recurrence in adulthood and have a higher familial loading for depression than child psychiatric controls.

Nevertheless, our findings suggest that there is probable heterogeneity in relation to several features. First, the epidemiological studies showed that age trends were much more striking for overt disorder reported at interview than for symptoms reported by questionnaire. The follow-up findings also underlined the need to distinguish between overt depressive disorders and other syndromes of negative mood. The risk of major depressive disorders in adult life was somewhat greater with the childhood disorders that approximated to adult patterns. Second, depressive disorder seems to have a different meaning when it occurs in conjunction with conduct disorder. In our study, "pure" depression had an outcome that was different from "pure" conduct disorder, with mixed disorders resembling conduct disorders. Third, there was evidence from both the longitudinal and family-genetic studies of important differences between prepubertal- and maturity-onset depressive disorders. Prepubertal-onset disorders were more likely to be associated with adverse family environments and with parental criminality or alcoholism than maturity-onset depressive conditions. However, they were less likely to have a poor outcome in adulthood.

The findings from the follow-up study also give rise to several conclusions about the pathways linking childhood psychopathology to later adverse outcomes. First, the pathways from childhood to adulthood for major depressive disorders and for conduct disorder are distinct. They do not seem to be part of the same underlying process. Second, however, pathways can also be indirect and there may be different pathways to the same outcome. Suicidal behavior, for example, can be reached by apparently different routes—one via depression and a different route through conduct disturbance. Third, continuities from childhood to adulthood also depend on what happens later in life. Childhood depression predicts a suicidal attempt in adulthood largely because of its association with depression in adult life. Fourth, the causal routes to major and minor depressive disorders appear to differ in some important respects. The latter involves conduct problems and personality disorder; whereas, these features seem less influential with severe depressive disorders. In conclusion, there appear to be diverse pathways from child to adult depression that are probably mediated by several mechanisms. Further research on these mechanisms is likely to have important implications for the treatment and prevention of a common and disabling disorder.

Further Research

Longitudinal research into linkages between early- and late-onset forms of depression is still at an early stage. Only a few studies have extended from childhood into adult life. Perhaps the most immediately pressing need is, therefore, for studies designed to replicate the main findings of the research-described above. Thus, it should be possible in the next few years to mount long-term, prospective follow-ups of children diagnosed as depressed, using standardized interviews and present-day diagnostic criteria. Such studies are already under way and, although they are expensive and difficult to undertake, they will teach us much about child-to-adult continuities.

Clearly, the starting point for these studies will need to be a reconsideration of some of the important issues that have been raised by the existing studies, such as the strength of the links between adolescent and adult depressive disorders and the impact of comorbidity on prognosis. It will continue to be important to control for symptomatology other than depression, as it is becoming clear that the effects of early depression need to be distinguished from the effects of comorbid difficulties. It will also be necessary to study potentially informative subgroups, of which two stand out as particularly in need of further investigation: (a) prepubertal depressed children and (b) children with depression and conduct disorder. Prepubertal depressed children are of interest not only in their own right, but also because of the finding that they seem to differ from depressed adolescents in respect of adult prognosis and family history. Children with depression and conduct disorder need to be studied further because of the uncertainties regarding the meaning of the overlap between these two conditions. Our own follow-up research produced the striking, apparently paradoxical, finding that the subgroup of depressed young people with the worst overall social outcome (namely those with comorbid conduct disorder) was at the *lowest* risk of recurrence of major depression. This surprising finding raises crucial questions about the developmental processes involved in the continuities between depressive disorders in children and adults. Future long-term follow-up studies clearly need to extend the questions from those of simple continuities and discontinuities over time to the nature of the mechanisms involved. To intervene effectively, we must know more about the factors that mediate the strong continuities found in previous research, rather than just the factors that predict continuity.

Three main groups of factors stand out as requiring further investigation. First, the recurrent nature of early-onset depressive disorders underlines the need to move beyond the study of the acute precipitants of one episode in order to study adversities as they occur over time. In particular, we need to know where the acute adversities that are highly prevalent in the lives of depressed children come from (Rutter, Champion, Quinton, Maughan, & Pickles, 1995). In a few children, depression occurs in response to acts of fate, such as disasters. However, a glance through lists of adverse events that have been studied in depressed young people (Goodyer, 1990) shows that very few of them can be regarded as completely independent of the child or his family. Some depressed children seem to act in ways that increases their likelihood of experiencing adversity. Second, more needs to be known about the role of *family factors* in determining the course of early-onset depressive disorders. There is some evidence pointing towards the importance of environmentally mediated mechanisms (see above), but much more also needs to be known about the role of genetic factors. Third, continuities of depressive disorder could be a function of personal qualities, such as neuroticism, dysfunctional cognitions or negative attributions, and low self-esteem. These have tended to be viewed as risk factors for depression, but they have also been found to vary with clinical state, and it may well be that they have a greater role in the persistence of depression than in its onset.

REFERENCES

American Psychiatric Association. (1994). *Diagnostic and statistical manual of mental disorders-DSM-IV* (4th ed.). Washington, DC: Author.

Angold, A., Costello, E. J., Pickles, A., & Winder, F. (1987). *The development of a questionnaire for use in epidemiological studies of depression in children and adolescents.* London: Medical Research Council Child Psychiatry Unit.

Angold, A., & Costello, E. J. (1995). A test–retest reliability study of child-reported psychiatric symptoms and diagnoses using the Child and Adolescent Psychiatric Assessment (CAPA–C). *Psychological Medicine, 25,* 755–762.

Angold, A., Costello, E. J., Messer, S. C., Pickles, A., Winder, F., & Silver, D. (1995). The development of a short questionnaire for use in epidemiological studies of depression in children and adolescents. *International Journal of Methods in Psychiatric Research, 5,* 237–249.

Angold, A., Prendergast, M., Cox, A., Rutter, M., & Harrington, R. (1995). The Child and Adolescent Psychiatric Assessment (CAPA). *Psychological Medicine, 25,* 739–753.

Angold, A., & Rutter, M. (1992). Effects of age and pubertal status on depression in a large clinical sample. *Development and Psychopathology, 4,* 5–28.

Brown, G. W., & Harris, T. (1978). *Social origins of depression.* London: Tavistock.

Champion, L. A., Goodall, G., & Rutter, M. (1995). Behaviour problems in childhood and stressors in early adult life. I. A 20-year follow-up of London school children. *Psychological Medicine, 25,* 231–246.

Eaves, L. J., Silberg, J. L., Meyer, J. M., Maes H. H., Simonoff, E., Pickles, A., Rutter, M. et al. (1996). *Genetics and developmental psychopathology: 2. The main effects of genes and environment on behavioral problems in the Virginia Twin Study of Adolescent Behavioral Development.* Manuscript submitted for publication.

Garber, J., Kriss, M. R., Koch, M., & Lindholm, L. (1988). Recurrent depression in adolescents: A follow-up study. *Journal of the American Academy of Child and Adolescent Psychiatry, 27,* 49-54.

Goodyer, I. M. (1990). *Life experiences, development, and childhood psychopathology.* Chichester: Wiley.

Harrington, R. C. (1993). *Depressive disorder in childhood and adolescence.* Chichester: Wiley.

Harrington, R. C. (1994). Affective disorders. In M. Rutter, E. Taylor, & L. Hersov (Eds.), *Child and adolescent psychiatry: Modern approaches.* 3rd ed., pp. 330–350. Oxford: Blackwell Scientific.

Harrington, R. C., & Shariff, A. (1992). Choosing an instrument to assess depression in young people. *News-letter of the Association for Child Psychology and Psychiatry, 14,* 279–282.

Harrington, R. C., Bredenkamp, D., Groothues, C., Rutter, M., Fudge, H., & Pickles, A. (1994). Adult outcomes of childhood and adolescent depression. III. Links with suicidal behaviours. *Journal of Child Psychology and Psychiatry, 35,* 1380–1391.

Harrington, R. C., Fudge, H., Rutter, M., Bredenkamp, D., Groothues, C., & Pridham, J. (1993). Child and adult depression: A test of continuities with data from a family study. *British Journal of Psychiatry, 162*, 627–633.

Harrington, R. C., Fudge, H., Rutter, M., Pickles, A., & Hill, J. (1990). Adult outcomes of childhood and adolescent depression: I. Psychiatric status. *Archives of General Psychiatry, 47*, 465–473.

Harrington, R. C., Fudge, H., Rutter, M., Pickles, A., & Hill, J. (1991). Adult outcomes of childhood and adolescent depression: II. Risk for antisocial disorders. *Journal of the American Academy of Child & Adolescent Psychiatry, 30*, 434–439.

Harrington, R. C., Hill, J., Rutter, M., John, K., Fudge, H., Zoccolillo, M., & Weissman, M. M. (1988). The assessment of lifetime psychopathology: A comparison of two interviewing styles. *Psychological Medicine, 18*, 487–493.

Harrington, R. C., Rutter, M., Pickles, A., Fudge, H., Groothues, C., & Bredenkamp, D. (1996a). *Age trends in depressive symptomatology during early adolescence: Comparison with other psychological symptoms.* Manuscript in preparation.

Harrington, R. C., Rutter, M., Weissman, M., Fudge, H., Groothues, C., Bredenkamp, D., Rende, R., Pickles, A., & Wickramaratne, P. (1996b). Psychiatric disorders in the relatives of depressed probands. I. Comparison of prepubertal, adolescent and early adult onset forms. *Journal of Affective Disorders.*

Hewitt, J. K., Silberg, J. L., Rutter, M., Simonoff, E., Meyer, J. M., Maes, H., Pickles, A., et al. (1996). *Genetics and developmental psychopathology. I. Phenotypic assessment in the Virginia Twin Study of Adolescent Behavioral Development.* Manuscript submitted for publication.

Hill, J., Fudge, H., Harrington, R., Rutter, M., & Pickles, A. (1995). The Adult Personality Functioning Assessment (APFA): Factors influencing agreement between subject and informant. *Psychological Medicine, 25*, 263–275.

Hill, J., Harrington, R. C., Fudge, H., Rutter, M., & Pickles, A. (1989). Adult Personality Functioning Assessment (APFA): An investigator based standardized interview. *British Journal of Psychiatry, 155*, 24–35.

Kandel, D. B., & Davies, M. (1986). Adult sequelae of adolescent depressive symptoms. *Archives of General Psychiatry, 43*, 255–262.

Pearce, J. B. (1974). *Childhood depression.* MPhil Thesis, Univ. of London.

Pearce, J. B. (1978). The recognition of depressive disorder in children. *Journal of the Royal Society of Medicine, 71*, 494–500.

Rao, U., Ryan, N. D., Birmaher, B., Dahl, R. E., Williamson, D. E., Kaufman, J., Rao, R., & Nelson, B. (1995). Unipolar depression in adolescence: clinical outcome in adulthood. *Journal of the American Academy of Child and Adolescent Psychiatry 34*, 566–578.

Rao, U., Weissman, M. M., Martin, J. A., & Hammond, R. W. (1993). Childhood depression and risk of suicide: preliminary report of a longitudinal study. *Journal of the American Academy of Child & Adolescent Psychiatry, 32*, 21–27.

Rutter, M. (1991). Childhood experiences and adult social functioning. In G. R. Bock & J. Whelan (Eds.), *The childhood environment and adult disease. Ciba Foundation Symposium No. 156* (pp. 189–200). Chichester: Wiley.

Rutter, M., Champion, L., Quinton, D., Maughan, B., & Pickles. A. (1995). Origins of individual differences in environmental risk exposure. In P. Moen, G. Elder, & K. Luscher (Eds.), *Examining lives in context: Perspectives on the ecology of human development* (pp. 61–93). Washington DC: American Psychological Association.

Rutter, M., Graham, P., Chadwick, O. F., & Yule, W. (1976). Adolescent turmoil: Fact or fiction? *Journal of Child Psychology and Psychiatry, 17*, 35–56.

Rutter, M., Harrington, R., Quinton, D., & Pickles. A. (1994). Adult outcome of conduct disorder in childhood: implications for concepts and definitions of patterns of psychopathology. In R. D. Ketterlinus & M. E. Lamb (Eds.), *Adolescent problem behaviors* (pp. 57–80). Hillsdale, NJ: Erlbaum.

Rutter, M., Tizard, J., & Whitmore, K. (Eds.). (1970). *Education, health, and behaviour.* London: Longmans.

Simonoff, E., Pickles, A., Meyer, J., Silberg, J., Maes, H., Loeber, R., Rutter, M., Hewitt, J., & Eaves, M. (1996). *Epidemiology of child psychopathology in the Virginia twin study of adolescent behavioral development: Influences of age, gender and impairment on rates of disorder.* Manuscript submitted for publication.

Smith, A. L., & Weissman, M. M. (1992). Epidemiology. In E. S. Paykel (Ed.), *Handbook of affective disorders* 2nd ed., (pp. 111–129). Edinburgh: Churchill Livingstone.

Spitzer, R. L., Endicott, J., & Robins, E. (1978). Research diagnostic criteria: Rationale and reliability. *Archives of General Psychiatry, 35,* 773–782.

Weissman, M. M., Gammon, G. D., John, K., Merikangas, K. R., Warner, V., Prusoff, B. A., & Sholomskas, D. (1987). Children of depressed parents: Increased psychopathology and early onset of major depression. *Archives of General Psychiatry, 44,* 847–853.

Zeitlin, H. (1986). *The natural history of psychiatric disorder in children.* Oxford: Oxford University Press.

14

Presentation and Course of Major Depressive Disorder During Childhood and Later Years of the Life Span

Maria Kovacs

School of Medicine Western Psychiatric Institute and Clinic, University of Pittsburgh

Objective: *To examine whether major depressive disorder (MDD) in childhood, adolescence, and adulthood represents essentially the same diagnostic entity.* **Method:** *Recent publications on clinically referred patients with MDD that met certain selection criteria were examined to abstract information on six phenomenological features of the disorder: episode number, symptom presentation, psychiatric comorbidity, recovery from the index episode, recurrence of MDD, and switch to bipolar illness. The studies included both inpatients and outpatients with an age range of 6 to 80+ years.* **Results:** *Synthesizing the information across broad age groups revealed that clinically referred depressed youths, compared with adults and the elderly, are almost exclusively first-episode probands, evidence comparable symptom pictures, have similar rates of psychiatric comorbidity, recover somewhat faster from their index episode of MDD, have a similar recurrence rate, and are at greater risk for bipolar switch.* **Conclusions:** *MDD in clinically referred youths is similar in many regards to MDD in adults and the elderly. However, the findings that the risk of recurrent MDD among children approximates the rate among adults but, on average, about 20 years earlier in their lives, and that youths with unipolar depression convert to bipolar illness more frequently than do adults, suggest that very early onset MDD is a particularly serious form of affective illness.*

During the past 15 years, the existence of major depressive disorder (MDD) among children and adolescents has been conclusively documented in clinical settings and the community (Angold, 1988; Fleming & Offord, 1990). Nonetheless, questions have arisen about the developmental psychopathology of depression, the validity of the diagnosis in the younger years, and whether the disorder represents the same condition among youths and adults (Angold, 1988; Jensen et al., 1993;

Reprint with permission from *J. Am. Acad. Child Adolesc Psychiatry*, 1996, Vol. 35(6), 705-715. Copyright © 1996 by the American Academy of Child and Adolescent Psychiatry.

A previous version of this article was delivered at the Plenary Session of the Fiftieth Annual Meeting of the Society of Biological Psychiatry, Miami, May 17–21, 1995.

Preparation of this article was supported by NIMH grant MH33990.

Rutter, 1986). Does the presentation of major depression vary as a function of age? Does the course of depression in youths differ from the course of the disorder in adults? Are clinical outcomes of children and adolescents with MDD similar to the outcomes of adults who have been depressed (Rutter, 1986)?

In the present article, the above-noted questions are considered by evaluating the relevant literature on MDD during childhood, adolescence, and the later years of the life span. To accomplish this goal, it was necessary to ensure some comparability among studies. Therefore, only studies of clinically referred samples were considered, with preference given to recent investigations in which operational psychiatric diagnostic criteria and systematic evaluations were used. Reports on the course and outcome of MDD were excluded from consideration if the initial diagnoses or later status of patients was based solely on reassessments of prior records (e.g., Black, Goldstein, Nasvallah, & Winokur, 1991). Nonetheless, relevant investigations did vary in the strategies that were used to ascertain patients, the proportion of inpatients versus outpatients, and the operational diagnostic schemas that were applied. Three related definitions of major depression have been used, based on the Research Diagnostic Criteria (RDC) (Feighner et al., 1972), *DSM-III* (American Psychiatric Association, 1980), and *DSM-III-R* (American Psychiatric Association, 1987).

Therefore, several assumptions were adopted in evaluating the literature. The first assumption was that MDD, identified through the RDC, *DSM-III*, or *DSM-III-R*, reflects essentially the same psychopathological entity. The second assumption was that it is feasible to synthesize findings from clinical descriptive studies of individuals in the same broad developmental stage, regardless of the setting in which patients were recruited. The third assumption was that if findings concerning aspects of depression across major developmental stages or age groups appear to differ substantially, then the trends may be attributed to age differences in the study cohorts.

To determine whether features of major depression vary across the age span, six phenomenological aspects of the disorder are considered: episode number, symptom constellation, psychiatric comorbidity, recovery from the index episode of MDD, recurrence of MDD, and switch from unipolar MDD to bipolar affective illness.

PRESENTATION OF THE INDEX EPISODE

The Episode Number

There is impressive evidence that children and adolescents with MDD in clinical settings represent almost exclusively first-episode probands. As the figures in Table 1 indicate, from 90% to almost 100% of depressed youths who have been studied were in their first episodes, regardless of setting (inpatient versus outpatient). In contrast, among adults as well as the elderly, only approximately one third of clinically referred patients presented in their first MDD episode (Table 1). The preponderance of "new" cases of depression among clinically referred youths has also made it possible for McCauley and associates (1993) to study solely first-episode patients.

The significance of the recency of illness onset among depressed youths derives from the fact that prognosis at presentation appears to be episode-dependent. For instance, among adults, multiple episodes of depression are associated with worse outcome with regard to remission and risk of recurrence (e.g., Keller, Lavori, Lewis, & Klerman 1983b). Furthermore, switching from unipolar to bipolar illness typically occurs after the patient has cycled through several episodes of depression (Akiskal et al., 1983). Thus, the prognosis for MDD in childhood would be expected to be considerably better than for MDD in the later years of the life span.

TABLE 1
Rate of First-Episode Major Depression in Clinically Referred Samples

Age Range of Sample	N	Recruitment Site	First-Episode Cases (%)	Reference
8–13	92	OP	95	(Kovacs et al., unpublished)
13–16	60	IP	97	(Strober and Carlson, 1982)
13–17	58	IP	90	(Strober et al., 1993)
17–79	431	IP/OP	37	(Keller et al., 1992)
18–60+	242	IP/OP	33	(Brodaty et al., 1991)
20–73	243	OP	26	(Rush et al., 1995)
60–+	127	IP	29	(Hinrichsen, 1992)

Note: For recruitment site, OP = outpatient setting and IP = inpatient setting.

Symptoms

It has long been posited that there exist age-related changes in the expression and rates of depressive symptoms (e.g., Poznanski, 1982). However, the descriptive information is sparse and does not readily lend itself to synthesis. Some symptoms (e.g., suicide attempt or suicide ideation) have been defined in various ways by different investigators. Furthermore, symptom prevalence can be affected by whether the ratings refer to patients' initial presentation, the worst point, or any point in the episode. Finally, even when differential rates in *specific* symptoms are evident across age groups, such trends may reflect age-related parameters, including changes in health status (Gallo, Anthony, & Muthen, 1994), rather than variable developmental expression of the disorder. Therefore, only very general statements may be made about symptom expression in MDD across the age span.

The most consistent empiric evidence regarding developmental changes in symptom presentation of MDD concerns hypersomnia. Children appear to be far less likely to evidence hypersomnia than adolescents, and the rate then increases in adulthood, but eventually the rate declines so that adults are more likely to have this form of sleep disturbance than the elderly (Brodaty et al., 1991; Kovacs & Gatsonis, 1989; Mitchell, McCauley, Burke, & Moss, 1988; Ryan et al., 1987). There also are indications that weight loss and appetite loss may be subject to developmental variation; in one group of depressed youths, most of whom were outpatients, few children had weight loss as compared with adolescents (Ryan et al., 1987), although in another group, children and adolescents had similarly low rates of this symptom (Mitchell et al., 1988). Elderly depressed patients appear to have the highest rates of appetite or weight loss and are much more likely to have these symptoms than young or middle-age depressed adults (Blazer, Bachar, & Hughes, 1987; Brodaty et al., 1991). The presence of delusion may also be developmentally mediated. Delusions in conjunction with MDD appear to be infrequent in younger patients, with children and adolescents possibly having similar rates (Chambers, Puig-Antich, Tabrizi, & Davies, 1982; Mitchell et al., 1988; Ryan et al., 1987). But once again, elderly patients with MDD seem to have higher rates of delusions than young or middle-age adults (Brodaty et al., 1991). Evidence regarding developmental changes in other symptoms of depression is unsystematic and inconclusive.

Comorbidity with Other Psychiatric Disorders

High rates of concurrent psychiatric disorders have been consistently detected in studies of depressed children and adolescents. The prevalence of psychiatric comorbidity among youths with MDD has led some investigators to question the validity of *DSM-III* or RDC for depression in younger age

TABLE 2
Rates of Comorbid Disorders in Clinically Referred Samples with Major Depression

Comorbid Disorder	Adults				Children			
	Ages	Recruitment Site	N	Rate (%)	Ages	Recruitment Site	N	Rate (%)
Any Axis I disorder	36(12)[a]	OP	197[1]	59	8–13	OP	62[8]	81
	38(11)[a,b]	OP	116[2]	88	11(4)[a,c]	OP	136[9]	96
Dysthymic disorder	17–79	IP/OP	316[3]	25	8–13	OP	87[10]	35
	29(7)[a,c]	OP	81[4]	38	6–13	IP	45[11]	40
	41(13)[a,c]	OP	101[5]	41	11(4)[a,c]	OP	136[9]	13
	24–87	IP/OP	113[6]	65	12–18	?	28[12]	21
	60+	IP	127[7]	9	7–17	IP/OP	95[13]	13
Anxiety disorder	29(7)[a,c]	OP	81[4]	58	8–13	OP	87[10]	51
	36(12)[a]	OP	197[1]	42	6–13	IP	45[11]	40
	38(11)[a,b]	OP	116[2]	47	12–18	?	28[12]	32
	41(13)[a,c]	OP	101[5]	34	12–18	IP	48[14]	23
	24–87	IP/OP	113[6]	73[d]	11(4)[a,c]	OP	136[9]	35[e]
Substance use disorder	29(7)[a,c]	OP	81[4]	35	12–18	IP	48[14]	4
	36(12)[a]	OP	197[1]	15				
	38(11)[a,b]	OP	116[2]	25				
Conduct disorder					8–13	OP	62[8]	15
					7–17	IP/OP	95[13]	15
					12–18	?	28[12]	7
					11(4)[a,c]	OP	136[9]	24
					6–18	IP/OP	187[15]	13

Note: For recruitment site, OP = outpatient setting and IP = inpatient setting.
[a]Mean (*SD*).
[b]Early history for early-onset cases.
[c]Estimated figure.
[d]Generalized anxiety disorder only.
[e]Overanxious disorder only.
[1]Sanderson et al., 1990; [2]Alpert et al., 1994; [3]Keller et al., 1983a; [4]Klein et al., 1988; [5]Levitt et al., 1991; [6]Hughes et al., 1993; [7]Hinrichsen, 1992; [8]Kovacs et al., 1988, 1989; [9]Biederman et al., 1995; [10]Kovacs et al., unpublished; [11]Ferro et al., 1994; [12]Rao et al., 1995; [13]Mitchell et al., 1988; [14]Shain et al., 1991; [15]Ryan et al., 1987.

groups (e.g., Angold, 1988). It also has been implicitly suggested that, given the comparative rarity of uncomplicated MDD among youths, depression in childhood may be a different clinical entity than depression in the later years. However, the literature reveals that, when full differential diagnoses of adult probands are conducted, high rates of nonaffective disorders are found in postadolescent age groups as well.

Table 2 presents rates of comorbidity of MDD with any other psychiatric disorder and with the most commonly reported specific diagnoses. The indications are that rates of comorbid psychiatric disorders among children and youths are similar to, or only slightly higher than, rates in adults and the elderly. Indeed, the data are remarkably consistent given that (1) comorbidity was defined in variable ways, including lifetime comorbidity, episode comorbidity, or comorbidity at clinical presentation; and (2) the samples differed in proportions of inpatients and outpatients.

Comorbidity with any Axis I or Axis II psychiatric disorder appears to characterize about 60% and 90% of depressed adults, and about 80% to 95% of children and youths (Table 2). Dysthymic disorder coexists with MDD in approximately 30% of youngsters and adults, with inconsistent data on rates in the elderly. In tabulating the data on comorbid anxiety disorders, preference was given to publications that included a summary figure for "any" anxiety disorder. The reason for this decision was that the various anxiety disorders themselves tend to be comorbid (Last, Hersen, Kazdin, Finkelstein, & Strauss, 1987), and listing the rates for specific anxiety diagnoses overestimates the number of cases with anxiety disorder.

It appears that slightly more than about one third of depressed juveniles suffer from anxiety disorders and that the rate may be somewhat higher, at around 40% to 50%, among depressed adults. Generalized anxiety disorder is the single most prevalent comorbid diagnosis among depressed adults (e.g., Sanderson, Beck, & Beck, 1990), and separation anxiety disorder is the most prevalent comorbid diagnosis among depressed children (Kovacs & Gatsonis, 1989). Substance use disorder, a comorbid condition in about one quarter of depressed adults, is not typically evident in younger probands owing to the stringent criteria that have to be met in *DSM-III* and *DSM-III-R*. However, conduct disorder, which is the closest "juvenile" equivalent of substance use–related diagnoses, is present in about 15% of depressed children. Therefore, overall, the indications are that comorbid psychiatric disorders with MDD occur at similar rates in children, adolescents, and adults, while data regarding the elderly are inconsistent.

CLINICAL COURSE

The three most commonly examined indices of the clinical course of depression have been recovery from the index episode (or its converse, chronicity), recurrence (or relapse into a further episode), and switch from unipolar to bipolar illness. It has been posited that the clinical course of depression may be affected by the age of the patient (e.g., Alexopoulos, Young, Abrams, Meyers, & Shamoian, 1989; Rutter, 1986). However, the effects of age on outcome are complicated by the fact that the older the patient, the greater the likelihood of having experienced multiple episodes of depression. In turn, a history of previous depression is known to influence prognosis of the index episode (Keller et al., 1982, 1992).

Recovery from the Index Episode of MDD

Recovery from an episode can be described as the rate of remission or the proportion of cases who went into remission at various points in time, as well as the duration of the episode. In general, the most useful information is the length of time from the *onset* of the episode until the patient meets criteria for having achieved remission.

Three types of data are needed to estimate the rate of remission or length of an episode: date of the onset of the episode, specific criteria for remission, and date of remission. Because some patients will discontinue participation in a study prior to recovery and some others may still be symptomatic at the last assessment, the most desirable way to report recovery data is by means of the Kaplan-Meier (K-M) estimator (Kalbfleish & Prentice, 1980). The K-M estimator is a longitudinal statistical approach that takes into consideration that patients may have been under observation for different time intervals and that only partial information is available on those who had not yet recovered from their depression at the last observation. Unfortunately, few reports include K-M statistics using the onset date of an episode. Typically, outcome is described since the time of clinical referral or admission up until a particular point, such as a 1- or 2-year follow-up evaluation (e.g., Keitner, Ryan, Miller, & Norman, 1992; Shain, King, Naylor, & Alessi, 1991).

Table 3 includes only studies in which recovery from the episode was defined in a diagnostic and categorical fashion, requiring that patients *maintain an essentially asymptomatic state for at least eight consecutive weeks*. The upper portion of Table 3 contains information on the cumulative probability of

TABLE 3

Recovery from Major Depression in Clinically Referred Samples

Time from Onset of Episode	Adults		Children	
	Index Episode	Prospective Episode	Index Episode	Index Episode
By 6 months	.34	.55	.33	.40
By 1 year	.50	.73	.69	.80
By 1.5 years	—	.78	.82	.95
By 2 years	.64	.83	.86	.98
Median (approx), months	12	4.4	9	7
Sample size	101[1]	359[2]	87[3]	100[4]
Age at entry, years	17–79	17–79	8–13	7–17
Recruitment site	IP/OP	IP/OP	OP	IP/OP
Time from Study Entry	Adults			Children
By 6 months	.54			.48
By 1 year	.70			.81
By 2 years	.81			.90
Median (approx), months	5–6			6
Sample size	431[5]			58[6]
Age at entry, years	17–79			13–17
Recruitment site	IP/OP			IP

Note: Figures are approximate because some of them represent extrapolations from published data or graphs. All figures are Kaplan-Meier estimates. For recruitment site, OP = outpatient setting and IP = inpatient setting.
[1]Keller et al., 1982; [2]Coryell et al., 1994; [3]Kovacs et al., unpublished; [4]McCauley et al., 1993; [5]Keller et al., 1992; [6]Strober et al., 1993.

recovery *from onset* of MDD, and the lower portion contains data on recovery estimated from the time of study entry or clinical referral. The indications are that among children and adolescents, time to recovery from onset of index MDD is shorter than among adults. Among youths, median time to recovery from MDD is approximately 7 to 9 months and the average length of depressive episode is about 9 months (McCauley et al., 1993). Among adults, median time to recovery is about 12 months (Table 3).

Recovery from the index episode, which prompted study entry and treatment, appears to differ from recovery from subsequently observed and not necessarily treated episodes. Confirming an early report of the National Institute of Mental Health (NIMH) collaborative study (Keller et al., 1986), a subsequent follow-up revealed that recovery from the first prospectively observed MDD episode was faster than recovery from the index MDD episode (Table 3; Coryell et al., 1994). A longitudinal study of initially clinically referred 8- to 13-year-old children revealed a similar trend: recovery was faster from the first prospectively observed MDD episode than the index MDD episode (Kovacs, unpublished data, 1994). It appears, therefore, that, *in the same patients,* treatment referral may indicate a more severe episode of depression.

In some studies, recovery was estimated from the time of clinical referral (rather than episode onset). However, this approach disregards the length of the disorder *prior* to referral, yields a biased estimate, and obscures apparent age-related differences. More specifically, the rate of recovery from study entry may look more favorable than the rate of recovery computed from episode onset. In the recent report of the NIMH collaborative study (Keller et al., 1992), 70% of the patients recovered by 1 year after study entry (Table 3, lower portion), compared with the 50% rate by 1 year from onset of index episode (Table 3, upper portion). A similarly positive outcome was reported for an elderly cohort (60 years or older) using the assessment methods of the collaborative study; 1 year past study admission, 72% of the patients recovered from their MDD (Hinrichsen, 1992).

The faster recovery rate, or shorter episode length in the younger years compared with adulthood (Table 3, upper portion), is obscured when remission is calculated from study entry or clinical referral (Table 3, lower portion). This appears to be due to the fact that youths present for clinical care earlier in their episodes of MDD than do adults. In the study by Strober, Lampert, Schmidt, & Morell (1993), cited in Table 3 (lower portion), the mean episode length at admission was 21 weeks, with a range from 6 to 50 weeks. In contrast, in the Keller et al. (1992) study, the median episode length for depressed adults was 30 weeks at study entry, with 13 weeks and 73 weeks corresponding to the lower and upper quartiles of illness duration.

Recurrence of an Episode of MDD

The recurrent nature of depressive illness has long been recognized (Kraepelin, 1968; Zis & Goodwin, 1979) and was generally identified when patients were rehospitalized. In more recent follow-up studies, however, recurrence was ascertained on the basis of prescheduled clinical examinations (as opposed to treatment seeking), yielding more accurate data on clinical course. Unfortunately, many publications on the outcome of depressed patients could not be included in the present overview for two reasons: (1) recurrence and relapse were not distinguished from one another, and (2) outcome was defined by means of unstandardized clinical judgement or cutoff scores on depressive symptom scales (e.g., Blackburn, Eunson, & Bishop, 1986).

Rates of recurrence are best conveyed by the K-M estimator, described in connection with recovery from an episode of MDD. However, in almost all articles, recurrence is reported as the proportion of patients from the initial sample who had a new episode of depression at follow-up. Percent figures are probably underestimates of the true rate of recurrence. Furthermore, methodological issues, such as differences in the definitions of the period of risk, also have to be taken into consideration as accounting for some of the variability in findings (see Belsher & Costello, 1988, for a discussion of methodological issues).

The data in Table 4 are grouped by length of follow-up, because recurrence is time-dependent. In the upper half of Table 4, the shortest observation interval is associated with the study by Shea et al. (1992), involving an 18-month naturalistic follow-up of patients after they finished a randomized treatment study. Overall, although rates of recurrence of MDD are somewhat lower in child and adolescent probands than adults, the variation across the age span is not substantial. On longer follow-up, spanning an average of approximately 7 years, up to 90% of initially clinically referred, depressed, adult patients have at least one recurrent episode of MDD. Over a much longer follow-up of 18 years (not cited in Table 4), 95% of a sample of 65 inpatients (ascertained at ages 16 to 75 years) were found to have recurrent depression (Lee & Murray, 1988). About 70% of previously clinically referred children and adolescents have a recurrent MDD when followed up for 5 or more years. At the time of their reassessment, most of the children and adolescents in the studies cited in Table 4 were in their early to mid-20s. Therefore, these initially first-episode cohorts convert to multiple episodes relatively early in their lives.

Switch from Unipolar MDD to Bipolar Disorder

The distinction between unipolar and bipolar illness has long been considered important with regard to affective disorders among adults. It is generally accepted that these two diagnostic entities

TABLE 4
Recurrent Major Depression in Clinically Referred Samples

Mean Follow-up	Adults				Children			
	Initial Age	Recruitment Site	N	Rate (%)	Initial Age	Recruitment Site	N	Rate (%)
Up to 3 years	17–79[1]	IP/OP	336	30	7–17[6]	IP/OP	65	54[a]
	19–60[2]	OP	41	32				
	21–60[3]	OP	76	38				
	37(9)[4,b]	OP	50	32				
5–7 years	17–79[5]	IP/OP	401	90	6–12[7]	IP	16	44
					8–13[8]	OP	102	40
					12–18[9]	?	26	69

Note: For each study, N refers to cases on whom follow-up information was available. For recruitment site, OP = outpatient setting and IP = inpatient setting.
[a] Kaplan-Meier estimate.
[b] Mean *(SD)*.
[1] Keller et al., 1986; [2] Gonzales et al., 1985; [3] Shea et al., 1992; [4] Thase et al., 1992; [5] Coryell et al., 1994; [6] McCauley et al., 1993; [7] Hughes et al., 1990; [8] Kovacs et al., 1994; [9] Rao et al., 1995.

are associated with differential familial aggregation of psychiatric disorders, differences in long-term clinical course, and different treatment needs (Gershon, Dunner, & Goodwin, 1971). However, among unipolar depressed probands who are predisposed to bipolarity, the probability of converting to bipolar illness is partly a function of time since the onset of the affective disorder and the number of episodes of depression (Dunner, Fleiss, & Fieve, 1976). Moreover, clinical experience with adults suggests that if a switch to bipolarity is to occur in a given episode of unipolar major depression, it will take place within a few months after the onset of that particular episode of MDD (e.g., Angst, 1987).

Information on rates of conversion from unipolar depression to bipolar illness has been somewhat muddled by disagreements as to whether the bipolar I (mania) and bipolar II (hypomania) forms reflect the same psychopathology (Endicott et al., 1985; Heun & Maier, 1993; Kupfer, Carpenter, & Frank, 1988). The disagreement has been fueled partly by the low rate of conversion from hypomania to mania in adults. However, estimates of the stability of polarity are influenced by the methods of computation. In one study, for example, about 13% of initially bipolar II patients were estimated to convert to mania when longitudinal statistical methods were used; but a cross-sectional summary revealed only a 7.5% conversion rate (Coryell et al., 1995).

In the younger ages, the bipolar I versus II distinction is still open to debate. In one study, 50% of the young patients who had bipolar II disorder (hypomania) developed frank manic illness or bipolar I disorder during an average follow-up period of 8 years (Kovacs & Pollock, 1995). However, in another investigation involving a 2- to 5-year follow-up, only 12% of the children with bipolar II diagnoses converted to bipolar I (Geller, Fox, & Clark, 1994). Possibly, during the juvenile years, the rate at which bipolar I disorder develops into bipolar II is time-dependent.

In Table 5, data are presented on the rate of switch or conversion from unipolar to bipolar illness in various samples of previously clinically referred depressed youths or adults. There are relatively few long-term naturalistic follow-up studies of large groups of patients with depressive disorders. Therefore, Table 5 includes information from two investigations in which clinical data were gathered prior to the use of research psychiatric interviews and operational diagnostic criteria (Angst, 1987; Winokur & Morrison, 1973). The figure cited from Angst (1987) concerns only the outcome of patients hospitalized from 1958 onward.

TABLE 5
Conversion from Unipolar Major Depression to Bipolar Disorder in Clinically Referred Samples
on Prospective Follow-up

Mean Follow-up	Adults				Children			
	Initial Age	Recruitment Site	N	Rate (%)	Initial Age	Recruitment Site	N	Rate (%)
Up to 5 years	"Adults"	IP	414[1]	4.6[a]	6–12	OP	79[6]	14.1[b]
	45 (median)	IP	212[2]	4.3	—	—	—[6]	36.8[a,b]
	14–67	OP	206[3]	19.9	7–17	IP/OP	65[7]	7.7[a]
	25(6)[c]	IP	49[4]	6.1	13–16	IP	60[8]	20.0
					13–17	IP	58[9]	8.6[a]
5–10 years	17–79	IP/OP	362[5]	4.1	8–13	OP	92[10]	21.0[a,b]
	—	—	—[5]	9.1[a]	12–18	?	26[11]	19.0

Note: For recruitment site, OP = outpatient setting and IP = inpatient setting.
[a]Bipolar I and II combined.
[b]Kaplan-Meier estimate.
[c]Mean (SD).
[1]Angst, 1987; [2]Winokur and Morrison, 1973; and Winokur et al., 1972; [3]Akiskal et al., 1983; [4]Goldberg et al., 1995; [5]Coryell et al., 1995; [6]Geller et al., 1994; [7]McCauley et al., 1993; [8]Strober and Carlson, 1982; [9]Strober et al., 1993; [10]Kovacs et al., 1994, and unpublished; [11]Rao et al., 1995.

The findings are striking in view of the fact that, across studies of adults as well as children, the assessment approaches and diagnostic strategies were variable. The inevitable conclusion is that very early onset depression is a marker of bipolar illness. As shown, the switch rate from unipolar depression to bipolar illness in adult cohorts is generally lower than 10%. In contrast, bipolar illness can be expected to develop in up to 20% to 30% of depressed children while they are still in their teens or early 20s. In the two studies of youths where the lowest switch rates of 7.7% (McCauley et al., 1993) and 8.6% (Strober et al., 1993) were found, the follow-up intervals were relatively short, with 3 years and 2 years of observation, respectively.

DISCUSSION

Is there evidence that the diagnosis of MDD in childhood and in the later years of the life span capture the same psychopathological entity? Are there significant developmental variations in illness expression as a function of age? Based on the present overview of recent literature, the answer appears to be "yes" to the first question, and a qualified "no" to the second question. Indeed, with a few notable exceptions, the most striking aspect of the literature is the similarity of features of MDD across groups of juveniles and older patients who typically differ in age by an average of about 20 years.

Episode Number and Symptoms of MDD

Given their youth, it is not surprising that children and adolescents with MDD in clinical settings represent almost entirely first-episode probands. This particular feature of depression in the younger age groups has a twofold significance. First, by prospectively following young patients with major depression, it becomes possible to characterize the course of this condition from the beginning and perhaps to identify early prognosticators of long-term outcomes. Second, because they are in their first episodes of depression, one would expect a better prognosis for depressed youths than depressed adults. However, such a positive expectation is weakly supported by the available information.

With regard to developmental variations in the features of MDD, there is no compelling evidence that the cardinal symptoms of MDD have significantly different rates of occurrence across the age span in clinically referred samples. A similar conclusion was reached by Ryan et al. (1987) in their study of depressed children and adolescents, most of whom were outpatients. Indeed, there was "relatively little variation" from childhood through adolescence (ages 6 through 18 years) in rates of RDC symptoms of major depression. The most consistent evidence regarding the effects of age on depressive symptoms concerns neurovegetative and severe cognitive problems. Variability in rates of neurovegetative symptoms across the age span could reflect the maturing of neuroendocrine systems, while increase in severe cognitive symptoms could reflect "cerebral aging" or changing brain functioning with age (Brodaty et al., 1991).

Psychiatric Comorbidity

Comorbidity has been documented in epidemiological surveys of youths as well as adults (Caron & Rutter, 1991; Robins & Regier, 1991). Although the existence of psychiatric comorbidity is now generally accepted, there are unresolved issues about its validity and significance (for an incisive discussion, see Caron & Rutter, 1991). Assuming that the coexistence of other disorders with depression is a valid phenomenon, two conclusions can be drawn from the literature. First, regardless of age, the vast majority of depressed patients have comorbid disorders. Second, also regardless of age, some type of anxiety disorder is the single most prevalent diagnosis in conjunction with depression.

However, comorbidity does entail different combinations and sequencing of specific disorders as a function of age. Among depressed youths, attention deficit disorder or enuresis-encopresis account for some of the overall comorbidity, whereas in the later years of the life span, other comorbid conditions such as panic disorder come into play. The anxiety disorder that predominates among clinically referred depressed children and young adolescents is separation anxiety disorder (Kovacs et al., 1989; Ryan et al., 1987), while among adults it is generalized anxiety disorder (e.g., Hughes, DeMallie, & Blazer, 1993; Sanderson et al., 1990). Moreover, among young patients with MDD and comorbid anxiety disorder, the anxiety disorder precedes the depression about two thirds of the time (Alpert, Maddocks, Rosenbaum, & Fava, 1994; Kovacs et al., 1989). However, among adults with comorbid MDD and anxiety, the converse has been observed, with depression having predated the anxiety disorder about two thirds of the time (Sanderson et al., 1990). Unfortunately, the significance of the temporal sequencing of comorbid disorders in depressed patients has not been well studied and its implications are not known.

Recovery and Recurrence

Clinically referred children and adolescents with MDD appear to recover somewhat faster from their index episode of depression than do adults. While it has been proposed that in elderly patients, poor medical health, social isolation, and other adverse correlates of advanced age would lead to more protracted depressions, the evidence has been equivocal (Alexopoulos et al., 1989). Although, in general, the length of the index MDD episode does not substantially differ across the age span, it is more than likely that predictors of recovery are related to a patient's developmental stage. However, in the studies that were reviewed, variability in the predictor sets precluded a cogent examination of this issue.

The positive short-term outcome for depressed children and adolescents is tempered by the fact that they have recurrent episodes relatively early in their lives. Because recent follow-up studies of clinically referred and operationally diagnosed youths have not yet extended into adulthood, the eventual recurrence rate of juveniles will probably equal the rate reported for adults, but at an earlier age. This expectation is supported by the findings of Harrington and associates (1990) on the outcome of symptomatically depressed children who were reassessed approximately 18 years after referal. The presenting diagnoses of the children were verified retrospectively, from clinical case records. On follow-up, the cumulative probability of an episode of depression was .60 (60%), a rate that was significantly higher than that among psychiatric controls. Furthermore, having had at least one new episode of depression after age 17 prognosticated a further episode almost 100% of the time.

Switch from Unipolar Depression to Bipolar Illness

Akiskal (e.g., Akiskal et al., 1983) has argued for many years that early age at onset of depressive disorder is a prognosticator of bipolar outcome. Recent prospectively gathered information does suggest that the risk of bipolar outcome is up to threefold higher in childhood-onset unipolar depression than in later-onset depression. Therefore, the indications are that very early onset depression portends a high propensity for *early* bipolar switch.

According to Akiskal et al. (1983), if onset of illness is identified as the first clinical depression (rather than first episode of endogenous or primary depression or first hospitalization), then patients who eventually switch polarity generally do so about 4 years after depression onset (median interval), and the switch is most likely to occur after two to four episodes of MDD. The latter information suggests an acceleration of bipolar course in more recently studied predisposed individuals, compared with cohorts who received their diagnosis several decades ago. For example, a record review of patients who were hospitalized during a period of several decades prior to 1982 (Angst, 1985) showed that in those earlier birth cohorts there was a fairly long time interval between illness onset and "switch" in polarity (a median of more than 10 years) and more intervening depressive episodes (median of seven).

According to studies of both clinically referred youths and adults, if a switch is to occur in a *given episode* of unipolar depression, it is likely to take place relatively early after the onset of that episode of depression. In one group of hospitalized adults (Angst, 1987), the median length of the index depressive episode was about 4 months when the "switch" occurred, with approximately 75% of the conversions having taken place by about 8 months after the onset of depression. Among 13- to 16-year-old adolescents, a subset of whom had mania on prospective follow-up, the switch occurred on an average of 28 weeks after index admission (Strober and Carlson, 1982). Therefore, if a switch from unipolar depression to bipolar illness is to occur in a given episode, its temporal unfolding seems to be very similar in youths and adults.

Clinical Implications

Mindful of differences in methodologies, ascertainment strategies, population samples, and reporting practices, the present overview of recent studies of clinically referred patients with MDD suggests that, while juvenile-onset depression is generally similar to depression in adulthood, early onset portends a worse course in several respects. The favorable initial likelihood of recovery from depression in childhood is followed by a high rate of recurrence. There also is a notable risk of conversion to bipolar illness. Just as it is in adulthood, the course of childhood-onset MDD is complicated by psychiatric comorbidity. The finding that similar clinical outcomes are observable among youths and adults, but, on average, about 20 years earlier in the life span, underscores the gravity of early diagnosis. The treatment and management of youths with MDD therefore presents a challenge and suggests the importance of *long-term*, continued monitoring, clinical care, and patient education.

REFERENCES

Akiskal, H. S., Walker, P., Puzantian, V. R., King, D., Rosenthal, T. L., & Dranon, M. (1983). Bipolar outcome in the course of depressive illness. Phenomenologic, familial, and pharmacologic predictors. *J. Affect. Disord., 5*, 115–128.

Alexopoulos, G. S., Young, R. C., Abrams, R. C., Meyers, B., & Shamoian, C. A. (1989). Chronicity and relapse in geriatric depression. *Biol. Psychiatry, 26*, 551–564.

Alpert, J. E., Maddocks, A., Rosenbaum, J. F., & Fava, M. (1994). Childhood psychopathology retrospectively assessed among adults with early onset major depression. *J. Affect. Disord., 31*, 165–171.

American Psychiatric Association (1980). *Diagnostic and statistical manual of mental disorders (DSM-III).* (3rd ed.). Washington, DC: American Psychiatric Association.

American Psychiatric Association (1987). *Diagnostic and statistical manual of mental disorders (DSM-III-R).* (3rd ed. rev.) Washington, DC: American Psychiatric Association.

Angold, A. (1988). Childhood and adolescent depression: II. Research in clinical populations. *Br. J. Psychiatry, 153*, 476–492.

Angst, J. (1985). Switch from depression to mania: A record study over decades between 1920 and 1982. *Psychopathology, 18*, 140–154.

Angst, J. (1987). Switch from depression to mania, or from mania to depression. *J. Psychopharmacol., 1*, 13–19.

Belsher, G., & Costello, C. G. (1988). Relapse after recovery from unipolar depression: A critical review. *Psychol. Bull., 104*, 84–96.

Biederman, J., Faraone, S., Mick, E., & Lelon, E. (1995). Psychiatric comorbidity among referred juveniles with major depression: Fact or artifact? *J. Am. Acad. Child Adolesc. Psychiatry, 34*, 579–590.

Black, D. W., Goldstein, R. B., Nasrallah, A., & Winokur, G. (1991). The prediction of recovery using a multivariate model in 1,471 depressed inpatients. *Eur. Arch. Psychiatry. Clin. Neurosci., 241*, 41–45.

Blackburn, I. M., Eunson, K. M., & Bishop, S. (1986). A two-year naturalistic follow-up of depressed patients treated with cognitive therapy, pharmacotherapy and a combination of both. *J. Affect. Disord., 10*, 67–75.

Blazer, D., Bachar, J. R., & Hughes, D. C. (1987). Major depression with melancholia: A comparison of middle-aged and elderly adults. *J. Am. Geriatr. Soc., 35*, 927–932.

Brodaty, H., Peters, K., Boyce, P. et al. (1991). Age and depression. *J. Affect. Disord., 23*, 137–149.

Caron, C., & Rutter, M. (1991). Comorbidity in child psychopathology: Concepts, issues and research strategies. *J. Child Psychol. Psychiatry, 32*, 1063–1080.

Chambers, W. J., Puig-Antich, J., Tabrizi, M. A., & Davies, M. (1982). Psychotic symptoms in prepubertal major depressive disorder. *Arch. Gen. Psychiatry, 39*, 921–927.

Coryell, W., Akiskal, H. S., Leon, A. C. et al. (1994). The time course of nonchronic major depressive disorder. Uniformity across episodes and samples. *Arch. Gen. Psychiatry, 51*, 405–410.

Coryell, W., Endicott, J., Maser, J. D., Keller, M. B., Leon, A. C., & Akiskal, H. S. (1995). Long-term stability of polarity distinctions in the affective disorders. *Am. J. Psychiatry, 152*, 385–390.

Dunner, D. L., Fleiss, J. L., & Fieve, R. R. (1976). The course of development of mania in patients with recurrent depression. *Am. J. Psychiatry, 133*, 905–908.

Endicott, J., Nee, J., Andreasen, N., Clayton, P., Keller, M., & Coryell, W. (1985). Bipolar II. Combine or keep separate? *J. Affect. Disord., 8*, 17–28.

Feighner, J. P., Robins, E., Guze, S. B., Woodruff, R. A., Winokur, G., & Munoz, R. (1972). Diagnostic criteria for use in psychiatric research. *Arch. Gen. Psychiatry, 26*, 57–63.

Ferro, T., Carlson, G. A., Grayson, P., & Klein, D. N. (1994). Depressive disorders: Distinctions in children. *J. Am. Acad. Child Adolesc. Psychiatry, 33*, 664–670.

Fleming, J. E., & Offord, D. R. (1990). Epidemiology of childhood depressive disorders: A critical review. *J. Am. Acad. Child Adolesc. Psychiatry, 29*, 571–580.

Gallo, J. J., Anthony, J. C., & Muthen, B. O. (1994). Age differences in the symptoms of depression: A latent trait analysis. *J. Gerontol, 49*, P251–P264.

Geller, B., Fox, L. W., & Clark, K. A. (1994). Rate and predictors of prepubertal bipolarity during follow-up of 6- to 12-year-old depressed children. *J. Am. Acad. Child Adolesc. Psychiatry, 33*, 461–468.

Gershon, E. S., Dunner, D. L., & Goodwin, F. K. (1971). Toward a biology of affective disorders. Genetic contributions. *Arch. Gen. Psychiatry, 25*, 1–15.

Goldberg, J. F., Harrow, M., & Grossman, L. S. (1995). Course and outcome in bipolar affective disorder: A longitudinal follow-up study. *Am. J. Psychiatry, 152*, 379–384.

Gonzales, L. R., Lewinsohn, P. M., & Clarke, G. N. (1985). Longitudinal follow-up of unipolar depressives: An investigation of predictors of relapse. *J. Consult. Clin. Psychol., 53*, 461–469.

Harrington, R., Fudge, H., Rutter, M., Pickles, A., & Hill, J. (1990). Adult outcomes of childhood and adolescent depression. I. Psychiatric status. *Arch. Gen. Psychiatry, 47*, 465–473.

Heun, R., & Maier, W. (1993). The distinction of bipolar II disorder from bipolar I and recurrent unipolar depression: Results of a controlled family study. *Acta. Psychiatr. Scand., 87*, 279–284.

Hinrichsen, G. A. (1992). Recovery and relapse from major depressive disorder in the elderly. *Am. J. Psychiatry, 149*, 1575–1579.

Hughes, C. W., Preskorn, S. H., Wrona, M., Hassanein, R., & Tucker, S. (1990). Followup of adolescents initially treated for prepubertal-onset major depressive disorder with imipramine. *Psychopharmacol. Bull., 26*, 244–248.

Hughes, D. C., DeMallie, D., & Blazer, D. G. (1993). Does age make a difference in the effects of physical health and social support on the outcome of a major depressive episode? *Am. J. Psychiatry, 150*, 728–733.

Jensen, P. S., Koretz, D., Locke, B. Z. et al. (1993). Child and adolescent psychopathology research: Problems and prospects for the 1990s. *J. Abnorm. Child Psychol, 21*, 551–580.

Kalbfleish, J. D., & Prentice, R. L. (1980). *The Statistical Analysis of Failure Time Data.* New York: John Wiley.

Keitner, G. I., Ryan, C. E., Miller, I. W., & Norman, W. H. (1992). Recovery and major depression: Factors associated with twelve-month outcome. *Am. J. Psychiatry, 149*, 93–99.

Keller, M. B., Lavori, P. W., Endicott, J., Coryell, W., & Klerman, G. L. (1983a). "Double depression": Two-year follow-up. *Am. J. Psychiatry, 140*, 689–694.

Keller, M. B., Lavori, P. W., Lewis, C. E., & Klerman, G. L. (1983b). Predictors of relapse in major depressive disorder. *JAMA 250*, 3299–3304.

Keller, M. B., Lavori, P. W., Mueller, T. I. et al. (1992). Time to recovery, chronicity, and levels of psychopathology in major depression. A 5-year prospective follow-up of 431 subjects. *Arch. Gen. Psychiatry, 49*, 809–816.

Keller, M. B., Lavori, P. W., Rice, J., Coryell, W., & Hirschfeld, R. M. A. (1986). The persistent risk of chronicity in recurrent episodes of nonbipolar major depressive disorder: A prospective follow-up. *Am. J. Psychiatry, 143*, 24–28.

Keller, M. B, Shapiro, R. W., Lavori, P. W., & Wolfe, N. (1982). Recovery in major depressive disorder. Analysis with the life table and regression models. *Arch. Gen. Psychiatry, 39*, 905–910.

Klein, D. N., Taylor, E. B., Harding, K., & Dickstein, S. (1988). Double depression and episodic major depression: Demographic, clinical, familial, personality, and socioenvironmental characteristics and short-term outcome. *Am. J. Psychiatry, 145*, 1226–1231.

Kovacs, M., Akiskal, H. S., Gatsonis, C., & Parrone, P. L. (1994). Childhood-onset dysthymic disorder. Clinical features and prospective naturalistic outcome. *Arch. Gen. Psychiatry, 51*, 365–374.

Kovacs, M., & Gatsonis, C. (1989). Stability and change in childhood-onset depressive disorders. Longitudinal course as a diagnostic validator. In L. N. Robins & J. E. Barrett, (Eds.), *The validity of psychiatric diagnosis* (pp. 57–75). New York: Raven Press.

Kovacs, M., Gatsonis, C., Paulauskas, S. L., & Richards, C. (1989). Depressive disorders in childhood. IV. A longitudinal study of comorbidity with and risk for anxiety disorders. *Arch. Gen. Psychiatry, 46*, 776–782.

Kovacs, M., Paulauskas, S., Gatsonis, C., & Richards, C. (1988). Depressive disorders in childhood. III. A longitudinal study of comorbidity with and risk for conduct disorders. *J. Affect. Disord., 15*, 205–217.

Kovacs, M., & Pollock, M. (1995). Bipolar disorder and comorbid conduct disorder in childhood and adolescence. *J. Am. Acad. Child Adolesc. Psychiatry, 34*, 715–723.

Kraepelin, E. (1968). *Lectures on clinical psychiatry*. New York: Hafner.

Kupfer, D. J., Carpenter, L. L., & Frank, E. (1988). Is bipolar II a unique disorder? *Compr. Psychiatry, 29*, 228–236.

Last, C. G., Hersen, M., Kazdin, A. E., Finkelstein, R., & Strauss, C. C. (1987). Comparison of *DSM-III* separation anxiety and overanxious disorders: Demographic characteristics and patterns of comorbidity. *J. Am. Acad. Child Adolesc. Psychiatry, 26*, 527–531.

Lee, A. S., & Murray, R. M. (1988). The long-term outcome of Maudsley depressives. *Br. J. Psychiatry, 153*, 741–751.

Levitt, A. J., Joffe, R. T., & MacDonald, C. (1991). Life course of depressive illness and characteristics of current episode in patients with double depression. *J. Nerv. Meut. Dis., 179*, 678–682.

McCauley, E., Myers, K., Mitchell, J., Calderon, R., Schloredt, K., & Treder, R. (1993). Depression in young people: Initial presentation and clinical course. *J. Am. Acad. Child Adolesc. Psychiatry, 32*, 714–722.

Mitchell, J., McCauley, E., Burke, P. M., & Moss, S. J. (1988). Phenomenology of depression in children and adolescents. *J. Am. Acad. Child Adolese. Psychiatry, 27*, 12–20.

Poznanski, E. O. (1982). The clinical phenomenology of childhood depression. *Am. J. Orthopsychiatry, 52*, 308–313.

Rao, U., Ryan, N. D., Birmaher, B. et al. (1995). Unipolar depression in adolescents: Clinical outcome in adulthood. *J. Am. Acad. Child Adolesc. Psychiatry, 34*, 566–578.

Robins, L. N., & Regier, D. A. (Eds.). (1991). *Psychiatric Disorders in America*. New York: Free Press.

Rush, A. J., Laux, G., Giles, D. E. et al. (1995). Clinical characteristics of outpatients with chronic major depression. *J. Affect. Disord., 34*, 25–32.

Rutter, M. (1986). Depressive feelings, cognitions, and disorders: A research postscript. In M. Rutter, C. E. Izard, & P. B. Read (Eds.), *Depression in young people* (pp. 491–519). New York: Guilford Press.

Ryan, N. D., Puig-Antich, J., Ambrosini, P. et al. (1987). The clinical picture of major depression in children and adolescents. *Arch. Gen. Psychiatry, 44*, 854–861.

Sanderson, W. C., Beck, A. T., & Beck, J. (1990). Syndrome comorbidity in patients with major depression or dysthymia: Prevalence and temporal relationships. *Am. J. Psychiatry, 147*, 1025–1028.

Shain, B. N., King, C. A., Naylor, M., & Alessi, N. (1991). Chronic depression and hospital course in adolescents. *J. Am. Acad. Child Adolesc. Psychiatry, 30*, 428–433.

Shea, M. T., Elkin, I., Imber, S. D. et al. (1992). Course of depressive symptoms over follow-up. Findings from the National Institute of Mental Health Treatment of Depression Collaborative Research Program. *Arch. Gen. Psychiatry, 49*, 782–787.

Strober, M., & Carlson, G. (1982). Bipolar illness in adolescents with major depression. Clinical, genetic, and psychopharmacologic predictors in a three- to four-year prospective follow-up investigation. *Arch. Gen. Psychiatry, 39*, 549–555.

Strober, M., Lampert, C., Schmidt, S., & Morrell, W. (1993). The course of major depressive disorder in adolescents: I. Recovery and risk of manic switching in a follow-up of psychotic and nonpsychotic subtypes. *J. Am. Acad. Child Adolesc. Psychiatry, 32*, 34–42.

Thase, M. E., Simons, A. D., McGeary, J. et al. (1992). Relapse after cognitive behavior therapy of depression: Potential implications for longer courses of treatment. *Am. J. Psychiatry, 149*, 1046–1052.

Winokur, G., & Morrison, (1973). The Iowa 500: Follow-up of 225 depressives. *Br. J. Psychiatry, 123*, 543–548.

Winokur, G., Morrison, J., Clancy, J., & Crowe, R. (1972). The Iowa 500. II. A blind family history comparison of mania, depression, and schizophrenia. *Arch. Gen. Psychiatry, 27*, 462–464.

Zis, A. P., & Goodwin, F. K. (1979). Major affective disorder as a recurrent illness: A critical review. *Arch. Gen. Psychiatry, 36*, 835–839.

Part IV

OTHER CLINICAL ISSUES: LARGE-*N* STUDIES

The papers in this section are illustrative of the many faces of large-*N* studies. In the first paper in this section, Lavigne et al. have determined the prevalence of *DSM–III–R* psychiatric disorder among preschool children in a primary care pediatric sample. The study used a standard two-stage design; initial screening by means of the Child Behavior Check List (CBCL), followed by direct examination of mothers and children. These procedures made it possible to characterize subjects diagnostically, as well as in terms of patterns of behavioral organization, dimensions of temperament, or the presence or absence of specific behavior problems.

Although not fully generalizable to the community at large, the findings of this study of 3,860 initially screened preschool children—drawn from 68 pediatric practices serving a wide range of SES and minority groups, 510 of whom received fuller evaluations—reveal a high prevalence of psychiatric problems among preschool children. However, the CBCL and clinician review of information obtained in the course of semistructured interviews with mothers and direct observations of the children yielded very different prevalence rates. "Probable" occurrence of an Axis I *DSM–III–R* disorder was 21.4 (9%) severe, a rate comparable to that found in older children. However, rates for behavior problems above the 90th percentile on the CBCL norms were approximately 8% to 10%, considerably lower than the occurrence of *DSM* diagnoses.

Developmental differences in prevalence rates between CBCL and *DSM* diagnoses were found as well. *DSM* disorders (primarily, oppositional defiant disorder) across all levels of severity increased significantly between 2 and 3 years of age, but changes from 3 to 5 years were not significant. For severe disorders, there was also an increase from ages 2 to 3 years and a significant decline in severe disorders from ages 4 to 5 years, suggesting that disorders with onset during this time period may not necessarily be prolonged. CBCL disorders increased in frequency only between ages 3 and 4 years; changes between 2 and 3 years and between 4 and 5 years were nonsignificant.

The results of this study suggest that the pediatric health care setting is a potentially important service delivery area for early mental health screening and intervention. Nevertheless, differences in ascertainment between the CBCL and the diagnoses of clinicians based on observation of children and talking directly with their parents suggest that appropriate screening measures to identify children with early manifestations of psychiatric disorder are not as yet at hand.

In the second paper, Caspi, Moffitt, Newman, and Silva use data derived from a longitudinal–epidemiologic study to test whether behavioral differences among children in the first 3 years of life are linked to specific adult psychiatric disorders: anxiety and mood disorders, antisocial personality disorder, recidivistic and violent crime, alcoholism, and suicidal behavior in early adulthood. Data derive from the Dunedin Multidisciplinary Health and Development Study, a longitudinal investigation of a complete cohort born between April 1, 1972, and March 31, 1973, in Dunedin, a city of approximately 120,000 in New Zealand. Perinatal data were obtained at delivery, and when the children were traced for follow-up at 3 years of age, 91% of the eligible births participated in the assessment, resulting in a base sample of 1,037 (52% male) from families representative of the social class distribution in the general population of similar age in New Zealand for longitudinal study. The Dunedin cohort has been reassessed at ages 3, 5, 7, 9, 11, 13, 15, 18, and now 21 years of age.

On the basis of behavioral observations at age 3 years, children were classified into one of five distinct groups. The undercontrolled group includes children who are impulsive, restless, and distractable; the inhibited group includes children who are shy, fearful, and easily upset. The well-adjusted type includes children who are capable of self-control when it is demanded of them, are adequately self-confident, and do not become unduly upset when confronting new people and situations. These three groups closely resemble the difficult, slow-to-warm-up, and easy groups identified by Chess and Thomas in their longitudinal studies of temperamental organization. Two additional types of children not anticipated by the Chess and Thomas studies were also described: the confident type that included children who at 3 years were zealous and friendly and the reserved type that included children who were somewhat overcautious. Ninety-two percent of the original sample were reassessed at 21 years of age, using standardized interviews based on *DSM–III–R* criteria. Additional information was obtained from an informant nominated by the study member as someone who knew them well and from a search of conviction records of all courts in New Zealand and Australia.

The results suggest that behavior styles observed in the third year of life are significantly related to mental health problems at age 21 years. Although effect sizes were small, undercontrolled children and inhibited children differed significantly from comparison children in young adulthood. Undercontrolled 3-year-olds were more likely at 21 years to meet diagnostic criteria for antisocial personality disorder and to be involved in crime. Inhibited 3-year-olds were more likely at 21 years to meet diagnostic criteria for depression, and both groups were more likely to attempt suicide. Boys in both groups displayed an increased frequency of alcohol-related problems. The findings were unaffected when social class was controlled.

Although previous longitudinal studies have demonstrated links between behavioral characteristics during childhood, and early and mid-adolescence, this report represents the first to consider relationships between the preschool period and early adulthood. The study combines long-term follow-up with an epidemiological sampling frame, making it possible to capture the full range of population variation in measures of toddler behavior and adult psychopathologic abnormality, adding to the generalizability of the findings. Because the time span is long and the behavioral observations relatively brief, these results provide a conservative estimate of the extent to which individual differences in early childhood influence adult mental health. That some forms of adult psychopathology are meaningfully linked to behavioral differences observed among children in the third year of life underscores the contribution of early temperamental attributes to emotional and behavioral organizations later in life. Nevertheless, while early-appearing behavioral differences may well act as a persisting risk factor for some forms of psychiatric disorder in adulthood, the modest effect sizes underscore the importance of intervening experience in potentially modifying outcome.

The final paper in the section, "Trends in a National Sample of Sexually Abusive Youths," is a large-*N* study of a different sort. The Uniform Data Callection system (UDCS) developed by the National Adolescent Perpetrator Network, provided data from 90 contributors in 30 states on more than 1,600 juveniles referred to them for specialized evaluation and/or treatment following a sexual offense.

The National Adolescent Perpetrator Network (NAPN) is an ongoing program supported by the C. Henry Kempe National Center for the Prevention and Treatment of Child Abuse and Neglect at the University of Colorado. The NAPN is a voluntary, multidisciplinary network of more than 900 persons from programs across the United States, Canada, and other countries who are providing interventions with juveniles who sexually abuse others. The UDCS, designed by a committee of network members, consists of four separate structured questionnaires that collect both factual information and clinical impressions. The four questionnaires include initial intake information, clinical impressions at the time of evaluation, treatment progress reports, and information at the time of exit from treatment. This report is based on voluntary reports, submitted on consecutive referrals. Cases included youths in a wide variety of settings, including outpatient program, specialized group homes, and residential and correctional treatment programs.

This paper summarizes information of the sociodemographic characteristics of abusive youth, prior history of abuse, nonsexual offense history, the nature of sexual offenses, the impressions of evaluating professionals, self ratings of clients, and recommendations for treatment. The reliability of the database is somewhat limited because reporters constitute a diverse group of people with different levels of training and experience, with different degrees of access to sources of information. Nevertheless, the availability of this database provides a rich source of information to support hypothesis generation and further empirical studies of an as yet only poorly characterized and understood group of children and adolescents.

15

Prevalence Rates and Correlates of Psychiatric Disorders Among Preschool Children

John V. Lavigne

Children Memorial Hospital

Robert D. Gibbons

University of Illinois, Chicago

Katherine Kaufer Christoffel, Richard Arend, Diane Rosenbaum, and Helen Binns

Children Memorial Hospital

Nichole Dawson, Hollie Sobel, and Crystal Isaacs

Northwestern University Medical Center

Objective: *To determine the prevalence and correlates of psychiatric disorders among preschool children in a primary care pediatric sample.* **Method:** *In a two-stage design, 3,860 preschool children were screened; 510 received fuller evaluations.* **Results:** *For quantitative assessment of disorder ($\geq$90th percentile), prevalence of behavior problems was 8.3%. "Probable" occurrence of an Axis I DSM-III-R disorder was 21.4% (9.1%, severe). Logistic regression analyses indicated significant demographic correlates for quantitative outcomes (older age, minority status, male sex, low socio-economic status, father absence, small family size) but not for DSM-III-R diagnoses. Maternal and family characteristics were generally not significant. Child correlates included activity level, timidity, persistence, and IQ.* **Conclusions:** *Overall prevalence of disorder was consistent with rates for older children; correlates varied by approach used for classification.*

Studies of the epidemiology of childhood disorders have concentrated on school-age children and adolescents. Early reviews estimated the prevalence of child psychiatric disorders at 11.8% (Gould, Wunsch-Hitzig, & Dohrenwend, 1981; Vikan, 1985). These estimates may be conservative (Links, 1983); recent studies have found prevalence rates for moderate/severe disorder of 16% to 20% (Anderson, Williams, McGee, & Silva, 1987; Bird, Gould, Yager, Staghezza, & Canino, 1989; Brandenburg, Friedman, & Silver, 1990; Costello, 1989; Costello et al., 1988a; Esser, Schmidt, & Woerner, 1990;

Reprinted with permission from *J. Am. Acad. Child Adolesc. Psychiatry*, 1996, Vol. 35(2), 204–214. Copyright © 1996 by the American Academy of Child and Adolescent Psychiatry.

This study was supported by grant MH46089 from the NIMH. The authors gratefully acknowledge the members of the Pediatric Practice Research Group who participated in this study.

McGee et al., 1990; Offord et al., 1987; Velez, Johnson, & Cohen, 1989), with higher rates when impairment is not considered (Giaconia et al., 1994). Comorbidity may be as high as 40% to 50% (Bird, Gould, & Staghezza, 1993; Offord et al., 1989; Rac-Grant, Thomas, Offord, & Boyle, 1989).

Little is known about the prevalence of *DSM-III* disorders among preschool children. Historically, studies of preschool children's problems have concentrated on a limited range of specific problem behaviors (Lapouse & Monk, 1958; Richman, Stevenson, & Graham, 1982; Thomas, Byrne, Offord, & Boyle, 1991) or examined quantitative outcome measures derived from behavior problem checklists (Campbell, 1995; Campbell, Breaux, Ewing, & Szumowski, 1986; Cornely & Bromet, 1986; Pianta & Castaldi, 1989; Pianta & Caldwell, 1990; Rose, Rose, & Feldman, 1989), often with small clinical or convenience samples. For *DSM* disorders, studies have used clinic samples (Cantwell & Baker, 1989; Hooks, Mayes, & Volkmar, 1988), but studies of community samples are scarce and limited. The Ontario Child Health Study (Offord et al., 1987) described the occurrence of specific behavior problems rather than disorders for children younger than age 5 years (Thomas et al., 1991), while Earls' (1982) Martha's Vineyard study identified 100 three-year-old children, of whom only 14 children were assigned a *DSM-III* diagnosis, too few to identify the range of possible disorders. A stronger empirical base is needed for understanding psychiatric disorders in children younger than 5 years of age (Costello, Burn, Angold, & Leaf, 1993; Loeber, Lahey, & Thomas, 1991; Rutter, 1988).

The present study is one of the first to examine the occurrence of preschool children's psychiatric disorders outside of a psychiatric or developmental clinic, recruiting subjects through primary care, pediatric settings. At present, there are two contrasting approaches to the categorization of childhood disorder, a taxonomic approach (e.g., *DSM-III*, *DSM-IV*) (American Psychiatric Association, 1987) and a quantitative approach, which views behavior problems as occurring along a continuum rather than dichotomously. Since the relative merits of the two approaches should be established empirically (Achenbach, 1990), both approaches to classification were used. Finally, few studies have examined the correlates of psychiatric disorder among preschool children. Lewis, Dlugokinski, Caputo, and Griffin (1988) have categorized types of risk factors for child/adolescent psychopathology as environmental factors, nuclear family factors, and child-based factors. The present study examined early correlates from each category.

METHOD

This report describes the prevalence and correlates of psychiatric disorder from the first year of a longitudinal study now in progress. The first year methodology was reported previously (Lavigne et al., 1993) and is summarized here.

Subjects

Subjects were recruited during a visit to one of 68 Chicago-area pediatricians. The pediatricians, members of a practitioner's research consortium (Christoffel et al., 1988), were similar to board-certified pediatricians nationally on personal and practice characteristics (Lavigne et al., 1993). Of the 4,891 children aged 2 through 5 years with an English-speaking mother who were study-eligible, 3,860 (79%) agreed to participate. Screened children did not differ from those whose parent declined screening on social class or child's age. Unmarried mothers, mothers of boys, and Hispanic mothers were more likely to refuse participation. Differences were small; statistical significance was achieved because of the large sample size. White and African-American mothers did not differ in participation rates.

At screening, mothers completed a Child Behavior Checklist (CBCL) (Achenbach, 1991, 1992). Mothers whose child "screened high" (≥90th percentile on the CBCL) were invited to the second-stage evaluation. Subsequently, children who screened low were matched with the child who screened high on age, sex, and race. Two children were then randomly selected (two children were selected to better identify the onset of disorder in the longitudinal study). If a mother declined, another child was randomly selected until two mothers agreed to participate.

There were 510 children who completed the second-stage evaluation; 191 (37.4%) had screened high, 319 (62.6%) screened low. Only 56.3% of the families with eligible children participated, but there were no differences between those who completed the second-stage evaluation and those who refused on age, sex, race, social class, marital status, or total problem score on the CBCL. Age distribution among participants was fairly uniform (age 2 years, 25.8%; 3 years, 24.3%; 4 years, 31.9%; 5 years, 18.0%). Almost two thirds were boys (boys, 59.9%; girls, 40.1%) and white (67.1%; African-Americans, 18.8%; Hispanic, 7.2%; other, 6.8%); the majority were from lower socioeconomic groups.

Measures

Demographic information. Mothers completed a questionnaire concerning socioeconomic status (SES) (Hollingshead, 1975), child's age, sex, race, family size and membership, and parents' marital status.

Child behavior checklist. The mothers completed the CBCL (Achenbach, 1991, 1992) both at screening and second-stage evaluation. Correlations between the two administrations were high on major scales (.84 to .87); screening test results were used for data analyses.

Rochester adaptive behavior inventory. This is a semistructured interview administered to parents of preschool children, yielding measures of child cooperation, friendships, timidity, fearfulness, activity level, imaginary play, symptomatic behavior, whininess, demanding attention, depression, and persistence (Jones, 1977; Seifer & Sameroff, 1981). Three of these characteristics, activity level, timidity, and persistence, are sometimes identified as temperamental characteristics (Thomas & Chess, 1984). Interrater reliability was .84 to .99.

Play observation. Each dyad was observed in child-directed and parent-directed activities (Forehand & McMahon, 1981). Videotapes were reviewed by the clinicians.

Developmental evaluation. An age-appropriate developmental test—either the Bayley Scales of Mental Development (Bayley, 1969) or the McCarthy Scales of Children's Abilities (McCarthy, 1972)— was administered to each child.

Moos family environment scale (FES). This 90-item measure provides 11 subscales assessing the family social environment (Moos and Moos, 1981).

Lanyon psychological screening inventory (PSI). This measure of adult psychological adjustment (Lanyon, 1978) was completed by participating mothers. Validity has been established through comparisons with various other personality inventories (Lanyon, 1978). The measure yields five indices of adjustment: alienation, social nonconformity, discomfort, expressiveness, and defensiveness.

Life events scale. This measure of child life stresses (Coddington, 1972) was completed by the child's mother. The sum of negative life events occurring in the year prior to the evaluation was used in data analysis.

Children's global assessment scale (C-GAS). The psychologists who assigned a diagnosis also provided a consensus rating of the child's overall level of impairment on the C-GAS (Shaffer et al., 1983). The scale allows for rating individuals from most severely impaired (0) to exhibiting superior functioning (100).

Procedure

Mothers were invited to participate at the time of a pediatric office visit. Those consenting completed a demographic questionnaire and the CBCL. Subsequently, participants who screened high on the CBCL and matched screen-low children were seen for the second-stage visit. A psychology graduate student administered the CBCL and Rochester Adaptive Behavior Inventory to the mother and conducted the play observation and developmental evaluation.

In the absence of a structured interview for preschool children, a "best estimate" based on clinicians' ratings was used for diagnosis (Weissman, Fendrich, Warner, & Wickramaratne, 1992). Two Ph.D.-level, licensed clinical child psychologists reviewed each protocol. Each psychologist independently assigned a *DSM-III-R* diagnosis (American Psychiatric Association, 1987), rated whether a diagnosis was absent, possible, or probable, and completed the C-GAS. The psychologists were asked to follow the guidelines of the *DSM-III-R* as closely as possible. The psychologists could assign multiple Axis I diagnoses; two diagnoses proved sufficient for this age group. Consensus diagnoses were achieved through regular conferences (Lavigne et al. 1994). The reliability of assigning diagnoses was moderately high (.62 to .99 for specific Axis I diagnoses) and comparable with those in studies of older children (Lavigne et al., 1994).

It was felt initially that time demands for interviewing would prevent mothers from completing any additional information. Experience, however, indicated that the mothers could complete some further information that would be helpful in identifying correlates of behavior problems. As a result, the second wave of the mothers ($n = 332$) who participated in the evaluation completed the FES, PSI, and Life Events Scale.

Statistical Analyses

Prevalence rates for the CBCL data could be calculated for the entire sample of children who participated in screening ($N = 3,860$). Following procedures reported by Verhulst and Van der Ende (1992), a child was considered a "case" based on CBCL data if he or she obtained a score at or above the 90th percentile on major scales. Prevalence rates were calculated for total behavior problems, "pure" internalizing problems (Internalizing scale score exceeded the 90th percentile while the Externalizing score was below the 90th percentile), "pure" externalizing problems (Externalizing scale score exceeded the 90th percentile while the Internalizing score was below the 90th percentile), and comorbidity (Externalizing and Internalizing scale scores both exceeded the 90th percentile).

Weighted prevalence rates for *DSM-III-R* disorders were calculated based on the second-stage evaluations and clinicians' ratings. Prevalence rates were calculated for the total screened sample of 3,860 by weighting the proportion of children who screened positive or negative in the second-stage sample of 510 by the appropriate sampling fraction. Only cases rated as "probable" were considered. Cases were considered severe if an Axis I disorder was present and there was a clinicians' consensus C-GAS rating of 60 or less. Confidence intervals (CIs) were calculated following procedures described by Lillienfield (1980).

Correlates of behavior problems were examined separately for CBCL outcomes and *DSM-III-R* diagnoses using logistic regression procedures. Because the occurrence of specific disorders is generally low, Axis I diagnoses were categorized as disruptive disorders (DD), emotional disorders (ED), and comorbid disorders (a disruptive disorder comorbid with either an emotional disorder or other disorder) to assess correlates of disorder.

RESULTS

Prevalence of CBCL Disorders

Table 1 presents the prevalence of problems for CBCL scores above the 90th percentile for total problems, "pure" internalizing problems, "pure" externalizing problems, and comorbid internalizing and externalizing problems.

TABLE 1

Prevalence Rates Derived from Quantitative (Child Behavior Checklist) Scale Scores above the 90th Percentile

	N^a	Total Behavior Problems		Internalizing		Externalizing		Comorbid	
		Prevalence[b]	95% CI[c]	Prevalence	95% CI	Prevalence	95% CI	Prevalence	95% CI
Age 2–5	3,860	8.3	0.9	3.7	0.6	3.7	0.6	3.3	0.6
2	1,210	4.7	1.2	1.2	0.6	2.6	0.9	1.6	0.7
3	1,052	7.3	1.6	4.1	1.2	3.5	1.2	1.6	0.8
4	846	13.2	2.4	5.8	1.6	5.0	1.5	6.4	1.7
5	752	10.0	2.2	4.9	1.6	4.3	1.4	5.1	1.6
Boy	1,967	10.0	1.4	3.9	0.8	5.5	1.0	4.3	0.8
Girl	1,893	6.6	1.0	3.6	0.8	1.8	0.6	2.3	0.6

[a]Total N for screening sample.
[b]Rates per 100, above the 90th percentile on Child Behavior Checklist norms.
[c]±95% Confidence interval.

Overall, the rate of disorder on the Total Behavior Problems scale was 8.3%. Rates were significantly higher for boys than girls (i.e., 95% CIs do not overlap). There was a significant increase between ages 3 and 4 years on the Total Behavior Problems scale, but changes between 2 and 3 years, and 4 and 5 years were nonsignificant.

The prevalence of pure internalizing and pure externalizing problems was 3.7% each; the comorbidity rate was 3.3%. With the three scales combined, the overall rate of problems (10.7%) is slightly higher than the rate on the Total Behavior Problems scale (8.3%). The sexes did not differ on internalizing problems, but boys were significantly more likely to exhibit total behavior problems, externalizing behavior problems, and comorbid disorders. There was a significant increase in internalizing problems from ages 2 to 3 years; the increase from age 3 to 4 years and the decline from 4 to 5 years were not significant. Age trends for externalizing disorders were not significant. Rates for comorbidity increased significantly between ages 3 and 4 years.

Prevalence of DSM Disorders

See Table 2 for prevalence rates of any *DSM-III-R* Axis I mental disorder based on consensus diagnoses. The overall rate prevalence of an Axis I disorder, including pure and comorbid cases, is 21.4%; for a single, "pure" diagnosis, 16%; for comorbidity, 5.4%. The prevalence of severe cases was 9.1% overall; severe, pure disorders occurred in 5.7%, and severe comorbid disorders, 3.4%. Boys were significantly more likely to exhibit any occurrence of disorder and pure disorder across all severity levels and for severe cases only. Sex differences for comorbidity were not significant.

A significant increase in disorder across all levels of severity occurred between ages 2 years to 3 years, but changes from 3 years to 5 years were nonsignificant. For severe disorders, there was also an increase from age 2 to 3 years and a significant decline in the severe disorders from ages 4 to 5 years. A similar increase occurred in rates of problems from ages 2 to 3 years for pure disorders at all levels of severity, followed by a decline at ages 4 to 5 years; more severe pure disorders showed an increase from ages 2 to 3 years. Comorbid disorders at all levels of severity showed an increase from ages 2 to 3 years. More severe levels of comorbid disorders declined from 4 to 5 years. The decline in severe disorders from ages 4 to 5 years is noteworthy. Prior to that time, severe disorders constitute one third to one half of all occurrences of disorder. At age 5 years, however, severe disorders constituted only one tenth of all the Axis I disorders and the pure disorders and only one fourth of the comorbid disorders.

Prevalence of Specific Disorders

Table 3 presents prevalence rates for specific Axis I disorders that exceeded 1%. In each instance, prevalence rates were included for overall rates of problems and for sexes separately; for two disorders showing significant age trends, rates were included for each age.

Disruptive disorders. By far the most common disorder was oppositional defiant disorder (ODD). ODD was present in 16.8% of the children aged 2 through 5 years; half of these cases (8.1%) were considered severe. Approximately one fourth of the children with ODD (or severe ODD) showed comorbidity with another Axis I disorder. Rates for any occurrence of ODD and for severe ODD were almost twice as high for boys than girls. Boys were significantly more likely to have a pure form of ODD, both for all levels of severity and for more severe impairment. In contrast, when comorbidity was present, rates were very similar for the sexes.

Age trends for ODD were notable. Prevalence rates were highest among 3-year-olds (the "terrible twos" should be the "terrible threes"). There was a significant decline in any occurrence of ODD and severe occurrences of ODD among 5-year-olds; rates of ODD dropped from a high of 22.5% at age

TABLE 2
Prevalence Rates for Overall Axis I Disorder

		All Occurrences				Pure Disorder				Comorbid Disorder			
		All Severity Levels		Severe Only[a]		All Severity Levels		Severe Only		All Severity Levels		Severe Only	
	N[b]	Prevalence[c]	95% CI[d]	Prevalence	95% CI	Prevalence	95% CI	Prevalence	95% CI	Prevalence	95% CI	Prevalence	95% CI
Age 2-5	166	21.4	1.3	9.1	0.9	16.0	1.2	5.7	0.7	5.4	0.7	3.4	0.6
2	26	13.6	2.0	7.1	1.5	12.2	1.9	5.8	1.4	1.4	0.7	1.2	0.6
3	51	26.5	2.3	14.0	2.1	19.2	2.4	7.2	1.6	7.4	1.6	6.8	1.6
4	57	25.0	3.0	10.5	2.1	19.0	2.7	7.1	3.1	6.0	1.6	3.4	0.2
5	32	21.9	3.0	2.8	1.2	13.2	2.5	1.0	2.1	8.8	2.1	1.8	1.0
Boy	112	25.3	2.0	11.1	1.4	19.0	1.8	7.5	1.2	6.3	1.1	3.6	0.8
Girl	54	16.0	1.7	6.5	1.1	11.7	1.5	3.4	0.8	4.3	1.0	3.1	0.8

[a] Severity based on clinicians' consensus Children's Global Assessment Scale rating of 60 or less.
[b] N of cases diagnosed in second-stage sample ($N = 510$).
[c] Rate per 100.
[d] ±95% Confidence interval.

TABLE 3
Prevalence Rates for Specific Axis I Disorders

	All Severity Levels			Severe Only		
	N	Prevalence[a]	95% CI	N	Prevalence	95% CI
ODD (313.81)						
Any occurrence						
Age 2–5	133	16.8	15.2–17.8	74	8.1	7.2–9.1
2	25	12.6	10.8–14.7	15	7.1	5.8–8.8
3	45	22.5	19.8–25.4	29	12.8	10.8–15.1
4	40	17.3	14.6–20.4	22	8.6	6.8–10.9
5	23	15.0	12.5–18.0	8	1.9	1.0–3.2
Boy	91	20.0	18.1–22.0	53	10.0	8.7–11.5
Girl	42	12.4	10.9–14.0	21	5.6	4.6–6.8
Pure disorder						
Age 2–5	57	12.5	11.4–13.6	30	5.2	3.6–4.8
2	10	11.2	9.4–13.2	8	5.8	4.6–7.4
3	20	16.5	14.2–19.1	11	7.2	5.6–9.0
4	19	12.8	10.5–15.6	9	5.5	4.0–7.4
5	8	8.7	6.8–11.0	2	0.5	0.4–0.7
Boy	39	15.5	13.9–17.4	23	7.1	6.0–8.4
Girl	18	8.4	7.2–9.8	7	2.6	1.9–3.4
Comorbid disorder						
Age 2–5	47	4.2	3.6–4.9	34	2.9	2.4–3.5
2	4	1.4	0.8–2.2	7	1.2	0.7–2.0
3	18	6.0	4.6–7.8	16	5.7	4.4–7.4
4	12	4.5	3.2–6.1	9	3.2	2.1–4.7
5	13	6.2	4.6–8.2	6	1.4	0.7–2.6
Boy	29	4.4	3.6–5.5	21	3.0	2.3–3.9
Girl	18	4.1	3.3–5.1	13	3.0	2.3–3.9
ADHD (314.01)						
Any occurrence						
Age 2–5	23	2.0	1.6–2.5	17	1.5	1.2–1.9
Boy	15	2.4	1.8–3.2	12	1.8	1.2–2.5
Girl	8	1.3	0.8–1.9	5	0.1	0.7–1.7
Pure disorder						
Age 2–5	3	0.1	0.04–0.33	3	0.1	0.04–0.33
Boy	2	0.2	0.05–0.51	2	0.2	0.05–0.51
Girl	1	0.1	0.08–0.36	1	0.1	0.08–0.36
Comorbid disorder						
Age 2–5	20	1.8	1.5–2.3	14	1.3	0.7–1.3
Boy	13	2.3	1.7–3.1	10	1.6	1.1–2.3
Girl	7	1.2	0.8–1.8	4	1.0	0.6–1.6
Parent–Child problem (V62.20)						
Any occurrence						
Age 2–5	27	4.6	4.0–5.3	8	1.1	0.80–1.6
2	13	9.2	7.6–11.2	4	2.2	1.4–3.2
3	6	4.0	2.8–5.4	1	—	
4	7	2.8	2.4–4.2	3	1.3	0.6–2.3
5	1	—		0	—	
Boy	18	4.7	3.8–5.8	8	1.9	1.3–2.5
Girl	9	4.5	3.6–5.6	0	—	

TABLE 3 (*Continued*)

	All Severity Levels			Severe Only		
	N	Prevalence[a]	95% CI	N	Prevalence	95% CI
Pure disorder						
Age 2–5	5	1.2	0.9–1.6	1	0.3	0.2–0.52
2	4	3.0	2.1–4.2	0	—	
3	0	—		0	—	
4	1	1.0	0.4–2.0	1	1.0	0.4–2.0
5	0	—		0	—	
Boy	1	0.5	0.2–0.9	1	0.5	0.2–0.9
Girl	4	2.2	1.6–3.0	0	—	
Comorbid disorder						
Age 2–5	22	3.4	2.9–4.0	7	0.8	0.5–1.1
2	9	6.2	4.9–7.9	4	2.2	1.4–3.2
3	6	4.0	2.8–3.0	1	0.2	0.1–0.3
4	6	1.9	1.1–3.0	2	0.4	0.3–0.6
5	1	0.4	0.3–0.6	0	—	
Boy	17	4.2	3.4–5.6	7	1.4	0.9–2.0
Girl	5	2.3	1.7–3.1	0	—	

Note: Severity based on clinicians' consensus Children's Global Assessment Scale rating of 60 or less. ODD = oppositional defiant disorder; ADHD = attention-deficit hyperactivity disorder; CI = confidence interval.
[a]Rate per 100.

3 years, to 15.0% at age 5 years. There were significant declines in severe, pure ODD but not comorbid ODD from age 4 to 5 years. Declines across all levels of severity were not significant for either pure or comorbid ODD.

Attention-deficit hyperactivity disorder (ADHD) was identified in 2% of this preschool samples. ADHD was almost always comorbid with some other condition, usually ODD. Undifferentiated attention deficit disorder (ADD) (*DSM-III-R* 314.00) occurred in 0.4% of the cases ($n = 3$ cases; 95% CI, 0.2% to 0.7%), while conduct disorder (*DSM-III-R* 312.00) occurred in 0.2% ($n = 4$ cases; 95% CI, 0.1% to 0.4%).

Emotional disorders. Prevalence rates for each ED were less than 1%: avoidant disorder (*DSM-III-R* 313.21), 0.7% ($n = 4$; 95% CI, 0.5% to 1.2%); separation anxiety disorder (309.21), 0.5% ($n = 6$; 95% CI, 0.3% to 0.8%); overanxious disorder (313.00), 0.7% ($n = 4$; 95% CI, 0.5% to 1.0%); simple phobia (300.29), 0.6% ($n = 2$; 95% CI, 0.4% to 0.9%); depression not otherwise specified (311.00), 0.3% ($n = 7$; 95% CI, 0.2% to 0.5%).

Other disorders. Prevalence rates were below 1% for each of the other Axis I disorders: sleepwalking (307.46), 0.2% ($n = 4$; 95% CI, 0.1% to 0.4%); functional enuresis (307.60), 0.7% ($n = 5$; 95% CI, 0.5% to 1.0%); stuttering (307.00), 0.3% ($n = 2$; 95% CI, 0.2% to 0.5%); posttraumatic stress disorder (309.89), 0.1% ($n = 2$; 95% CI, 0.03% to 0.3%); dream anxiety disorder (307.47), 0.1% ($n = 5$; 95% CI, 0.03% to 0.3%); adjustment disorder with mixed emotions and conduct (309.40), 0.4% ($n = 4$; 95% CI, 0.2% to 0.7%); The prevalence of one V code category, parent–child problems, was also calcualted because such problems may be associated with the later development of regular Axis I disorders in this age group (Table 3). The prevalence of parent–child problems was 4.6% overall. In a majority of cases, the parent–child problem was comorbid with another *DSM* diagnosis. Age trends in parent–child problems are notable for being the only diagnosis to show a significant decline from age 2 to 3 years, accompanied by further significant decline through age 5 years.

Correlates of Disorder

Demographic correlates. Data collection and analyses of the correlates of disorder differed across subsets of subjects. Information on demographic correlates and the CBCL were obtained at screening; statistical analyses were conducted on the entire screening sample ($N = 3, 860$). Analyses of demographic information and *DSM-III-R* diagnoses were conducted on the entire second-stage sample ($N = 510$). In the second-stage sample, statistical analyses were conducted on the 343 subjects in the cohort who were administered all family and maternal measures ($N = 343$).

Significant odds ratios (ORs) (only ORs significant at $p \leq .05$ are reported) for the CBCL Total Behavior Problems scale were obtained for older age (OR = 1.40), minority status (OR = 1.44), male sex (OR = 1.27), low SES (OR = 1.18), father absence (OR = 1.30), and smaller family size (OR = 1.28). Correlates of internalizing problems included older age (OR = 1.54) and minority status (OR = 1.64). For externalizing problems, significant correlates were older age (OR = 1.25) and male sex (OR = 1.77). For comorbid internalizing and externalizing disorders, significant correlates were older age (OR = 1.68), minority status (OR = 1.41), male sex (OR = 1.36), low SES (OR = 1.36), father absence (OR = 1.54), and smaller family size (OR = 1.57).

In analyses of any *DSM-III-R* disorder (defined as any case with an Axis I disorder), DD, and comorbid disorders, only subjects for whom a problem was rated as probable were considered cases. For ED, the number of "probables" was very small, and data were analyzed for probables and possibles, following a procedure suggested by Weissman et al. (1992) for inclusion of subthreshold diagnoses for relatively rare conditions.

For the analysis of *DSM* disorders and demogrpahics, age, race, and sex were not included among the demographic variables because these variables had been used to match subjects who screened high versus low on the CBCL initially. Marital status, SES, father absence, and crowdedness were not significantly related to the presence of a DD, comorbid disorders, or overall "caseness" (i.e., the presence of any disorder, regardless of diagnosis). For ED, risk increased for children whose mothers were unmarried (OR = 2.33; 95% CI, ±0.33; $p < .01$).

Family correlates. Prior to the analyses of family and maternal correlates of disorder, FES and PSI data were reduced through principal-components analyses with varimax rotation of factors. The FES yielded three factors: (1) cohesiveness/expressiveness/vigorous; (2) inhibited/controlling; (3) unconflicted/cohesive/organized. The PSI yielded two factors: anxious/depressed and nonconforming/alienated. To assess factor validity, the FES family factors and PSI maternal characteristics were correlated. Significant correlations were obtained: lower family cohesion was associated with maternal anxiety/depression ($r = -.34$, $p < .01$) and maternal alienation ($r = -.18$, $p < .05$), while lower family conflict and greater organization were associated with maternal anxiety/depression ($r = -.32$, $p < .01$) and alienation ($r = -.22$, $p < .01$). These correlations seemed reasonable, and factor scores were used in further analyses.

Logistic regression analyses then were conducted to examine the relationship between family and maternal correlates, negative life events, and CBCL psychopathology. In these analyses, none of the family variables were associated with CBCL-derived total behavior problems, internalizing problems, or comorbid problems. There was a small but significant correlation between externalizing problems and nonconforming/alienated maternal personality (OR = 1.06; 95% CI, ±0.03; $p < .01$).

For *DSM* disorders, none of the family, maternal, or negative life event variables were associated with ED, comorbid disorders, or presence of any disorder. Greater family conflict and lower family cohesiveness (OR = 1.03; 95% CI, ±0.01; $p < .02$) were associated with the presence of a DD. Contrary to expectations, fewer negative life events in the prior year were associated with DD (OR = 1.43; $p < .03$).

Child correlates. A logistic regression model was developed for predictors of emotional status based on child characteristics of IQ and temperamental characteristics of activity level, timidity, and persistence.

For CBCL-derived disorders, only a lower level of persistence (OR = 1.96) was significantly associated with total behavior problems. Lower activity level (OR = 3.85) was associated with internalizing problems, while both higher activity levels (OR = 5.37) and lower levels of persistence (OR = 1.85) were associated with externalizing problems. For comorbid problems, higher activity level (OR = 2.41), lower IQ (OR = 1.02), and lower levels of persistence (OR = 2.08) were associated with comorbidity.

In the analyses of child variables and *DSM* disorders, ratings of temperament and IQ scores entered into these logistic regression equations were also used by the reviewers to assign diagnoses. Thus, the correlates and diagnoses were not entirely independent (as they were in examining the CBCL-derived diagnoses). As a result, the analyses of *DSM*-derived diagnoses were considered exploratory and were included because the results could be compared to the analyses for CBCL ratings. The occurrence of any *DSM* Axis I disorder was associated with lower IQ (OR = 1.03), less persistence (OR = 1.77), and higher activity levels (OR = 3.10) and ratings of timidity (OR = 3.09). ED was associated with higher ratings of timidity (OR = 8.30). DD was associated with lower IQ (OR = 1.03), less persistence (OR = 2.04), higher activity level (OR = 5.25), and timidity (OR = 3.03); for comorbidity, significant correlates were the same (IQ, OR = 1.03; persistence, OR = 1.72; activity, OR = 3.10; timidity, OR = 3.14).

DISCUSSION

For Axis I disorders, the overall prevalence rate was 21.4% (9.1% for severe Axis I disorders). Comparison with other studies of preschool children is difficult because the only available community study (Earls, 1982) included a very small sample of children, and there are no other primary care studies. The overall prevalence, however, is comparable with that for older children, although rates of severe disorder among preschool children may be somewhat lower. In contrast, the prevalence of comorbidity was considerably lower among preschool children. This may be attributable to the low rates of disorders other than ODD in this study, decreasing the likelihood of identifying comorbidity. In addition, the present study used bestestimate clinician diagnoses rather than structured interviews, and there may be systematic differences in the likelihood of identifying comorbidity using the two procedures.

Rates for behavior problems above the 90th percentile on CBCL norms were approximately 8% to 10%, considerably lower than the occurrence of *DSM* diagnoses. While identifying 10% of a sample exceeding the 90th percentile is expectable, a primary care study with older children found that almost 25% of the sample exceeded that cutoff (Costello et al., 1988b). In addition, secular trends primarily among older children reflect an increase in CBCL-reported problem behaviors (Achenbach & Howell, 1993). If there is a tendency for CBCL-identified problem behaviors to be increasing or occurring at a higher rate in pediatric samples, the trend does not appear to begin among preschool children.

Why the *DSM*-based disorders would be more common than CBCL-identified problems depends on the interrelationship between the two diagnostic systems. Arend et al. suggest that most preschool children scoring above the 90th percentile on the CBCL are assigned a *DSM-III-R* diagnosis, usually a DD (Arend, Lavigne, Rosenbaum, Binns, & Christoffel, unpublished). A substantial number of false-negatives, however, do occur; i.e., many children with a CBCL score below the 90th percentile appear to have a *DSM* disorder when the parent is interviewed and the child is observed. The implications of differences in case identification between quantitative and taxonomic systems are potentially important; studies that identify children based on *DSM* versus CBCL criteria in this age group may be examing rather different samples of children.

Consistent with reports of older children, prevalence rates for both CBCL- and *DSM*-derived disorders indicated higher rates of overall problems and externalizing problems for boys. Unlike older children, the children in this study showed no sex differences in rates of CBCL internalizing problems; this finding raises the question why older girls are at greater risk for (or boys are more protected from) developing such disorders.

There were developmental differences in prevalence rates between CBCL and *DSM* diagnoses. The increase in the prevalence of disorder from ages 2 to 3 years was significant for *DSM* disorders but not CBCL-derived disorders. This increased prevalence of disorder at 2 to 3 years suggests that this may be a critical period for understanding the onset of early disorder in the preschool years. There were also nonsignificant changes from ages 4 to 5 years on the CBCL, while disruptive disorders, chiefly ODD, declined. Prior work (Loeber et al., 1991) suggested a decline in oppositional behavior between ages 4 and 9 years; the present study suggests there is a major change in the earliest portion of that age range. Although disruptive behavior problems in preschool children may be troubling for families, the decline in frequency of problems, especially severe problems, suggests that the disorders occurring at that time may not necessarily be prolonged. It is not surprising that some disorders would be limited to a specific developmental period; of greater interest is determining which factors contribute to persistent disorder for early-onset problems.

By far the most common Axis I disorders were disruptive disorder, particularly ODD. Rates of ADHD and ADD were lower than ODD rates but were similar to the rates of ADHD and ADD in school-age children reported by Costello et al. (1988a). Parent–child problems showed the only decline in occurrence from age 2 to 3 years and beyond. This can be constrated with the increase at 2 to 3 years of most other problems, particularly ODD, suggesting the possibility that some early parenting difficulties become solidified in an Axis I disorder.

Rates of ED were low in this sample. Campbell (1995) argues that difficulties in detecting internalizing disorders in this age group have resulted in relatively few studies of these disorders in preschool children. This study made a concerted effort to identify such disorders, and we found that the rates are low for those meeting *DSM-III-R* criteria. Of interest, the rates for *DSM* EDs are lower than expected based on prevalence among older children; however, rates of high levels of internalizing symptoms based on CBCL ratings are not different from rates of externalizing symptoms for preschool children in this sample. This raises the possibility of developmental changes in the organization of such symptoms; possibly, internalizing symptoms are present but not organized clearly into patterns recognizable at this age, while externalizing symptoms have been organized into more recognizable patterns in some instances.

Certain demographic correlates for the quantitative outcomes were consistent with those noted in other studies with older children (including lower SES, minority status, male gender, and father absence) (Costello, 1989; Rae-Grant et al., 1989; Rutter, 1989) and with preschool children (low SES, single-parent homes) (Campbell, 1995; Thomas et al., 1991). In the present study, most of the same demographic factors (low SES, sex differences, father absence) were correlates of behavior problems derived from the CBCL. Larger family size has been associated with increased problems in older children (Hetherington, 1989), but in this study the presence of fewer children in the home was associated with problem behaviors. It is possible that among preschool children, smaller family size allows caretakers to devote more attention to the children, increasing the likelihood of problem detection.

There do not appear to be other studies that have examined demographic or other correlates of *DSM*-derived diagnoses among preschool children. Demographic correlates of *DSM* disorders differed from those identified for quantitative ratings in prior work. Because of the study design, age, sex, and race, which have been identified as risk factors examined in other studies, could not be studied because they were used in subject matching. Other variables, however, including marital status, were not correlates of *DSM* diagnoses.

Certain family characteristics, notably marital conflict, maternal psychopathology, and life stresses, have been identified as correlates of disorder in prior studies, but not in the present study. This may be in part due to differences in methodology, with some studies identifying these correlates among clinic-referred children or children nominated for participation because they had problems (e.g., Campbell, March, Pierce, Ewing, & Szumowski, 1991) rather than using community samples to identify cases. Marital status, child's gender, father absence, crowdedness, family characteristics, and maternal psychopathology were not correlates of *DSM* disorders in the present study. Other studies using community samples and quantitative outcome measures did not find certain risk factors to be associated with child behavior problems, including maternal depression, parental health, sibship size, domestic violence, and early childhood problems in young children (Thomas et al., 1991).

Child temperament and IQ showed stronger associations with both CBCL-based and *DSM*-based disorders in this preschool sample than either maternal, child, or demographic variables. While clinicians who provided the *DSM*-based diagnoses had temperament and IQ data available to them possibly contaminating their ratings, this is not true for CBCL-based diagnoses. Since the patterns of response were similar for both types of ratings, the confound of temperament and *DSM* diagnoses alone cannot account for the strong associations. It is possible that temperament is most closely tied to early-onset behavior problems, while other family and maternal personality characteristics show stronger associations with long-term prognosis or with problems of later onset. As with certain other issues raised in this report, fuller information will only be available with longitudinal studies.

Limitations to this study are several. First, the subjects from the study were drawn from a primary care pediatric sample. While children in the sample came from a wide range of SES and minority groups, and included clinics that primarily served lower SES families, it was not a randomly selected community sample. At present it is not known how such primary care samples differ from community samples, and direct comparisons to community demographics are difficult to make because of the wide range of suburbs in which these subjects lived. Nonetheless, children who are receiving no health care at all are underrepresented. Similarly, children from entirely Spanish-speaking families were excluded because funding limitations precluded the necessary development and standardization of measures and hiring of bilingual staff; as a result, the present study underrepresented Hispanic children. Although there were relatively few systematic differences between participants in the second-stage evaluation and those who declined participation, the participation rate was low; distance from the data collection center contributed to this, but other, undetected biases may also have been present. Finally, there are limitations in the use of best-estimate diagnostic procedures such as those employed in the study which may have affected the prevalence estimates. Other limitations were present in certain scales used to assess family climate and maternal personality because of the absence of standardization data with Hispanic samples.

This study demonstrates that the prevalence of disorder in young children is significant and comparable with that of older children. In many instances, however, the child's disorder may be less severe. There are several implications of these findings, both for further research and for clinical service. Research is needed to address the prevalence of children's problems directly in a community sample. Ideally such studies would use structured-interview procedures that are comparable with those used in epidemiological studies with older children. Second, this cross-sectional study suggests that there is a reduction in certain kinds of problems around age 5 years, but further research is needed to examine the stability and patterns of change that occur among individuals with a wide range of disorders that have their onset in the preschool years. Finally, further research is needed to delineate the degree to which the correlates of disorder identified in this study serve as risk factors for the onset or maintenance of disorders within a longitudinal framework.

Clinically, the high prevalence of psychiatric problems in preschool children in primary care offices and clinics suggests that the pediatric health care setting is a potentially important service delivery area for early mental health screening and intervention. Pediatricians tend to underidentify the problems that are present among preschool children in their practices (Lavigne et al., 1993), and collaborative work between pediatricians and mental health professionals may be important for developing appropriate screening measures to identify children with early manifestations of psychiatric disorder. As further research helps to delineate which problems are relatively stable, collaborative interventions between pediatricians, developmental pediatricians, and mental health professionals will become increasingly important.

REFERENCES

Achenbach, T. M. (1990). "Comorbidity" in child and adolescent psychiatry: Categorical and quantitative perspectives. *J. Child Adolesc. Psychopharmacol., 14*, 271–278.

Achenbach, T. M. (1991). *Manual for the child behavior checklist/4–18 and 1991 profile.* Burlington: University of Vermont Department of Psychiatry.

Achenbach, T. M. (1992). *Manual for the child behavior checklist/2–3 and 1992 profile.* Burlington: University of Vermont Department of Psychiatry.

Achenbach, T. M., & Howell, C. T. (1993). Are American children's problems getting worse? A 13-year comparison. *J. Am. Acad. Child Adolesc. Psychiatry, 32*, 1145–1154.

American Psychiatric Association (1987). *Diagnostic and statistical manual of mental disorders, 3rd edition-revised (DSM-III-R).* Washington, DC: American Psychiatric Association.

Anderson, J. C., Williams, S. M., McGee, R. O., & Silva, P. A. (1987). *DSM-III* disorders in preadolescent children. *Arch. Gen. Psychiatry, 44*, 69–76.

Bayley, N. (1969). *Manual of the Bayley Scales of mental development.* New York: Psychological Corporation.

Bird, H. R., Gould, M. S., & Staghezza, B. (1993). Patterns of diagnostic comorbidity in a community sample of children aged 9 through 16 years. *J. Am. Acad. Child Adolesc. Psychiatry, 32*, 361–368.

Bird, H. R., Gould, M. S., Yager, T., Staghezza, B., & Canino, G. (1989). Risk factors for maladjustment in Puerto Rican children. *J. Am. Acad. Child Adolesc. Psychiatry, 28*, 847–850.

Brandenburg, N. A., Friedman, R. M., & Silver, S. (1990). The epidemiology of childhood psychiatric disorders. *J. Am. Acad. Child Adolesc. Psychiatry, 29*, 76–83.

Campbell, S. B. (1995). Behavior problems in preschool children: A review of recent research. *J. Child Psychol. Psychiatry, 36*, 113–149.

Campbell, S., Breaux, A. M., Ewing, L. J., & Szumowski, E. K. (1986). Correlates and predictors of hyperactivity and aggression: A longitudinal study of parent-referred problem preschoolers. *J. Abnorm. Child Psychol., 14*, 217–234.

Campbell, S. B., March, C. L., Pierce, E. W., Ewing, L. J., & Szumowski, E. K. (1991). Hard-to-manage preschool boys: Family context and the stability of externalizing behavior. *J. Abnorm. Child Psychol., 19*, 301–318.

Cantwell, D. P., & Baker, L. (1989). Stability and natural history of *DSM-III* childhood diagnoses. *J. Am. Acad. Child Adolesc, Psychiatry, 28*, 691–700.

Christoffel, K. K., Binns, H. J., Stockman, J. A. et al. (1988). Practice-based research: Opportunities and obstacles. *Pediatrics, 82*, 399–406.

Coddington, R. D. (1972). The significance of life events as etiological factors in the diseases of children: II. A study of a normal population. *J. Psychosom. Res. 16*, 205–213.

Cornely, P. & Bromet, E. (1986). Prevalence of behavior problems in three-year-old children living near Three Mile Island: A comparative analysis. *J. Child Psychol. Psychiatry, 27*, 489–498.

Costello, E. J. (1989). Developments in child psychiatric epidemiology *J. Am. Acad. Child Adolesc. Psychiatry, 28*, 836–841.

Costello, E. J., Burns, B. J., Angold, A., & Leaf, P. J. (1993). How can epidemiology improve mental health services for children and adolescents? *J. Am. Acad. Child Adolesc. Psychiatry, 32*, 1106–1117.

Costello, E. J., Costello, A. J., Edelbrock, C. et al. (1988a). Psychiatric disorders in pediatric primary care: Prevalence and risk factors. *Arch. Gen. Psychiatry, 45*, 1107–1116.

Costello, E. J., Edelbrock, C., Costello, A. J., Dulcan, M. K., Burns, B. J., & Brent, D. (1988b). Psychopathology in pediatric primary care: The new hidden morbidity. *Pediatrics, 82*, 415–424.

Earls, F. (1982). Application of *DSM-III* in an epidemiological study of preschool children. *Am. J. Psychiatry, 139*, 242–243.

Esser, G., Schmidt, M. H., & Woerner, W. (1990). Epidemiology and course of psychiatric disorders in school-age children: results of a longitudinal study. *J. Child. Psychol. Psychiatry, 31*, 243–263.

Forehand, R. L., & McMahon, R. J. (1981). *Helping the noncompliant child.* New York: Guilford.

Giaconia, R. M., Reinberg, H. Z., Silverman, A. B., Pakiz, B., Frost, A. K., & Cohen, E. (1994). Age on onset of psychiatric disorders in a community population of older adolescents. *J. Am. Acad. Child Adolesc. Psychiatry, 33*, 706–717.

Gould, M. S., Wunsch-Hitzig, R., & Dohrenwend, B. (1981). Estimating the prevalence of childhood psychopathology. *J. Am. Acad. Child Psychiatry, 20*, 462–476.

Hetherington, E. M. (1989). Coping with family transitions: Winners, losers, and survivors. *Child Dev., 60*, 1–14.

Hollingshead, A. B. (1975). *Four-factor index of social position.* New Haven, CT: Yale University Department of Sociology.

Hooks, M. Y., Mayes, L. C., & Volkmar, F. R. (1988). Psychiatric disorders among preschool children. *J. Am. Acad. Child Adolesc. Psychiatry, 27*, 623–627.

Jones, F. H. (1977). The Rochester adaptive behavior inventory: A parallel series of instruments for assessing social competence during early and middle childhood and adolescence. In J. S. Strauss & H. M. Babigian (Eds.), *The Origins and Course of Psychopathology* (pp. 249–281). New York: Plenum.

Lanyon, R. I. (1978). *Manual for the psychological screening inventory.* Los Angeles: Western.

Lapouse, R., & Monk, M. (1958). An epidemiological study of behavior characteristics in children. *Am. J. Public Health, 48*, 1134–1144.

Lavigne, J. V., Arend, R., Rosenbaum, D. et al. (1994). Interrater reliability of the *DSM-III-R* with preschool children. *J. Abnorm. Child Psychol., 22*, 679–690.

Lavigne, J. V., Binns, H. J., Christoffel, K. K. et al. (1993). Behavioral and emotional problems among pre-school children in pediatric primary care: Prevalence and pediatrician's recognition. *Pediatrics, 91*, 649–655.

Lewis, R. J., Dlugokinski, E. L., Caputo, L. M., & Griffin, R. B. (1988). Children at risk for emotional disorders: Risk and resource dimensions. *Clin. Psychol. Rev., 8*, 417–440.

Lillienfield, D. E. (1980). *Foundations of epidemiology.* New York: Oxford.

Links, P. (1983). Community surveys of the prevalence of childhood psychiatric disorders: A review. *Child Dev., 54*, 531–548.

Loeber, R., Lahey, B. B., & Thomas, C. (1991). Diagnostic conundrum of oppositional defiant disorder and conduct disorder. *J. Abnorm. Psychol., 100*, 379–390.

McCarthy, D. (1972). *Manual for the McCarthy scales of children's abilities.* New York: Psychological Corporation.

McGee, R., Feehan, M., Williams, S., Partridge, F., Silva, P. A., & Kelly, J. (1990). *DSM-III* disorders in a large sample of adolescents. *J. Am. Acad. Child Adolesc. Psychiatry, 29*, 611–619.

Moos, R. H., & Moos, B. S. (1981). *Family environment scale manual.* Palo Alto, CA: Consulting Psychologists Press.

Offord, D., Boyle, M., Fleming, J. et al. (1989). Ontario child health study. *Can. J. Psychiatry, 34*, 483–491.

Offord, D., Boyle, M. H., Szatmari, P. et al. (1987). Ontario child health study II: Six-month prevalence rates and service utilization. *Arch. Gen. Psychiatry, 44*, 832–836.

Pianta, R. C., & Caldwell, C. B. (1990). Stability of externalizing symptoms from kindergarten to first grade and factors related to instability. *Dev. Psychopathol., 2*, 246–258.

Pianta, R. C., & Castaldi, J. (1989). Stability of internalizing symptoms from kindergarten to first grade and factors related to instability. *Dev. Psychopathol., 1*, 305–316.

Rae-Grant, N., Thomas, B. H., Offord, D. R., & Boyle, M. H. (1989). Risk, protective factors, and the prevalence of behavioral and emotional disorders in children and adolescents. *J. Am. Acad. Child Adolesc. Psychiatry, 28*, 262–268.

Richman, N., Stevenson, J., & Graham, P. J. (1982). *Pre-school to school: A behavioral study*. London: Academic Press.

Rose, S. L., Rose, S. A., & Feldman, J. F. (1989). Stability of behavior problems in very young children. *Dev. Psychopathol., 1*, 5–19.

Rutter, M. (1988). Epidemiological approaches to developmental psychopathology. *Arch. Gen. Psychiatry, 45*, 486–495.

Rutter, M. (1989). Isle of Wight revisited: Twenty-five years of child psychiatry epidemiology. *J. Am. Acad. Child Adolesc. Psychiatry, 28*, 633–659.

Seifer, R., & Sameroff, A. J. (1981). Multiple determinants of risk and invulnerability. In E. J. Anthony & B. J. Cohler (Eds.), *The invulnerable child* (pp. 51–69). New York: Guilford.

Shaffer, D., Gould, M. S., Brasic, J. et al. (1983). A children's global assesment scale (CGAS). *Arch. Gen. Psychiatry, 40*, 1228–1231.

Thomas, B. H., Byrne, C., Offord, D. R., & Boyle, M. H. (1991). Prevalence of behavioral symptoms and the relationship of child, parent, and family variables in 4- and 5-year-olds: Results from the Ontario Child Health Study. *J. Dev. Behav. Pediatr., 12*, 177–184.

Thomas, A., & Chess, S. (1984). *Origins and evolution of behavior disorders: From, infancy to early adult life*. New York: Brunner/Mazel.

Velez, C. N., Johnson, J., & Cohen, P. (1989). A longitudinal analysis of selected risk factors for childhood psychopathology. *J. Am. Acad. Child Adolesc. Psychiatry, 28*, 861–864.

Verhulst, F. C., & Van der Ende, J. (1992). Six-year developmental course of internalizing and externalizing problem behaviors. *J. Am. Acad. Child Adolesc. Psychiatry, 31*, 941–950.

Vikan, A. (1985). Psychiatric epidemiology in a sample of 1,510 ten-year-old children. *J. Child Psychol. Psychiatry, 26*, 55–76.

Weissman, M. M., Fendrich, M., Warner, V., & Wickramaratne, P. (1992). Incidence of psychiatric disorder in offspring at high and low risk for depression. *J. Am. Acad. Child Adolesc. Psychiatry, 32*, 640–648.

16

Behavioral Observations at Age 3 Years Predict Adult Psychiatric Disorders: Longitudinal Evidence from a Birth Cohort

Avshalom Caspi, Terrie E. Moffitt, and Denise L. Newman
Department of Psychology, University of Wisconsin, Madison

Phil A. Silva
Dunedin Multidisciplinary Health and Development Unit, University of Otago Medical School, Dunedin, New Zealand

Background: *This study provides, to our knowledge, the first empirical test of whether behavioral differences among children in the first 3 years of life are linked to specific adult psychiatric disorders: anxiety and mood disorders, antisocial personality disorder, recidivistic and violent crime, alcoholism, and suicidal behavior.* **Methods:** *In a longitudinal-epidemiological study, 3-year-old children were classified into groups based on examiner observations of their behavior. At age 21 years, they were reassessed for psychopathologic functioning using standardized interviews based on DSM-III-R criteria.* **Results:** *Although effect sizes were small, undercontrolled (includes children who are impulsive, restless, and distractible) and inhibited (includes children who are shy, fearful, and easily upset) children differed significantly from comparison children in young adulthood. Under-controlled 3-year-olds were more likely at 21 years to meet diagnostic criteria for antisocial personality disorder and to be involved in crime. Inhibited 3-year-olds were more likely at 21 years to meet diagnostic criteria for depression. Both groups were more likely to attempt suicide, and boys in both groups had alcohol-related problems. Controls for family social class did not change the findings.* **Conclusion:** *Some forms of adult psychopathologic abnormality are meaningfully linked, albeit weakly, to behavioral differences observed among children in the third year of life.*

Reprinted with permission from *Arch. Gen. Psychiatry*, 1996, Vol. 53, 1033–1039.

This research was supported by grants MH-49414 (Dr. Caspi) and MH-45070 (Dr. Moffitt) from the National Institute of Mental Health, Bethesda, Md; the William T. Grant Foundation, New York, NY; and the William Freeman Vilas Trust, University of Wisconsin, Madison. The Dunedin Multidisciplinary Health and Development Research Unit is supported by the Health Research Council of New Zealand.

We thank the Dunedin Unit investigators and staff, the New Zealand Police, and the study members and their families.

Developmental theories hypothesize that the origins of many adult mental disorders can be identified in behavioral characteristics that appear already in the first few years of life (Goldsmith et al., 1987; Rothbart & Ahadi, 1994). A scientific test of this hypothesis is difficult because it requires costly longitudinal studies from birth to adulthood. Thus, empirical evidence about continuities from bahavioral characteristics in early childhood—from the first 3 years of life—to psychopathologic abnormality in adulthood is practically nonexistent (Halverson, Kohnstamm, & Martin, 1994). Several longitudinal studies have linked behavioral characteristics in late childhood to adult adjustment problems (Caspi, Bem, & Elder, 1989; Huesmann, Eron, Lefkowitz, & Walder, 1984; Magnusson, 1988; Pulkkinen, 1988; Robins, 1966). Other longitudinal studies, involving preschool samples followed up into adolescence, have linked behavioral characteristics in early childhood to adjustment problems in early-adolescence (Tremblay, Pihl, Vitaro, & Dobkin, 1994) and mid-adolescence (Block, Block, & Keyes, 1988). As part of a longitudinal investigation of a large representative sample of children studied from age 3 to 21 years, this article provides, to our knowledge, the first empirical test of whether behavioral differences in early childhood are differentially linked to specific adult psychiatric disorders: anxiety, depression, mania, antisocial personality disorder, recidivistic and violent crime, alcoholism, and suicidal bahavior.

The predictor variables for this study were introduced previously (Caspi & Silva, 1995). We reported that, on the basis of behavioral observations at age 3 years, children in our study could be reliably classified into 1 of 5 distinct groups. The first 3—labeled *undercontrolled, inhibited,* and *well-adjusted*—resemble groups identified by Chess and Thomas (1987) in their pioneering studies of child temperament. The undercontrolled type, resembling the Chess–Thomas *difficult* type, includes children who are impulsive, restless, and distractible. The inhibited type, resembling the Chess–Thomas *slow-to-warm-up* type, includes children who are shy, fearful, and easily upset. The well-adjusted type, resembling the Chess–Thomas *easy* type, includes children who are capable of self-control when it is demanded of them, are adequately self-fonfident, and do not become unduly upset when confronting new people and situations. Typological research has identified these 3 types of children using different sources of information (e.g., parent reports or observations), different statistical methods (e.g., inverse factor analysis or cluster analysis), in different parts of the world (e.g., United States, the Netherlands or New Zealand), and in different age groups (e.g., early childhood or early adolescence) (Robins, John, Caspi, Moffitt, & Resilient, 1996), suggesting that these 3 types are the best candidates for inclusion in a generalizable classification of temperament. We also found 2 types of children not anticipated by Chess and Thomas: the *confident* type that included children who at 3 years were zealous and friendly and the *reserved* type that included children who at 3 years were slightly cautious.

We previously reported that these behavior styles at age 3 years predict personality traits at age 18 years, (Block, 1993), adding to a growing body of longitudinal research about the coherence of personality development beginning in early childhood (Block, 1993; Kagan, 1994). At 18 years, undercontrolled children described themselves as danger-seeking, impulsive, prone to respond with strong negative emotions to everyday events, and enmeshed in adversarial relationships. At 18 years, inhibited children described themselves as overcontrolled, harm-avoidant, and nonassertive. The behavior style of well-adjusted 3-year-olds was still discernible at 18 years, when, statistically, they defined normal, average young adults. The confident and reserved children resembled the well-adjusted children in their personality profile at age 18 years.

This article extends the study of development and tests 2 hypotheses about links between behavior styles at age 3 years and psychopathologic abnormality at 21 years. First, we tested whether undercontrolled and inhibited children are more likely to have psychiatric problems than other children. This hypothesis follows Thomas, Chess, and Birch (1970), who reported that of the 141 children in their study, difficult and slow-to-warm-up children required more psychiatric attention by early adolescence than easy children. Second, we tested whether behavioral characteristics of 3-year-olds provide discriminant validity in predicting specific psychiatric outcomes in adulthood (Bates, Wachs, & Emde, 1994). We expected that inhibited children would be at risk for anxiety disorders and for depressive disorders. We expected that undercontrolled children would be at risk for antisocial personality disorder and criminal behavior. Regarding alcohol-related problems and suicidal behavior, we expected that both undercontrolled and inhibited children would be at increased risk, although for different reasons. Research suggests that undercontrolled children may be attracted to the "good time" they associate with alcohol's disinhibiting effects, whereas inhibited children may use alcohol as a "self-medicating" strategy, to escape dysphoria (Weinberger & Bartholomew, 1996). This hypothesis is consistent with the notion that there may be at least two distinct temperamental-developmental pathways to adult alcohol problems (Cloninger, 1987; Zucker, Fitzgerald, & Moses, 1995). Similarly, research has shown that impulsive behavior and depressive disorders are independently linked to suicide attempts, suggesting that undercontrolled and inhibited childhood behaviors may also represent distinct risks for suicidal behavior in later life (Andrews & Lewinsohn, 1992; Virkkunen, De Jong, Bartko, & Linnoila, 1989).

The current study offers several advantages for testing these hypotheses. First, it combines long-term following with an epidemiological sampling frame. We can thus capture the full range of population variation on measures of toddler behavior and adult psychopathologic abnormality. Previous shorter-term studies have examined small or homogeneous samples, or clinic-referred samples, and the generalizability of results from such studies may be compromised by their selectivity (Cohen & Cohen, 1984). Second, the current study uses a well-established diagnostic interview enabling us to differentiate between adult psychiatric outcomes. Previous shorter-term studies have focused on nonspecific measures of psychopathologic functioning or on global measures of maladjustment, which may obscure meaningful differences in the developmental importance of distinct behavior styles (McDevitt, 1986). Third, the current study uses multiple data sources to test longitudinal predictions. Studies that rely on a single data source to measure both predictor and outcome variables cannot separate true prediction from confounded method variance. The only unconfounded strategy is to gather data from different sources at different ages (Bank & Patterson, 1992). We use bahavioral observations at age 3 years to predict outcomes at age 21 years, measured via self-reports, informant reports, and official records.

With independent data sources, we offer the first test in an epidemiological sample of the hypothesis that behavior in early childhood is linked to adult psychopathologic functioning. Our study constitutes a rigorous test in that it spans 18 years, uses independent data sources, and seeks to predict specific psychiatric disorders at age 21 years from behavioral observations made by an examiner after only 90 minutes of interaction with each child at age 3 years. Because the time span is long and the behavioral observations brief, this test provides a conservative estimate of the extent to which individual differences in early childhood influence adult mental health, and we expected modest effect sizes.

SUBJECTS AND METHODS

Sample

Participants are members of the Dunedin Multidisciplinary Health and Development Study. Silva (1990) has described the study's history. It is a longitudinal investigation of a complete cohort born between April 1, 1972, and March 31, 1973, in Dunedin, a city of approximately 120,000 on New Zealand's South Island. Perinatal data were obtained at delivery, and when the children were traced for follow-up at age 3 years, 91% of the eligible births participated in the assessment, providing a base sample of 1,037 (52% male) for longitudinal study. The children's fathers were representative of the social class distribution in the general population of similar age in New Zealand. The study members were of predominantly European ancestry. Fewer than 7% identified themselves as Maori or Polynesian, which matches the ethnic distribution of the South Island.

The Dunedin cohort has been reassessed at ages 3, 5, 7, 9, 11, 13, 15, 18, and 21 years. The basic procedure involves bringing participants to the research unit within 60 days of their birthday for a full day of individual data collection. The various research topics are presented as standardized modules, each administered by a different trained examiner in counterbalanced order (e.g., physical examination, mental health interview, delinquency interview, injury risk assessment). At each assessment, interview data are supplemented by a search of official records and questionnaires are mailed to informants who know each study member well.

Assessment of behavior styles in 3-year-olds. At age 3 years, children participated in a 90-minute testing session involving cognitive and motor tasks. Each child was tested by 1 of 10 examiners who had no knowledge of the child's behavioral history. Following the testing, the examiner rated the child's behavior on 22 behavioral characteristics, based on scales derived from the Collaborative Study on Cerebral Palsy, Mental Retardation, and Other Neurological Disorders of Infancy and Childhood (Caspi, Henry, McGee, Moffitt, & Silva, 1990). Factor- and cluster-analyses of the examiners' behavioral ratings revealed 5 reliable, homogeneous, and mutually exclusive clusters of children at age 3 (Caspi & Silva, 1995; Caspi, Henry, McGee, Moffitt, & Silva, 1990). Undercontrolled children ($n = 106$, 62% male) were described as irritable, impulsive, and impersistent; they had difficulty sitting still, were rough and uncontrolled in their behavior, and labile in their emotional responses. Inhibited children ($n = 80$, 40% male) were socially reticent (fearful and limited communication), inhibited in the testing situation, upset by strangers, and had difficulty concentrating on tasks. The behavior of well-adjusted children ($n = 405$, 48% male) was rated by examiners as within normal limits for their age. Confident children ($n = 281$, 52% male) were zealous, eager to explore the testing materials, and adjusted to the testing situation quickly. Reserved children ($n = 151$, 48% male) were timid and somewhat uncomfortable in the testing session; however, unlike inhibited children, their response disposition was not extreme, and their caution did not interfere with their task orientation.

Assessment of mental health problems at age 21 years: Psychiatric diagnosis. The Diagnostic Interview Schedule (DIS), developed by the National Institute of Mental Health for the Epidemiological Catchment Area program (Robins & Regier, 1991), was used to obtain diagnoses of mental disorder in the last 12 months. The Dunedin version of the DIS was modified to use only those items that were criteria for *DSM-III-R* (American Psychiatric Association, 1987) classifications to omit lifetime prevalence questions, and to score items as 0, no; 1, sometimes; and 2, yes, definitely. In identifying disorder, only scores of 2 were used to indicate a symptom (commensurate with a 5 in the original DIS). Diagnoses were determined by computerassisted algorithms that followed explicit criteria specified by *DSM-III-R*. The measurement and prevalence of mental disorders in the Dunedin study is reported elsewhere (Newman et al., 1996).

For this study, we examined the following groupings of psychiatric disorder: (1) anxiety disorders ($n = 195$) consisting of generalized anxiety disorder, obsessive-compulsive disorder, panic disorder, agoraphobia, social phobia, simple phobia, or any combination of these disorders; (2) depressive disorders ($n = 172$) consisting of major depressive episode, dysthymia, or both; (3) manic episode ($n = 19$), consisting of study members who experienced a manic episode in the past 12 months; (4) antisocial personality disorder ($n = 31$); and (5) alcohol dependence ($n = 94$).

Clinical significance of impairment associated with mental-health problems. Using a reporting period of the past 12 months, we assessed 6 indexes of impairment associated with mental health problems. These included reports of treatment seeking for psychiatric symptoms, hospitalizations for psychiatric symptoms, use of psychotropic medication, reports of suicide attempts, and court convictions for criminal offenses exclusive of traffic violations. In addition, respondents who reported symptoms in any of the modules of the DIS reported whether they experienced functional interference in work and daily activities associated with those symptoms. We created an overall impairment scale by summing these 6 indexes of impairment.

Informant index of mental health. This index was based on the endorsement of symptoms of mental-health problems in a mailed questionnaire completed by a significant other nominated by the study member as someone who knew them well. Of the 961 participants at age 21 years, 914 (95.1%)-nominated informants returned valid questionnaires. The questionnaire asked the informant to rate the study member on a series of positive and negative attributes. Thirteen of the items represented signs of mental disorders for each of the major categories of the DIS, worded in a general manner such as "Feeling depressed, miserable, sad or unhappy," or "Problems related to the use of alcohol" (Newman et al., 1996). Informants rated items as 0, does not apply; 1, applies somewhat; and 2, definitely applies.

Measures of criminality. Computerized records of participants' cumulative court convictions at all courts in New Zealand and Australia were obtained by searching the central computer systems of the New Zealand police. Conviction records excluded traffic offenses, with the exception of driving under the influence of alcohol or criminally negligent driving. Informed consent for the search was obtained at age 21 years. For this study, we examined 2 variables. The criminal recidivism group ($n = 80$) included individuals who had been convicted of 2 or more criminal offenses. The violent offender group ($n = 44$) included individuals who had been convicted of at least 1 of the following offenses: inciting violence, cruelty to an animal, using an attack dog on a person, possession of an offensive weapon, threatening a police officer, rape, manual assault, assault on a police officer, assault with a deadly weapon, manslaughter, and aggravated robbery.

Suicidality. As part of the mental-health interview, participants were asked about suicide attempts they had made during the past 12 months. Attempts were counted whether or not they had required medical attention.

Attrition. At age 21 years, mental-health interviews were missing for 76 members (7.3%) of the original sample of 1037; 17 persons died since age 3 years, 9 persons were not located, 19 refused to participate, and 31 were interviewed by telephone, but were not asked questions about mental health. The 76 nonrespondents did not differ from the 21-year-old participants on family social class ($t[939] = 1.35$, $P = .18$), race ($\chi^2[1] = .41$, $P = .52$), or sex ($\chi^2[1] = 1.26$, $P = .26$). Missing data were not disproportionately concentrated among any of the 5 temperament groups ($\chi^2[4] = 6.25$, $P = .18$). These results suggest that our findings are not compromised by attrition bias.

Statistical Analysis

Contingency tables and analyses of variance (ANOVA) were used to test the hypothesis that undercontrolled and inhibited 3-year-olds would have more mental health problems at age 21 years than other types of children. In addition, multivariate logistic regressions were used to examine specific continuity between behavior styles at age 3 years and particular types of adult psychiatric disorders at 21 years. Each regression equation contained a dummy variable representing undercontrolled children and a dummy variable representing inhibited children. The contrast or reference group in each regression equation was the well-adjusted group. After entering these 2 main effects and the main effect of sex, we added 2 interaction terms to test whether the association between undercontrolled and inhibited behavior at age 3 years and specific disorders at 21 years differed for male subjects and female subjects. We examined whether a model with sex interaction terms yielded significant improvements in the fit of the model to the data than a model with main effects only. In presenting the results, we report odds ratios (ORs) and the P values associated with the regression coefficients for the undercontrolled and inhibited dummy variables. The ORs indicate the factor by which the odds of a specific outcome occurring increased for undercontrolled and inhibited children relative to well-adjusted children. When there was no significant sex-by-temperament interaction effect, we report combined results for male and female subjects because this model constitutes a better form for the estimation of relative risk for undercontrolled and inhibited children. When there was a significant interaction at $P < .05$, results are reported separately by sex. To establish that the associations between behavior styles at age 3 years and adult disorders are independent of the family circumstances in which the study members grew up, we included a measure of family social class (Elley & Irving, 1985) as a covariate in all regression models. All reported ORs are adjusted for family social class. All significance tests are 2 tailed.

In performing the regression analyses we had to choose between a reference group of well-adjusted children or a reference group combining well-adjusted, reserved, and confident children. We performed the analyses using both options and the statistical and substantive findings did not change significantly. We report analyses using well-adjusted children as the reference group because, as noted in the introduction, this group provides an interpretive fit with previous studies about the structure of temperament. In contrast, the generality of additional types, such as the reserved and confident groups, has yet to be replicated in other samples to test whether they constitute independent types or whether they can be subsumed within the 3 replicable types.

RESULTS

Are Undercontrolled and Inhibited Children More Likely to Have Psychiatric Problems?

Table 1 gives the association between behavior styles at age 3 years and mental health problems at age 21 years. As shown in the table, the 1-year prevalence rate of psychiatric disorder, assessed by diagnostic interview at age 21 years, was 40%. This estimate is consistent with prevalence data for this age group in the National Comorbidity Survey (Kessler et al., 1994), in which the 12-month prevalence rate of any psychiatric disorders among 15- to 24-year-olds was 37%.

The table also shows that, as predicted, undercontrolled and inhibited children were the most likely to have a psychiatric disorder, and were also the most severely impaired by their condition. The likelihood of any psychiatric disorder at 21 years was weakly linked to behavior styles at age 3 years (χ^2 [4] = 8.5, $P = .07$). As expected, undercontrolled (46%) and inhibited (53%) children were the most likely to be diagnosed with a psychiatric disorder. The likelihood of multiple disorders at 21 years was significantly linked to behavior styles at age 3 years, ($\chi^2[4] = 12.4$, $P = .01$). Undercontrolled (27%) and inhibited (29%) children were significantly more likely to suffer from multiple disorders. An ANOVA of the impairment scale at age 21 years, with the behavior styles at age 3 years as the independent factor, also revealed a significant effect [$F(4,947) = 3.14$, $P = .01$]. Undercontrolled and inhibited children were the most impaired. Finally, an ANOVA of the informant reports of mental health problems at age 21 years, with the behavior styles at age 3 years as the independent factor, revealed a significant effect [$F(4,878) = 2.76$, $P = .03$]. According to informants, undercontrolled and inhibited children had the most mental health problems at age 21 years, corroborating the results based on clinical interviews with the sample members themselves.

In summary, across 18 years and across three different data sources—observer ratings, diagnostic interviews, and informant reports—the results provide support for the hypothesis that undercontrolled and inhibited children are at increased risk of psychiatric problems. By contrast, well-adjusted, reserved, and confident children were not distinguishable and had better mental health outcomes at age 21 years.

Do Behavior Styles at Age 3 Years Predict Specific Adult Psychiatric Outcomes?

Anxiety disorders. Figure 1 shows the association between behavior styles at age 3 years and anxiety disorders at 21 years. The figure shows the 1-year prevalence rates (i.e., cohort base rates) of specific

TABLE 1

Behavior Styles at 3 Years of Age and *DSM-III-R* Diagnoses, Level of Impairment Associated with Psychiatric Symptoms, and Informant-Observed Problems at 21 Years of Age

Outcome at Age 21 Years	Sample Base Rate at Age 21 Years	Behavior Styles at Age 3 Years*					χ^2 or F (P)
		Well-adjusted ($n = 375$)	Undercontrolled ($n = 94$)	Inhibited ($n = 73$)	Reserved ($n = 142$)	Confident ($n = 268$)	
Any disorder (%)	40	38[a]	46	53[b,c]	37[a]	42	$\chi^2 = 8.5$ (.07)
Multiple disorders (%)	19	15[a,d]	27[b]	29[b,e]	21	18[a]	$\chi^2 = 12.4$ (.01)
Mean (SD) impairment scale	0.76 (0.98)	0.65 (0.83)[a,d,e]	0.99 (1.27)[b,c]	0.93 (1.12)[b]	0.70 (0.94)[d]	0.81 (1.01)[b]	$F = 3.14$ (.01)
Mean (SD) informant scale	3.90 (3.67)	3.75 (3.37)[d]	4.82 (4.12)[b,e]	4.69 (4.11)[e]	3.87 (3.67)	3.58 (3.74)[a,d]	$F = 2.76$ (.03)

*Although 961 sample members participated in the mental health interview at 21 years of age, a few were missing complete information across all the Diagnostic Interval Schedule modules; hence $N = 952$.

[a] $P < .05$, pairwise contrast with the inhibited group.
[b] $P < .05$, pairwise contrast with the well-adjusted group.
[c] $P < .05$, pairwise contrast with the reserved group.
[d] $P < .05$, pairwise contrast with the undercontrolled group.
[e] $P < .05$, pairwise contrast with the confident group.

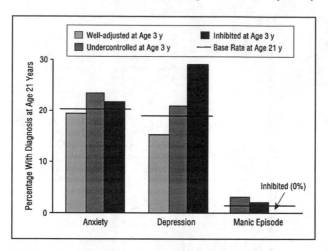

Figure 1. The association between behavior styles at age 3 years and adult anxiety and mood disorders.

disorders in the Dunedin sample as a whole, and the rates for well-adjusted, undercontrolled, and inhibited children. Because the sample is an unselected birth cohort, the sample rates may be treated as estimates of population rates among young adults in New Zealand.

Figure 1 shows that behavior styles at age 3 years could not significantly distinguish persons at risk for developing an anxiety disorder. However, before concluding that behavior styles do not constitute risk for anxiety disorders we conducted 3 additional tests. First, we tested the possibility that behavior styles at age 3 years could distinguish persons at risk for developing 2 or more anxiety disorders, but this test was not significant. Second, we tested whether behavior styles at age 3 years could predict specific subtypes of anxiety disorders (e.g., social phobia, agoraphobia, or obsessive-compulsive disorder), but these tests were not significant. Third, because categorical data are less sensitive than continuous measures, we examined scores on an anxiety symptom scale, consisting of 19 items from the DIS. An ANOVA of the number of anxiety symptoms at age 21 years did not show the predicted relation between inhibited behavior at age 3 years and anxiety at age 21 years. Rather, there was weak indication that, relative to well-adjusted children (mean $\pm$ *SD*, 2.6 $\pm$ 5.2), undercontrolled (mean $\pm$ *SD*, 3.9 $\pm$ 6.9) and inhibited (mean $\pm$ *SD*, 3.6 $\pm$ 6.7) children had slightly elevated anxious symptomatology [$F(2,538) = 2.54$, $P = .08$]. This association was not conditioned by sex [$F(2,538) = 0.66$, insignificant].

Mood disorders. The center panel in Fig. 1 shows the link between behavior styles at age 3 years and depressive disorders at 21 years. As predicted, inhibited children were significantly more likely to be diagnosed with depression at age 21 years (OR = 2.2, $P < .01$, 95% confidence interval [CI] = 1.2–3.9). Undercontrolled children were not significantly more likely to be diagnosed with depression. Although manic episodes could not be predicted from behavior styles at age 3 years, none of the inhibited children experienced mania, which is characterized by symptoms of increased activity, inflated self-esteem, and impulsive behaviors. Thus, inhibition showed predictive specificity within the family of mood disorders. There were no significant interaction effects between behavior style and sex in predicting mood disorders.

Antisocial behavior and criminality. Figure 2 shows the association between behavior styles at age 3 years and antisocial outcomes at age 21 years. As predicted, undercontrolled children were significantly overrepresented in every outcome examined. They were 2.9 times as likely to be diagnosed

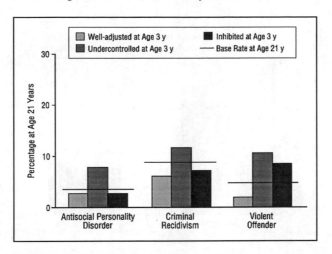

Figure 2. The association between behavior styles at age 3 years and adult criminal behavior.

with antisocial personality disorder ($P < .05$, 95% CI, 1.1–8.1), 2.2 times as likely to be recidivistic offenders ($P < .05$, 95% CI, 1.1–4.7), and 4.5 times as likely to be convicted for a violent offense ($P < .01$, 95% CI, 1.8–10.9). There were no sex interaction effects.

Unexpectedly, inhibited children were also significantly more likely to be convicted for a violent offense (OR = 2.9, $P < .05$, 95% CI, 1.0–8.4). However, this association was moderated by an interaction effect; inhibited boys (OR = 5.7, 95% CI, 1.6–20.1), but not girls (OR = 0.84, 95% CI, 0.09–7.9), were more likely to have been convicted for a violent offense.

Alcohol-related problems. Figure 3 shows the association between behavior styles at age 3 years and alcohol dependence at age 21 years. Undercontrolled children were 2.2 times as likely to be diagnosed

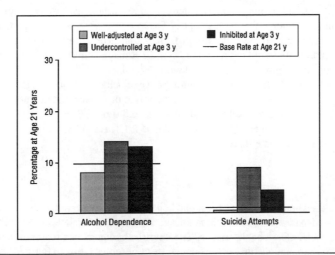

Figure 3. The association between behavior styles at age 3 years and adult alcohol dependence and suicide attempts.

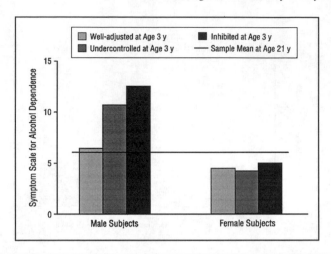

Figure 4. Scores on Diagnostic Interview Schedule alcohol abuse symptom scale at age 21 years as a function of behavior styles at age 3 years and sex.

with alcohol dependence ($P < .05$, 95% CI, 1.1–4.4). However, this association was moderated by an interaction effect; undercontrolled boys (OR = 2.7, 95% CI, 1.2–6.2), but not girls (OR = 0.53, 95% CI, 0.06–4.4), were more likely to have alcohol dependence. As predicted, inhibited children also had elevated rates of alcoholism, but this result did not attain statistical significance (OR = 1.8, $P = .15$, 95% CI, 0.80–4.1).

To further explore the relation between childhood behavior styles and alcohol-related problems, we examined scores on an alcohol abuse symptom scale, consisting of 23 items from the DIS. An ANOVA of the number of alcohol symptoms at age 21 years, with behavior styles at age 3 years as the independent factor, revealed a significant effect [$F(2,531) = 6.72$, $P = .01$]. Both undercontrolled and inhibited children had significantly more alcohol-related problems. However, this main effect was moderated by an interaction effect with sex [$F(2,531) = 5.80$, $P = .01$]. As shown in Fig. 4, both undercontrolled and inhibited boys, but not girls, had significantly more alcohol-related problems. Thus, whereas inhibited boys did not meet the *DSM-III-R* diagnostic cut-off for alcohol dependence, they did experience more problems associated with alcohol.

Suicide attempts. Figure 3 shows the association between behavior styles at age 3 years and suicide attempts at 21 years. Suicide attempts were significantly more concentrated among undercontrolled and inhibited children; undercontrolled children were 16.8 times ($P < .01$, 95% CI, 3.5–81.7) and inhibited children were 6.5 times as likely ($P < .05$, 95% CI, 1.1–39.8) to report attempting suicide. There were no sex interaction effects.

COMMENT

Results from the Dunedin study suggest that behavior styles observed in the third year of life are significantly related to mental-health problems at age 21 years. These relations were obtained even with adjustments for social class characteristics. The empirical connections represent small effect sizes, but they span 18 years and distinct data sources, from observer ratings after a 90-minute exposure to the child at age 3 years to mental health information gathered from clinical interviews with the sample members at 21 years. Although small cell sizes in some analyses may render some statistical estimates unstable, the patterns of associations reported were corroborated across independent data sources such as clinical interviews, informant reports, and official records. Still, the present results should be regarded with caution until they are replicated in other samples.

The results provide evidence that specific behavior styles in early childhood are connected to specific psychiatric problems in adulthood. Undercontrolled children were characterized by an impulsive, undercontrolled behavior style at age 3 years. At 21 years, they were more likely to meet the criteria for antisocial personality disorder and to be involved in criminal activities. Inhibited children were shy, fearful, and easily upset in novel settings at age 3 years. At 21 years, they were significantly more likely to meet diagnostic criteria for depression.

There were also similarities between the undercontrolled and inhibited groups. suggesting that children with different behavior styles may be at general risk for similar adult outcomes. Both groups were significantly more likely to attempt suicide, and both groups of boys were more likely to report alcohol-related problems. The latter finding is consistent with causative accounts that posit 2 pathways to alcohol-related problems: one associated with under-socialized behavior, the other with neurotic-depressive behavior (Cloninger, 1987). That the relation between both behavior styles and alcohol-related problems was confined to boys is consistent with evidence that enduring, heritable behavior traits may play a more important role in alcohol-related problems among males than females (McGue, Pickens, & Svikis, 1992).

There was 1 unexpected finding and 1 negative finding in our study. The unexpected finding was that inhibited boys, like undercontrolled children, were more likely to have been convicted for a violent offense. However, they were not more likely to be recidivistic offenders; they appeared in court records only once. Nor did they meet the diagnostic criteria for antisocial personality disorder. This suggests that inhibited boys who had been convicted for violence may have committed a single offense that was uncharacteristic of their usual behavior. The negative finding was that inhibited children were not, as predicted, at increased risk for anxiety disorders. This finding is inconsistent with shorter-term studies linking behavioral inhibition to anxiety problems (Biederman et al., 1990; Hirshfeld et al., 1992). However, those studies relied on very small samples and found differences only for specific subsets of extremely inhibited children, for example, children who showed a stable pattern of inhibition at four assessment ages or children with a family history of psychiatric disorder. It is thus possible that inhibited childhood behavior is a risk factor for anxiety disorders among a specific segment of children who have a family history of anxiety or who experience chronic family stress (Bernstein & Borchardt, 1991).

Although specific episodes of psychiatric disorders may be transient, documentation of a link between behavior styles in early childhood and psychopathologic abnormality in adulthood, paired with knowledge about the consistency of personality from childhood through adulthood (Caspi & Bem, 1990), suggests that, in the absence of significant characterological change, early-appearing behavioral differences may act as a persisting risk factor for some forms of psychiatric disorders.

REFERENCES

American Psychiatric Association. (1987). *Diagnostic and statistical manual of mental disorders* (3rd ed., rev.) Washington, DC: American Psychiatric Association.

Andrews, J. A., & Lewinsohn, P. M. (1992). Suicidal attempts among older adolescents: Prevalence and co-occurrence with psychiatric disorders. *J. Am. Acad. Child Adolesc. Psychiatry, 31*, 655–662.

Bank, L., & Patterson, G. R. (1992). The use of structural equation modeling in data from differnt types of assessments. In J. C. Rosen & P. McReynolds (Eds.), *Advances in psychological assessment* (pp. 41–74). New York: Plenum Press.

Bates, J. E., Wachs, T. D., & Emde, R. N. (1994). Toward, practical uses for biological concepts of temperament. In J. E. Bates & T. D. Wachs (Eds.), *Temperament: Individual differences at the interface of biology and behavior* (pp. 275–306). Washington, DC: American Psychological Association.

Bernstein, G. A., & Borchardt, C. M. (1991). Anxiety disorders of childhood and adolescence: A critical review. *J. Am. Acad. Child Adolesc. Psychiatry, 30*, 519–532.

Biederman, J., Rosenbaum J. F., Hirshfeld, D. R., Faraone, S. V., Bolduc, E. A., Gersten, M., Meminger, S. R., Kagan, J., Snidman, N., & Reznick, S. (1990). Psychiatric correlates of behavioral inhibition in young children of parents with and without psychiatric disorders. *Arch. Gen. Psychiatry, 47*, 21–26.

Block, J. (1993). Studying personality the long way. In D. Funder, R. D. Parke, C. Tomlinson-Keasey, & K. Widaman (Eds.), *Studying lives through time: Personality and development* (pp. 9–41). Washington, DC: American Psychological Association.

Block, J., Block, J. H., & Keyes, S. (1988). Longitudinally foretelling drug usage in adolescence: early childhood personality and environmental precursors. *Child Dev., 59*, 336–355.

Caspi, A., & Bem, D. J. (1990). Personality continuity and change across the life course. In L. Pervin (Ed.), *Handbook of personality: Theory and research* (pp. 549–575). New York: Guilford Press.

Caspi, A., Bem, D. J., & Elder, G. H. (1989). Continuities and consequences of interactional styles across the life course. *J. Pers., 57*, 375–406.

Caspi, A., & Silva, P. A. (1995). Temperamental qualities at age 3 predict personality traits in young adulthood: Longitudinal evidence from a birth cohort. *Child Dev., 66*, 486–498.

Caspi, A., Henry, B., McGee, R., Moffitt, T. E., & Silva, P. A. (1990). Temperamental origins of child and adolescent behavior problems: From age three to age fifteen. *Child Dev., 66*, 55–68.

Chess, S., & Thomas, A. (1987). *Origins and evolution of behavior disorders.* Cambridge, MA: Harvard University Press.

Cloninger, C. R. (1987). Neurogenetic adaptive mechanisms in alcoholism. *Science, 36*, 410–416.

Cohen, P., & Cohen, J. (1984). The clinician's illusion. *Arch. Gen. Psychiatry, 41*, 1178–1182.

Elley, W. B., & Irving, J. B. (1985). The Elley-Irving Socio-Economic Index 1981 census revision. *N. Z. J. Educ. Stud., 20*, 115–128.

Goldsmith, H. H., Buss, A. H., Plomin, R., Rothbart, M., Thomas, A., Chess, S., Hinde, R. A., & McCall, R. B. (1987). Roundtable: What is temperament? four approaches. *Child Dev., 58*, 505–529.

Halverson, C. F., Kohnstamm, G. A., & Martin, R. P. (Eds.). (1994). *The developing structure of temperament and personality from infancy to adulthood.* Hillsdale, NJ: Lawrence Erlbaum Associates.

Hirshfeld, D. R., Rosenbaum, J. F., Biederman, J., Bolduc, E. A., Faraone, S. V., Snidman, N., Reznick, J. S., & Kagan, J. (1992). Stable behavioral inhibition and its association with anxiety disorder. *J. Am. Acad. Child Adolesc. Psychiatry, 31*, 103–111.

Huesmann, L. R., Eron, L. D., Lefkowitz, M. M., & Walder, L. O. (1984). Stability of aggression over time and generations. *Dev. Psychol., 20*, 1120–1134.

Kagan, J. (1994). *Galen's prophecy.* New York: Basic Books.

Kessler, R. C., McGonagle, K. A., Zhoa, S., Nelson, C. B., Hughes, M., Eshleman, S., Wittchen, H. U., & Kendler, K. S. (1994). Lifetime and 12-month prevalence of *DSM-III-R* psychiatric disorders in the United States: Results from the National Comborbidity Study. *Arch. Gen. Psychiatry, 51*, 8–19.

Magnusson, D. (1988). *Individual development from an interactional perspective.* Hillsdale, NJ: Lawrence Erlbaum Associates.

McDevitt, S. C. (1986). Continuity and discontinuity of temperament in infancy and early childhood: A psychometric perspective. In R. Plomin & J. Dunn (Eds.), *The study of temperament: Changes, continuities, and challenges* (pp. 27–39). Hillsdale, NJ: Lawrence Erlbaum Associates.

McGue, M., Pickens, R. W., & Svikis D. S. (1992). Sex and age effects on the inheritance of alcohol problems: A twin study. *J. Abnorm. Psychol., 101*, 3–17.

Newman, D. L., Moffitt, T. E., Caspi, A., Mogdal, L., Silva, P. A., & Stanton, W. (1996). Psychiatric disorder in a birth cohort of young adults: Prevalence, comorbidity, clinical significance, and new case incidence from age 11 to 21. *J. Consult. Clin. Psychol., 105*, 299–312.

Pulkkinen L. (1988). The role of impulse control in the development of antisocial and prosocial behavior. In D. Olweus, J. Block, & M. Radke-Yarrow (Eds.), *Development of antisocial and prosocial behavior* (pp. 149–175). New York: Academic Press.

Robins, L. (1966). *Deviant children grown up*. Baltimore, MD: Williams & Wilkins.

Robins, L. N., & Regier, D. A. (Eds.). (1991). *Psychiatric disorders in America*. New York: Free Press.

Robins, R. W., John, O. P., Caspi, A., Moffitt, T. E., & Stouthamer-Loeber, M. (1996). Resilient, overcontrolled, and undercontrolled children: Three replicable personality types. *J. Pers. Soc. Psychol., 70*, 157–171.

Rothbart, M., & Ahadi, S. (1994). Temperament and the development of personality. *J. Abnormal Psychol., 103*, 55–66.

Silva, P. A. (1990). The Dunedin Multidisciplinary Health and Development study: A fifteen-year longitudinal study. *Pediatr. Perit. Epidemiol., 4*, 96–127.

Thomas, A., Chess, S., & Birch, H. G. (1970). The origins of personality. *Sci. Am., 223*, 102–109.

Tremblay, R. E., Pihl, R. O., Vitaro, F., & Dobkin, P. L. (1994). Predicting early onset of male antisocial behavior from preschool behavior. *Arch. Gen. Psychiatry, 51*, 732–739.

Virkkunen, M., De Jong, J., Bartko, J., & Linnoila, M. (1989). Psychobiological concomitants of history of suicide attempts among violent offenders and impulsive fire setters. *Arch. Gen. Psychiatry, 46*, 604–606.

Weinberger, D. A., & Bartholomew, K. (1996). Social-emotional adjustment and patterns of alcohol use among young adults. *J. Pers., 64*, 495–527.

Zucker, R. A., Fitzgerald, H. E., & Moses, H. D. (1995). Emergence of alcohol problems and the several alcoholisms. In D. Cicchetti & D. J. Cohen (Eds.), *Developmental Psychopathology* (pp. 677–711). New York: John Wiley & Sons.

17

Trends in a National Sample of Sexually Abusive Youths

Gail Ryan

*National Adolescent Perpetrator Network, C. Henry Kempe National Center for the
Prevention and Treatment of Child Abuse and Neglect, and Department of
Pediatrics, University of Colorado Health Sciences Center*

Thomas J. Miyoshi and Jeffrey L. Metzner

University of Colorado Health Sciences Center

Richard D. Krugman

*University of Colorado School of Medicine, University of Colorado Health
Sciences Center*

George E. Fryer

University of Colorado Health Sciences Center

Objective: *To describe sociodemographic factors pertinent to sexually abusive youths,
to define common characteristics of the offending behaviors and victims, and to identify
issues relevant to treatment recommendations.* **Method:** *The Uniform Data Collection
system (UDCS), developed by the National Adolescent Perpetrator Network, provided
data from 90 contributors in 30 states on more than 1,600 juveniles referred to them for
specialized evaluation and/or treatment following a sexual offense. The UDCS comprises
four separate structured questionnaires that collect both factual information and clinical
impressions.* **Results:** *Physical and sexual abuse, neglect, and loss of a parental figure
were common in these youths' histories. Twenty-two percent of the youths, who had
been victims of sexual abuse, reported that the perpetrator of their own sexual abuse
was female. The youths committed a wide range of sexual offenses, with twice as many
of the referring offenses involving female victims than male victims.* **Conclusion:** *The
discovery of sexually abusive youths across both urban and rural areas supports the
need for comprehensive service delivery and a continuum of treatment services to be
available in all communities.*

Reprinted with permission from *J. Am. Acad. Child Adolesc. Psychiatry,* 1996, Vol. 35(1), 17–25. Copyright
© 1996 by the American Academy of Child and Adolescent Psychiatry.

The authors thank the many individuals who support the Uniform Data Collection System: the Development
Committee, the contributors, and the membership of the National Adolescent Perpetrator Network. Special thanks
to Mildred TeSelle, Brandt Steele, the National Task Force on Juvenile Sexual Offending, and the Kempe Center
for financial contributions.

As the taboo that prevented the disclosure of the sexual abuse of children has dissipated, it has become known that many of the perpetrators of sexual abuse are themselves children. The 1990 Uniform Crime Reports indicated that 15% of the arrests for forcible rape (excluded by definition were statutory rape without force and other sex offenses) were committed by youths younger than 18 years old (Federal Bureau of Investigation, 1990). Studies of adult offenders reveal that a significant proportion of persons with a paraphiliac disorder develop deviant sexual arousal patterns before the age of 18 years (Abel, Rouleau, Cunningham-Rathner, 1986; Longo & Groth, 1983; Marshall, Barbaree, & Eccles, 1991).

Historically, the sexual offenses of juveniles were often denied and there was little accountability for the nature or impact of such behavior. Fear of labeling and the stigma associated with perversion supported denial of the sexual and criminal nature of some juvenile behavior. However, as specialized programs have developed to treat sexually abusive youths, identification and referrals have increased and it becomes more possible to describe the characteristics and crimes of these youths. Various clinicians have demonstrated that deviant sexual behaviors exhibited by adolescents are not the exploration of the inexperienced (Becker, Cunningham-Rathner, & Kaplan, 1986; Groth, 1977). The objective of this study was to define sociodemographic factors pertinent to sexually abusive youths, to define common characteristics of the offending behaviors and victims, and to identify issues relevant to treatment recommendations.

METHOD

The Uniform Data Collection System (UDCS) is a function of the National Adolescent Perpetrator Network (NAPN), which is an ongoing program supported by the C. Henry Kempe National Center for the Prevention and Treatment of Child Abuse and Neglect (Department of Pediatrics, University of Colorado Health Sciences Center, Denver). The NAPN is a voluntary, multidisciplinary network of more than 900 persons from programs across the United States, Canada, and some other countries who are providing interventions with juveniles who sexually abuse others. Approximately 90 members of the NAPN in 30 states have contributed data on more than 1,600 juveniles referred to them for specialized evaluation and/or treatment following a sexual offense. These contributions were voluntary and were submitted on consecutive referrals. Cases included youths in a wide variety of settings including smaller outpatient programs, special group homes, and larger residential and correctional treatment programs. Analyses of differences between various programs or contributors have not been done.

The UDCS was designed by a committee of network members in Denver during 1986. After collection of data on approximately 1,000, cases the UDCS was revised in 1989 to its current form. The UDCS comprises four separate structured questionnaires that collect both factual information and clinical impressions. Contributors submit data over time as new referrals come to them and are able to access their own data at a later date. The four questionnaires include initial intake information, clinical impressions at the time of evaluation, treatment progress reports, and information at the time of exit from treatment. The contributors' commitment of time to the submission of such data is extraordinary, as is their dedication to work with this difficult population.

Such a database provides a rich source of information to support hypothesis generation and further empirical studies in this field. This article will summarize information and clinical impressions obtained during the initial intakes and evaluations of a sample of 1,616 youths. Except where otherwise stated, the reader may assume an N of 1,616. Some subsets of data are smaller because they have been derived from the original 1,000 cases prior to (or the 616 cases following) revision of the instruments. Variations of these numbers (totals) are caused by the nonreporting by contributors on specific items.

RESULTS

Sociodemographics

The age range of sexually abusive youths in this sample is 5 to 21 years, with 90% between 10 and 18 years of age. The modal age is 14 years. Race, income, and religion are very similar to the general population. Males represent 97.4% and females 2.6% of the sample. These youths ($n = 1,000$) have been discovered in all areas of the country, with 27.4% living in rural areas with populations of less than 15,000, 21.0% in communities with populations between 15,000 and 50,000, 18.6% in cities with populations of more than 50,000 but less than 250,000, 16.1% in suburbs near large cities, and 16.9% in cities with populations of more than 250,000.

Most were living in a parent's home (84.9%), 6.3% in the home of a relative, and 8.8% in placements with unrelated caregivers at the time of discovery of their abusive behaviors. In 97.0% of the homes, one or more other juveniles were present. Only 53.9% were living with two parents (27.8% were living with both natural parents and 26.1% with one natural parent and one stepparent), 23.1% were with only a mother, 3.2% were with only a father, 6.3% were with a parent and the parent's housemate, and 15.1% were living with neither parent. In the general population, 70.7% of children younger than 18 years old were living with both parents, 23.3% with mother only, 3.3% with father only, and only 2.6% with neither parent (US Bureau of the Census, 1993). In 71.9% of the households ($n = 1,000$) the head of the house was employed; 20.3% were receiving either aid to dependent children or social security support.

Only 5% of this sample were elementary school students, 53.7% were in junior high school (grades 7, 8, 9), and 42.4% were attending high school (grades 10, 11, 12). Seventy percent maintained at least a C average in school, with 23% having a grade point average of more than 3.0. Most attended regular public schools; 6.8%, 0.5%, and 1.8% of the sample attended alternative schools, private schools, and church-affiliated schools, respectively. In spite of reasonable academic success, a large number (60%) of these youths were known to have truancy, learning disabilities, and/or behavior problems at school. Only 28% were reported as having no record of problems at school.

History of Abuse

Traumatic experiences were common in the histories or these youths. At the point of intake (before further disclosures or discoveries during the treatment process), it was known that 41.8% had been victims of physical abuse and 39.1% of sexual abuse. Neglect was also recorded in 25.9%. In 63.4%, the youth had witnessed some form of family violence in the home (i.e., spouse abuse, abuse of a sibling), 27.9% had some indication of substance abuse, and 45.6% had previously been referred for some type of therapy. Of those known to have been abused during childhood, only 16.9% of the physical abuse complaints and only 37.0% of the sexual abuse complaints had resulted in adjudication (i.e., a final judgment of the court).

Fifty-seven percent had experienced the loss of a parental figure and 13.6% the loss of some other significant person. In 12% of these cases of parental loss, the loss was the result of the death of one or both parents; another 34.2% of these losses were accounted for by out-of-home placements during chilhood. Other losses occurred with the termination of parent–child relationships due to abuse interventions, abandonment, or desertion associated with parental divorce.

Nonsexual Offense History

Nonsexual offenses known at the point of intake were present in 63% of these cases; 27.8% were known for more than three nonsexual offenses. The nonsexual offenses included the full range of delinquent behaviors (Table 1).

TABLE 1
Nonsexual Offenses ($N = 1,616$)

Offense	%
Shoplifting	41.4
Theft	30.7
Burglary	17.1
Assault	26.4
Vandalism	20.4
Arson	15.3
Runaway	26.0
Animal cruelty	8.1

In response to nonsexual offenses, 25.0% of those involved had been adjudicated delinquent, 17.5% had been referred to diversion programs, and 31.5% had been on probation. For 27.3% of those involved in delinquent behavior, placement in either a group home, treatment facility, or state correctional facility had occurred previously in response to nonsexual misbehavior.

Sexual Offenses

These youths had committed a wide range of sexual offenses. Ninety-one percent of their victims were between 3 and 16 years of age; 63% were younger than age 9 years. The most frequently reported victim was 6 years old, and a small number (2.6%) were infants and toddlers younger than age 2 years. Twice as many of the referring offenses involved female victims compared to male victims. The average number of victims known at the time of intake was 7.7, 38.8% of whom were blood relations of the young offender from the same household. Sexual abuse of a peer accounted for 10% of the offenses, sexual victimization of strangers was 6%, and only 4.5% were sexual abuse of an adult.

Many referring offenses (35.4% of $n = 741$) involved one or more types of vaginal or anal penetration without oral-genital contact, 14.7% involved one or more types of oral-genital contact, and 17.9% involved both penetration and oral-genital contact; thus 68% involved penetrating and/or oral-genital behavior.

The offenses of these youths included verbal coercion (57%), threats (24.5%), and physical force (31.7%). In the revised instrument data ($n = 616$), it was known at intake that 25.9% of those referred after age 12 had committed some sexually abusive behavior before age 12.

For some of these youths, the referring offense was a hands-off offense (Table 2). Many of these youths were already known to have committed one or more prior hands-off offenses, and a large portion of those referred for hands-off offenses were known (at the time of the intake) to have also sexually abused a child.

Only 7.5% of this sample had previously been charged with a sexual offense. Regarding the referring offense, 1.1% were charged as adults in criminal court, 82.9% were charged in juvenile court, and 3.8% were referred to family courts. Forty-seven percent were found guilty as charged. Some had plea bargained to nonsexual or less serious charges and some had been referred to diversion programs.

Professional and Client Impressions

Information was obtained concerning the process of evaluation and assessment on more than 75% of the sample. This information has been analyzed in 774 cases from the original 1,000 cases. Payment for these evaluations came from the following sources: courts (39.3%), grant funds (16.9%), social

TABLE 2

Hands-Off Offense History for Youths Whose Referral Was
Precipitated by a Hands-Off Offense ($N = 1,000$)

History of	n	Known Priors (%)	Also Sexual Abuse of a Child (%)
Exhibitionism	161	33	35
Voyeurism	48	75	50
Obscene calls	32	87	40
Stealing underwear	29	65	40

services (16.7%), client's family (15.9%), and medical insurance (4.0%). Less than 1% were paid for by either Medicaid or Civilian Health and Medical Program of the Uniformed Services (CHAMPUS). Referrals came from juvenile courts (65.4%), probation (25.8%), and social services (15.9%). Public defenders and private attorneys originated 3% of the referrals, and only 3.5% were referrals by the client and/or family themselves. More than 7% came from multiple referral sources. The purpose of most referrals was to determine "amenability for treatment" (81.8%) and treatment needs (90.8%). Other referral questions included issues related to dangerousness (52.5%), dispositional recommendations (49.7%), placement decisions (28.8%), and verification of what had occurred during the offense (20%).

Most evaluators (95.3%) had access to at least some corroborating sources of information; 76.7% had current offense reports, 40.3% had probation reports, and 57.4% had access to victim statements. Approximately one third had school records, medical and/or prior psychological reports, and/or prior offense reports. Many evaluators used one or more testing instruments in the assessment: MMPI (58.9%), WISC-R or WAIS-R (34.4%); slightly fewer than 30% used the Thematic Apperception Test, Bender Gestalt, or Draw-A-Person, and Rorschach (23%). More than 70% reported that these measures were helpful in their evaluations. In data ($n = 774$) received between 1986 and 1988, only 12.3% had used a sexual interest cardsort. Several additional measures were used in the more recent sample: Multiphasic Sexual Inventory (21.5%), Program for Healthy Adolescent Sexual Expression (PHASE) Typology (7.49%), and Wenet-Clark Risk Criteria (15.0%).

Impressions from the Clients

Evaluators rated the youths' empathy, remorse, sense of responsibility, and levels of denial. Eighty-six percent of these youths were admitting at the time of initial assessment that a sexual offense had, in fact, occurred, although 5% of those did not admit being present, and 13% of those who thought an offense had occurred denied being a participant. Only 19.4% were accepting full responsibility, while 32.8% attributed little or no responsibility to themselves. Sixty-two percent were rated as expressing little or no empathy for the victim of their offense, and 51% expressed little or no remorse or guilt. Although nearly two thirds (63.6%) said they blamed themselves for the offense, one third blamed the victim, and some dispersed the blame among coparticipants (12.0%), parents (9.8%), or drug/alcohol use (5.3%). A few (4.4%) attributed their offense to "being sick," and 14.1% blamed their own past experience. Many cases dispersed blame among more than one source.

Slightly more of the youths (45.3%) reported having been beaten by a household member than the physical abuse of record (41.8%), and slightly fewer (33.6%) reported a history of sexual abuse than the prevalence of record (39.1%). Of those who had experienced beatings at home, more than half said they had "deserved" to be beaten. Forty-two percent reported being left home either alone or in charge of younger siblings before age 10 years. Of the youths who acknowledged having been sexually abused, 25.4% said the perpetrator was less than 5 years older and a total of 50.8% said the perpetrator was less than 10 years older than themselves. More than 22% said the perpetrator of their own sexual abuse was female and only 10% were strangers.

Only 57.8% of these youths perceived themselves as sexually "normal/adequate," 14.7% said they were sexually "mature," and 25.2% reported feeling inadequate or different from others. Only 1.9% identified themselves as homosexual. Forty percent reported having had an "age-appropriate" sexual relationship at some time. Only half as many of the youths known to have been sexually abused reported feeling sexually "normal or adequate"; two times as many of those youths also felt "different or inadequate"; and two and one half times as many identified themselves as homosexual (still less than 4%). Of the 774 evaluation cases, 664 responded to the question of masturbation, and 587 (88%) of those clients said they do masturbate, although 46.4% said "less than once per week"; 45.4% reported masturbating to a sexual fantasy and 33.2% of those thought their fantasies were deviant. Only about 10% denied ever masturbating.

Some of these young offenders said they think of sex as a way to "hurt/degrade/punish" (8.4%), dissipate anger (9.4%), and control/feel powerful (23.5%). Only about one third thought of sex as a way of showing love or caring for another person. More than half (55.9%) viewed aggression as a way to protect themselves and felt it was an expected masculine trait.

In the initial evaluation, 45.6% were able to report some "trigger" feeling or situation which they believed was associated with their offending behavior. These were most frequently described as anger, boredom, or family problems. Many disclosed to the evaluator additional sexual offenses not previously reported (21.3%), with 11.8% reporting "several" and 4.6% "a lot."

Clinicians' Impressions of the Clients

Based on all sources of information, evaluators reported their impressions of several factors along a continuum and their belief regarding prognosis. Although the impressions were clearly subjective, the data suggest that the young offenders in this sample may be less assertive, less mature, and less educated about sexual matters than their peers. For example, 65% of the sample were rated as having a maturity level less than was age appropriate and almost 70% were described as demonstrating sexual knowledge that was either less than average or distorted. Family function and individual social competence appeared problematic despite the sociodemographic variables such as race, religion, geography, and parental income being very similar to the general population (Ryan, Davis, Miyoshi, Lane, & Wilson, 1987). In most cases (72.0%), the evaluator felt the client was "treatable," although in 23.8% the evaluator was uncertain. Only 4.2% marked "no." At the same time, only 36.2% felt sure the client was "motivated" to change, 43.8% said "maybe," and 14.4% reported "no."

Evaluators' Recommendations

In light of the nature of this sample, it is not surprising that most of the evaluators had some treatment options available. Seventy-seven percent had the option of specialized group treatment for sexually abusive youths available, and 87.5% of those recommended group therapy, either alone or in conjunction with other treatment options (e.g., family therapy and/or individual psychotherapy). Only 44.4% had an option of secure residential placements and only slightly more than half of those included offense-specific treatment; 22.9% made recommendations for secure residential placements, with approximately three quarters of those placements including specialized treatment. Only 37.7% had open residential facilities as an option, although fewer than half of those offered offense-specific treatment;

16.7% recommended this option. Seventy percent had outpatient treatment available, although not all were offense specific; 46.4% recommended outpatient treatment (usually offense specific).

It was expected that treatment would be paid for by the court (29.8%), social services (19.1%), family (18%), medical insurance (5.3%), and in some instances, through grants or contracts. In 73% of the cases, evaluators expected to be involved in the ongoing treatment.

DISCUSSION

The limits of a database such as the UDCS include the following:

1. Data are contributed by a diverse group of people who may have different levels of training and experience, and may define terminology differently. Interrater reliability is certainly questionable.

2. The reported data are from a group of youths who are alleged to have committed sexual offenses and have been referred to programs offering specialized services. It is unknown how this group as a whole may vary from youths who have engaged in sexually abusive behavior and have either remained undetected or been referred to routine counseling or correctional systems.

3. The sources of data available to the contributors are not entirely consistent or defined, although it is known that only 5% of the entries relied solely on the self-reports of the juveniles and their family and that 75% had accessed police or court records for corroboration of offense details. It is not possible, however, to know the interplay between various sources of information and how contributors record information in the face of conflicting reports.

Although it is clear that such data have some limitations, several strengths of the system help to mitigate the weaknesses:

1. Great care was taken in designing the data collection instruments to make each item as clear and explicit as possible, and each choice of answer, when provided, mutually exclusive. Thus, although interrater reliability is a concern, much effort was expended to lessen its impact.

2. The large number of contributors ($N = 90$) lessens the influence of individual cases ($N = 1,616$) and differences by providing a broad-based sample.

3. The fact that it is a national sample from 30 states also lessens the impact of policy and system differences because many geographic areas are represented.

4. The clinician-provided data suggest greater access to and knowledge of the juveniles in this sample than might be available or possible through a retrospective records-based data process.

5. The combination of factual and perceptual data suggests trends in both the identification and description of these youths and the clinical understanding of this population.

The age range and modal age of identified sexually abusive youths during the 1980s is very similar to those reported elsewhere. Studies conducted in Washington, Michigan, California, Oregon, Vermont, and Canada have each shown very similar findings in regard to modal age of juvenile offenders, types of offenses, and number of victims (Chabot, 1987; Department of Youth Authority, 1986; Farrell & O'Brien, 1988; Mathews & Stermac, 1989; Wasserman & Kappel, 1985; Wheeler, 1986). It is not yet possible to know how increased awareness and reporting of sexually abusive behavior in the 1990s among preadolescents will impact this description. Remembering that these data come from providers working with sexually abusive youths, it is not surprising that few had been found not guilty or had charges dismissed; only 6.3% had been referred for pretrial evaluation, 35.6% had been referred for evaluation prior to sentencing, and the balance were referred for intake into treatment.

The represenᴛation of females who are sexually abusive in this sample (2.6%) is similar to the proportion reported by other programs (Grayson, 1989), although there continues to be some debate regarding the proportion of females among juvenile sex offenders (Barbaree, Hudson, & Seto, 1993). The lower representation of female offenders in all data may be symptomatic of an overall reticence to identify the sexually abusive behavior of females because of its dissonance with cultural expectations, or it may represent a truly lower incidence. However, more than 22% of these youths reported that the perpetrator of their own abuse was female. Anecdotally, programs offering treatment for both male and female sexually abusive youths do report a somewhat higher proportion of female referrals.

Disruptions in early childhood care are evident in the data on family constellations and dysfunctions. The small number (27.8%) of intact families and high incidence of parental loss (57%) support the finding of "inconsistent care" reported by Prentky et al. (1989) as a significant developmental factor in an adult sample of sexual offenders. At the same time, in considering the high incidence of out-of-home placements (34.2%) and family disruption during childhood, the reader is cautioned that it is not possible with these data to separate the effect of out-of-home placement and family breakdowns from the effect of those factors that led to such conditions. Additional family dysfunction appeared to be related to the presence of substance abuse and family violence.

Although the prevalence of physical and sexual abuse of these youths is known at the time of initial evaluation to be considerably higher than is reported in the general population (Finkelhor, Hotaling, Lewis, & Smith, 1990), the history of sexual abuse (39.1%) appears lower than is frequently suggested by sex offender therapists, who routinely report that 60% to 80% of these clients have experienced childhood sexual abuse prior to offending (Burgess, Hazelwood, Rokous, Hartman, & Burgess 1988; Longo, 1982). This discrepancy may be related to the client's initial lack of definition of sexual abuse: just as these youths often do not recognize or understand the abusive nature of their own sexual behavior, they have often failed to define the abusive nature of their own childhood experiences. The "normalization" of harmful, nonempathic interpersonal interactions may help explain the "contagious" aspects of sexual abuse as well as resistance to change. Denial and misattribution are common characteristics of sexual abuse. It is not surprising that as sexually abusive youths are held accountable for sexually abusive behavior and learn to correctly define sexual abuse, many discover that earlier experiences of their own were abusive, and the reported incidence of victimization in the history of this population rises. It may also be suggested that male socialization discourages male disclosures of sexual victimization and that these disclosures are facilitated by the treatment process.

Of special concern is the low rate of adjudication in cases of known physical and sexual abuse of these clients during childhood. For most, the perpetrator(s) of their abuse had not been held accountable, which describes a lack of protection, validation, and empathy in the experience of these youths. It is not unexpected, therefore, that many of these youths do not have either a moral or legal sense of responsibility for their own abusive behavior. Fifty-one percent of the youths in this sample, known to have been victims of sexual abuse in their own childhood, were sexually abused by a perpetrator who was less than 5 years older. This finding directly parallels the incidence of perpetration by adolescents in studies of sexually abused boys (Rogers & Terry, 1984; Showers, Faber, Joseph, Oshins, & Johnson, 1983).

Kobayashi, Sales, Becker, Figueredo, and Kaplan (1995) described the results of a theoretical model tested on 117 juvenile male sexual offenders that indicated physical abuse by the father and sexual abuse by males increase sexual aggression by adolescents. Sexual aggression by adolescents was decreased by bonding to the adolescent's mother. A number of explanations were provided by the authors for their findings, although they seem to favor a social modeling theory to explain the behavioral development of juvenile sex offenders. This theory hypothesizes that sexual abuse by females would not be relevant for social modeling (as those behaviors would not be sexually appropriate to a developing male) and that deviant patterns of sexual behavior were apparently modeled based on such experiences with other males. This theory does not adequately address hypotheses regarding the importance of attachments, which are primarily the product of the maternal-child relationships (Marshall, Hudson, & Hodkinson, 1993). There are obviously a variety of other factors relevant to the etiology of deviant sexual aggression by adolescents (Ryan, 1991). Our data certainly support the commonsense hypotheses that issues pertinent to the development of empathy should be further studied with this adolescent population (Marshall, Hudson, Jones, & Fernandez, 1994; Pithers, 1994).

The amount of nonsexual offending in this sample is significant. Remembering that studies of adult sex offenders report that fewer than 10% are psychotic, approximately 30% are considered antisocial, and more than 60% have primarily paraphilic disorder (Knopp, 1984), it is reasonable to hypothesize that the 27.8% of this juvenile sample who are known to have been identified with three or more nonsexual offenses might be considered conduct-disordered and may constitute the antisocial group of offenders as they become adults. Other studies (Kavoussi, Kaplan, & Becker, 1988; Shaw et al., 1993) have reported a high incidence (48% and 81%, respectively) of conduct disorders in a population of adolescent sex offenders. Further analysis of the subgroup demonstrating multiple nonsexual offending may have important implications for criminal justice prevention and intervention efforts (Metzner & Ryan, 1995).

Sexual attitudes demonstrated by this sample seem to reflect extreme experiences and confusion. However, although sexual preference, gender identity, and homophobic issues have been described as major treatment concerns by Breer (1987) and others, only a very small percentage of these youths (1.9%) identify themselves as homosexual and only one third believe their sexual fantasies are deviant. The levels of denial, lack of empathy, and projection of blame parallel the thinking errors, generalized defenses, and externalized control issues reported in much of the descriptive literature (Ward, Hudson, & Marshall, 1995). The evaluators' assessments concerning treatability appear to support the belief that most of these youths have the potential to benefit from treatment, but require a court order to encourage compliance, which is similar to assessments of many adult offenders (Travin, 1994).

The wide range of sexual offenses committed by this sample seems to parallel the findings of research with adult offenders, which indicates that many sexual offenders exhibit more than one type of sexually deviant behavior (Abel et al., 1986). This finding of multiple paraphilias suggests that the same individual may be raping, exposing, peeping, and/or molesting children within a single period of time or progressing from one type of abusive behavior to another over time. While more than half of the referring offenses were known to have included the more intrusive acts of penetration and/or oral-genital contact, even the less intrusive "hands-off" referrals were often known to have also committed hands-on offenses. Only a small portion of this sample had been referred for a single incident of the less intrusive behavior. That there were reports of multiple victims points out the chronic nature of these youths' sexual problems.

The use of force in more than 30% of the referring offenses is of concern because it is usually not necessary to use force in order to gain the compliance of vulnerable victims, especially children. These findings contradict the assertions of critics who suggest that juveniles are being labeled sex offenders and ordered into treatment for minor misbehavior. In this sample, the sexual offenses most frequently reported by the press (assault on an adult by a juvenile) represent the smallest portion of their crimes (4.5%). The only area of sexual offending receiving significant attention in direct education with teenagers (acquaintance rape) is also less frequent (10%). The sexual abuse of small children by older children is still largely unrecognized by the public, even though it has been reported in the literature since 1984 that more than half of the sexual abuse of boys and 15% to 25% of the sexual abuse of girls is committed by older juveniles (Rogers & Terry, 1984; Showers et al., 1983).

Our sample's history of early childhood disruptions, significant prevalence of physical and sexual abuse, nonsexual offending, and sexual attitudes that seem to reflect extreme experiences and confusion all have important treatment implications. These findings support the recommendation by the National Task Force on Juvenile Sexual Offending (1993) that certain definable issues, which have been identified as a result of clinical experience, should be addressed in the treatment process of every sexually abusive youth. These include victimization issues for the offender, sexual identity, identification (and the remediation to the extent possible) of family issues or dysfunction that support offending behaviors, development of prosocial relationship skills with peers, and remediation of skill deficits that interfere with successful functioning. Our findings are also consistent with the National Task Force's recommendations that treatment emphasize acceptance of responsibility for behavior, identification of a pattern or cycle of offense behavior, development of empathy with others, and identification of cognitive distortions related to offending behaviors.

The discovery of sexually abusive youths across both urban and rural areas parallels the prevalence of child sexual abuse in the United States (Finkelhor et al., 1990) and supports the need for comprehensive service delivery and a continuum of treatment services to be available in all communities (Bengis, 1986). Recognition of the very young onset of sexually abusive behaviors in this sample has important implications for future service delivery. Although only 10% of this sample were referred before age 10 years, it was known that one fourth of the older referrals had committed sexually abusive acts before age 12 years. It may be expected that prepubescent referrals will increase in response to the more recent recognition of childhood perpetration (Cantwell, 1988; Gil & Johnson, 1993; Isaac, 1987; Johnson, 1987; Ryan et al., 1989). It is also hoped that in future samples, the 45.6% who had previously been referred for counseling will begin to drop as those earlier referrals begin to provide more effective interventions. Although the UDCS does not document the referral questions or type of treatment in these earlier referrals, anecdotal information from young offenders and their parents suggests that often their earlier experiences in counseling were triggered by concern about sexual issues or behavior, but that mental health professionals rarely addressed sexuality directly in sessions.

Less than 40% of the sexual abuse in this sample is clearly incestuous. In many areas, social service systems decline to investigate or intervene in reports of extrafamilial sexual abuse. Although referral of these cases to law enforcement authorities may be very appropriate (National Task Force on Juvenile Sexual Offending, 1993), the social and familial problems of these young offenders may also benefit from social service interventions. The need to provide adequate intervention with sexually abusive youths following early referrals has important implications in preventing the sexual abuse of additional victims.

The prevalence of specialized group treatment as both an option and a recommendation reflects the same consensus set forth in the revised report from the National Task Force on Juvenile Sexual Offending (1993). At the same time, the desirability of adjunct therapies including individual and family work is also evident in these recommendations to a much lesser extent. It is not known to what extent treatment recommendations are shaped by lack of financial resources, although it is likely that options are heavily influenced by such resources.

Although the juveniles described by these data are a select group, referred to specialists for evaluation and treatment, this information confirms the findings of many smaller samples and provides a basis for comparison. Further analysis of variables and subgroups is desirable in order to refine the development of hypotheses and promote sound empirical research. Such analysis will occur as time and funds allow. Areas of interest include (1) comparison of certain offense variables with specific personal variables; (2) comparisons between offenders using physical force and less violent offenders as well as the relationship, if any, to rates of offense behaviors; (3) comparison of sibling offenses to extrafamilial offenses; (4) relationships among initial self-statements of the youth, length of treatment, and exit variables; and (5) relationships between characteristics of these youths' offenses and their own victimization. Additional data collection will be considered as an avenue for comparisons over time and relevant to discrete variables of interest.

REFERENCES

Abel, G., Rouleau J., & Cunningham-Rathner, J. (1986). Sexually aggressive behavior. In W. Curran, A. McGarry, & S. Shah, (Eds.), *Forensic psychiatry and psychology: Perspectives and standards for interdisciplinary practice* (pp. 289–314). Philadelphia: FA Davis.

Barbaree, H. E., Hudson, F. M., & Seto, M. C. (1993). Sexual assault in society: The role of the juvenile offender. In H. E. Barbaree, W. L. Marshall, & S. M. Hudson, (Eds.), *The juvenile sex offender* (pp. 1–24). New York: Guilford Press.

Becker, J. V. Cunningham-Rathner, J., & Kaplan, M. S. (1986). Adolescent sexual offenders: Demographics, criminal and sexual histories: Recommendations for reducing future offenses. *J. Interpersonal Violence, 1*, 431–445.

Bengis, S. (1986). *Comprehensive service delivery and a continuum of care.* Orwell, VT: Safer Society Press.

Breer, W. (1987). *The adolescent molester.* Springfield, IL: Charles, C. Thomas.

Burgess, A., Hazelwood, R., Rokous, F., Hartman, C., & Burgess, A. (1988). Serial rapists and their victims: Re-enactment and repetition in human sexual aggression: Current perspectives. *Ann. NY Acad. Sci., 528*, 277–295.

Cantwell, H. (1988). Child sexual abuse: Very young perpetrators. *Child Abuse Negl., 12*, 579–582.

Chabot, H. (1987). Interdisciplinary cooperation. In *Juvenile justice's approach to child sexual abuse: Final report.* Pierce Country, WA: Juvenile Sexual Assault Unit, pp. 1–46.

Department of Youth Authority, Task Force on Sex Offenders (1986). *Sex offender task force report.* California Department of Youth Authority.

Farrell, K. J., & O'Brien, B. (Eds.). (1988). *Sexual offenses by youths in Michigan: Data, implications, and policy recommendations.* Detroit: Safer Society Resources.

Federal Bureau of Investigation (US Department of Justice) (1990). *Uniform crime reports of the United States*, Washington, DC: US Government Printing Office.

Finkelhor, D., Hotaling, G., Lewis, I. A., & Smith, C. (1990). Sexual abuse in a national survey of adult men and women: Prevalence, characteristics, and risk factors. *Child Abuse Negl., 14*, 19–28.

Gil, E., & Johnson, T. (1993). *Sexualized children.* Rockville, MD: Launch Press.

Grayson, J. (1989). Female sex offenders. *Virginia child protection newsl., 28*, 1–12.

Groth, A. N. (1977). The adolescent sex offender and his prey. *Int. J. Offender Ther. Comp. Criminol., 21*, 249–254.

Isaac, C. (1987). Identification and interruption of sexually offending behaviors in prepubescent children. Presented at the Sixteenth Annual Child Abuse & Neglect Symposium, Keystone, CO.

Johnson, T. (1987). Child Perpetrators: Children who molest children. *Child Abuse Negl., 12*, 219–230.

Kavoussi, R. J., Kaplan, M., & Becker, J. V. (1988). Psychiatric diagnoses in adolescent sex offenders. *J. Am. Acad. Child Adolesc. Psychiatry, 27*, 241–242.

Knopp, F. H. (1984). *Retraining adult sex offenders: Methods and models.* Syracuse, NY: Safer Society Press.

Kobayashi, J., Sales, B. D., Becker, J. V., Figueredo, A. J., & Kaplan, M. S. (1995). Perceived parental deviance, parent type and child bonding, child abuse, and child sexual aggression. *Sex Abuse J. Res. Treat, 7*, 25–44.

Longo, R. (1982). *Child molestation: The offender and the assault.* Presented to American Correctional Association, 112th Annual Congress, Toronto.

Longo, R. E., & Groth, A. N. (1983). Juvenile sexual offenses and the histories of adult rapists and child molesters. *Int. J. Offender Ther. Comp. Criminol., 27*, 150–155.

Marshall, L. L., Barbaree, H. E., & Eccles, A. (1991). Early onset and deviant sexuality in child molesters. *J. Interpersonal Violence, 6*, 323–336.

Marshall, W., Hudson, S., Jones, R., & Fernandez, Y. (1994). *Empathy in sex offenders.* Presented at the 13th Annual Research and Treatment Conference of the Association for the Treatment of Sexual Abusers, San Francisco.

Marshall, W. L., Hudson, S. M., & Hodkinson, S. (1993). The importance of attachment bonds in the development of juvenile sex offending. In H. E. Barbaree, W. L. Marshall, & S. M. Hudson (Eds.), *The juvenile sex offender* (pp. 164–181). New York: Guilford Press.

Mathews, F., & Stermac, L. (1989). *A Tracking study of adolescent sex offenders.* Toronto: Central Toronto Youths Services.

Metzner, J., & Ryan, G. (1995). Sexual abuse perpetration. In G. P. Sholevar (Ed.), *Conduct disorders in children and adolescents* (pp. 119–142). Washington, DC: American Psychiatric Press.

National Task Force on Juvenile Sexual Offending (1993). The revised report from the National Task Force on Juvenile Sexual Offending, 1993 of the National Adolescent Perpetrator Network. *Juvenile Fam. Court J.*, *44*, 1–120.

Pithers, W. (1994). Process evaluation of group theory component to enhance sex offenders' empathy. *Behav. Res. Ther.*, *32*, 565–570.

Prentky, R. A., Knight, R. A., Sims-Knight, J. E., Straus, H., Rokous, F., & Cerce, D. (1989). Developmental antecedents of sexual aggression. *Dev. Psychopathol.*, *1*, 153–169.

Rogers, C. M., & Terry, I. (1984). Clinical intervention with boy victims of sexual abuse. In I. R. Stuart & J. G. Greer (Eds.), *Victims of sexual aggression* (pp. 99–103). New York: Nostrand Reinhold.

Ryan, G. (1991). Theories of etiology. In G. Ryan & S. Lane (Eds.), *Juvenile sexual offending: Causes, consequences, and correction* (pp. 41–55). Lexington, MA: Lexington Books.

Ryan, G., Blum, J., & Law, S. et al. (1989). *Understanding and responding to the sexual behavior of children: Trainer's manual*, Denver: Kempe National Center.

Ryan, G., Davis, J., Miyoshi, T., Lane, S., & Wilson, K. (1987). *Getting at the facts: The first report from the uniform data collection system, interchange (NAPN).* June, pp. 5–7.

Shaw, J. A., Campo-Bowen, A. E., Applegate, B. et al. (1993). Young boys who commit serious sexual offenses: Demographics, psychometrics, and phenomenology. *Bull. Am. Acad. Psychiatry Law*, *21*, 399–408.

Showers, J., Farber, E. D., Joseph, J. A., Oshins, L., & Johnson, D. F. (1983). The sexual victimization of boys: A three year survey. *Health Values: Achieving High Level Wellness*, *7*, 15–18.

Travin, S. (1994). Sex offenders: Diagnostic assessment, treatment, and related issues. In R. Rosner (Ed.), *Principles and practice of forensic psychiatry* (pp. 528–534). New York: Chapman and Hall.

US Bureau of the Census (1993). *Statistical abstract of the United States* (113th ed.). Washington, DC: US Government Printing Office.

Ward, T., Hudson, S. M., & Marshall, W. L. (1995). Cognitive distortions and affective deficit in sex offenders: A cognitive deconstructionist interpretation. *Sex Abuse J. Res. Treat*, *7*, 67–82.

Wasserman, J., & Kappel, S. (1985). *Adolescent sex offenders in vermont 1985.* Burlington: Vermont Department of Health.

Wheeler, J. R. (1986). *Final evaluation of the snohomish county prosecutor's juvenile sex offender project.* Olympia, WA: Juvenile Justice Section, Department of Social and Health Services.

Part V

TREATMENT ISSUES

The papers in this section address a range of issues relevant to the treatment of psychiatrically disturbed children and adolescents. Wilens and colleagues review available evidence concerning tricyclic antidepressant (TCA)–associated cardiovascular effects in children and adolescents. TCAs play an important role in the treatment of a range of pediatric psychiatric disorders. Efficacy has been established for the treatment of enuresis, obsessive–compulsive disorder, and attention deficit disorder; is less convincing for anxiety and tic disorders; and is as yet unproven for major depression. Nevertheless, as many as 10% of children in the United States may have a potentially TCA-responsive disorder. Despite widespread clinical use, concerns about their possible cardiovascular risk have arisen following the publication of several accounts of sudden death associated with TCA use in children.

Twenty-four studies involving a total of 730 children and adolescents receiving imipramine, amitriptyline, desipramine, or nortriptyline were reviewed, providing the basis for the development of guidelines for their use in pediatric populations. Wilens et al. further note that available information on sudden death in TCA-treated children suggests that, if it is more than a coincidence, this phenomenon is almost certainly idiosyncratic, bringing into question the preventative effectiveness of current dose, serum level, and ECG guidelines for monitoring children receiving TCAs. Nevertheless, the authors emphasize that although TCA treatment in children and adolescents, like that in adults, is generally associated with cardiovascular changes of uncertain, but probably minor, clinical significance, the risk-to-benefit ratio of the TCAs must be weighed carefully before prescribing. Most particularly, TCA treatment needs to be carefully considered in cases of a personal or family history of premature cardiac disease as well as in the presence of clinically significant conduction defects such as atrioventricular block, complete intraventricular conduction delay, Wolff-Parkinson-White or other reentry disturbances, cardiac structural anomalies, and clinically significant rhythm disturbances. Parents and children need to be informed regarding the adverse effects of TCAs, including the potential association with sudden death, and made aware of the need for close medical supervision and monitoring of ECG and TCA levels. This thoughtful review of the cardiovascular effects of tricyclic antidepressants in children, together with guidelines for use, is an invaluable source of clinically relevant information.

Although childhood-onset schizophrenia is a rare form of the disorder, it is often severe and refractory to treatment. The study reported by Kumra and colleagues is the first reported controlled trial of the effectiveness of atypical neuroleptics in children and adolescents. In it the efficacy and adverse effects of clozapine and haloperidol were compared in a sample of 21 patients with a mean age of 14.0 years ($SD = 2.3$ years) who met $DSM–III–R$ criteria for the diagnosis of schizophrenia that began by age 12 years and who had been nonresponsive to typical neuroleptics in the past. Patients were randomized to a 6-week double-blind parallel comparison of clozapine or haloperidol. Both efficacy and adverse effects were carefully monitored. Results indicated that clozapine was superior to haloperidol on all measures of psychosis. Both positive and negative symptoms of schizophrenia improved. Although the adverse effect profiles of the two medications were similar with respect to such measures as weight, pulse, temperature, and blood pressure and differed only slightly with regard to drowsiness and salivation (greater with clozapine) and insomnia (greater with haloperidol), more serious adverse events were causes of concern throughout the trial. Neutropenia and seizures were major concerns, and one third of the group has discontinued using clozapine.

345

Although pediatric populations may indeed be more prone to increased clozapine toxicity and close monitoring for adverse effects is essential, the superior efficacy of clozapine for the treatment of childhood-onset schizophrenia is welcome news. When schizophrenia begins during the developmental period, social disability tends to be more severe, and the amelioration of symptoms during this period may well contribute to improvements in long-term outcome. In addition, the absence of tardive dyskinesia during clozapine treatment reduces the 4% risk of this complication experienced by those who receive long-term treatment with typical neuroleptics. For these reasons, the judicious use of clozapine for selected severely ill children and adolescents is clearly a major advance in the therapeutics of this most severe and debilitating illness.

As Diamond and colleagues note in their report on the current status of family-based outcome and process research, family therapy initially evolved outside of research centers and universities and consequently failed to develop a strong research tradition. It is only recently that researchers have accumulated enough information about family-based therapies to evaluate their efficacy. This review provides a concise and thoughtful summary of selected studies of the outcome of family-based treatment of schizophrenia, depression, anxiety, eating disorders, ADHD, conduct disorder, and substance abuse. In addition, several process research and meta-analytic studies are considered.

As Diamond et al. point out, three family-oriented treatment traditions—behavioral, psychoeducational, and systems therapies—have all contributed to the growing body of available research data. Despite differences in theoretical orientation and focus, all three approaches hold that family interaction may cause, maintain, or exacerbate child symptomatology. Moreover, if appropriately mobilized, family relationships can also be a potent therapeutic agent for symptom reduction and the prevention of relapse. In addition, these three initially separate therapeutic tradition have increasingly borrowed therapy and technique from each other, leading to more integrative psychotherapeutic models.

The studies reviewed in this article serve to indicate that family-based treatment models are effective in the treatment of schizophrenia, conduct disorder, and substance abuse. In addition, several process studies have identified and validated core therapeutic ingredients that contribute to these outcomes. These studies have refined treatment models and intervention targets at a much higher level of specificity through, for example, the use of treatment manuals, than has previously occurred in many family treatment models. Given the potency of family relationships both for precipitating and maintaining child psychopathology and for promoting prosocial development, the systematic study of family-based treatment models is of undeniable importance. Diamond et al.'s succinct summary provides a valuable introduction to the current "state of the art" of family-based therapy research.

The final paper in this section, "A Continuum of Care: More Is Not Always Better," considers the treatment of psychiatric disorders in children and adolescents from a very different perspective. Rather than focusing on the effectiveness of one or another specific treatment modality, this report examines both the cost-effectiveness and the clinical effectiveness of different models of service delivery. Concerns about large expenditures for mental health services and about the quality of care received by children and adolescents is an issue of increasing concern to both providers and consumers of mental health services. It has long been suggested that the availability of "a continuum of care" designed to deliver coordinated mental health services on an individualized basis by using case management and interdisciplinary treatment teams to integrate and facilitate transition between services would result in improved treatment outcomes at less cost. The importance of the opportunity to test this proposition cannot be overstated.

The Fort Bragg Child and Adolescent Mental Health Demonstration provided just such an opportunity. Blickman's careful and detailed description of the project includes a full discussion of the theory underlying the design of the continuum of care. The evaluation consisted of four substudies: (a) the implementation study, (b) the quality study, (c) the mental health outcome study, and

(d) the cost–utilization study. Overall, the study showed that an integrated continuum was successfully implemented, and that it provided better access, greater continuity of care, and more client satisfaction while treating children in less restrictive environments. However, the cost was higher, and clinical outcomes were not better than those at the comparison site.

Blickman points out that the findings of this and similar research suggest that the mental health field has moved directly from laboratory-based treatment efficacy studies to system reform efforts without sufficiently studying the effectiveness of clinical services as delivered in community settings. He concludes that although system reform can be expected to influence access, cost, and satisfaction, system reform alone will not improve clinical outcome. The significant questions about the validity of widely held beliefs regarding the cost-effectiveness as well as the clinical effectiveness of services delivered under a continuum of care raised by the results of this study must be seriously considered by all those responsible for the planning and delivery of services to children and adolescents.

PART V: TREATMENT ISSUES

18

Cardiovascular Effects of Therapeutic Doses of Tricyclic Antidepressants in Children and Adolescents

Timothy E. Wilens, and Joseph Biederman
Pediatric and Adult Psychopharmacology Units, Massachusetts General Hospital, Harvard Medical School

Ross J. Baldessarini
Pediatric and Adult Psychopharmacology Units and Department of Psychiatry and Neuroscience-McLean Division, Massachusetts General Hospital, Harvard Medical School

Barbara Geller
Department of Psychiatry, Washington University School of Medicine, St. Louis

David Schleifer and Thomas J. Spencer
Pediatric and Adult Psychopharmacology Units, Massachusetts General Hospital, Harvard Medical School

Boris Birmaher
Western Psychiatric Institute and Clinic, University of Pittsburgh

Alan Goldblatt
Division of Pediatric Cardiology, Massachusetts General Hospital, Harvard Medical School

Objective: *Tricyclic antidepressants (TCAs) play an important role in the treatment of pediatric psychiatric disorders. Despite widespread clinical use, concerns about their possible cardiovascular risk have arisen following several published reports of sudden death associated with their use in children. Accordingly, available evidence concerning TCA-associated cardiovascular effects in children and adolescents was surveyed.*

Reprinted with permission from *J. Am. Acad. Child Adolesc. Psychiatry*, 1996, Vol. 35(11), 1491–1501. Copyright ©1996 by the American Academy of Child and Adolescent Psychiatry.

This work was supported in part by NIMH grants MH-01175 (Dr. Wilens), MH-31154 and MH-47370 (Dr. Baldessarini), MH-40273 and MH-40646 (Dr. Geller), and the Anderson, Corneel, Temte, & Whalin Funds (Dr. Baldessarini).

Method: *A systematic literature search from 1967 to 1996 identified relevant pediatric studies that evaluated cardiovascular effects of TCAs.* **Results:** *Twenty-four studies involving 730 children and adolescents given imipramine, amitriptyline, desipramine, or nortriptyline were found. TCA treatment was associated with minor increases in systolic and diastolic blood pressure, in heart rate, and in the electrocardiographic (ECG) conduction parameters PR, QRS, and QT_c. Holter ECG monitoring and exercise testing also revealed minor treatment effects. Some ECG changes related to specific TCAs emerged. Few age-related ECG differences in TCA-treated children, adolescents, or adults were detected. Associations of ECG abnormalities and relatively higher serum TCA levels were found.* **Conclusion:** *TCA treatment in children and adolescents, like that in adults, is associated with cardiovascular changes of uncertain, but probably minor, clinical significance. More information is needed on the contribution of other physiological conditions on the cardiovascular system during exposure to TCAs. Guidelines for using TCAs in children and adolescents are presented.*

Tricyclic antidepressants (TCAs) have played an important role in the pharmacotherapy of pediatric psychiatric disorders over the past three decades. Their efficacy has been established in the treatment of enuresis (Poussaint & Ditman, 1965), obsessive-compulsive disorder (Leonard et al., 1989), and attention-deficit hyperactivity disorder (ADHD) (Spencer et al., 1996), with less convincing evidence in anxiety (Bernstein & Borchardt, 1991) and tic disorders (Singer et al., 1995) and yet unproven efficacy in major depression (for reviews see Ambrosini, Bianchi, Rabinovich, & Elia, 1993; Bernstein & Borchardt, 1991; Leonard & Rapoport, 1989; Poussaint and Ditman, 1965; Singer et al., 1995; Spencer et al., 1996). Considering the current epidemiological estimates of the prevalence of child and adolescent mental disorders, as many as 10% of children in this country may have a potentially TCA-responsive disorder (Anderson, Williams, McGee, & Silva, 1987; Costello, 1989).

Whereas early studies focused on the tertiary-amine TCAs amitriptyline (AMI) and imipramine (IMI) (Krawkowski, 1965; Preskorn, Weller, & Weller, 1982; Rapoport, 1965), more recently the secondary-amine TCAs desipramine (DMI) and nortriptyline (NT) have been used because of their generally more favorable side effect profile (Baldessarini, 1996). Within adult psychiatry, extensive clinical and research experience with the TCAs has provided abundant information about their adverse effects (Giardina, Bigger, Glassman, Perel, & Kantor, 1979; Glassman, Roose, Giardina, & Bigger, 1987; Roose and Glassman, 1989; Ziegler, Co, & Biggs, 1977). However, their potential cardiac depressant effects have long been of concern in children (Hayes, Panitch, & Barker, 1975; Silber & Katz, 1975; Winsberg, 1975) because of their similarities with the type IA antiarrhythmics (Giardina et al., 1979). The type IA antiarrhythmics can induce a wide array of adverse effects including hypotension, excessive depression of conduction indices on the electrocardiogram (ECG), and rare, paradoxical arrhythmias (Giardina et al., 1979).

Concerns about TCA-associated adverse cardiovascular effects in pediatric groups increased greatly following published reports of sudden death in four children, and possibly one additional child, aged 8 to 12 years during routine treatment with presumably therapeutic doses of DMI (*Medical Letter*, 1990; Popper, 1993; Riddle, Geller, & Ryan, 1993). These deaths may have been related to sudden-onset cardiac arrhythmias, although this cause was not established (Biederman, 1991; Geller, 1991; *Medical Letter*, 1990; Riddle et al., 1991, 1993). Inasmuch as all four of the reported sudden deaths in children involved DMI, it follows that concerns of possible serious cardiovascular events have focused largely on DMI, limiting its clinical utility (Biederman, 1991; *Medical Letter*, 1990; Riddle et al., 1991, 1993). However, there remains a paucity of studies examining the other TCAs for similar cardiovascular effects or risks. The purpose of this report is to survey the literature to assess the known cardiovascular effects associated with clinical doses of specific TCAs in children and adolescents.

METHOD

A literature search was performed on *Medline*, using Medical Subject Headings (MeSH) to identify available studies on the cardiovascular effects of TCAs on children or adolescents from 1967 to 1996. The search included the terms children, adolescents, pediatric, cardiovascular, or ECG; these were cross-referenced with TCA and specific TCA agents. The search was limited to available systematic studies and large case series. For the purposes of this review, 5- to 12-year-olds were defined as children, and 13- to 18-year-olds were defined as adolescents.

On the basis of previously suggested guidelines in pediatrics (Biederman et al., 1989; Park, 1988; Ryan et al., 1987b), abnormalities in conduction were defined by the following ECG criteria: A heart rate ≥ 100 beats/min was considered *sinus tachycardia*; PR intervals ≥ 200 ms were considered *first-degree atrioventricular block*; QRS intervals of 100 through 119 ms were considered *incomplete intraventricular conduction delay*; QRS intervals ≥ 120 ms were considered *complete intraventricular conduction delay*; and QT_c intervals ≥ 440 ms were considered to represent prolonged repolarization phases. ECG changes were determined as values for TCA-treated ECG intervals compared to baseline intervals. New onset of an ECG abnormality was defined as onset during treatment that was not present at baseline.

To assess abnormal cardiovascular function, systolic and diastolic blood pressure >118 and >78 mm Hg (95th percentile), respectively, were considered to represent *hypertension* in children; >136 and >86 mm Hg, respectively, were the corresponding criteria for adolescents (Park, 1988). *Hypotension* in children was defined as systolic and diastolic pressure <78 and <46 mm Hg, respectively (95th percentile), or <96 and <50 mm Hg in adolescents (Park, 1988).

For the comparison of ECG indices among the TCAs, all mean values in the individual studies were weighted by the number (N) of subjects evaluated. Studies in which data were not available were not included in the calculation of weighted means. In cases of missing body weight, estimates from the 50th percentile for age were used (Baldessarini, 1996).

RESULTS

Our survey yielded 24 human studies involving a total of 730 children and adolescents receiving TCAs. Investigations specifically addressing 12-lead ECG findings included 8 studies with IMI ($N = 181$ subjects), 7 studies with DMI ($N = 271$), 4 studies with NT ($N = 119$), 1 study with AMI ($N = 18$), and I study with clomipramine (CMI) ($N = 47$) for a total of 20 studies involving 636 children and adolescents. The daily doses of NT ranged from 0.6 to 2.0 mg/kg, and the other TCAs from 0.7 to 5 mg/kg (mean 3.7 mg/kg).

ECG Findings

Few studies in children and adolescents compared ECG findings in subjects treated with a placebo and a TCA, and in such studies, few differences were found. For example, Geller et al. (1990, 1992) reported significant differences only in heart rate differences in NT-treated youths. Studies varied in duration, with only a minority of subjects receiving TCAs over a long period of time (Biederman, Gastfriend, Jellinek, & Goldblatt, 1985; Leonard et al., 1995; Wilens et al., 1993a, 1993b). Of interest, one study comparing children at 5 weeks and again at 1 year found no difference in the short- versus long-term ECG effects of CMI (Leonard et al., 1995).

A minority of studies assessed ECGs before and during treatment. Studies assessing predrug ECGs indicated that at baseline 5% to 15% of children had sinus tachycardia, up to 10% had an incomplete intraventricular conduction delay, and 5% to 15% had a prolonged QT_c interval (Bartels, Verley, Mitchell, & Stamm, 1991; Biederman et al., 1989; Geller et al., 1985b, 1990, 1992; Leonard et al., 1995; Wilens et al., 1993a, 1993b). Moreover, 27% of children in one study were found to have unspecified ECG abnormalities prior to TCA treatment (Bartels et al., 1991). It is noteworthy that in three separate studies of normal untreated children, even larger proportions showed ECG abnormalities: 100% had evidence of sinus arrhythmias, 26% had junctional escape beats, 23% had premature atrial contractions, and 24% had single premature ventricular contractions (Dickinson & Scott, 1984; Scott, Williams, & Fiddler, 1980; Southall, Johnston, Shinebourne, & Johnston, 1981).

ECG changes in children and adolescents receiving TCAs included elevations in heart rate and lengthening of the PR, QRS, and QT_c conduction (Table 1). The PR interval, which reflects depolarization of the atria, was consistently prolonged by 5% to 10% with TCA treatment. The PR interval has been reported to be the index most positively correlated with serum TCA levels (Leonard et al., 1995; Preskorn, Weller, Weller, & Glotzbach, 1983; Wilens et al., 1993a).

First-degree atrioventricular block (PR $\geq$200 ms) was reported in only 0.9% of TCA-treated children. However, in studies using 180 ms as the defining criterion, atrioventricular block was reported in from 10% to 14% of IMI-treated children (Bartels et al., 1991; Preskorn et al., 1983; Winsberg, Bialer, Kupietz, & Tobias, 1972). There were similarities in the incidence of atrioventricular block among the various TCAs.

There appears to be a qualitatively greater increase in the QRS duration with IMI (24% increase over baseline) than with DMI or NT in children and adolescents (7% and 11%, respectively) (Table 1). Complete intraventricular conduction delay with TCA treatment (QRS >200 ms) was rare (incidence <0.5%) (Biederman et al., 1989; Wilens et al., 1993a, 1993b). In contrast, incomplete intraventricular conduction delay of the right bundle branch type (QRS = 100 to 120 ms) was found in 9% of the cases (Table 1). The incidence of an incomplete intraventricular conduction delay was less commonly reported in children and adolescents given IMI (3%) than in those given NT (14%) or DMI (19%) (Table 1).

There remains much concern regarding the clinical utility and findings of electrical ventricular depolarization (QRS) and repolarization (T wave) of the myocardium, the combination that is referred to as the QT interval which is corrected for cardiac rate (QT_c). The QT_c interval is associated with a 4% (DMI, NT, and CMI) to 10% (IMI) average increase in duration with TCA treatment. The incidence of QT_c prolongation (>440 ms) has varied widely in the pediatric literature from none (IMI) (Bartels et al., 1991; Martin and Zaug, 1973) to 48% (IMI and DMI) (Ryan et al., 1987b; Wilens et al., 1993a). Overall there appeared to be higher rates of QT_c >440 ms with DMI (30%) compared with IMI (16%), NT (17%), and CMI (11%). Although Wilens et al., (1993a) reported that 35% of DMI-treated patients had a new onset of QT_c >440 ms, only 18% had a QT_c $\geq$450 ms, and 8% had a more clinically meaningful QT_c $\geq$460 ms (unpublished data).

An inverse relationship between ECG parameters before versus during TCA treatment has been reported in studies of children, adolescents, and young adults. In studies of NT (Geller et al., 1985b, 1990, 1992), DMI (Leonard et al., 1995; Wilens et al., 1993a), CMI (Leonard et al., 1995), and IMI (Saraf, Klein, Gittelman-Klein, Gootman, & Greenhill, 1978), juveniles with the longest pretreatment conduction times manifested the *least* change with TCA treatment. Conversely, children with lower pretreatment indices (heart rate and ECG conduction intervals) had the *largest* change in their ECG indices. It may be that this phenomenon represents a sampling effect with a tendency for nonspecific regression to the mean (Fava & Rosenbaum, 1992). Further complicating the matter, data on the effect of TCAs in children with a baseline "abnormal ECG" remains sketchy, with one study indicating higher rates of ECG abnormalities in IMI-treated children with baseline abnormal ECGs (Bartels et al., 1991).

TABLE 1

Summary of the Effects of TCAs on the ECGs of Children and Adolescents

Agent	N Studies	Mean Age: Years (Range)	Diagnosis	TCA Dose (mg/kg)	[TCA] (ng/ml)	ECG Changes on TCAs: Δ (%)				Rates of ECG Abnormality (%)			
						Rate	PR	QRS	QT_c	Sinus Tachycardia	AV Block	Incomplete IVCD	Prolonged QT_c
CMI	47 (1)	14 (7–17)	OCD	3.1	NA	92 (17)	148 (0)	89 (3)	419 (5)	36	None	2	11
AMI	18 (1)	16 (13–18)	MDD	3.4	242	98	170	80	380	28	None	NA	11
IMI	181 (8)	12 (5–18)	MDD ADHD ODD	3.8	145	98 (20)	149 (10)	93.0 (24)	432 (10)	16	1.8	3	16
NT	119 (4)	11 (5–18)	ADHD MDD	1.5	96.0	102 (24)	147 (7)	84.0 (7)	422 (4)	61	None	14	17
DMI	271 (7)	12 (5–18)	Multiple	3.6	173	99 (20)	145 (5)	95.0 (11)	427 (3)	38	0.9	19	30

Note: ECG intervals are expressed in milliseconds; HR per minute. New-onset sinus tachycardia = HR ≥100 beats/min; first-degree AV block = PR ≥200 ms; incomplete IVCD = QRS 100 to 120 ms; and prolonged QT_c = QT_c ≥440 ms. TCA = tricyclic antidepressant; ECG = electrocardiogram; AV = atrioventricular; IVCD = intraventricular conduction defect; CMI = clomipramine; AMI = amitriptyline; IMI = imipramine; NT = nortriptyline; DMI = desipramine; OCD = obsessive-compulsive disorder; MDD = major depressive disorder; ODD = oppositional defiant disorder; ADHD = attention-deficit hyperactivity disorder.

Twenty-Four-Hour Ambulatory ECG Monitoring

While single, routine ECG assessments can be informative, they may not detect intermittent disturbances of cardiac rhythm. For this reason, 24-hour Holter ECG monitoring has been studied in IMI- and DMI-treated children. In a naturalistic Holter monitor study of 71 pediatric psychiatric patients aged 5 to 17 years who were receiving DMI (mean daily doses = 3.5 mg/kg), Biederman et al. (1993) reported that DMI-treated children had a significantly lower incidence of atrioventricular block, sinus pauses, and junctional rhythm compared to data from three studies of normal children (Dickinson & Scott, 1984; Scott et al., 1980; Southall et al., 1981). DMI-treated children also had asymptomatic but significantly higher rates of single and paired premature atrial and ventricular contractions, unifocal ventricular contractions, and runs of supraventricular tachycardia than historical controls (Biederman et al., 1993). It is noteworthy that in cases with positive Holter findings, the corresponding standard 12-lead ECGs were normal (Biederman et al., 1993).

In a prospective study, repeated Holter monitoring showed an asymptomatic, advanced Mobitz type II second-degree atrioventricular block (periodic block of atrioventricular conduction) in 1 (5%) of 23 behaviorally disordered children with normal baseline studies who received doses of IMI of up to 5 mg/kg per day (Fletcher, Case, Sallee, Hand, & Gillette, 1993). Although the mean heart rate increased by an average of 18 beats/min, there was no increase in the frequency of premature ventricular or supraventricular beats with IMI treatment. One child was not treated with IMI, because ventricular tachycardia was found during baseline Holter ECG monitoring (Fletcher et al., 1993).

Graded Exercise Tests

There has been concern that TCA-associated cardiovascular abnormalities may be more evident during exercise or other stress-related conditions, based in part on information that two of the four reported cases of pediatric sudden deaths associated with DMI had involved exercising (running and playing tennis) prior to collapse (Riddle et al., 1991, 1993). Moreover, exercise in adults is associated with an increase in sympathetic activity, cardiac arrhythmias, and risk of sudden death (approximately 1 in 200,000 athletes) (Wight & Salem, 1995). Unfortunately, there are few data available to assess cardiovascular effects of exercise on children or adolescents receiving a TCA.

In the only systematic investigation on TCAs and graded exercise testing, Fletcher and associates (1993) studied 23 children aged 5 to 15 years with normal baseline Holter studies who received IMI (3 to 5 mg/kg per day). No dysrhythmias or abnormal ECGs were found during exercise or shortly thereafter (Fletcher et al., 1993). Similarly, no ECG abnormalities were found after exercise testing in three children receiving DMI (Biederman & Wilens, unpublished data). In addition, Holter monitoring that included periods of exercise in 94 children aged 6 to 17 years receiving either IMI or DMI (3 to 5 mg/kg per day) also showed no elevated incidence of dysrhythmias (Biederman et al., 1993; Fletcher et al., 1993).

TCA Dose and Serum Levels

The relationships of drug doses and serum TCA levels to ECG parameters in pediatric patients have also been examined. In early studies of IMI given at relatively low doses (25 to 50 mg daily) for enuresis in children, no ECG abnormalities were reported (Martin & Zaug, 1973; Poussaint & Ditman, 1965). More recent studies using larger doses of TCAs have reported minor relationships between cardiovascular changes and TCA dose or serum levels (Biederman et al., 1989; Leonard et al., 1995; Wilens et al., 1993a, 1993b). ECG evidence of TCA-associated prolongation of cardiac conduction parameters has been reported more consistently at doses of DMI or IMI >3.5 mg/kg, and NT >1.0 mg/kg (Biederman et al., 1989; Geller et al., 1985b, 1990, 1992; Preskorn et al., 1983; Puig-Antich et al., 1987; Ryan et al., 1987a; Saraf et al., 1978; Wilens et al., 1993a, 1993b; Winsberg, 1975).

Overall, the available reports on TCA-treated children and adolescents suggest at least trends for higher heart rates, diastolic blood pressure, and intracardiac conduction intervals at relatively high serum TCA concentrations (IMI, DMI, or their sum >250 ng/ml, NT >150 ng/ml) (Biederman et al., 1989, 1993; Preskorn et al., 1982, 1983; Wilens et al., 1993a, 1993b). Conversely, in the presence of abnormal ECGs, trends to higher TCA levels have been found (Biederman et al., 1989; Wilens et al., 1993a, 1993b). Likewise, Holter monitor data indicate that children with relatively high serum DMI levels had higher rates of paired premature atrial contractions and supraventricular tachycardia than those with lower levels (Biederman et al., 1993).

Hydroxy-TCA Metabolites

In addition to the parent TCA, the pharmacologically active, hydroxylated metabolites are putative contributors to adverse cardiac effects. When given intravenously to laboratory animals, the hydroxy-TCA metabolites reduce left ventricular function and cardiac output (Jandhyala, Steenberg, Perel, Manian, & Buckley, 1977) and induce arrhythmias (Pollock & Perel, 1989). For IMI and DMI, serum hydroxy-TCA concentrations range from 43% to 52% of the parent compound in children and adolescents. Despite higher weight-corrected doses, children and adolescents tend to have relatively *lower* levels of circulating hydroxy-TCA metabolites than adults, suggesting rapid metabolic clearance of these products and their precursors in children (Dell, Hein, Ramakrishnan, Puig-Antich, & Cooper, 1990; Morselli, 1977; Wilens, Biederman, Baldessarini, Puopolo, & Flood, 1992). For NT, wide interindividual variation has been reported, with the hydroxy metabolite-to-parent NT concentrations reported at a mean of 230% in children (Geller et al., 1992) to a mean of 90% in adolescents (Geller et al., 1990). In addition to the preponderance of trans- versus cishydroxy NT at any age, higher ratios of the hydroxy metabolite-to-parent NT have been reported with relatively older versus younger adults (Bertilsson, Mellstrom, & Sjoqvist, 1979; Young et al., 1984). Reports on 12-lead ECG studies in children, adolescents, and adults receiving IMI, NT, or DMI indicate minor, generally insignificant associations between metabolite levels and ECG changes (Geller et al., 1990, 1992; Ryan et al., 1987b; Wilens et al., 1993a). Associations between serum hydroxy-TCA metabolites and the ECG have been similar, but less robust, than those associated with the parent compound (Geller et al., 1990; Ryan et al., 1987b; Wilens et al., 1993a). Likewise, the combination of the metabolites and the parent TCA add little cardiovascular information compared with the TCA alone (Geller et al., 1990, 1992; Ryan et al., 1987b; Wilens et al., 1993a).

Age Effects

In studies of DMI and NT, few clinically meaningful age-related differences in ECG, pulse, or blood pressure have been found between TCA-treated prepubertal and adolescent children (Biederman et al., 1989; Geller et al., 1990, 1992; Wilens et al., 1993b). Confounding these comparisons, baseline differences in ECG parameters in untreated children and adolescents at baseline have been reported: children have higher heart rates than adolescents, whereas adolescents have longer conduction intervals than children (Biederman et al., 1989; Geller et al., 1990, 1992; Wilens et al., 1993a, 1993b). More *change* in heart rate from baseline has been reported in adolescents compared with children given NT or DMI (Biederman et al., 1989; Geller et al., 1990, 1992). In a prospective investigation of the ECG in DMI-treated subjects, higher heart rates were found in children whereas relatively greater lengthening of ECG indices were noted in adults (Wilens et al., 1993a). In laboratory animals of varying ages, no developmental differences were found in the transmembrane action potentials of cardiac Purkinje fibers that were superfused with differing concentrations of IMI (Fletcher et al., 1992). Overall, there is little evidence to suggest clinically meaningful developmental differences in the cardiovascular effects of the TCAs.

Vital Signs

Investigations of TCA-related changes in pulse and blood pressure have not found clinically significant effects but have reported statistically significant increases in heart rate and both systolic and diastolic blood pressure during TCA treatment (IMI, DMI ≥2.5 mg/kg per day; NT >1 mg/kg per day) (Bartels et al., 1991; Biederman et al., 1985, 1989; Donnelly, Zametkin, & Rapoport, 1986; Geller et al., 1985b, 1990, 1992; Preskorn et al., 1983; Puig-Antich et al., 1987; Ryan et al., 1987a; Schroeder et al., 1989; Winsberg, 1975). Increases in heart rate ranged from 8% to 30% (Table 1), resulting in heart rates of 92 to 105 beats/min, well within the normal ranges in pediatric populations (Park, 1988; Garson, Bricker, & McNamara, 1990). If one applies the adult criterion of sinus tachycardia (ventricular rate ≥100 beats/min) to children, from 16% to 61% (pooled mean = 36%) of TCA-treated children manifest tachycardia (Table 1); however, only 0.5% of children taking IMI, DMI, or NT developed a more clinically relevant level of tachycardia ≥140 beats/min (Biederman et al., 1989; Garson et al., 1990; Wilens et al., 1993a, 1993b).

Systematic studies with IMI and DMI have reported mild elevations in both systolic and diastolic blood pressures (2 to 5 mm Hg), with few differences between children and adolescents (Biederman et al., 1985, 1989; Donnelly et al., 1986; Preskorn et al., 1983; Rapoport, Quinn, Bradbard, Riddle, & Brooks, 1974). In studies of NT versus placebo, significant treatment-related differences in diastolic blood pressure (4 mm Hg greater with NT) were found in children only (Geller et al., 1990, 1992). No significant orthostatic blood pressure changes have been reported in studies of children or adolescents receiving NT or IMI (Fletcher et al., 1993; Geller et al., 1990, 1992). It is noteworthy that in one study, the majority of DMI-associated vital sign changes observed during the initial stages of dosing were reported to diminish during prolonged treatment (Schroeder et al., 1989). Despite group data indicating only minor TCA-treatment effects, there have been a few reported cases of changes in blood pressure that were great enough to require TCA discontinuation in children and adolescents (Bartels et al., 1991; Waizer, Hoffman, & Polizos, 1974). For example, in one report a 9-year-old girl receiving 50 mg of IMI developed hypotension associated with first-degree atrioventricular block, both of which abated with drug discontinuation (Waizer et al., 1974).

DISCUSSION

A survey of the available literature reveals that treatment of children and adolescents with TCAs results in consistent but mild increases in systolic and diastolic blood pressure, heart rate, and the ECG conduction parameters PR, QRS, and QT_c, at therapeutic doses and serum levels. Findings on dynamic measures including 24-hour Holter monitoring and ECG with graded exercise also reveal minor asymptomatic treatment effects. Only weak associations have been found between typical TCA doses or serum levels and ECG indices; however, more robust relationships to ECG abnormalities have emerged at relatively high TCA doses or serum levels. There appear to be few differences in the magnitude or incidence of ECG changes between children and adolescents, particularly when age-related normal standards for ECG parameters, pulse, and blood pressure are considered. The survey literature on ECG data reviewed here suggests general similarities among the various TCAs with some possible differences: IMI may be associated with lower rates of sinus tachycardia and intraventricular conduction than the other TCAs, and DMI may be associated with higher rates of

QT prolongation than the other TCAs. To some extent, however, these comparisons may be biased by the variability in data presentation, study methodologies, and differing dosing and serum levels in the studies surveyed.

The aggregate literature indicates that blood pressure changes in TCA-treated children and adolescents appear to be minimal. In most studies, TCA treatment was associated with asymptomatic, minor, but statistically significant increases in heart rate and ECG measures of cardiac conduction times consistent with the adult literature (Giardina et al., 1979; Glassman et al., 1987; Roose & Glassman, 1989; Ziegler et al., 1977). The pediatric literature reviewed indicates that TCA treatment was rarely associated with clinically symptomatic adverse cardiac effects. By a conservative definition of a heart rate >100 beats/min (Park, 1988), sinus tachycardia was found in up to 18% of children at predrug baseline (Biederman et al., 1989; Wilens et al., 1993a, 1993b) and in one-third of TCA-treated children and adolescents. Heart rates of less than 130 beats/min in children, and 120 beats/min in adolescents, are considered normal and are not known to have any short-term clinical or hemodynamic significance (Garson et al., 1990). Heart rates persistently above these values are of greater concern (Garson et al., 1990) but are less common. However, the effect of sustained elevations of heart rates, by even 10% above pre-TCA treatment rates, are not known.

The PR interval appears to be best correlated with TCA dose and serum concentration (Leonard et al., 1995; Wilens et al., 1993a). However, first-degree atrioventricular block is infrequent (<1/100 of cases), and second- or third-degree atrioventricular block is rare during TCA treatment in children (Fletcher et al., 1993).

New manifestations of incomplete intraventricular conduction delay during TCA treatment are common and have been noted in up to one quarter of pediatric patients. The incomplete intraventricular conduction delay reported with TCA treatment is generally of the right bundle branch type, with delay in depolarization of the right ventricle relative to the left ventricle. Although the clinical significance of incomplete intraventricular conduction delay is unclear, theoretical risks of a QRS interval of 100 to 120 ms include progression of excessive prolongation to complete intraventricular conduction block, impaired depolarization of both ventricles, reduction in cardiac output, or potentially dangerous idioventricular rhythms (Garson et al., 1990). Complete intraventricular conduction block (QRS ≥200 ms) is rare in children with or without TCA treatment (<1/200 cases).

The available data also indicate a mild TCA effect on myocardial repolarization as evidenced by QT lengthening. Since the QT interval normally rises with heart rate (Garson et al., 1990; Park, 1988), and the heart rate is increased by TCA treatment, it is not surprising that the QT_c is mildly prolonged with TCA treatment. It has been speculated that severe QT_c prolongation (>440 ms) associated with DMI treatment may predict serious arrhythmias (Riddle et al., 1991). If this view is valid, it may be important that a qualitatively higher incidence of QT_c prolongation is observed with DMI than with other TCAs (Table 1). However, comparing the QT_c interval during TCA treatment to the baseline interval, IMI apparently has the greater *increase from baseline* in the QT_c interval than with treatment with other TCAs. Moreover, in the case of a child who died suddenly while taking DMI, the QT_c on the ECG was normal during resuscitation in the emergency room (Biederman, 1991).

Despite similarities in the general direction of cardiovascular findings of various TCAs in pediatric subjects, evidence that there may be differential cardiotoxicity between specific TCAs remains elusive. It has been proposed that, because of its potent and selective inhibition of norepinephrine reuptake compared with the other TCAs, DMI may preferentially increase noradrenergic neurotransmission, circulating catecholamines, and cardiac sympathetic tone more than other TCAs (Riddle et al., 1991, 1993; Walsh, Giardina, Sloan, Greenhill, & Goldfein, 1994). Findings in bulimic adolescents and adults include highly variable heart rate and calculated alterations in the sympathetic to parasympathetic input to the heart during DMI treatment (Walsh et al., 1994). These findings may be of particular relevance as it has been suggested that increased sympathetic tone may predispose vulnerable individuals to myocardial conduction and repolarization aberrancies, ventricular tachyarrhythmias, syncope, and cardiac arrest (Meredith, Broughton, Jennings, & Esler, 1991; Van Ravenswaaij-Arts, Kollee, Hopman, Stoelinga, & Van Geijn, 1993; Zipes, 1991).

If a difference exists in the arrhythmogenic potential of specific TCAs, this might be reflected in the ECG. In the current survey, the greater *changes from baseline* in the ECG were observed with IMI compared with the other TCAs (Table 1); however, higher rates of incomplete intraventricular conduction were noted in DMI-and NT-treated children than in children treated with either CMI or IMI. There appeared to be qualitatively more repolarization delays with DMI compared with the other TCAs. These observations are similar to a recent controlled study showing DMI to manifest higher rates of incomplete intraventricular conduction delays than CMI (Leonard et al., 1995). Comparisons of the ECG of IMI- and DMI-treated children and adolescents are of interest as IMI is rapidly demethylated to DMI in children (Dell et al., 1990; Potter et al., 1982); accordingly, treatment with either IMI or DMI should theoretically place children at a similar risk for cardiovascular adverse effects.

Epidemiological data concerning the risk of fatal arrhythmias (sudden death) with DMI or other TCAs also remain controversial. Whereas unpublished data in children and adolescents indicate a higher relative risk of sudden death with DMI compared with IMI, AMI, or NT (Riddle, 1994), the systematic assessment of deaths of children receiving DMI completed by a task force of the American Academy of Child and Adolescent Psychiatry does not support such an association (Biederman, Thisted, Greenhill, & Ryan, 1995). This task force, using comparisons of baseline rates of sudden unexplained death in 5- to 14-year-old children, concluded that the evidence of DMI and sudden death is "weak," with a relative risk (odds ratio) of 2.5 (95% confidence interval = 0.5 to 15) over the annual population base rate of 4.2 deaths/million in the United States (Biederman et al., 1995).

Although not indicative of risks at therapeutic doses, TCA data in large groups of adults (Kapur, Mieczkowski, & Mann, 1992) and children (Popper, 1993) suggest a fatality rate of 1% associated with TCA overdose, primarily due to cardiovascular and CNS events. There is a statistically significant higher relative risk of fatality reported with DMI compared with the other TCAs in adults (odds ratio = 2.4) (Kapur et al., 1992). In addition, further concerns have been raised that the occurrence of sudden death may be underreported or erroneously attributed to overdose in some cases (Popper & Elliot, 1993). Until further studies are undertaken to directly compare the various TCAs in large numbers of individuals, there are inadequate data on cardiovascular risk factors to support or reject the notion of clinically significant differences between TCAs in rates of adverse cardiac effects with therapeutic dosing.

The literature surveyed here indicates that at "therapeutic" dosing, within individual studies there were few associations between ECG measures and TCA dose or serum concentration. Likewise, no differences in ECG measures were reported in IMI-treated adolescents dosed once versus three times a day (Ryan et al., 1987b). However, there were trends for greater ECG effects in studies using relatively high TCA doses or when ECG data were stratified by dose or serum levels in individual studies (Biederman et al., 1989, 1993; Preskorn et al., 1982, 1983; Wilens et al., 1993a, 1993b). Likewise, in the presence of TCA-induced ECG abnormalities, there is a trend to higher serum TCA levels. Elevated risk with high TCA levels is of particular concern in the approximately 10% of pediatric patients receiving TCAs who are slow hydroxylators and yield serum TCA levels that are two- to three-fold higher than predicted (Geller et al., 1985a; Potter et al., 1982; Wilens et al., 1992).

Given the wide application of TCA treatment in prepubertal children and concerns about a possible risk of sudden death in children receiving DMI, there has been an interest in evaluating age-specific adverse ECG effects of the TCAs. Although the findings are limited by low effect sizes and large variance, *few* consistent differences were found between children and adolescents in blood pressure changes, heart rate increases, or intraventricular conduction lengthening with TCA treatment

(Biederman et al., 1989; Geller et al., 1990, 1992; Wilens et al., 1993a, 1993b). In addition, the aggregate pediatric ECG findings are consistent with those reported in TCA-treated adults (Giardina et al., 1979; Glassman et al., 1987; Roose & Glassman, 1989; Ziegler et al., 1977) and do not support a differential risk between age groups as assessed clinically by the ECG (Wilens et al., 1993a).

Recent interest has focused on potential interactions of psychopathology, age, and medication on autonomic nervous system functioning. For instance, drug-free adults with depression or anxiety may have greater QT_c duration, more heart rate variability, and higher rates of cardiac disease than nondepressed controls (Pfeifer et al., 1983; Roose & Glassman, 1989). Similarily, children with psychiatric disorders have been reported to have increased glucocorticoid secretion, catecholaminergic activity, and autonomic reactivity (Kagan, Reznick, & Snidman, 1987; Ryan & Dahl, 1993). Although reduced sympathetic and parasympathetic functioning has been reported with increasing age in adults (Pfeifer et al., 1983), the potential of a developmental interaction of psychopathology and the autonomic effects of the TCAs in children and adults remains unclear (Walsh et al., 1994). For example, children with ADHD may show an exaggerated cardiovascular response to stimulants in those with versus without comorbid anxiety disorders (Urman, Ickowicz, Fulford, & Tannock, 1995). However, in the current review we found no support for developmental changes in ECG responses with TCA treatment. It may be that, in psychiatrically ill individuals, some ECG changes may be due to the TCA effects coupled with increased baseline sympathetic tone in the otherwise untreated state (Biederman et al., 1993; Pfeifer et al., 1983; Walsh et al., 1994; Zipes, 1991).

Guidelines for the use of TCAs in children and adolescents have been proposed (Biederman et al., 1989; Puig-Antich et al., 1979; Rosenberg, Holttum, & Gershon, 1994; Winsberg, 1975), but their stringent application may leave a number of cases untreated, particularly since normative ECG parameters found in the literature have often exceeded recommended exclusion criteria. Moreover, the predictive power for avoiding adverse events by suggested guidelines is not clear.

Given our current understanding, it appears reasonable to routinely obtain baseline ECGs and recheck them after several days of reaching daily doses of 2.5 mg/kg per day (NT doses of 1.0 mg/kg per day) and after each dose increase of 50 to 100 mg/day thereafter, and to avoid daily doses of more than 5 mg/kg in ordinary clinical practice. With suggestive clinical symptoms such as lightheadedness or headaches, vital signs should be assessed. Steady-state serum TCA levels should be checked when the ECG is repeated, and both TCA level and ECG should be repeated with the addition of agents suspected to interact pharmacokinetically with the TCAs.

We propose tentative guidelines that are based on established age-dependent normative values (Garson et al., 1990; Park, 1988) coupled with parameters adapted in ongoing pharmacological trials and our clinical experience with large numbers of children and adolescents given TCAs (Table 2). As are the limitations of previous guidelines, these parameters are not empirically derived, nor have they undergone the rigor of scientific testing to determine their predictability in identifying potentially dangerous cardiovascular states. ECG findings such as a persistent tachycardia, significant intraventricular conduction delays, or QT_c >460 ms necessitate reassessment. In cases of abnormal ECGs, the response to the TCA needs to be evaluated. If the medication has been beneficial, attempts to reduce the dose without loss of benefit, while rechecking the ECG, should be undertaken. If the ECG abnormality continues, another TCA or alternative agents should be considered. In cases with ECG perturbations that persist despite dose reductions, or when cardiovascular symptoms arise, we suggest consideration of closely monitored dose discontinuation, 24-hour Holter monitoring, and referral to a pediatric cardiologist. Similarly, in the presence of a family history of premature cardiovascular problems, or a personal history of cardiac disease, pediatric cardiology consultation is recommended.

The available information on sudden death in TCA-treated children suggests that, if it is more than a coincidence, this phenomenon is almost certainly idiosyncratic (Biederman et al., 1995), further bringing into question the preventive effectiveness of current dose, serum level, and ECG guidelines

TABLE 2
Suggested Guidelines for Monitoring Electrocardiograms and
Vital Signs of Children and Adolescents Receiving
Tricyclic Antidepressants

Parameter	Children	Adolescents
Vital signs		
Heart rate	$\leq$110–130 beats/min[a]	$\leq$110–120 beats/min[a]
Blood pressure	<120/80 mm Hg	<140/90 mm Hg
Electrocardiogram		
PR interval	<200 ms	<200 ms
QRS interval	$\leq$120 ms $\pm$ >30% over baseline	$\pm$120 ms
QT$_c$ interval	$\leq$460–480 ms	$\leq$460–480 ms

[a]For two consecutive weeks.

for monitoring children receiving TCAs. The number of potential adverse cardiac outcomes prevented by stringent monitoring of TCA use and the cost-to-benefit ratio of such procedures are unknown, and the nature of rare and idiosyncratic events such as malignant arrhythmias makes proof of the preventive efficacy of guidelines very difficult. However, given our current understanding of the TCAs in children and adolescents, some guidelines appear prudent. The risk-to-benefit ratio of the TCAs needs to be weighed carefully in consideration of their treatment efficacy. Whereas some argue that certain TCAs should not be used in children or adolescents (Werry, 1995), reviews by Ambrosini et al. (1993), Bernstein and Borchardt (1991), and Spencer et al. (1996) would support that the TCAs remain an important second-line class of medications for ADHD, obsessive-compulsive disorder (CMI only), tic disorders, enuresis, and, more distantly, anxiety and depressive disorders; this issue is beyond the scope of this report. Likewise, TCA treatment needs to be carefully considered in cases of a personal or family history of premature cardiac disease as well as in the presence of clinically significant conduction defects such as atrioventricular block, complete intraventricular conduction delay, Wolff-Parkinson-White or other re-entry disturbances, cardiac structural anomalies, and clinically significant rhythm disturbances. In discussions with parents and children regarding the adverse effects of the TCAs, we include the potential association of TCAs with sudden death and outline the need for close medical supervision and monitoring of ECG and TCA levels.

The results of this review of the literature should be viewed in light of their substantial methodological limitations. Dosing conditions and reporting of cardiovascular data varied between studies. The literature reviewed here may have been overrepresented by positive cardiovascular findings associated with TCAs, as negative reports in general are underrepresented in the literature. The use of earlier definitions of ECG abnormalities may have resulted in overinterpretation of ECG abnormalities. To define drug-related risk rates versus untreated risk and to assess differences between TCAs more accurately, studies using larger numbers of children under more controlled conditions are necessary.

In summary, TCA treatment in children and adolescents appears to produce predictable and generally minor cardiovascular changes. We recommend routine monitoring of the ECG at baseline and use of TCA assays and repeated ECG after significant dose increases and routinely when robust daily doses are administered. By the nature of infrequent serious adverse events, it is unclear whether stringent monitoring of TCA treatment can reduce the risk of sudden death during TCA treatment and, indeed, the contribution of TCAs to such dire events remains unclear. Given emerging data on the use of alternative treatments for certain disorders, further analysis of the risk-to-benefit ratio of TCA treatment needs to be undertaken. Future studies should compare cardiovascular risk factors of various agents under varying physiological conditions including graded exercise testing. The role of psychopathology and its interaction with the various TCAs on measures of autonomic cardiac tone, as well as potential contribution to cardiac rhythm disturbances, also needs to be evaluated further.

REFERENCES

Ambrosini, P. J., Bianchi, M. D., Rabinovich, H., & Elia, J. (1993). Antidepressant treatments in children and adolescents: I. Affective disorders. *J. Am. Acad. Child Adolesc. Psychiatry, 32*, 1–6.

Anderson, J. C., Williams, S., McGee, R., & Silva, P. A. (1987). *DSM-III* disorders in preadolescent children. *Arch. Gen. Psychiatry, 44*, 69–76.

Baldessarini, R. J. (1996). *Chemotherapy in psychiatry* Cambridge, MA: Harvard University Press.

Bartels, M. G., Varley, C. K., Mitchell, J., & Stamm S. J. (1991). Pediatric cardiovascular effects of imipramine and desipramine. *J. Am. Acad. Child Adolesc. Psychiatry, 30*, 100–103

Bernstein, G. A., & Borchardt, C. M. (1991). Anxiety disorders of childhood and adolescence: A critical review. *J. Am. Acad. Child Adolesc. Psychiatry, 30*, 519–532.

Bertilsson, L., Mellstrom, B., & Sjoqvist, F. (1979). Pronounced inhibition of noradrenaline uptake by 10-hydroxy-metabolites of nortriptyline. *Life Sci. 25*, 1285–1292.

Biederman, J. (1991). Sudden death in children treated with a tricyclic antidepressant. *J. Am. Acad. Child Adolesc. Psychiatry, 30*, 495–498.

Biederman, J., Baldessarini, R. J., Goldblatt, A., Lapey, K. A., Doyle, A., & Hesslein P. S. (1993). A naturalistic study of 24-hour electrocardiographic recordings and echocardiographic findings in children and adolescents treated with desipramine. *J. Am. Acad. Child Adolesc. Psychiatry, 32*, 805–813.

Biederman, J., Baldessarini, R. J., Wright, V., Knee, D., Harmatz, J. S., & Goldblatt A. (1989). A double-blind placebo controlled study of desipramine in the treatment of ADD: II. Serum drug levels and cardiovascular findings. *J. Am. Acad. Child Adolesc. Psychiatry, 28*, 903–911.

Biederman, J., Gastfriend, D., Jellinek, M. S., & Goldblatt, A. (1985). Cardiovascular effects of desipramine in children and adolescents with attention deficit disorder. *J. Pediatr., 106*, 1017–1020.

Biederman, J., Thisted, R. A., Greenhill L., & Ryan, N. (1995). Estimation of the association between desipramine and the risk for sudden death in 5- to 14-year old children. *J. Clin. Psychiatry, 56*, 87–93.

Costello, E. J. (1989). Developments in child psychiatry epidemiology. *J. Am. Acad. Child Adolesc. Psychiatry, 28*, 836–841.

Dell, R. B., Hein, K., Ramakrishnan, R., Puig-Antich, J., & Cooper, T. (1990). Model for the kinetics of imipramine and its metabolites in adolescents. *Ther. Drug Monit., 12*, 450–459.

Dickinson, D. F., & Scott, O. (1984). Ambulatory electrocardiographic monitoring in 100 healthy teenage boys. *Br. Heart J. 51*, 179–183.

Donnelly, M., Zametkin, A. J., & Rapoport, J. L. (1986). Treatment of childhood hyperactivity with desipramine: Plasma drug concentration, cardiovascular effects, plasma and urinary catecholamine levels, and clinical response. *Clin. Pharmacol. Ther. 39*, 72–81.

Fava, M., & Rosenbaum, J. F. (1992). *Research designs and methods in psychiatry*. New York: Elsevier.

Fletcher, S. E., Case, C. L., Sallee, F. R., Hand, L. D., & Gillette, P. C. (1993). Prospective study of the electrocardiographic effects of imipramine in children. *J. Pediatr. 122*, 652–654.

Fletcher, S. E., Case, C. L., Williamson, C. E., Gillette, P. C., Bucklee, D. S., & Hewett, K. W. (1992). *Developmental electrophysiologic properties of imipramine*. Presented at American Heart Association, 65th Annual Scientific Sessions, New Orleans.

Garson, A., Bricker, J. T., & McNamara, D. G. (1990). *The science and practice of pediatric cardiology*, Vols 1–3. Philadelphia: Lea & Febiger.

Geller, B. (1991). Commentary on unexplained deaths of children on Norpramin. *J. Am. Acad. Child Adolesc. Psychiatry, 30*, 682–684.

Geller, B., Cooper, T. B., & Chestnut, E. C. (1985a). Serial monitoring and achievement of steady state nortriptyline plasma levels in depressed children and adolescents. *J. Clin. Psychopharmacol., 5*, 213–216.

Geller, B., Cooper, T. B., Graham, D. L., Fetner, H. H., Marsteller, F. A., & Wells, J. M. (1992). Pharmacokinetically designed double-blind placebo-controlled study of nortriptyline in 6- to 12-year-olds with major depressive disorder. *J. Am. Acad. Child Adolesc. Psychiatry, 31*, 34–44.

Geller, B., Cooper, T. B., Graham, D. L., Marsteller, F. A., & Bryant, D. M. (1990). Double-blind placebo-controlled study of nortriptyline in depressed adolescents using a "fixed plasma level" design. *Psychopharmacol. Bull., 26*, 85–90.

Geller, B., Farooki, Z. Q., Cooper, T. B., Chestnut, E. C., & Abel, A. S. (1985b). Serial ECG measurements at controlled plasma levels of nortriptyline in depressed children. *Am. J. Psychiatry, 142*, 1095–1097.

Giardina, E. V., Bigger, T. J., Glassman, A. H., Perel, J. M., & Kantor, S. J. (1979). The electrocardiographic and antiarrhythmic effects of imipramine hydrochloride at therapeutic plasma concentrations. *Circulation, 60*, 1045–1052.

Glassman, A. H., Roose, S. P., Giardina, E. V., & Bigger, J. T. (1987), Cardiovascular effects of tricyclic antidepressants. In: H. Y. Meltzer (Ed.), *Psychopharmacology: The third generation of progress* (pp. 1437–1442). New York: Raven Press.

Hayes, T. A., Panitch, M. L., & Barker, E. (1975). Imipramine dosage in children: A comment on imipramine and electrocardiographic abnormalities in hyperactive children. *Am. J. Psychiatry, 132*, 545–547.

Jandhyala, B. S., Steenberg, M. L., Perel, J. M., Manian, A. A., & Buckley, J. P. (1977). Effects of several tricyclic antidepressants on the hemodynamics and myocardial contractibility of the anesthetized dogs. *Eur. J. Pharmacol., 42*, 403–410.

Kagan, J, Reznick, J. S., & Snidman, N. (1987). The physiology and psychiatry of behavioral inhibition in children. *Child Dev., 58*, 1459–1473.

Kapur, S., Mieczkowski, T., Mann, J. (1992). Antidepressant medications and the relative risk of suicide attempt and suicide. *JAMA, 268*, 5441–5445.

Krawkowski, A. J. (1965). Amitriptyline in treatment of hyperkinetic children. *Psychosomatics, 6*, 611–614.

Leonard, H. L., Meyer, M. C., Swedo, S. E. et al. (1995). Electrocardiographic changes during desipramine and clomipramine treatment in children and adolescents. *J. Am. Acad. Child Adolesc. Psychiatry, 34*, 1460–1468.

Leonard, H. L., & Rapoport, J. L. (1989). Pharmacotherapy of childhood obsessive-compulsive disorder. *Psychiatr. Clin. North Am. 12*, 963–970.

Leonard, H. L., Swedo, S. E., Rapoport, J. L. et al. (1989). Treatment of obsessive-compulsive disorder with clomipramine and desipramine in children and adolescents. *Arch. Gen. Psychiatry, 46*, 1088–1092.

Martin, G. I., & Zaug, P. J. (1973). ECG monitoring of enuretic children given imipramine. *JAMA, 224*, 902–903.

Medical Letter (1990). Sudden death in children treated with a tricyclic antidepressant. *32*, 53.

Meredith, I. T., Broughton, A., Jennings, G. L., & Esler, M. D. (1991). Evidence of a selective increase in sympathetic activity in patients with sustained ventricular arrhythmias. *N. Engl. J. Med., 325*, 618–624.

Morseili, P. L. (1977). Psychotropic drugs. In P. Morselli (Ed.), *Drug disposition during development*, (pp. 431–474). New York: Spectrum.

Park, M. K. (1988). *Pediatric cardiology for practitioners*. Chicago: Year Book Medical Publishers.

Pfeifer, M. A., Weinberg, C. R., Cook, D., Best, J. D., Reenan, A., & Halter, J. B. (1983). Differential changes of autonomic nervous system function with age in man. *Am. J. Med., 75*, 249–258.

Pollock, B. G., & Perel. J. M. (1989). Hydroxy metabolites of tricyclic antidepressants: Evaluation of relative cardiotoxicity. In S. G. Dahl, & L. F., *Clinical Pharmacology in Psychiatry (Psychopharmacology Series 7)* (pp. 232–236). Berlin: Springer-Verlag.

Popper, C. (1993). Simon Wile Symposium: Sudden death on antidepressants. *Scientific Proceedings of the American Academy of Child and Adolescent Psychiatry*, San Antonio, TX, *9*, 24.

Popper, C., & Elliot, G. R. (1993). Postmortem pharmacokinetics of tricyclic antidepressants: Are some deaths during treatment misattributed to overdose? *J. Child. Adolesc. Psychopharmacol., 3*, 10–12.

Potter, W. Z., Calil, H. M., Sutfin, T. A. et al. (1982). Active metabolites of imipramine, and desipramine in man. *Clin. Pharmacol. Ther., 31*, 393–401.

Poussaint, A. F., & Ditman, K. S. (1965). A controlled study of imipramine (Tofranil) in the treatment of childhood enuresis. *J. Pediatr., 67*, 283–289.

Preskorn, S. H., Weller, E. B., & Weller, R. A. (1982). Depression in children: Relationship between plasma imipramine levels and response. *J. Clin. Psychiatry, 43*, 450–453.

Preskorn, S. H., Weller, E. B., Weller, R. A., & Glotzbach, E. (1983). Plasma levels of imipramine and adverse effects in children. *Am. J. Psychiatry, 140*, 1332–1335.

Puig-Antich, J., Perel, J. M., Lupatkin, W. et al. (1979). Plasma levels of imipramine (IMI) and desmethylimipramine (DMI) and clinical response in prepubertal major depressive disorder. *J. Am. Acad. Child Psychiatry, 18*, 616–627.

Puig-Antich, J., Perel, J. M., Lupatkin, W. et al. (1987). Imipramine in prepubertal major depressive disorders. *Arch. Gen. Psychiatry, 44*, 81–89.

Rapoport, J. (1965), Childhood behavior and learning problems treated with imipramine. *Int. J. Neuropsychiatry, 1*, 635–642.

Rapoport, J. L., Quinn, P. O., Bradbard, G., Riddle, D., & Brooks, E. (1974). Imipramine and methylphenidate treatments of hyperactive boys. *Arch. Gen. Psychiatry, 30*, 789–793.

Riddle, M. (1994). *Forensic issues in tricyclic antidepressants in children and adolescents.* Institute on Advanced Topics in Psychopharmacology. Presented at the Annual Meeting of the American Academy of Child and Adolescent Psychiatry, New York, October.

Riddle, M., Geller, B., & Ryan, N. (1993). Another sudden death in a child treated with desipramine. *J. Am. Acad. Child Adolesc. Psychiatry, 32*, 792–797.

Riddle, M. A., Nelson, J. C., Kleinman, C. S. et al. (1991). Sudden death in children receiving Norpramin: A review of three reported cases and commentary. *J. Am. Acad. Child Adolesc. Psychiatry, 30*, 104–108.

Roose, S. P., & Glassman, A. H. (1989). Cardiovascular effects of tricyclic antidepressants in depressed patients. *J. Clin. Psychiatry, 7*, 1–18.

Rosenberg, D., Holttum, J., & Gershon, S. (1994). *Textbook of pharmacotherapy for child and adolescent psychiatric disorders.* New York: Brunner/Mazel.

Ryan, N. D., & Dahl, R. E. (1993). Neurobiology of depression in children and adolescents. *Clin. Neurosci., 1*, 108–112.

Ryan, N., Puig-Antich, J., Ambrosini, P. et al. (1987a). The clinical picture of major depression in children and adolescents. *Arch. Gen. Psychiatry, 44*, 854–861.

Ryan, N. D., Puig-Antich, J., Cooper, T. B. et al. (1987b). Relative safety of single versus divided dose imipramine in adolescent major depression. *J. Am. Acad. Child Adolesc. Psychiatry, 26*, 400–406.

Saraf, K. R., Klein, D. F., Gittelman-Klein, R., Gootman, N., & Greenhill, P. (1978). EKG effects of imipramine treatment in children. *J. Am. Acad. Child Psychiatry, 17*, 60–69.

Schroeder, J. S., Mullin, A. V., Elliott, G. R. et al. (1989). Cardiovascular effects of desipramine in children. *J. Am. Acad. Child Adolesc. Psychiatry, 28*, 376–379.

Scott, O., Williams, G. J., & Fiddler, G. I. (1980). Results of 24-hour ambulatory monitoring of electrocardiogram in 131 healthy boys aged 10 to 13 years. *Br. Heart. J. 44*, 304–308.

Silber, E. N., & Katz, L. N. (1975). *Heart disease.* New York: MacMillan.

Singer, H. V., Brown, J., Quaskey, S., Rosenberg, L. A., Mellits, E. D., & Denckla, M. (1995). The treatment of attention-deficit hyperactivity disorder in Tourette's syndrome: A double-blind placebo controlled study with clonidine and desipramine. *Pediatrics 95*, 74–81.

Southall, D. P., Johnston, F., Shinebourne, E. A., & Johnston, P. G. (1981). 24-Hour electrocardiographic study of heart rate and rhythm patterns in population of healthy children. *Br. Heart. J. 45*, 281–291.

Spencer, T., Biederman, J., Wilens, T., Harding, M., O'Donnell, D., & Griffin, S. (1996), Pharmacotherapy of attention-deficit hyperactivity disorder across the life cycle. *J. Am. Acad. Child Adolesc. Psychiatry, 35*, 409–432.

Urman, R., Ickowicz, A., Fulford, P., & Tannock, R. (1995). An exaggerated cardiovascular response to methylphenidate in ADHD children with anxiety. *J. Child. Adolesc. Psychopharmacol., 5*, 29–37.

Van Ravenswaaij-Arts, C. M. A. , Kollee, L. A. A., Hopman, J. C. W., Stoelinga, G. V. A., & Van Geijn, H. P. (1993). Heart rate variability. *Ann. Intern. Med. 118*, 436–447.

Waizer, J., Hoffman, S. P., & Polizos, P. (1974). Outpatient treatment of hyperactive school children with imipramine. *Am. J. Psychiatry, 131*, 587–591.

Walsh, B. T., Giardina, E. V., Sloan, R. P., Greenhill, L., & Goldfein, J. (1994). Effects of desipramine on autonomic control of the heart. *J. Am. Acad. Child Adolesc. Psychiatry, 33*, 191–197.

Werry, J. (1995). Cardiac arrhythmias make desipramine an unacceptable choice in children. *J. Am. Acad. Child Adolesc. Psychiatry, 35*, 1239–1241.

Wight, J. N., & Salem, D. (1995). Sudden cardiac death and the "athlete's heart." *Arch. Intern. Med., 155*, 1473–1480.

Wilens, T. E., Biederman, J., Baldessarini, R. J., Puopolo, P., & Flood, J. (1992). Developmental changes in serum concentrations of desipramine and 2-hydroxydesipramine during treatment with desipramine. *J. Am. Acad. Child Adolesc. Psychiatry, 31*, 691–699.

Wilens, T. E., Biederman, J., Baldessarini, R. J., Puopolo, P. R., & Flood, J. G. (1993a). Electrocardiographic effects of desipramine and 2-hydroxydesipramine in children, adolescents, and adults treated with desipramine. *J. Am. Acad. Child Adolesc. Psychiatry, 32*, 798–804.

Wilens, T. E., Biederman, J., Spencer, T., & Geist, D. E. (1993b). A retrospective study of serum levels and electrocardiographic effects of nortriptyline in children and adolescents. *J. Am. Acad. Child Adolesc. Psychiatry, 32*, 270–277.

Winsberg, B. G. (1975). Imipramine and electrocardiographic abnormalities in hyperactive children. *Am. J. Psychiatry, 132*, 542–547.

Winsberg, B. G., Bialer, I., Kupietz, S., & Tobias, J. (1972). Effects of imipramine and dextroamphetamine on behavior of neuropsychiatrically impaired children. *Am. J. Psychiatry, 128*, 1425–1431.

Young, R. C., Alexopoulos, G. S., Shamoian, C. A., Manley, M. W., Dhar, A. K., & Kutt, H. (1984). Plasma 10-hydroxynortriptyline in elderly depressed patients. *Clin. Pharmacol. Ther., 35*, 540–544.

Ziegler, V. E., Co, B. T., & Biggs, J. H. (1977). Plasma nortriptyline levels and ECG findings. *Am. J. Psychiatry, 134*, 441–443.

Zipes, D. P. (1991). Sympathetic stimulation and arrhythmias. *N. Engl. J. Med. 325*, 656–657.

19

Childhood-Onset Schizophrenia: A Double-Blind Clozapine-Haloperidol Comparison

Sanjiv Kumra
Child Psychiatry Branch, National Institute of Mental Health

Jean A. Frazier
Harvard University School of Medicine

Leslie K. Jacobsen
Child Psychiatry Branch, National Institute of Mental Health

Kathleen McKenna
Northwestern University School of Medicine

Charles T. Gordon
University of Maryland School of Medicine

Marge C. Lenane, Susan D. Hamburger, Amy K. Smith, Kathleen E. Albus, Javad Alaghband-Rad, and Judith L. Rapoport
Child Psychiatry Branch, National Institute of Mental Health

Background: *Childhood-onset schizophrenia is a rare but severe form of the disorder that is often treatment-refractory. In this study, the efficacy and adverse effects of clozapine and haloperidol were compared for children and adolescents with early-onset schizophrenia.* **Methods:** *Twenty-one patients (mean [±SD] age, 14.0±2.3 years) with onset of Diagnostic and Statistical Manual of Mental Disorders, Revised 3rd ed.–defined schizophrenia that began by age 12 years and who had been nonresponsive to typical neuroleptics participated in the study. Patients were randomized to a 6-week double-blind parallel comparison of clozapine (mean [±SD] final dose, 176 ± 149 mg/d), or haloperidol, (16 ± 8 mg/d).* **Results:** *Clozapine was superior to haloperidol on all measures of psychosis (P = .04–.002). Positive and negative symptoms of schizophrenia improved. However, neutropenia and seizures were major concerns. To date, one third*

Reprinted with permission from *Arch. Gen. Psychiatry*, 1996, Vol. 53, 1090–1097.

We thank Eric Goldstein, PharmD; Sandoz Pharmaceuticals Corp, Hanover, NJ; and Pharmaceutical Developmental Services Clinical Section at the National Institutes of Health, Bethesda, MD, for their assistance in the provision of the blinded medications used in this study. We also thank Barbara Karp, MD, Dale Grothe, PharmD, David Pickar, MD, and Alan Breier, MD, for their support of and consultation to this project and the nurses of the Child Psychiatry Branch Inpatient Unit at the National Institutes of Health who cared for the patients in this study.

of the group has discontinued using clozapine. **Conclusions:** *Clozapine has striking superiority for positive and negative symptoms in treatment-refractory childhood-onset schizophrenia. However, due to possibly increased toxic effects in this pediatric population, close monitoring for adverse events is essential.*

Childhood-onset schizophrenia is a chronic disorder accompanied by a significant deterioration in adaptive functioning from already-impaired premorbid levels (McClellan & Werry, 1994; Asarnow, Tompson, & Goldstein, 1994; Green, Gayol, Hardesty, & Bassiri, 1992; Alaghaband-Rad et al., 1995; Gordon et al., 1994). Some evidence suggests that these children are less responsive to typical neuroleptic agents and more sensitive to extrapyramidal adverse effects (Green, Gayol, Hardesty, & Bassiri, 1992; Campbell & Spencer, 1988; Realmuto, Erickson, Yellin, Hopwood, & Greenberg, 1984; Keepers, Clappison, & Casey, 1983). Thus, the enhanced therapeutic effects of clozapine for nonresponders and the absence of risk for tardive dyskinesia may have special importance for early-onset cases. Because of the considerable morbidity this illness carries for children, the possible usefulness of atypical neuroleptics for childhood-onset schizophrenia is of great interest.

Research in this field has been limited. Only 2 controlled trials of typical neuroleptics have been done in children with schizophrenia. The first, by Pool, Bloom, Mielke, Roniger, and Gallant, 1976, supported a modest but significant superiority of loxiapine (Loxitane) and haloperidol (Haldol) over placebo for 75 adolescents with schizophrenia. More recently, a placebo-controlled trial of haloperidol in children with schizophrenia found haloperidol superior to placebo on several measures (Spencer, Kafantaris, Padron-Gayol, Rosenberg, & Campbell, 1992; Spencer & Campbell, 1994).

No controlled trials of atypical neuroleptics have been done in children or adolescents. Two large open-label, retrospective medical chart studies indicated that two thirds to three fourths of adolescents with treatment-refractory schizophrenia showed some degree of clinical improvement, and that 11% of adolescents showed a complete remission of symptoms during clozapine treatment. Clozapine seemed helpful for positive and negative symptoms, although, as with adult patients, certain negative symptoms such as energy, mutism, and thought-blocking were less responsive to treatment (Carpenter, Conley, Buchanan, Breier, & Tamminga, 1995). About one fourth of these adolescent patients discontinued taking clozapine due to insufficient antipsychotic efficacy, deterioration of symptoms, or severe adverse effects (Schmidt, Trott, Blanz, & Nissen, 1989; Remschmidt, Schulz, & Martin, 1994). These findings were limited by diagnostic heterogeneity, administration of clozapine with additional psychotropic drugs, inclusion of some adult patients, lack of a control group, and lack of standardized ratings.

A systematic, prospective, open trial of clozapine in 11 treatment-refractory adolescents with childhood-onset schizophrenia carried out at the National Institute of Mental Health (NIMH) rated the conditions of 75% of patients as improved compared with their condition on admission medication. Clozapine improved positive and negative symptoms, although sedation, hypersalivation, and weight gain were troublesome (Frazier et al., 1994).

To our knowledge, our study is the first double-blind study of clozapine for treatment-refractory children and adolescents with early-onset schizophrenia. We hypothesized that clozapine would be superior to haloperidol for this group. The adverse effects of both drugs also were compared.

SUBJECTS AND METHODS

Study Design

Children and adolescents aged 6 to 18 years who had been diagnosed as having schizophrenia were sought by national recruitment through professional and patient advocacy organizations. Subjects were screened by at least 2 child psychiatrists (S.K., J.A.F., L.K.J., K.M., C.T.G., J.A.-R., or J.L.R.) at the Clinical Center of the National Institutes of Health, Bethesda, MD (McKenna et al., 1994).

Inclusion criteria were diagnosis of schizophrenia defined by the *Diagnostic and Statistical Manual of Mental Disorders, Revised Third Edition* (American Psychiatric Association, 1987), with documented psychotic symptoms by age 12 years; intolerance, nonresponse, or both to at least 2 different neuroleptic drugs; and a full-scale IQ of 70 or higher. Exclusionary criteria were neurologic or medical disease. During a screening evaluation, children and families were interviewed for historical data, including a detailed developmental history. Diagnosis was determined using previous records and clinical and structured interviews, which included the Schedule for Affective Disorders and Schizophrenia for School-Age Children—Epidemiologic Version (Orvaschell, Tabrizi, & Chambers, 1987) and the Diagnostic Interview for Children and Adolescents—Revised (Reich & Welner, 1988).

The protocol was approved by the Institutional Review Board at the NIMH, and each parent and child gave informed consent or assent before the child was entered into the study.

The study sample consisted of 21 patients (11 boys and 10 girls). Five of the 10 patients given clozapine and 6 of the 11 patients given haloperidol were boys. The group had considerable previous hospitalization and neuroleptic exposure (Table 1). On average, patients were receiving mean ($\pm SD$) 2.1 ± 1.8 medications at the time of admission to the study. Most of the patients had received high doses of standard neuroleptics, risperidone, and several augmenting agents, including mood stabilizers and antidepressants. Almost all of the patients were pubertal at the time of the study. Other demographic and past psychiatric characteristics of the 2 groups are given in Table 1.

The mean ($\pm SD$) full-scale IQ, based on the best premorbid IQ or testing done at the NIMH, for the subjects who were testable ($n = 18$) was 79 ± 12. Many of the children were acutely ill at the time of testing, so these data are an underestimation of their true abilities based on earlier educational and developmental history. Three subjects could not be tested adequately due to the severity of their illness

TABLE 1

Patient Characteristics for Clozapine-Haloperidol Comparison Trial*

Characteristic	Treatment Group	
	Clozapine	Haloperidol
Schizophrenia subtype		
Disorganized	5	5
Undifferentiated	5	5
Paranoid	0	1
Sex		
Male	5	6
Female	5	5
Age, (yr)		
At time of NIMH study	14.40 (2.95)	13.73 (1.62)
At onset of psychosis	9.60 (2.22)	10.36 (1.36)
At first hospitalization	11.50 (3.17)	11.67 (2.00)
Duration of Illness, (yr)	4.75 (1.93)	3.42 (1.64)
Months of hospitalization	12.80 (16.91)	6.05 (7.38)
Months of neuroleptic treatment	28.70 (16.54)	17.73 (13.45)
Tanner stage	4.05 (1.12)	3.55 (1.13)

*Values are given as number of patients and mean ($\pm SD$). No significant statistical differences were seen between groups. NIMH indicates National Institute of Mental Health.

and inability to comply, although all had shown normal educational and developmental achievement before onset of psychosis.

Procedure

On admission to the hospital, all medications were tapered during a 2-week period, followed by a 4-week drug-free interval as tolerated. A neurologic examination, medical and developmental evaluation, and psychometric testing and structured psychiatric interviews were carried out. Laboratory measures included an electroencephalogram (EEG), electrocardiogram, magnetic resonance imaging of the cerebrum, complete blood cell count, thyroid functions, liver chemistries, human immunodeficiency virus serologic tests, hepatitis screen, platelet serotonin levels, prolactin, lead levels, rapid plasma reagin, sedimentation rate, creatine kinase, toxicology screen, pregnancy test, and 24-hour urine collection for catecholamine metabolities. A lumbar puncture was performed and cerebrospinal fluid collected for analysis of monoamines and metabolites, antinuclear antibodies, and herpes simplex titers.

The 21 patients entering the double-blind study were randomly assigned to a 6-week parallel treatment trial of clozapine (up to 525 mg/d) or haloperidol (up to 27 mg/d), as clinically indicated. Randomization was done by the National Institute of Health pharmacy using a table of random numbers. In addition to coded antipsychotic medication, patients prophylactically received benztropine mesylate tablets up to 6 mg/d (haloperidol group) or identical placebo tablets (clozapine group) to enhance the double-blind study. Dosing was done by the treating physician; physicians and nurses were unaware of the treatment assignment of each patient. A doctor of pharmacy with specialty training in psychiatry was aware of the treatment assignment and served as the clinical monitor for the study.

Clozapine doses were prescribed by the treating physician at 6.25 to 25 mg/d or haloperidol at 0.25 to 1.0 mg/d depending on the patient's weight. The smallest individual pill strength for clozapine was 6.25 mg and for haloperidol, 0.25 mg. Doses could be increased every 3 to 4 days by 1 to 2 times the starting dose on an individual basis.

Evaluation of Efficacy

Weekly behavioral ratings were completed by a psychiatrist (S.K., J.A.F., L.K.J., C.T.G., or K.M.) during the course of the double-blind treatment (Table 2), using the Brief Psychiatric Rating Scale (BPRS) (Overall & Gorham, 1961), and the Bunney-Hamburg Psychosis Rating Scale (Bunney & Hamburg, 1963). During weeks 1 and 4 of the drug-free baseline period and weeks 2 and 6 of the medication phase, additional rating instruments were completed, including the Children's Global Assessment Scale (Shaffer et al., 1983), the Clinical Global Impressions (CGI) Scale (Guy, 1976), the BPRS for Children (BPRS-C) (Overall & Pfefferbaum, 1984), the Scale for the Assessment of Positive Symptoms (Andreasen, 1984), and the Scale for the Assessment of Negative Symptoms (Andreasen, 1983).

The 11 patients who were initially randomly assigned to haloperidol treatment subsequently received an open trial of clozapine and were rated in a similar fashion. Data for the CGI Scale and serious adverse effects for these patients is reported herein. All patients were contacted by telephone at regular intervals after discharge from the hospital and were seen in person after 2 years for a follow-up evaluation.

Evaluation of Adverse Effects and Vital Signs

Adverse effects were evaluated weekly by the Subjective Treatment Emergent Symptoms Scale (Campbell & Palig, 1985), which was modified to include adverse events known to be associated with clozapine (Kane, Honigfeld, Singer, & Meltzer, 1988). Extrapyramidal symptoms and involuntary

TABLE 2

Clinical Ratings for Children and Adolescents with Childhood-Onset Schizophrenia at Baseline and During Clozapine and Haloperidol Treatment*

Measure	Baseline		Week 6		ANCOVA		
	Clozapine (n = 10)	Haloperidol (n = 11)	Clozapine (n = 10)	Haloperidol (n = 11)	F	df	P
Brief Psychiatric Rating Scale	83.7 (14.0)	84.7 (17.6)	52.5 (12.6)	64.7 (18.1)	5.1	2,20	.04[a]
Bunney–Hamburg Rating Scale	19.4 (2.8)	20.1 (6.0)	11.7 (3.3)	15.3 (3.8)	6.1	2,20	.02[a]
Scale for the Assessment of Negative Symptoms	77.9 (36.0)	83.0 (26.1)	46.0 (30.3)	72.2 (24.7)	13.4	2,16	.002[a]
Scale for the Assessment of Positive Symptoms	53.9 (25.8)	59.0 (24.9)	19.1 (11.7)	35.9 (15.6)	10.0	2,16	.01[a]
Children's Global Assessment Scale	26.3 (11.9)	23.2 (12.5)	44.9 (9.5)	27.9 (12.1)	9.2	2,16	.01[b]
Abnormal Involuntary Movement Scale	14.7 (15.5)	14.0 (5.8)	12.1 (4.8)	12.2 (3.5)	0.01	2,15	.91
Simpson–Angus Neurological Rating Scale	12.1 (1.7)	11.9 (2.1)	12.0 (1.6)	13.9 (3.5)	1.6	2,15	.23

*Except where indicated, values are given as mean (±SD). No significant differences were found between the 2 medication groups, except for the Bunney–Hamburg Rating Scale, for which the variance for the haloperidol group is greater than the clozapine group. ANCOVA indicates analysis of covariance.

[a]Week 6 clozapine < week 6 haloperidol.

[b]Week 6 clozapine > week 6 haloperidol.

movements were rated on the Abnormal Involuntary Movement Scale (Rapoport, Connors, & Reatig, 1985) and the Simpson-Angus Neurological Rating Scale (Simpson & Angus, 1970). In addition, weekly complete blood cell counts with differential, liver function tests, an encephalogram, and an electrocardiogram were done at baseline and at week 6.

Data Analysis

Analysis of covariance, using baseline measures as the covariate, was used to examine the differences between drug treatments at week 6 for all efficacy variables, using an SAS analysis of covariance program (SAS Institute, 1989). An "intent-to-treat" analysis was carried out for all patients who had a baseline assessment and at least 1 assessment after randomization, with the last observation carried forward, on the BPRS, Bunney–Hamburg Psychosis Rating Scale, and the Subjective Treatment Emergent Symptoms Scale. Incidents of adverse reactions were compared across groups using the χ^2 statistic. A t test was used to compare demographic data, baseline ratings, week 6 CGI Scale, and vital sign variables. Analysis of variance was used to compare the variances for all efficacy variables at baseline. All P values are 2-tailed, and statistical significance was set at the 5% level ($P < .05$).

RESULTS

Twenty-one patients enrolled in the study, of whom 20 completed the 4-week washout-baseline phase of the study; 1 patient required randomization to blinded medication after 1 week of the taper period due to clinical deterioration. Ten patients were randomly assigned to clozapine, 11 to haloperidol. The 2 medication groups did not differ significantly with respect to any demographic variables (Table 1). No significant differences were seen between clozapine and haloperidol baseline ratings, with the exception that the Bunney–Hamburg Rating Scale total score baseline variance was greater for the haloperidol group than for the clozapine group ($P < .03$) (Table 2).

Four patients did not complete the 6-week double-blind medication trial due to serious adverse events. Three patients discontinued taking medication during the fourth week of medication (2 receiving clozapine and 1 receiving haloperidol), and an additional patient interrupted clozapine treatment during week 5. For each of these patients, the final scores for the Bunney–Hamburg Psychosis Rating Scale, BPRS, and the Subjective Treatment Emergent Symptoms Scale were carried forward in the analysis of the data.

For the 21 patients, the mean ($\pm SD$) dose of medication at the last treatment week for haloperidol was 16 ± 8 mg/d (range, 7–27 mg/d), or 0.29 ± 0.19 mg/kg per day (range, 0.08–0.69 mg/kg per day) and clozapine, 176 ± 149 mg/d (range, 25–525 mg/d) or 3.07 ± 2.59 mg/kg per day (range, 0.34–7.53 mg/kg per day). The dose of medication at the last treatment week for the 7 patients receiving clozapine who successfully completed the treatment trial was 239 ± 134 mg/d (range, 125–525 mg/d). Adverse effects that limited dose increase for both medication groups included tachycardia and sedation.

Clinical Response

In spite of small numbers, several end-point measures showed significant differences favoring clozapine. For the 4 overall indexes of improvement, clozapine was superior to haloperidol (Table 2 and Table 3). Clozapine also significantly decreased positive and negative symptoms of schizophrenia as measured on the Scale for the Assessment of Positive Symptoms and the Scale for the Assessment of Negative Symptoms. Cluster analysis of the BPRS-C (Table 3) disclosed a marked improvement in depression, social withdrawal, and thinking disturbance and a trend toward improvement in behavioral problems for the clozapine group.

TABLE 3

Test Results for Children and Adolescents with Childhood-Onset Schizophrenia: Change Score
from Weeks 0 to 6 of Medication Trial*

| | Treatment Group | | | | |
| | Clozapine | Haloparidol | | | |
Measure	($n = 6$)	($n = 10$)	t	P	Comments
Brief Psychiatric Rating Scale					
Depression[a]	2.50 (2.59)	−0.60 (2.17)	2.58	.02	C>H
Thinking disturbance[a]	6.00 (2.45)	3.00 (2.83)	2.15	.05	C>H
Withdrawal[a]	4.50 (2.81)	1.00 (2.71)	2.47	.03	C>H
Anxiety	5.00 (2.53)	4.30 (3.50)	0.43	.68	C=H
Behavior problems	4.17 (3.49)	0.80 (3.22)	1.96	.07	C=H
Motor agitation	2.50 (1.64)	3.30 (3.02)	−0.59	.56	C=H
Organicity	2.00 (1.41)	0.60 (3.92)	1.02	.33	C=H
Total[a]	**26.67** (9.07)	**12.40** (12.08)	2.49	.03	C>H
Clinical Global Improvement Index[b]	2.00 (0.58)	3.30 (1.49)	−2.50	0.03	C>H

*C indicates clozapine group; H, haloperidol group. Except where indicated, values are given as mean (±SD).
[a]Baseline score were subtracted from week 6 scores of medication trial.
[b]For clozapine group, $n = 7$.

The CGI Scale was also used to analyze the complete sample of patients in the study (open and double-blind trials of clozapine, $n = 21$) for global improvement after 6 weeks of treatment with clozapine. This index uses a 7-point scale from 1, indicating very much improved, to 7, indicating very much worse to assess how much patients have benefited from a clozapine trial compared with their clinical condition at admission to the project. Of the 21 patients who had an open or blinded clozapine trial, the conditions of 2 (9.5%) were rated as very much improved, 11 (52.4%) as much improved, 7 (33%) as minimally improved, and 1 (4.8%) as worse.

Evaluation of Adverse Effects and Vital Signs

Adverse reactions seen during the double-blind medication phase of the trial are given in Table 4; only the adverse effects that differed between the 2 drugs ($P < .05$) are reported. The adverse effect profiles of the 2 medications were similar except that drowsiness ($P < .04$) and salivation ($P < .02$) were greater with clozapine, while haloperidol produced more insomnia ($P < .03$). Weight, pulse temperature, and blood pressure did not differ. Presumably, the extrapyramidal adverse effects of haloperidol were masked by the prophylactic benztropine. On the Simpson–Angus Neurological Rating Scale, only salivation was seen to increase, and only for the clozapine group. Similarly, the total score on the Abnormal Involuntary Movement Scale did not change for either group from baseline to the end of the medication phase of the trial.

More serious adverse events, however, were causes for concern throughout the trial (Table 3). Although no cases of agranulocytosis occurred, hematopoietic toxic effects were a major issue for clozapine. Five patients who received clozapine experienced a drop in the absolute neutrophil count below 1500 mm³; for 3 of these patients, the white blood cell count normalized spontaneously. Two patients had to be dropped from the double-blind protocol at week 4 after neutropenia recurred with rechallenge. Although 1 of these patients was of Ashkenazi Jewish descent, the human lymphocyte antigen phenotype did not match the phenotypes that are known to be associated with an increased risk of clozapine-induced agranulocytosis (Alvir, Lieberman, Safferman, Schwimmer, & Schaaf, 1993). Both of these patients were taking concomitant antibiotic medications during the medication phase

TABLE 4

Most Frequent Side Effects and Adverse Reactions of Children and Adolescents with Childhood-Onset
Schizophrenia During the 6-Week Double-Blind Clozapine-Haloperidol Comparison Study*

Variable	Treatment Group		P	Comments
	Clozapine (n = 10)	Haloperidol (n = 11)		
No. (%) of side effects				
Drowsiness	9 (90)	3 (27)	.04	C>H
Insomnia	0 (0)	4 (36)	.03	H>C
Salivation	7 (70)	2 (18)	.02	C>H
No. (%) of adverse reactions				
Tachycardia (resting heart rate of ≥100 bpm)	7 (70)	5 (45)	.26	
Dorp in absolute neutrophil count	4 (40)	0 (0)	.02	C>H
Neuroleptic malignant syndrome	0 (0)	1 (9)	.33	
Seizures	1 (10)	0 (0)	.28	
Mean (±SD) vital signs[a]				
Weight change (kg)	0.90 (6.47)	0.94 (2.89)	.986	
Blood pressure change (mm Hg)				
Systolic	−1.6 (12.9)	3.27 (17.6)	.487	
Diastolic	−4.4 (14.3)	−7.00 (13.3)	.671	

*Only side effects in which $P \leq .05$ are included from the Subjective Treatment Emergent Symptoms Scale (modifed version).
All 21 subjects were included in the analysis of side effects and adverse events. C indicates clozapine group; H, haloperidol group.
[a]Last week receiving drug minus baseline.

of the study; 1 had been receiving amoxicillin before the first drop in absolute neutrophil count, and the other was receiving penicillin during the first rechallenge.

Two patients in the double-blind clozapine trial had clinically significant seizure activity: the first experienced myoclonus at the end of week 4 while receiving 400 mg/d of clozapine, followed by a tonic-clonic seizure the next day. Clozapine dosage was reduced and 3 different anticonvulsants were tried sequentially. No further seizures occurred, but the EEG continued to show epileptiform spikes, and use of clozapine was discontinued. A second patient experienced bifrontal and posterior delta-frequency slowing on the EEG at week 5. Three weeks after discharge from the hospital, this patient experienced tonic-clonic seizures while receiving 275 mg/d of clozapine. Clozapine dosage was lowered and valproate sodium was given, but the patient continued to have petit mal seizures, so use of clozapine was discontinued. Neither patient had preexisting epilepsy.

Of the 11 patients who received an open trial of clozapine, 3 required prophylactic anticonvulsant treatment. In each case, the child experienced EEG abnormalities in association with clinical deterioration (i.e., increased aggression, psychosis, or irritability). After the clozapine dose was lowered and valproate was added, symptoms improved for 2 patients. The third patient, however, experienced facial myoclonus with associated cortical spikes on EEG and clinical deterioration, necessitating discontinuation of clozapine treatment.

Other adverse effects during clozapine treatment included one instance of 2- to 3-fold elevation in hepatic enzymes that was judged clinically significant. Two patients experienced a sinus tachycardia while receiving clozapine (heart rate >100 bpm) documented by electrocardiogram. Most patients tolerated the increase in heart rate, but 1 patient required the addition of atenolol during the open trial of clozapine.

One patient was dropped from the study in the fifth week of haloperidol treatment because of early signs of neuroleptic malignant syndrome. During a 48-hour period, liver transaminase levels were elevated (aspartate transaminase, 1083 U/L; alanine transaminase, 313 U/L; lactic dehydrogenase, 4030 U/L); the creatine kinase level rose to 83000 U/L, and, when fractionated, was found to be 100% muscle; blood pressure was labile; confusion increased; no other neurologic symptoms were observed. With haloperidol discontinuation and supportive measures, vital signs and laboratory values normalized within a few days.

COMMENT

To our knowledge, this is the first controlled study of clozapine for children and adolescents with schizophrenia. Compared with patients who have later-onset schizophrenia, these patients have more severe premorbid abnormalities in language and motor development, premorbid psychiatric disorders, lower performance IQ, and a more severe and chronic course (Alaghaband-Rad et al., 1995; Gordon et al., 1994; Yang, Liu, Chiang, Chen, & Lin, 1995). All had been nonresponsive to at least 2 typical neuroleptics.

Consistent with the greater disease severity experienced by this group, the level of baseline psychopathologic characteristics was higher than that previously reported for adult subjects of inpatient studies. For example, the mean ($\pm SD$) baseline BPRS total score in the present study was 84.2 ± 15.6, whereas the mean baseline BPRS total scores in the studies by Kane et al. (1988) and Pickar et al. (1992) were 61 ± 12 and 62 ± 16, respectively.

The results of our study indicate that clozapine is superior to haloperidol for positive and negative symptoms in this population. In addition, we believe that clozapine was effective for primary negative symptoms, because our group had a low baseline level of extrapyramidal symptoms, yet we still observed a striking improvement in negative symptoms as measured by the Scale for the Assessment of Negative Symptoms. Our findings are consistent with the adult literature and the open and retrospective reports on clozapine for adolescents with treatment-refractory schizophrenia (Schmidt, Trott, Blanz, & Nissen, 1989; Remschmidt, Schulz, & Martin, 1994; Kane, Honigfeld, Singer, & Meltzer, 1988; Pickar et al. 1992; Breier et al. 1994; Jacobsen, Walker, Edwards, Chappell, & Woolston, 1994; Birmaher, Baker, Kapur, Quintana, & Ganguli, 1991; Meltzer, 1992; Mozes et al., 1994). We believe that our sample is representative of treatment-refractory childhood schizophrenia reported in the literature (Green, Gayol, Hardesty, & Bassiri, 1992; Yang, Liu, Chiang, Chen, & Lin, 1995; Jacobsen, Walker, Edwards, Chappell, & Woolston, 1994; Mozes et al., 1994; Towbin, Dykens, & Pugliese, 1994; Remschmidt, Schulz, Martin, Warnke, & Trott, 1994). The superiority of clozapine in this clinical trial is especially impressive in view of the small sample and severity of this group's illness.

Two children experienced a true awakening from their thought disorder and psychotic symptoms. One of these children, who had delusions, auditory hallucinations, multilated himself, and had other severe negative symptoms, had a complete remission of psychosis and behavioral problems after receiving clozapine and conversed in sentences for the first time in years. He now lives with his family, attends a day program regularly, and has been able to maintain friendships. Last year he successfully participated in 2 chess tournaments and enjoys taking nature walks.

For most children and adolescents in the study, clozapine improved interpersonal functioning and enabled a return to a less restrictive setting. Based on our continued monthly telephone contacts and interim history at 2-year follow-up, we believe that for some patients, maximal clozapine effects may not be seen until after 6 to 9 months of treatment, as reported for adults (Meltzer, 1992; Meltzer, 1995; Kane et al., 1996). One child entered the project catatonic, internally preoccupied, and requiring constant highly skilled supervision to remain safe. She gradually responded to clozapine during the course of a year and became more spontaneously verbal, attended school regularly, and went shopping and on passes outside her residential treatment center to visit her mother.

Children and adolescents treated with clozapine need to be carefully monitored. We have continued to follow up the patients in this study. Thirteen patients have continued taking clozapine therapy for an additional mean ($\pm SD$) 30 ± 15 months after completion of the study. Clozapine therapy has been stopped in 8 of our 21 patients because of seizures ($n = 3$), hematological abnormalities ($n = 2$), or treatment nonresponse ($n = 3$). Two large, open, retrospective series of adolescents with schizophrenia report a dropout rate of 5% to 17% because of similar adverse events (Schmidt, Trott, Blanz, & Nissen, 1989; Remschmidt, Schulz, & Martin, 1994). Whether our 38% dropout rate is a chance event or reflects the younger mean age of our sample with associated greater susceptibility to toxic effects of the drugs cannot be determined.

To date, 5 (24%) of the 21 patients enrolled in this study have experienced mild to moderate neutropenia. In adult patients, a cumulative risk of 1.5% to 2.0% of neutropenias has been estimated (Gerson, 1993). The risk for agranulocytosis has been reported to be higher in patients younger than 21 years compared with those between 21 and 40 years old (Alvir, Lieberman, Safferman, Schwimmer, & Schaaf, 1993). The pharmacokinetics of clozapine metabolism also may be different for children compared with adults and may explain the differential incidence of toxic effects. When children metabolize clozapine, higher concentrations are produced of the metabolite N-desmethylclozapine, which has been associated with hematopoietic toxicity (Piscitelli et al., 1994; Gerson, Arce, & Meltzer, 1994).

As reported for adults (Safferman, Lieberman, Alvir, & Howard, 1992), 2 of our patients who were rechallenged with clozapine experienced a recurrence of neutropenia, which tended to happen more rapidly with rechallenge. Both patients were treated with concomitant penicillin or penicillin-related antibiotics during the course of clozapine treatment. One patient had received antibiotics before the first drop in the absolute neutrophil count, and the second patient received antibiotics during the first rechallenge. This suggests a possible drug interaction between clozapine and certain antibiotics, as has been previously suggested (Krassner, 1995) and that caution must be used when treating patients receiving clozapine with other medications that can cause neutropenia.

Children and adolescents with schizophrenia treated with clozapine need to be carefully monitored for seizures. In a review by Freedman et al. (Freedman, Wirshing, Russell, Bray, & Unutzer, 1994), 3 (4%) of 80 clozapine-treated adolescents had seizures, while 32 (60%) of 53 patients experienced mild to marked epileptiform changes on EEG. To date, 6 (29%) of the 21 children in our sample required the addition of an anticonvulsant agent; 2 of these patients experienced tonic-clonic seizures. Devinsky and Pacia (1994) reported that 1.3% of adult patients treated with clozapine had generalized tonicclonic seizures during the first 6 months of therapy, and that myoclonic movements could progress to tonicclonic seizures (Devinsky, Honigfeld, & Patin 1991; Pacia, & Devinsky, 1994).

Three patients in our study were given anticonvulsants after they became more irritable and aggressive and experienced epileptiform changes on EEG. These patients responded behaviorally to a lower dose of clozapine and the addition of valproate. Thus, in children, the EEG may be a sensitive indicator of clozapine toxicity as previously reported in adult studies (Welch, Manschreck, & Redmond 1994). In our study, none of the patients had a history of epilepsy. The rate of titration of clozapine in our study was comparable with the open and retrospective reports of clozapine for adolescents with treatment-refractory schizophrenia (Schmidt, Trott, Blanz, & Nissen, 1989; Remschmidt, Schulz, & Martin, 1994; Jacobsen, Walker, Edwards, Chappell, & Woolston, 1994; Birmaher, Baker, Kapur, Quintana, & Ganguli, 1991; Mozes et al., 1994; Towbin, Dykens, & Pugliese, 1994).

The third major adverse effect of clozapine in our sample was weight gain. Adult patients treated with clozapine experience a significant weight gain during short- and long-term treatment with clozapine (Leadbetter et al., 1992; Umbricht, Pollack, & Kane, 1994). Our trial was too short to detect such a change, because weight gain was reported to be evident during weeks 8 to 16 of the clozapine trial (Leadbetter et al., 1992). Although our sample is small, the 2 best responders in the double-blind clozapine trial were the patients who had gained the most weight during the trial, consistent with similar reports in adults of an association between weight gain and improvement in BPRS score (Leadbetter et al., 1992).

Children and adolescents may be sensitive to the adverse effects of neuroleptics (Keepers, Clappison, & Casey, 1983; Campbell, Baldessarini & Teicher, 1988; Baldessarini, & Teicher, 1995). Supporting this hypothesis is evidence from open clinical trials with pediatric populations receiving risperidone (daily dose, 2–6 mg), which found that the incidence of serious adverse effects, including extrapyramidal side effects, weight gain, and galactorrhea, is high (Mandoki, 1995).

Although the mean dose in this study for the haloperidol group is high compared with other reports (range, 1.80–9.8 mg/d)(Pool, Bloom, Mielke, Roniger, & Gallant, 1976; Spencer, Kafantaris, Padron-Gayol, Rosenberg, & Campbell, 1992; Spencer & Campbell, 1994), our sample was unique in that all patients were treatment-refractory to typical neuroleptics, including haloperidol. The mean drug doses are not equivalent (by adult equivalence standards) because of an increased rate of tachycardia and serious adverse effects in the clozapine group, which lowered the overall mean dose of clozapine, and clinical nonresponse for positive symptoms in the haloperidol group, which resulted in a higher mean dose. The relatively high mean haloperidol dose could have mitigated the improvement in negative symptoms in the haloperidol group, but did not result in an increase in extrapyramidal adverse effects.

In summary, the superior efficacy of clozapine for the treatment of childhood-onset schizophrenia has considerable clinical importance. Childhood-onset schizophrenia is still poorly understood, but data from clinical phenomenology, smooth-pursuit eye movements, autonomic activity, and anatomic brain imaging suggest continuity with later-onset schizophrenia (Zahn et al., in press; Jacobsen et al., in press; Frazier et al., 1996). For children and adolescents with schizophrenia, the onset of their illness occurs during a period in which social and cognitive development is unfinished, resulting in more severe social disability (Hafner, & Nowotny, 1995; Benes, Turtle, Khan, & Farol, 1994). The enhanced therapeutic effects for some and the beneficial adverse effect profile of clozapine has led to meaningful improvements in the course of their illnesses and long-term outcome (Breier, Schreiber, Dyer, & Pickar, 1991). Because children with schizophrenia who are receiving long-term treatment with typical neuroleptics risk up to a 4% chance of experiencing tardive dyskinesia (Levkovitch et al., 1995; Gualtieri, Quade, Hicks, Mayo, & Schroeder, 1984), the absence of tardive dyskinesia during clozapine treatment is a major advance (Casey, 1989; Kane, Woerner, Pollack, Safferman, & Lieberman, 1993). For these reasons, the judicious use of clozapine for selected severely ill children and adolescents with schizophrenia is warranted. Ideally, benefits seen with clozapine treatment in children with schizophrenia will be maintained in the presence of even greater safety with some of the newer atypical antipsychotic drugs. Currently, the NIMH Childhood-Onset Schizophrenia Project is conducting clinical trials with these agents to test this hope.

REFERENCES

Alaghaband-Rad, J., McKenna, K., Gordon, C., Albus, K., Hamburger, S., Rumsey, J., Frazier, J., Lenane, M., & Rapoport, J. (1995). Childhood-onset schizophrenia: The severity of premorbid course. *J. Am. Acad. Child Adolesc. Psychiatry, 34*, 1273–1283.

Alvir, J. M., Lieberman, J. A., Safferman, A. Z., Schwimmer, J. L., & Schaaf, J. A. (1993). Clozapine-induced agranulocytosis. *N. Engl. J. Med., 329*, 162–167.

American Psychiatric Association (1987). *Diagnostic and statistical manual of mental disorders* (3rd ed., rev.). Washington, DC: American Psychiatric Association.

Andreasen, N. C. (1983). *The scale for the assessment of negative symptoms (SANS)*. Iowa City: The University of Iowa.

Andreasen, N. C. (1984). *The scale for the assessment of positive symptoms (SAPS)*. Iowa City: The University of Iowa.

Asarnow, J., Tompson, M., & Goldstein, M. (1994). Childhood-onset schizophrenia: A follow-up study. *Schizophr Bull., 20,* 599–617.

Baldessarini, R. J., & Teicher, M. H. (1995). Dosing of antipsychotic agents in pediatric populations. *J. Child Adolesc. Psychopharmacol., 5,* 1–4.

Benes, M., Turtle, M., Khan, Y., & Farol, P. (1994). Myelination of a key relay zone in the hippocampal formation occurs in the human brain during childhood, adolescence, and adulthood. *Arch. Gen. Psychiatry, 51,* 477–484.

Birmaher, B., Baker, R., Kapur, S., Quintana, H., & Ganguli, R. (1991). Clozapine for the treatment of adolescents with schizophrenia. *J. Am. Acad. Child Adolesc. Psychiatry, 31,* 160–164.

Breier, A., Buchanan, R. W., Kirkpatrick, B., Davis, O. R., Irish, D., Summerfelt, A., & Carpenter, W. T. (1994). Effects of clozapine on positive and negative symptoms in outpatients with schizophrenia. *Am. J. Psychiatry, 151,* 20–26.

Breier, A., Schreiber, J., Dyer, J., & Pickar, D. (1991). National Institute of Mental Health Longitudinal Study of Chronic Schizophrenia: Prognosis and predictors of outcome. *Arch. Gen. Psychiatry, 48,* 239–246.

Bunney, W. E., & Hamburg, D. A. (1963). Methods for reliable longitudinal observation of behavior. *Arch. Gen. Psychiatry, 9,* 280–294.

Campbell, A., Baldessarini, R. J., & Teicher, M. H. (1988). Decreasing sensitivity to neuroleptic agents in developing rats: Evidence for a pharmacodynamic factor. *Psychopharmacology, 94,* 46–51.

Campbell, M., & Palig, M. (1985). Subjective treatment emergent symptoms scale (STESS). *Psychopharmacol Bull., 21,* 1063–1082.

Campbell, M., & Spencer, E. (1988). Psychopharmacology in child and adolescent psychiatry: A review of the past five years. *J. Am. Acad. Child Adolesc. Psychiatry, 27,* 269–279.

Carpenter, W. T., Conley, R. R., Buchanan, R. W., Breier, A., & Tamminga, C. A. (1995). Patient response and resource management: Another view of clozapine treatment of schizophrenia. *Am. J. Psychiatry, 152,* 827–832.

Casey, D. (1989). Clozapine: Neuroleptic-induced EPS and tardive dyskinesia. *Psychopharmacology (Berl.), 99* (suppl.), 47–53.

Devinsky, O., Honigfeld, G., & Patin, J. (1991). Clozapine-related seizures. *Neurology, 41,* 369–371.

Devinsky, O., & Pacia, S. (1994). Seizures during clozapine therapy. *J. Clin. Psychiatry, 55,* 153–156.

Frazier, J., Giedd, J., Hamburger, S., Albus, K., Kaysen, D., Vaituzis, A., Rajapaske, J., Lenane, H., McKenna, K., Jacobsen, L., Gordon, C., Breier, A., & Rapoport, J. (1996). Brain anatomic magnetic resonance imaging in childhood-onset schizophrenia. *Arch. Gen. Psychiatry, 53,* 617–624.

Frazier, J. A., Gordon, C. T., McKenna, K., Lenane, M. C., Jih, D., & Rapoport, J. L. (1994). An open trial of clozapine in 11 adolescents with childhood-onset schizophrenia. *J. Am. Acad. Child Adolesc. Psychiatry, 33,* 658–663.

Freedman, J., Wirshing, W., Russell, A., Bray, M., & Unutzer, J. (1994). Absence status seizures during successful long-term clozapine treatment of an adolescent with schizophrenia. *J. Child Adolesc. Psychopharmacol, 4,* 53–62.

Gerson, S. L. (1993). Clozapine: Deciphering the risks. *N. Engl. J. Med., 329,* 204–205.

Gerson, S. L., Arce, C., & Meltzer, H. Y. (1994). N-desmethyclozapine: A clozapine metabolite that suppresses hemapoiesis. *Br. J. Haemotol., 85,* 123–125.

Gordon, C., Frazier, J., McKenna, K., Giedd, J., Zametkin, A., Zahn, T., Hommer, D., Hong, W., Kaysen, D., Albus, K., & Rapoport, J. (1994). Childhood-onset schizophrenia: An NIMH study in progress. *Schizophr Bull., 20,* 697–712.

Green, W., Gayol, M., Hardesty, A., & Bassiri, M. (1992). Schizophrenia with childhood onset: A phenomenological study of 38 cases. *J. Am. Acad. Child Adolesc. Psychiatry, 31,* 968–976.

Gualtieri, C., Quade, D., Hicks, R., Mayo, J., & Schroeder, S. (1984). Tardive dyskinesia and other clinical consequences of neuroleptic treatment in children and adolescents. *Am. J. Psychiatry, 141,* 20–23.

Guy, W. 1976. *ECDEU assessment manual for psychopharmacology.* Rockville, MD: US Dept of Health and Human Services.

Hafner, H., & Nowotny, B. (1995). Epidemiology of early-onset schizophrenia. *Eur. Arch. Psychiatry Clin. Neurosci., 245,* 80–92.

Jacobsen, L., Hong, W., Hommer, D., Frazier, J., Giedd, J., Gordon, C., Karp, B., McKenna, K., & Rapoport, J. (in press). Smooth pursuit eye movements in childhood-onset schizophrenia: comparison with ADHD and normal controls. *Biol. Psychiatry.*

Jacobsen, L., Walker, M., Edwards, J., Chappell, P., & Woolston, J. (1994). Clozapine in the treatment of a young adolescent with schizophrenia. *J. Am. Acad. Child Adolesc. Psychiatry, 33,* 645–650.

Kane, J., Honigfeld, G., Singer, J., & Meltzer, H. (1988). Clozapine for the treatment-resistant schizophrenia: A double-blind comparison with chlorpromazine. *Arch. Gen. Psychiatry, 45,* 789–796.

Kane, J. M., Schooler, N., Marder, S., Wirshing, W., Ames, D., Umbricht, D., Safferman, A., Baker, R., & Ganguli, R. (1996). Efficacy of clozapine vs. haloperidol in a long-term clinical trial. *Schizophr Res., 18,* 127. Abstract.

Kane, J., Woerner, M., Pollack, S., Safferman, A., & Lieberman, J. (1993). Does clozapine cause tardive dyskinesia? *J. Clin. Psychiatry, 54,* 327–330.

Keepers, G., Clappison, V., & Casey, D. (1983). Initial anticholinergic prophylaxis for acute neuroleptic induced extrapyramidal syndromes. *Arch. Gen. Psychiatry, 40,* 1113–1117.

Krassner, M. (1995). *Sandoz pharmaceuticals corporation brochure on possible drug interactions with clozapine.* East Hanover, NJ: Pharmaceutical Safety Division, Sandoz Pharmaceuticals Corp.

Leadbetter, R., Shutty, M., Pavalonis, D., Vieweg, V., Higgins, P., & Downs, M. (1992). Clozapine-induced weight gain: Prevalence and clinical relevance. *Am. J. Psychiatry, 149,* 68–72.

Levkovitch, Y., Kronenberg, J., Kayser, N., Zvyvagelski, M., Gaoni, B., & Gadoth, N. (1995). Clozapine for tardive dyskinesia in adolescents. *Brain Dev., 17,* 213–215.

Mandoki, M. (1995). Risperidone treatment of children and adolescents: Increased risk of extrapyramidal side effects? *J. Child Adolesc. Psychopharmacol, 5,* 49–67.

Meltzer, H. Y. (1992). Treatment of the neuroleptic nonresponsive schizophrenic patient. *Schizophr Bull., 18,* 515–542.

Meltzer, H. Y. (1995). Clozapine: Is another view valid? *Am. J. Psychiatry, 152,* 821–825.

McClellan, J., & Werry, J. (1994). Practice parameters for the assessment and treatment of children and adolescents with schizophrenia. *J. Am. Acad. Child Adolesc. Psychiatry, 33,* 616–635.

McKenna, K., Gordon, C., Lenane, M., Kaysen, D., Fahey, K., & Rapoport, J. (1994). Looking for childhood-onset schizophrenia: The first 71 cases screened. *J. Am. Acad. Child Adolesc. Psychiatry 33,* 636–644.

Mozes, T., Toren, P., Chernauzen, N., Mester, R., Yoran-Hagesh, R., Blumensohn, R., & Weizman, A. (1994). Clozapine treatment in very early onset schizophrenia. *J. Am. Acad. Child Adolesc. Psychiatry, 33,* 65–70.

Orvaschell, H., Tabrizi, M., & Chambers, W. (1987). *Schedule for affective disorders and schizophrenia for school-age children-epidemiologic version (Kiddie-SADS-E).* Philadelphia: Medical College of Pennsylvania, Eastern Pennsylvania Psychiatric Institute.

Overall, J. E., & Gorham, D. E. (1961). The brief psychiatric rating scale. *Psychol Rep., 10,* 799–812.

Overall, J., & Pfefferbaum, B. (1984). A brief psychiatric rating scale for children. *Innovations, 3,* 264.

Pacia, S. V., & Devinsky, O. (1994). Clozapine-related seizures: Experience with 5629 patients. *Neurology, 44,* 2247–2249.

Pickar, D., Owen, R. R., Litman, R. E., Konicki, E., Gutierrez, R., & Rapoport, M. H. (1992). Clinical and biologic response to clozapine in patients with schizophrenia: Crossover comparison with fluphenazine. *Arch. Gen. Psychiatry, 49,* 345–353.

Piscitelli, S. C., Frazier, J. A., McKenna, K., Albus, K. E., Grothe, D. R., Gordon, C. T., & Rapoport, J. L. (1994). Plasma clozapine and haloperidol concentrations in adolescents with childhood-onset schizophrenia: Association with response. *J. Clin. Psychiatry 55,* 94–97.

Pool, D., Bloom, W., Mielke, D. H, Roniger, J. J., & Gallant, D. M. (1976). A controlled evaluation of loxitane in 75 adolescent schizophrenic patients. *Curr. Ther. Res., 19*, 99–104.

Rapoport, J., Connors, C., & Reatig, N. (1985). Rating scales and assessment instruments for use in pediatric psychopharmacology research. *Psychopharm. Bull., 21*, 713–1111.

Realmuto, G. M., Erickson, W. D., Yellin, A. M., Hopwood, J. H., & Greenberg, L. M. (1984). Clinical comparison of thiothixene and thioridazine in schizophrenic adolescents. *Am. J. Psychiatry, 141*, 440–442.

Reich, W., & Welner, Z. (1988). *DICA-RC (DSM-III-R Version)*. St. Louis, Mo: Washington University.

Remschmidt, H., Schulz, E., & Martin, M. (1994). An open trial of clozapine in 36 adolescents with schizophrenia. *J. Child Adolesc. Psychopharmacol., 4*, 31–41.

Remschmidt, H. E., Schulz, E., Martin, M., Warnke, A., & Trott, G. (1994). Childhood-onset schizophrenia: History of the concept and recent studies. *Schizophr. Bull., 20*, 727–745.

Safferman, A., Lieberman, J., Alvir, J., & Howard, A. (1992). Rechallenge in clozapine-induced agranulocytosis. *Lancet., 339*, 1296–1297.

SAS Institute. *SAS language and procedures: Usage, version 6* (1st ed.) Cary, NC: SAS Institute Inc. 1989.

Schmidt, M., Trott, G., Blanz, B., & Nissen, G. (1989). Clozapine medication in adolescents. In: C., Stefanis, A., Rabavilas, C., Soldatos, (Eds.), *Psychiatry: A world perspective*. Proceedings of the VIII World Congress of Psychiatry (Vol. 1, pp. 1100–1104) Belle Mead, NJ: Excerpta Medica-Princeton.

Shaffer, D., Gould, M. S., Brasic, J., Ambrosini, P., Fisher, P., Bird, H., & Aluwahlia, S. (1993). A children's global assessment scale (CGAS). *Arch. Gen. Psychiatry, 40*, 1228–1231.

Simpson, G., & Angus, J. (1970). A rating scale for extrapyramidal side effects. *Acta. Psychiatr. Scand.* (suppl 212), 9–11.

Spencer, E. K., & Campbell, M. (1994). Children with schizophrenia: Diagnosis, phenomenology, and pharmacotherapy. *Schizophr Bull., 20*, 713–725.

Spencer, E. K., Kafantaris, V., Padron-Gayol, M. V., Rosenberg, C. R., & Campbell, M. (1992). Haloperidol in schizophrenic children: Early findings from a study in progress. *Psychopharmacol Bull., 28*, 183–186.

Towbin, K. E., Dykens, E. M., & Pugliese, R. G. (1994). Case study: Clozapine for early developmental delays with childhood-onset schizophrenia: Protocol and 15-month outcome. *J. Am. Acad. Child Adolesc. Psychiatry, 33*, 651–658.

Umbricht, D., Pollack, S., & Kane, J. (1994). Clozapine and weight gain. *J. Clin. Psychiatry, 55* (suppl B, part 9), 157–160.

Welch, J., Manschreck, T., & Redmond D. (1994). Clozapine-induced seizures and EEG changes. *J. Neuropsychiatry Clin. Neurosci., 6*, 250–256.

Yang, P. C., Liu, CY., Chiang, S. Q., Chen, J. Y., & Lin, T. S. (1995). Comparison of adult manifestations of schizophrenia with onset before and after 15 years of age. *Acta. Psychiatr. Scand., 91*, 209–212.

Zahn, T., Jacobsen, L., Gordon, C., McKenna, K., Frazier, J. A., & Rapoport, J. (in press). Autonomic nervous system markers of psychopathology in childhood-onset schizophrenia. *Arch. Gen. Psychiatry*.

20

Current Status of Family-Based Outcome and Process Research

Guy S. Diamond

Department of Psychiatry, University of Pennsylvania School of Medicine, Philadelphia, and Clinical Director of Outpatient Services, Philadelphia Child Guidance Center (PCGC)

Alberto C. Serrano

Psychiatry and Pediatrics, University of Pennsylvania School of Medicine, and Medical Director of PCGC

Mitchell Dickey

Marriage and Family Therapy Department, Southern Connecticut State University, New Haven

William A. Sonis

Psychiatry and Pediatrics, University of Pennsylvania School of Medicine, and PCGC

Objective: *To review family-based treatment research. A growing body of research and several meta-analytic reviews demonstrate that family-based treatments are effective for a variety of child and adolescent disorders. In addition, an emerging tradition of family-based process research has begun to identify important ingredients of effective family psychotherapy. This article reviews these advances and their implications for future research.* **Method:** *Selected studies on the treatment of schizophrenia, depression, anxiety, eating disorders, attention deficit, conduct disorder, and substance abuse are reviewed, as well as several process research and meta-analytic studies.* **Results:** *Family-based therapies have been shown to be effective for treating schizophrenia, conduct disorder, and substance abuse. Some data support their effectiveness in the treatment of eating disorders. Few studies have targeted internalizing disorders. A process research tradition is emerging, but it is in need of methodological advances. Meta-analytic studies suggest that family-based therapies are as effective as other models.* **Conclusions:** *More well-designed studies with diverse populations are needed to assess accurately the effectiveness of this increasingly popular treatment approach.*

Reprinted with permission from *J. Am. Acad. Child Adolesc. Psychiatry*, 1996, Vol. 35(1), 6–16. Copyright © 1996 by the American Academy of Child and Adolescent Psychiatry.
The authors thank Maria Belecanech for her assistance in the preparation of this manuscript.

Forty years of research has shown several individual psychotherapy models to be effective in treating adults and children with a variety of psychiatric problems (Garfield & Bergin, 1994; Weisz, Weiss, Alicke, & Klotz, 1987a). Only recently have researchers accumulated enough information about family-based therapies to accurately evaluate their efficacy. After a brief history, we review the findings on the treatment of several major disorders. Each section begins with a brief review of the family risk factors associated with the disorder. Treatments that address these underlying interpersonal deficits are more likely to produce positive and enduring changes. We then review selected process research studies that examine client and therapist behaviors and their association with outcome. We conclude with a review of several meta-analytic studies.

HISTORICAL CONTEXT OF FAMILY THERAPY RESEARCH

Family therapy first emerged in the context of several research projects headed for the most part by psychiatrists studying schizophrenic patients and their families (e.g., Lidz & Lidz, 1949; Wynne, Ryckoff, Day, & Hirsch, 1958). Shunned by the psychoanalytically dominated, mainstream psychiatric community, family therapy gained prominence in community psychiatry and in private training centers, such as the Mental Research Institute, the Ackerman Institute, and the Philadelphia Child Guidance Center. As part the "undeclared war" between family therapy and child psychiatry (McDermott & Char, 1974), family therapists rejected the traditional cause-and-effect logic of the scientific method, claiming it was epistemologically inconsistent with a systems approach (Tomm, 1983). As a result of these organizational and theoretical clashes, family therapy evolved outside of research centers and universities and consequently failed to develop a strong research tradition. For three decades, however, family therapy did enjoy the invigorating creativity that often characterizes rebels with a cause (i.e., bringing systemic thinking to mental health).

Since the late 1970s, several developments have helped family therapy shed its marginal status. On the ideological front, leaders within the field have challenged family therapy's antiempirical values (e.g., Bednar, Burlingam, & Masters, 1988; Liddle, 1991). On the research front, several developmental and psychopathology researchers have found substantial empirical evidence to support a systemic or contextual view of mental disorders (see Sameroff & Emde, 1989, or Cummings & Davies, 1994). On the organizational front, the National Institute on Drug Abuse funded the first psychotherapy research center focusing on family-based treatments (Liddle & Dakof, 1994). These developments indicate that empirical values have reentered the family systems tradition.

Before reviewing the empirical studies, one point of clarification should be made. Throughout this article, we use the term "family-based therapy" instead of "family therapy." This term reflects the increasing integration of three family-oriented treatment traditions: behavioral, psychoeducational, and systems therapies. *Behavioral* models are based on learning theory and operant conditioning (e.g., Patterson, 1982; Sanders & Dadds, 1983). They typically focus on the parent–child dyad and seek to improve parenting skills such as the use of behavioral contingencies and reinforcement. *Psychoeducational* models traditionally focus on altering negative attributions about patient illness, teaching coping skills, and providing support to both patient and family (e.g., Goldstein, 1991). *Systems* models view dysfunctional family relationships as causing or reinforcing child symptoms. Consequently, systems therapists attempt to restructure maladaptive patterns of family interaction. For example, they seek to reestablish parental hierarchy, detriangulate a child from parental conflicts, and modify weak or rigid boundaries (e.g., Minuchin, 1974).

All three approaches hold that family interaction may cause, maintain, or exacerbate child symptomatology. If appropriately mobilized, family relationships can also be a potent therapeutic agent for reducing symptoms and preventing relapse. In addition, these three traditions have increasingly borrowed theory and technique from each other, leading to more integrative psychotherapy models (e.g., Henggeler & Borduin, 1990; Liddle, Dakof, & Diamond, 1991). Given this trend, the term "family-based" therapies best represents the scope and intent of this body of work.

OUTCOME RESEARCH

Schizophrenia

In the last decade, important advances have been made in understanding and treating families with a schizophrenic adolescent or young adult. Early family systems theories of the double bind (Bateson, Jackson, Haley, & Weakland, 1956) and the schizophrenogenic mother (e.g., Fromm-Reichmann, 1948) have not been empirically tested and have been discarded. Family treatment approaches became important, however, when in the late 1960s and early 1970s, deinstitutionalization of psychiatric patients increased the families' burden to care for patients.

FAMILY RISK FACTORS. Basic research on interaction patterns in families of schizophrenics has greatly influenced the development of family treatments. For example, a parent's negative attributions about a patient's illness, high levels of parental hostility or criticism, and overinvolvement (Expressed Emotion (EE)) have been shown to predict adolescent onset of schizophrenia (Doane, West, Goldstein, Rodnick, & Jones, 1981) and to increase rates of relapse after discharge (e.g., Vaughn & Leff, 1981). Reduction of EE during treatment has also shown to reduce the likelihood of relapse (e.g., Goldstein et al., 1978).

TREATMENT. Several psychoeducational approaches to treating this disorder have been well studied and are extremely successful. These programs focus on reducing EE and increasing family coping skills. To accomplish this, these programs train family members in communication and problem-solving skills in order to reduce negative affect (such as confusion, guilt, and blame) and to create a more structured and predictable home environment. In addition, family members are taught to recognize early signs of relapse and to use booster therapy sessions for crisis intervention (see Goldstein, 1991, for a summary of programs). Brief (4–6 hr) educational and didactic approaches have demonstrated limited benefits, while extended intervention programs (often lasting a year or longer) have demonstrated impressive results. The longer programs generally combine psychoeducation with a systems approach and emphasize the need for changes between all family members.

Five rigorous clinical trials testing long-term treatment programs have demonstrated that medication, plus a psychosocial intervention, provide a better prophylactic against rehospitalization than medication alone (Falloon et al., 1982; Goldstein et al., 1978; Hogarty et al., 1986; Leff, Kuipers, Berkowitz, Eberlein-Vries, & Sturgeon, 1982; Tarrier et al., 1988). Figure 1 summarizes relapse rates in these studies. These programs have proven so successful that current research no longer questions whether family-based treatments for this population are effective. Instead, current studies examine interactions among dosage, phase of illness, and intensity and duration of treatment (Schooler, Keith, & Severe, 1989). Although several questions remain regarding the contribution of family environment to this disorder, programs targeting the improvement of family relationship have become an important component of treatment for schizophrenia.

Depression

FAMILY RISK FACTORS. Four family factors have repeatedly been highly associated with the onset of a depressive illness. These factors include (1) neglect and poor child–parent attachment (e.g., Lefkowitz & Tesiny, 1985; Orvaschel, Weissman, & Kidd, 1980); (2) criticism and hostility between

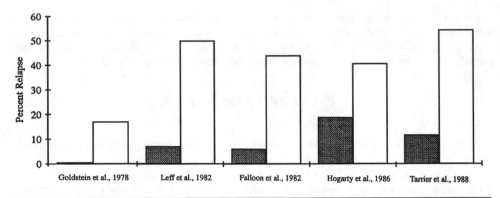

Figure 1. Follow-up relapse rates of schizophrenic patients treated with family therapy plus medication (*shaded bars*) and those treated with medication alone (*white bars*).

parent and child (e.g., Asarnow, Goldstein, Tompson, & Guthrie, 1993); (3) parental psychopathology, particularly depression (Downey and Coyne, 1990); and (4) ineffective parenting (e.g., Radke-Yarrow, Ricters, & Wilson 1988). While some of these factors are also associated with externalizing disorders, they are all highly predictive of depression (e.g., Dadds, Sanders, Morrison, & Rebgetz, 1992).

TREATMENT. Studies of depressed youth remain sparse. Kazdin, Bass, Ayers, and Rodgers, (1990) reported that only 4 (1.8%) of 233 child treatment studies addressed mood and depression. Although two studies included parent training (Lewinsohn, Clarke, Hops, & Andrews, 1990; Stark, 1990), only one (Brent, Holder, & Kolko, 1993) has specifically targeted family relationships as a primary treatment focus. Given increasing evidence that interpersonal factors, particularly family relations, play a critical role in the development and maintenance of child and adolescent depression (Burbach & Borduin, 1986; Puig-Antich et al., 1985; Rutter, 1988), the paucity of family-focused treatments is surprising.

Anxiety
FAMILY RISK FACTORS. Family-based psychopathology and treatment studies on anxiety are lacking as well. Existing studies demonstrate that a parent with an anxiety disorder increases the likelihood that his or her offspring will manifest similar problems (Klein & Last, 1989). In addition, the way parents focus a child's attention on threatening experiences, and the way they reinforce a child's avoidance, differentiate anxious children from control groups. Given the high comorbidity rate of anxiety and depression, many family factors are common for both groups (see Dadds, 1995).

TREATMENT. Several behavioral and/or cognitive programs have trained parents to administer or reinforce an intervention package for the treatment of fears and anxiety (e.g., Graziano & Mooney, 1980). Only one study has compared family-based and individual-based treatment for this disorder. Barrett, Dadds, Rapee, and Ryan (1993) compared cognitive-behavioral treatment (CBT) to CBT plus a family intervention for the treatment of overanxious and avoidant disorders. At termination, 61% of children who received CBT alone, 88% who received the combined treatment, and 30% of those on a waiting list no longer met *DSM-III-R* criteria for anxiety. These findings are promising and encourage further family-based research with this disorder.

Eating Disorders
Anorexia nervosa and bulimia nervosa
FAMILY RISK FACTORS. In a recent review of 19 studies, Humphrey (1994) differentiated subgroups of families in which a child had an eating disorder, and she identified differences between these families

and controls. She concluded that families with a bulimic or bulimic/anorectic child function worse than families of restricting anorectic children: more hostility, chaos, isolation, and less nurturance and empathy. In contrast, families with restricting anorectic children report less disturbance and more satisfaction, yet more dependency and rigidity.

TREATMENT. In 1978, Minuchin et al. conducted the first study (open trial) of a family-based treatment (structural family therapy) for this disorder and produced an 86% improvement rate. However, only one controlled clinical trial has been completed. Russell, Szmukler, Dare, and Eister (1987) randomly assigned 80 patients with anorexia ($n = 57$) and bulimia ($n = 23$) to 1 year of family therapy or individual supportive therapy after discharge from inpatient medical treatment. Family therapy produced better maintenance of weight gains and better menstrual functioning for adolescents (younger than 18 years) when problems had developed within the last 3 years. In contrast, adult patients (older than 18; mean $= 27.8$ years) improved more from individual therapy. Both groups had an equal number of patients living with parents. These results were essentially the same at a 5-year follow-up (Russell, Dare, Eisler, & Le Grange, 1994).

Obesity

TREATMENT. Programs for obesity are most often behavioral and involve parents in varying degrees. Some studies have shown parental involvement to have no effect (e.g., Kingsley & Shapiro, 1977), whereas others have yielded a positive effect (e.g., Brownell, Kelman, & Stunkard, 1983) on short-term weight loss. Although results across studies are mixed, one study was exemplary. Epstein, Wing, Koeske, Andrasik, and Ossip (1981) randomly assigned 76 obese parents and their overweight children (aged 6–12 years) to three conditions: parents and child treated separately (group 1), child treated alone (group 2), and child treated alone focusing on nonspecific factors (group 3). Treatment consisted of 14 sessions over a period of 8 months. All children showed a decrease in percent overweight.

After 5 years, however, group 1 maintained changes while groups 2 and 3 returned to pretreatment levels of obesity (Epstein, Wing, Koeske, & Valoski, 1987). Even after 10 years, group 1 continued to decrease percent overweight while children treated alone increased. Parents in group 1 did not maintain their own improvement (Epstein, Valoski, Wing, & McCurley, 1990). Epstein and colleagues suggest that parental modeling may facilitate skill acquisition (e.g., weight management techniques) with young children but may not be as important as other factors (e.g., peer influences) for maintaining these skills.

Attention Deficit Disorder

RISK FACTORS. Family-based research on family risk factors for attention-deficit hyperactivity disorder (ADHD) is lacking. Two studies, however, suggest that families with a child with ADHD, when comorbid with oppositional defiant disorder, display greater conflict, anger, and rebelliousness, along with more aversive, negative communication (e.g., insults, commands, complaints, and defensiveness) (Barkley, Anastopoulos, Guevremont, & Flecther, 1992; Weiss & Hechtman, 1986).

TREATMENT. Relative to a wait-list control, behavioral parent-training programs have proven successful in reducing ADHD (e.g., Anastopoulos, Shelton, DuPaul, & Guevremont, 1993). In a comparison of three different brief family-based models, Barkley et al. (1992) found equal improvement in family communication, school behavior, and maternal depression. However, clinically significant improvement (i.e., the number of cases no longer meeting criteria for diagnosis) was minimal (5%–30%). Although the results are often conflictual, stimulant medication alone has generally proven more successful than family-based behavioral treatments alone, or in combination with medications, for short-term symptom reduction (e.g., Horn et al., 1991). However, Satterfield and colleagues (1987) demonstrated that stimulant medication in combination with a long-term (2–3 year) intensive multimodal, psychosocial treatment had significantly better outcome (i.e., better performance at home and school and fewer arrests) than did long-term medication treatment alone. These results were maintained at a

9-year follow-up assessment, suggesting that intensive, comprehensive, long-term treatment may be cost-effective in preventing future delinquency (Satterfield, Satterfield, & Schell, 1987).

Conduct and Oppositional Defiant Disorders

FAMILY RISK FACTORS. A relative abundance of research on family and individual processes exists for conduct and oppositional disorders. For example, parental psychopathology (e.g., depression, antisocial behavior, aggression), harsh and inconsistent discipline, poor parental supervision, marital discord, single parenthood, and lower socioeconomic status have all been linked to conduct disorder (see Kazdin, 1987, for a review).

Based on several years of systematic research, Patterson (1982) described a pattern of parent–child interaction that exacerbates conduct problems. Typically, parents of these children ignore low levels of aversive or demanding child behaviors. As a child's noncompliance increases (e.g., temper tantrums), parents either withdraw or punish the child harshly. Thus, the child learns that increased demanding behavior will produce "negative attention," and parents learn that harsh punishment provides temporary relief. This interaction sets up a cycle of reciprocal coercion which reinforces aggressive and negative child behavior and harsh and inconsistent discipline by the parent.

TREATMENT. Parent management training (PMT) attempts to alter these specific family interactions. PMT teaches parents to monitor, discipline, and reward child behaviors more consistently. Not only has PMT been successful in bringing child behavior within normal ranges (e.g., Eisenstadt, Eyberg, McNeil, Newcomb, & Funderburk, 1993), but treatment gains have generalized to improvements in school performance, siblings' behavior, and maternal stress and depression (e.g., Patterson & Fleischman, 1979). Fourteen-year follow-up studies have found PMT to have long-term benefits as well (see McMahon, 1994, for a review).

Targeting the entire family, Alexander and colleagues (Alexander, 1988) have developed functional family therapy (FFT). FFT views a child's symptoms as serving a psychological function for the family, such as regulating emotional distance among family members or avoiding interpersonal conflict. Rather than focus on the presenting problem (e.g., child's negative behavior), the FFT therapist focuses on reorganizing family relationships so that individual needs can be met in more constructive ways. Treatment attempts to reduce defensiveness, blame, and scapegoating and establish a receptive foundation for learning and practicing more health-promoting behavioral and interpersonal skills. The direct teaching of parenting skills is also an active component of FFT. Several studies have demonstrated that improvement in family interaction (decreased defensiveness and increased supportiveness) is associated with treatment gains and lower relapse rates in juvenile delinquents (Klein, Alexander, & Parsons, 1977; Parsons and Alexander, 1973).

Henggeler and colleagues (see Henggeler & Borduin, 1990) have developed an integrative, broad-band, home-based treatment. Multisystemic family therapy (MST) targets many family and extrafamilial factors associated with juvenile delinquency (e.g., peers, school, neighborhood). As with a growing number of empirically based family approaches, MST integrates knowledge of both child development and cognitive-behavioral techniques into a family-based approach. In an impressive series of clinical trials, MST has been effective in reducing rates of rearrest for both serious delinquents and sex offenders (Borduin, Henggeler, Blaske, & Stein, 1990; Henggeler, Borduin, Melton, Mann, & Smith, 1991) and for treating child abuse and neglect (Brunk, Henggeler, & Whelan, 1987).

Finally, family-based treatments have also augmented the effectiveness of well-established individual and group treatments. For example, Dadds, Schwartz, and Sanders (1987) added a couple's component to individual child therapy. They found that children whose maritally distressed parents had received the parenting component showed greater retention of treatment gains at follow-up than did children treated alone. Similarly, Kazdin, Bass, Siegel, and Thomas (1989) found that the combination of PMT and individual treatment produced better outcomes for child problems at posttreatment and at 1-year follow-up than did treatments aimed at either parents or children alone.

Drug Abuse

FAMILY RISK FACTORS. Given the high rates of comorbidity, it is not surprising that adolescent drug abuse and delinquency share common family risk factors. Family problems such as poor parenting, poor parent–child bonding, and chronic family conflict are highly associated with adolescent drug abuse (see Liddle & Dakof, 1994). Parents' and siblings' own substance use is also predictive of adolescent use (McDermott, 1984).

TREATMENT. Based on work by Minuchin (1974) and Haley (1976), the Addicts and Families Project (Stanton & Todd, 1982) applied structural-strategic family therapy to patients who were receiving methadone. Patients who received family therapy had more drug-free days during the year after treatment than did control groups. Since this initial work by Stanton and Todd, five studies have demonstrated the superiority of brief (10–16 session) family treatment over individual and group treatments for reducing drug use (Friedman, 1989; Henggeler et al., 1991; Joanning, Quinn, Thomas, & Mullen, 1992; Lewis, Piercy, Sprenkle, & Trepper, 1990; Liddle, Dakof, Parker, Diamond, & Garcia, 1995). Family treatments also had attrition rates between 11% and 30% versus 49% to 56% for peer groups. Furthermore, Szapocznik et al. (1988) demonstrated that a family-based strategy to engage patients in treatment increased attendance at first sessions by nearly 40%. These are impressive results given the difficult challenge of engaging this population.

In 1992, the National Institute on Drug Abuse funded the Center for Research on Adolescent Drug Abuse (CRADA) at Temple University (Liddle & Dakof, 1994). CRADA is a three-site center, conducting both randomized clinical trials and process research, with minority, urban families. This is the first federally funded research center dedicated to family-based treatment research, and it represents a landmark in the empirical development of family-based treatment.

Meta-Analytic Reviews

When treatment modalities mature, overall evaluations of efficacy are often conducted with meta-analyses. Meta-analysis is a statistical method in which results from each study are standardized and then combined to yield an average effect size (ES). ES is calculated by subtracting differences in treatment gains among groups and then dividing by the standard deviation. For instance, the gains achieved by individual child therapy might be compared to (i.e., subtracted from) the gains achieved by family-based treatments. ESs of .50 are generally considered moderate, and .80 is a large effect.

To date, three meta-analytic studies have been published on family treatments (Fig. 2). Hazelrigg, Cooper, and Borduin (1987) found an overall ES of .45 for family interactions and an ES of .50 for behavioral ratings. Markus, Lange, and Pettigrew (1990) found an ES equal to .70. Shadish, Montgomery, Wilson, Bright, and Okwumabua (1993), using conservative criteria, found an overall ES of .51. These findings demonstrate that, on average, families treated with family-based treatments improved more than at least 67% of families treated with alternative treatments or no treatment.

Meta-analyses conducted on other models have shown comparable effects. For instance, when controlling for outcomes that were very similar to actual interventions, family-based treatments fared about as well as cognitive-behavioral (ES = .56), behavioral (ES = .61), and nonbehavioral treatments (ES = .51) (Fuhrman & Lampman, 1991; Weisz et al., 1987a). However, meta-analytic reviews of child treatment in general found ESs of .80 (see Weisz, Weiss, & Donenberg, 1992, for a review).

Several reasons may account for this difference. First, many family treatment studies, particularly the systems models, lack the methodological sophistication (i.e., manuals, adherence measures) common to modern-day clinical trials for other models. Second, as Henggeler, Borduin, and Mann

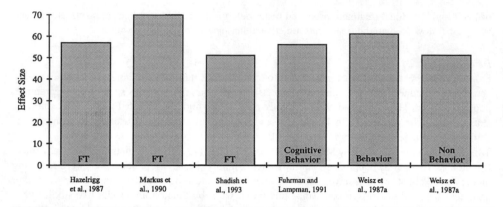

Figure 2. Comparison of three family therapy (FT) and two individual child therapy meta-analyses of outcome research.

(1993) point out, studies of externalizing disorders are overrepresented in the family meta-analyses, thereby limiting the interpretation of these reviews. Third, important procedural variations between individual studies and between meta-analytic reviews themselves (e.g., variable selection, types of outcome measures, statistical procedures, etc.) make comparisons difficult and subject to interpretation. More valid estimates of efficacy can only be derived from a larger sample of well-designed studies, addressing a number of disorders.

FAMILY-BASED PROCESS RESEARCH

Process research has reemerged as an essential component of contemporary psychotherapy research (Russell, 1994). In contrast to outcome studies that test an overall treatment "package," process research examines how specific processes or components of therapy contribute to outcome. Process researchers examine which interventions, with which patients, at what stage of treatment would be most effective. This investigation strategy increases our understanding of the "thought rules" that guide therapists through the labyrinth of clinical phenomena. Systematically developing a taxonomy of patient conditions, problem states, intervention strategies, and contextual factors will enhance our ability to deliver effective treatment and assess its impact.

Early efforts in this tradition primarily relied on analyzing static variables across sessions (e.g., patient talk time as predictive of outcome) or analog studies (i.e., laboratory simulations). In the last decade researchers have begun to investigate specific, highly defined, in-session change events or good moments (Mahrer, 1988; Rice & Greenberg, 1984). Focusing on "discovery" rather than hypothesis-testing, these studies examine patterns of patient-therapist interactions that lead to small, within-session moments of change (e.g., precursors and antecedents of an intervention). This research design leads to highly refined, descriptive models of essential mechanisms of change within and across therapy models. Although few family-based process studies have been conducted, some important findings have emerged (see Friedlander, Wildnan, Heatherington, & Skowron, 1994).

Tenets, Techniques, and Good Moments

Process researchers have made some advances in operationalizing and validating the basic tenets and techniques of family therapy. For instance, Mann, Borduin, Henggeler, and Blaske (1990) found that cross-generational coalitions (e.g., mother–adolescent) were associated with child behavioral problems and that improvement in parental communication and cooperation lead to a decrease in child symptomatology. Schmidt, Liddle, and Dakof (in press) found that improving parenting skills during treatment was highly predictive of good treatment outcome with substance-abusing delinquents. In an important series of studies, Alexander and colleagues (e.g., Morris, Alexander, & Turner, 1991) explored how reframing (creating a more positive attributional set about a presenting problem) influences in-session behavior and outcome. The results of these studies are mixed but provocative. Shoham-Solomon and Jancourt (1985) demonstrated that paradoxical interventions were effective with highly resistant clients. In families with a drug-abusing adolescent, Diamond and Liddle (in press) found that shifting therapeutic focus from organizational problems (e.g., curfew) to broader interpersonal/relational problems (e.g., neglect) helped to resolve a therapeutic impasse and momentarily to improve general family functioning. In a similar study, Heatherington and Friedlander (1990) found similar results. Although several other intervening variables may influence these types of outcomes, mapping in-session therapy sequences and tying them to outcome represent a clear advance in our ability to study therapy.

General Skills

Several studies have investigated supportiveness and directiveness. For example, Alexander et al. (1976) found that supportive skills such as humor and warmth accounted for 45% of the variance in outcome in a sample of delinquent adolescents. In one study, husbands rated therapist's nurturance and competence as beneficial, whereas wives rated them as neutral (Holtzworth-Munroe, Jacobson, Deklyen, & Whisman, 1989). Findings regarding structuring statements (e.g., confrontation or making attributions about client's motivations early in therapy) are less consistent. Structuring skills detracted from outcome in several studies (e.g., Green & Herget, 1991; Shields, Sprenkle, & Constantine, 1991) and predicted improvement in others (e.g., Alexander, Barton, Schaivo, & Parsons, 1976; Holtzworth-Munroe et al., 1989). Taken together, these studies encourage therapists to be more attentive to their stylistic variations and to family members' reactions to them.

The effectiveness of specific therapeutic techniques has been found to interact with therapists' level of experience. Experienced therapists may intervene more often and with greater directness than trainees (Pinsof, 1986), but they chose less directive techniques than did trainees when family conflict was high (Dickey, 1992). When conflict was low, experience did not make a difference. It remains to be seen whether experienced therapists achieve better outcomes.

Several studies examining early termination have yielded mixed findings. For example, Weisz, Weiss, and Langmeyer (1987b) found that client demographic factors and psychopathology did not predict outcome. In a sample of children with conduct disorder, Kazdin (1990b) found that premature terminators were no different from completers with respect to the sex, age, IQ, child diagnosis, maternal psychopathology, or number of parents in the home. However, terminating families had more child conduct and delinquency problems, lower socioeconomic status, and higher parenting stress. Gould, Shaffer, and Kaplan (1985) found that parental psychopathology and a school-initiated referral predicted early termination.

Limitations and Future Directions of Process Research

Although therapy process studies are illuminating, they frequently have methodological problems. Investigators typically rely on small, heterogeneous samples, use different definitions of similar constructs and investigator-specific instruments, depend too much on correlational designs, lack control groups, and conduct few replication studies (Diamond & Dickey, 1993; Garfield, 1990). Future studies would benefit from addressing these problems, as well as by using specific populations with specific disorders and obtaining more information on the client's subjective experience of the therapy.

CONCLUSIONS: IMPLICATIONS AND FUTURE DIRECTIONS

Family-based treatments are gaining empirical support from a young, yet evolving research tradition. Several outcome studies, focusing on specific disorders with standardized treatment models, have demonstrated the effectiveness of this approach. In addition, several process studies have identified and validated core therapeutic ingredients that contribute to these outcomes. These studies have refined treatment models and intervention targets at a much higher level of specificity (i.e., treatment manuals) than has previously occurred in many family treatment models. In this regard, the empirical tradition represents a leading creative edge in the current evolution of family-based therapies.

While these advances are promising, several areas are in need of attention. First, in addition to replications of previous studies, more studies are needed with diverse populations, such as obsessive-compulsive disorder (de Haan & Hoogduin, 1992), and particularly with internalizing disorders (e.g., anorexia, depression, anxiety). Second, more programmatic research is needed which uses knowledge from basic psychopathology and process research to inform the development of treatment models (Forgatch, 1991). Interventions built on empirically tested theories and techniques should produce more consistent and robust results. Third, the absence of reliable, valid, and treatment-sensitive family assessment tools seriously inhibits the advancement of basic and treatment family research (see Grotevant & Carlson, 1989; Touliatos, Perlmutter, & Straus, 1990, for source books on family assessment).

Fourth, more investigators should explore the effectiveness of their treatment models in community settings. Current data suggest a large discrepancy between outcomes achieved in the "laboratory" and in "real" world clinical settings (Weisz et al., 1992). Fifth, parental psychopathology and marital conflict should be studied as primary intervention targets and outcome criteria. These problems pose serious risks for child psychopathology and impede treatment efficacy. Although these limitations need to be addressed, our current knowledge base suggests several emerging trends about family-based treatments.

Emerging Trends

INTEGRATIONISM. The emphasis on "schoolism" has given way to theoretical integration and technical eclecticism (Liddle, 1991). Family psychotherapists now tailor a full range of clinical theory and techniques to a continuum of clinical problems (Alexander, 1988; Gotlib & Colby, 1987; Henggeler & Borduin, 1990; Liddle et al., 1991). Within a single treatment course, a therapist may work with individual family members, attend to historical material, enact in-session behavioral changes, and teach parenting skills. This trend provides clinicians with a broader set of intervention strategies and greater choice about when to intervene at the individual, family, or social system levels.

ETIOLOGY. Empirical findings have broadened our understanding of etiology. In contrast to ascribing all pathology to family interaction or parental conflict, contemporary researchers generally adhere to some variation of a diathesis-stress model. This model suggests that children have a temperamental and genetic predisposition to certain vulnerabilities. These vulnerabilities can be aggravated by internal or external stressors (e.g., maturational processes or family conflict), or contained by internal or external supports (e.g., cognitive development or adequate caregiving). Once activated, however, these vulnerabilities (i.e., symptoms) have a negative impact on the family (and social) system surrounding the patient (see Cook, 1994).

INTERVENTION IMPLICATIONS. Family-based therapies attempt to establish, or reestablish, a developmental context that will help contain or manage the child's symptoms. Family treatments promote normative family processes that foster healthy child or adolescent development. Medication and adjunctive treatments (e.g., hospitalization) are used as needed (Clarkin et al., 1990; Coyne, 1987). All intervention strategies, however, are considered from the perspective of promoting family competency and growth.

The therapeutic value of this "corrective development experience" is supported by extensive developmental research which indicates that healthy parent–child relationships have a positive impact on child and adolescent development in a variety of domains (e.g., attachment, ego development, self-esteem, social adjustment) (e.g., Grotevant & Cooper, 1983; Steinberg, 1990). Given the potency of family relationships for precipitating and maintaining child psychopathology, and for promoting prosocial development (Maccoby & Martin, 1983), several prominent researchers have strongly encouraged the further exploration of family-based treatment models for children and adolescents (Kazdin, 1990a; Kendall & Morris, 1991; Kovacs, Feinberg, Crouse-Novak, Paulauskas, & Finkelstein, 1984; Rutter, 1988).

REFERENCES

Alexander, J. F. (1988). Phases of family therapy process: A framework for clinicians and researchers. In L. C. Wynne (Ed.), *The state of the art in family therapy research*. New York: Family Process Press.

Alexander, J. F., Barton, C., Schaivo, R. S., & Parsons, B. V. (1976). Systems-behavioral intervention with families of delinquents: Therapist characteristics, family behavior, and outcome. *J. Consult. Clin. Psychol., 44*, 656–664.

Anastopoulos, A. D., Shelton, T. L., DuPaul, G. T., & Guevremont, D. C. (1993). Parent training for attention-deficit hyperactivity disorder: Its impact on parent functioning. *J. Abnorm. Child Psychol., 21*, 581–596.

Asarnow, J. R., Goldstein, M. J., Tompson, M., & Guthrie, D. (1993). One-year outcomes of depressive disorders in child psychiatric in-patients: Evaluation of the prognostic power of a brief measure of expressed emotion. *J. Child Psychol. Psychiatry, 34*, 129–137.

Barkley, R. A., Anastopoulos, A. D., Guevremont, D. C., & Flecther, K. E. (1992). Adolescents with attention deficit hyperactivity disorder: Mother–adolescent interactions, family beliefs and conflicts and maternal psychopathology. *J. Abnorm. Child Psychol., 20*, 263–288.

Barrett, P. M., Dadds, M. R., Rapee, R. M., & Ryan, S. (1993, November). *Cognitive-behavioral and family therapy for childhood anxiety disorders: A controlled trial*. Presented at the annual convention of the Association for the Advancement of Behavioral Therapy, Atlanta.

Bateson, G., Jackson, D. D., Haley, J., & Weakland, J. (1956). Toward a theory of schizophrenia, *Behav. Sci., 1*, 251–264.

Bednar, R. L., Burlingam, G. M., & Masters, K. S. (1988). Systems of family treatment: Substance or semantics? *Annu. Rev. Psychol., 39*, 401–434.

Borduin, C. M., Henggeler, S. W., Blaske, D. M., & Stein, R. (1990). Multisystemic treatment of adolescent sexual offenders. *Int. J. Offender Ther. Comp. Criminol, 34*, 105–113.

Brent, D., Holder, D., & Kolko, D. (1993). *A psychotherapy treatment for depresed adolescents: Models and treatment integrity*. Panel presentation at the Society for Psychotherapy Research, Pittsburgh.

Brownell, K., Kelman, J., & Stunkard, A. (1983). Treatment of obese children with and without their mothers: Changes in weight and blood pressure. *Pediatrics, 71*, 515–523.

Brunk, M., Henggeler, S. W., & Whelan, J. P. (1987). Comparison of multisystemic therapy and parent training in the brief treatment of child abuse and neglect. *J. Consult. Clin. Psychol., 55*, 171–178.

Burbach, D. J., & Borduin, C. M. (1986). Parent–child relations and the etiology of depression: A review of methods and findings. *Clin. Psychol., Rev., 6*, 133–153.

Clarkin, J. F., Glick, I. D., Haas, G. L. et al. (1990). A randomized clinical trial of inpatient family intervention. *J. Affect. Disord., 18*, 17–28.

Cook, W. L. (1994). A structural equation model of dyadic relationships within the family system. *J. Consult. Clin. Psychol., 62*, 500–509.

Coyne, J. (1987). Depression, biology, marriage and marital therapy. *J. Marital. Fam. Ther., 13*, 393–407.

Cummings, E. M., & Davies, P. (1994). *Children and marital conflict*. New York: Guilford Press.

Dadds, M. R. (1995). *Families, children and the development of dysfunction*. Newbury Park, CA: Sage.

Dadds, M. R., Sanders, M. R., Morrison, M., & Rebgetz, M. (1992). Child depression and conduct disorder II: An analysis of family interactions in the home. *J. Abnorm. Psychol., 101*, 505–513.

Dadds, M. R., Schwartz, S., & Sanders, M. R. (1987). Marital discord and treatment outcome in behavioral treatments for child conduct disorders. *J. Consult. Clin. Psychol., 55*, 396–403.

de Haan, E., & Hoogduin, C. A. (1992). The treatment of children with obsessive-compulsive disorder. *Acta Paedopsychiatr., 55*, 93–97.

Diamond, G., & Dickey, M. S. (1993). Process research: Its history, intent and findings. *Fam. Psychol., 9*(2), 23–25.

Diamond, G., & Liddle, H. A. (in press). Resolving a therapeutic impasse between parents and adolescents. *J. Consult. Clin. Psychol.*

Dickey, M. H. (1992, June). *Therapist experience and family conflict as predictors of therapist emotion and intervention*. Presented at the Annual Meeting of the Society for Psychotherapy Research, Berkeley, CA.

Doane, J. A., West, K. L., Goldstein, M. J., Rodnick, E. H., & Jones, J. E. (1981). Parental communication deviance and affective style. Predictors of subsequent schizophrenia spectrum disorders in vulnerable adolescents. *Arch. Gen. Psychiatry, 38*, 685–697.

Downey, G., & Coyne, J. C. (1990). Children of depresed parents: An integrative review. *Psychol. Bull., 108*, 50–76.

Eisenstadt, T. H., Eyberg, S., McNeil, C. B., Newcomb, K., & Funderburk, B. (1993). Parent–child interaction therapy with behavior problem children: Relative effectiveness of two stages and overall treatment outcome. *J. Clin. Child Psychol., 22*, 42–51.

Epstein, L., Valoski, A., Wing, R., & McCurley, J. (1990). Ten-year follow-up of behavioural, family-based treatment for obese children. *JAMA 264*, 2519–2523.

Epstein, L., Wing, R., Koeske, R., Andrasik, F., & Ossip, D. (1981). Child and parent weight loss in family-based behavior modification programs. *J. Consult. Clin. Psychol., 49*, 674–685.

Epstein, L., Wing, R., Koeske, R., & Valoski, A. (1987). Long-term effects of family-based treatment of childhood obesity. *J. Consult. Clin. Psychol., 55*, 91–95.

Falloon, I. R. H., Boyd, J. L., McGill, C. W., Razani, J., Moss, H. B., & Gilderman, A. M. (1982). Family management in the prevention of exacerbations of schizophrenia: A controlled study. *N. Engl. J. Med., 306*, 1437–1440.

Forgatch, M. S. (1991). The clinical science vortex: Developing a theory for antisocial behavior. In D. Pepler & K. H. Rubin (Eds.), *The development and treatment of childhood aggression* (pp. 291–315). Hillsdale, NJ: Lawrence Erlbaum.

Friedlander, M. L., Wildman, J., Heatherington, L., & Skowron, E. A. (1994). What we do and don't know about the process of family therapy. *J. Fam. Psychol., 8*, 390–416.

Friedman, A. S. (1989). Family therapy vs parent groups: Effects on adolescent drug abusers. *Am. J. Fam. Therapy, 17*, 335–347.

Fromm-Reichmann, F. (1948). Notes on the development of treatment of schizophrenics by psychoanalytic psychotherapy. *Psychiatry, 11*, 263–273.

Fuhrman, D. L., & Lampman, T. C. (1991). Effectiveness of cognitive-behavioral therapy for maladapting children: A meta-analysis. *Psychol. Bull., 110*, 204–214.

Garfield, S. L. (1990). Issues and methods in psychotherapy process research. *J. Consult. Clin. Psychol., 58*, 273–280.

Garfield, S. L., & Bergin, A. E. (1994). *Handbook of psychotherapy and behavior change*. New York: John Wiley.

Goldstein, M. J. (1991). Psychosocial (non-pharmacological) treatments for schizophrenia. In A. Tazman & S. M. Goldfinger (Eds.), *Review of Psychiatry* (pp. 116–135). Washington, DC: American Psychiatric Association.

Goldstein, M. J., Rodnick, E. H., Evans, J. R., Philip, R. A., May, R. A., & Steinberg, M. R. (1978). Drug and family therapy in the aftercare of acute schizophrenics. *Arch. Gen. Psychiatry, 35*, 1169–1177.

Gotlib, I. H., & Colby, C. A. (1987). *Treatment of depression: An interpersonal systems approach.* New York: Pergamon Press.

Gould, M. S., Shaffer, D., & Kaplan, D. (1985). The characteristics of dropouts from a child psychiatry clinic. *J. Am. Acad. Child Psychiatry, 24,* 316–328.

Graziano, A. M., & Mooney, K. C. (1980). Family self-control instructions for children's nighttime fear reduction. *J. Consult. Clin. Psychol., 48,* 206–213.

Green, R. J., & Herget, M. (1991). Outcome of systemic/strategic team consultation: III. The importance of therapist warmth and active structuring. *Fam. Proc., 30,* 321–336.

Grotevant, H. D., & Carlson, C. I. (1989). *Family assessment: A guide to methods and measures.* New York: Guilford Press.

Grotevant, H. D., & Cooper, C. R. (Eds.). (1983). *Adolescent development in the family.* San Francisco: Jossey-Bass.

Haley, J. (1976). *Problem-solving therapy.* New York: Harper & Row.

Hazelrigg, M. D., Cooper, H. M., & Borduin, C. M. (1987). Evaluating the effectiveness of family therapies: An integrative review and analysis. *Psychol. Bull., 101,* 4228–4442.

Heatherington, L., & Friedlander, M. L. (1990). Complementarity and symmetry in family therapy communication. *J. Counseling Psychol., 37,* 261–268.

Henggeler, S. W., & Borduin, C. M. (1990). *Family therapy and beyond: A multisystemic approach to treating the behavior problems of children and adolescents.* Pacific Grove, CA: Brooks/Cole.

Henggeler, S. W., Borduin, C. M., & Mann, B. J. (1993). Advances in family therapy: Empirical foundations. In T. H. Ollendick & R. J. Prinz (Eds.), *Advances in clinical child psychology.* New York: Plenum Press.

Henggeler, S. W., Borduin, C. M., Melton, G. B., Mann, B. J., & Smith, L. A. (1991). Effects of multisystemic therapy on drug use and abuse in serious juvenile offenders: A progress report from two outcome studies. *Fam. Dynamics Addict. Q, 1,* 40–51.

Hogarty, G. E., Anderson, C. M., Reiss, D. J. et al. (1986). Family education, social skills training, and maintenance chemotherapy in the aftercare of schizophrenia. *Arch. Gen. Psychiatry, 43,* 633–642.

Holtzworth-Munroe, A., Jacobson, N. S., DeKlyen, M., & Whisman, M. A. (1989). Relationship between behavioral marital therapy outcome and process variables. *J. Consult. Clin. Psychol., 57,* 658–662.

Horn, W. F., Lalong, N. S., Pascoe, J. J. et al. (1991). Additive effects of psychostimulants, parent training and self-control therapy with ADHD children. *J. Am. Acad. Child Adolesc. Psychiatry, 30,* 233–240.

Humphrey, L. L. (1994). Family relationships. In K. A. Halmi (Eds.), *Psychobiology and treatment of anorexia nervosa and bulimia nervosa* (pp. 263–282). Washington, DC: American Psychiatric Press.

Joanning, H., Quinn, W., Thomas, F., & Mullen, R. (1992). Treating adolescent drug abuse: A comparison of family systems therapy, group therapy, and family drug education. *J. Marital Fam. Ther., 18,* 345–356.

Kazdin, A. (1990a). Psychotherapy for children and adolescents. *Annu. Rev. Psychol., 41,* 21–54.

Kazdin, A. E. (1987). *Conduct disorder in childhood and adolescents.* Newbury Park, CA: Sage.

Kazdin, A. E. (1990b). Premature termination from treatment among children referred for antisocial behavior. *J. Child Psychol. Psychiatry, 31,* 415–425.

Kazdin, A. E., Bass, D., Ayers, W. A., & Rodgers, A. (1990). Empirical and clinical focus of child and adolescent research. *J. Consult. Clin. Psychol., 58,* 729–740.

Kazdin, A. E., Bass, D., Siegel, T., & Thomas, C. (1989). Cognitive-behavioral therapy and relationship therapy in the treatment of children referred for antisocial behavior. *J. Consult. Clin. Psychol., 57,* 522–535.

Kendall, P. C., & Morris, R. J. (1991). Child therapy: Issues and recommendations. *J. Consult. Clin. Psychol., 59,* 777–784.

Kingsley, R. G., & Shapiro, J. M. (1977). A comparison of three behavior programs for the control of obesity in children. *Behav. Ther., 8,* 30–36.

Klein, N. C., Alexander, J. F., & Parsons, B. V. (1977). Impact of family systems intervention on recidivism and sibling delinquency: A model of primary prevention and program evaluation. *J. Consult. Clin. Psychol., 45,* 469–474.

Klein, R. G., & Last, C. G. (1989). *Anxiety disorders in children.* Newbury Park, CA: Sage.

Kovaes, M., Feinberg, T. L., Crouse-Novak, M. A., Paulauskas, S. L., & Finkelstein, R. (1984). Depressive disorders in childhood: A longitudinal prospective study of characteristics and recovery. *Arch. Gen. Psychiatry, 41,* 229–237.

Leff, J., Kuipers, L., Berkowitz, R., Eberlein-Vries, R., & Sturgeon, D. (1982). A controlled trial of social intervention in the families of schizophrenia patients. *Br. J. Psychiatry, 141,* 121–134.

Lefkowitz, M. M., & Tesiny, E. P. (1985). Rejection and depression: Prospective and contemporaneous analyses. *Dev. Psychol., 20,* 776.

Lewinsohn, P. M., Clarke, G. N., Hops, H., & Andrews, J. (1990). Cognitive-behavioral treatment for depressed adolescents. *Behav. Ther., 21,* 385–401.

Lewis, R. A., Piercy, F. P., Sprenkle, D. H., & Trepper, T. S. (1990). Family-based intervention for helping drug-abusing adolescents. *J. Adolesc. Res., 50,* 82–95.

Liddle, H. A. (1991). Empirical values and the culture of family therapy. *J. Marital Fam. Ther., 17,* 327–348.

Liddle, H. A., & Dakof, G. (1994). Family-based treatment for adolescent drug use: State of the science. In E. Rahdert (Ed.), *Adolescent drug abuse: Assessment and treatment (NIDA Research Monograph).* Rockville, MD: National Institute on Drug Abuse.

Liddle, H. A., Dakof, G., & Diamond, G. (1991). Adolescent substance abuse: Multidimensional family therapy in action. In E. Kaufman & P. Kaufman (Eds.), *Family therapy approaches with drug and alcohol problems.* Boston: Allyn & Bacon.

Liddle, H. A., Dakof, G., Parker, K., Diamond, G., & Garcia, R. (1995). *A clinical trial of family therapy for the treatment of adolescent drug abuse.* Presentation at the Society for Psychotherapy Research, Santa Fe, NM, 1994.

Lidz, R. W., & Lidz, T. (1949). The family environment of schizophrenia patients. *Am. J. Psychiatry, 106,* 332–345.

Maccoby, E. E., & Martin, J. A. (1983). Socialization in the context of the family: Parent–child interaction. In E. M. Heatherington (Ed.), *Handbook of child psychology, Vol 4: socialization, personality, and social development.* New York: John Wiley.

Mahrer, A. R. (1988). Discovery-oriented psychotherapy research: Rationale, aims, and methods. *Am. Psychol., 43,* 694–702.

Mann, B. J., Borduin, C. M., Henggeler, S. W., & Blaske, D. M. (1990). An investigation of systemic conceptualizations of parent–child coalitions and symptom change. *J. Consult. Clin. Psychol., 58,* 336–344.

Markus, E., Lange, A., & Pettigrew, T. F. (1990). Effectiveness of family therapy: A meta-analysis. *J. Fam. Ther. 12,* 205–221.

McDermott, D. (1984). The relationship of parental drug use and parents' attitude concerning adolescent drug use to adolescent drug use. *Adolescence, 19,* 89–97.

McDermott, J., & Char, W. (1974). The undeclared war between child and family therapy. *J. Am. Acad. Child Psychiatry, 13,* 422–436.

McMahon, R. (1994). Diagnosis assessment and treatment of externalizing problems in children: The role of longitudinal data. *J. Consult. Clin. Psychol., 62,* 901–917.

Minuchin, S. (1974). *Families and Family Therapy.* Cambridge, MA: Harvard University Press.

Minuchin, S., Rosman, B. L., & Baker, L. (1978). *Psychosomatic families: Anorexia nervosa in context,* Cambridge, MA: Harvard University Press.

Morris, S. B., Alexander, J. F., & Turner, C. W. (1991). Does retribution of delinquent behavior reduce blame? *J. Fam. Psychol., 5,* 192–203.

Orvaschel, H., Weissman, M. M., & Kidd, K. K. (1980). Children and depression: The children of depressed parents; the childhood of depressed patients; depression in children. *J. Affect. Disord., 2,* 1–16.

Parsons, B. V., & Alexander, J. F. (1973). Short-term family intervention: A therapy outcome study. *J. Consult. Clin. Psychol., 41,* 195–201.

Patterson, G. R. (1982). *Coercive family process*. Eugene, OR: Castalia.

Patterson, G. R., & Fleischman, M. J. (1979). Maintenance of treatment effects: Some considerations concerning family systems and follow-up data. *Behav. Ther., 10*, 168–185.

Pinsof, W. (1986). The process of family therapy: The development of the family therapist coding system. In L. Greenberg & W. Pinsof (Eds.), *The psychotherapeutic process: A research handbook*. New York: Guilford Press.

Puig-Antich, J., Lukens, E., Davies, M., Goetz, D., Brennan-Quattrock, J., & Todak, G. (1985). Psychosocial functioning in prepubertal major depressive disorders: II. Interpersonal relationships after sustained recovery from affective episode. *Arch. Gen. Psychiatry, 42*, 500–507.

Radke-Yarrow, M., Ricters, J., & Wilson, W. E. (1988). Child development in a network of relationships. In R. Hinde & J. Stevenson-Hinde (Eds.), *Individuals in a network of relationships*, Cambridge, England: Cambridge Press.

Rice, L. N., & Greenberg, L. S. (1984). *Patterns of change*. New York: Guilford Press.

Russell, G. F. M., Dare, C., Eisler, I., Le Grange, P. D. F. (1994). Controlled trials of family treatment of anorexia nervosa. In K. A. Halmi (Ed.), *Psychobiology and treatment of anorexia nervosa and bulimia nervosa* (pp. 237–262). Washington, DC: American Psychiatric Press .

Russell, G. F. M., Szmukler, G., Dare, C., & Eisler, I. (1987). An evaluation of family therapy in anorexia nervosa and bulimia nervosa. *Arch. Gen. Psychiatry, 44*, 1047–1056.

Russell, R. L. (Ed.). (1994). *Reassessing psychotherapy research*. New York: Guilford Press.

Rutter, M. (1988). Depressive disorders. In M. Rutter, A. H. Tuma, & I. S. Lann (Eds.), *Assessment and diagnosis in child psychopathology*. New York: Guilford Press.

Sameroff, A. J., & Emde, R. N. (1989). *Relationship disturbances in early childhood: A developmental approach*. New York: Basic Books.

Sanders, M. R., & Dadds, M. R. (1983). *Behavioral family intervention*. New York: Longwood.

Satterfield, J. H., Satterfield, B., Schell, A. M. (1987). Therapeutic interventions to prevent delinquency in hyperactive boys. *J. Am. Acad. Child Adolesc. Psychiatry, 26*, 56–64.

Schmidt, S., Liddle, H. A., Dakof, G. (in press). Changes in parenting practice in multidimensional family therapy. *J. Fam. Psychol.*

Schooler, N., Keith, S., Severe, J. (1989). Acute treatment response and short term outcome in schizophrenia: First results of the NIMH treatment strategies in schizophrenia study. *Psychopharmacol. Bull., 25*, 331–335.

Shadish, W. R., Montgomery, L. M., Wilson, P., Bright, I., & Okwumabua, T. (1993). Effects of family and marital psychotherapies: A meta-analysis. *J. Consult. Clin. Psychol., 61*, 992–1002.

Shadish, W. R., & Sweeney, R. B. (1991). Mediators and moderators in meta-analysis: There's a reason we don't let dodo birds tell us which psychotherapies should have prizes. *J. Consult. Clin. Psychol., 59*, 883–893.

Shields, C., Sprenkle, D. H., & Constantine, J. A. (1991). Anatomy of an initial interview: The importance of joining and structuring skills. *Am. J. Fam. Ther., 19*, 3–18.

Shoham-Solomon, V., & Jancourt, A. (1985). Differential effectiveness of paradoxical interventions for more versus less stress-prone individuals. *J. Counseling Psychol., 32*, 499.

Stanton, M. D., & Todd, T. C. (1982). *The family therapy of drug abuse and addiction*. New York: Guilford Press.

Stark, K. (1990). *Childhood depression: School-based intervention*. New York: Guilford Press.

Steinberg, L. (1990). Autonomy, conflict, and harmony in the family relationship. In S. S. Feldman & G. R. Elliot (Eds.), *At the threshold: The developing adolescent*. Cambridge, MA: Harvard University Press.

Szapocznik, J., Perez-Vidal, A., Brickamen, A. L. et al. (1988). Engaging adolescent drug abusers and their families in treatment. *J. Consult. Clin. Psychol., 36*, 552–557.

Tarrier, N., Barrowclough, C., Vaughn, C. et al. (1988). The community management of schizophrenia: A controlled trial of a behavioral intervention with families to reduce relapse. *Br. J. Psychiatry, 153*, 532–542.

Tomm, L. (1983). The old hat doesn't fit. *Family Therapy Networker, 7*, 39–41.

Touliatos, J., Perlmutter, B. F., & Straus, M. A. (Eds.). (1990). *Handbook of family measurement techniques.* Newbury Park, CA: Sage.

Vaughn, C. E., & Leff, J. P. (1981). Patterns of emotional response in relatives of schizophrenic patients. *Schizophr. Bull., 7*, 43–44.

Weiss, G., & Hechtman, T. L. (1986). *Hyperactive children grown up.* New York: Guilford Press.

Weisz, J. R., Weiss, B., Alicke, M. D., & Klotz, M. L. (1987a). Effectiveness of psychotherapy with children and adolescents: A meta analysis for clinicians. *J. Consult. Clin. Psychol., 55*, 542–549.

Weisz, J. R., Weiss, B., & Donenberg, G. R. (1992). The lab versus the clinic: Effects of child and adolescent psychotherapy. *Am. Psychol., 47*, 1578–1585.

Weisz, J. R., Weiss, B., & Langmeyer, D. B. (1987b). Giving up on child psychotherapy: Who drops out? *J. Consult. Clin. Psychol., 55*, 916–918.

Wynne, L. C., Ryckoff, I., Day, J., & Hirsch, S. I. (1958). Pseudo-mutuality in the family relationships of schizophrenics. *Psychiatry, 21*, 205–220.

21

A Continuum of Care: More Is Not Always Better

Leonard Bickman

Vanderbilt University

This article describes an $80-million project designed to test whether a continuum of mental health and substance abuse services for children and adolescents is more cost-effective than services delivered in the more typical fragmented system. The study showed that an integrated continuum was successfully implemented that had better access, greater continuity of care, more client satisfaction, and treated children in less restrictive environments. However, the cost was higher, and clinical outcomes were no better than those at the comparison site. The article concludes that reform of mental health systems alone is unlikely to affect clinical outcomes. Cooperation is needed between mental health providers and researchers to better understand how to improve services delivered in the community.

No controlled studies report on the cost, quality, and mental health outcomes for any of the varieties of mental health systems for children and adolescents. The Fort Bragg Evaluation is the first study to examine what may be considered one type of system of care, the provision of a full continuum of services to children and adolescents with mental health and substance abuse problems. This article first summarizes key aspects of that complex study and then discusses the implications of the findings.[1]

An integrated and comprehensive system of care has been proposed for improving the availability and delivery of mental health services for children. Stroul and Friedman (1986) outlined the basic principles and components of an accessible, least restrictive, and cost-effective system of care for children. A key aspect of such a system is the availability of a full range of mental health services tailored to the needs of children. This range of services has been termed a *continuum of care* (Behar,

Reprinted with permission from *American Psychologist*, 1996, Vol. 51(7), 689–701. Copyright © 1996 by the American Psychological Association, Inc.

This research was supported by the U.S. Army Health Services Command Grant DADA 10-89-C-0013 as a subcontract from the North Carolina Department of Human Resources, Division of Mental Health, Developmental Disabilities, and Substance Abuse Services; and from Grant R01MH-46136-01 from the National Institute of Mental Health.

This five-year project was the work of many individuals and organizations. I would like to especially recognize Lenore Behar for her initiative in conceptualizing the Demonstration and her strong support for an independent evaluation, and the contributions of the Vanderbilt management team: Pam Guthrie, Michael Foster, Warren Lambert, Tom Summerfelt, Carolyn Breda, and Craig Anne Heflinger. The feedback on a draft of this article from Carolyn Breda, Michael Foster, Craig Anne Heflinger, C. Deborah Laughton, and Laura Scaramella is very much appreciated.

[1]This article can only provide an overview of the methods and results of this large-scale study. More information about the Fort Bragg study can be found in Bickman, Guthrie et al. (1995).

1985; Stroul & Friedman, 1986) and includes residential, intermediate, and nonresidential services. The continuum of care aims to deliver coordinated services on an individualized basis using case management and interdisciplinary treatment teams to integrate and facilitate transition between services. The continuum is designed to be community-based, involving various agencies pertinent to children's needs.

Concerns about large expenditures for mental health services and about the quality of care, especially for children and adolescents, prompted Congress and the Department of Defense to implement several demonstrations of different ways of managing service delivery. The Fort Bragg Child and Adolescent Mental Health Demonstration and the Fort Bragg Evaluation Project were designed to "demonstrate that this continuum of services [would] result in improved treatment outcomes while the cost of care per client is decreased when compared to current CHAMPUS[2] costs."[3] This $80-million Demonstration provided a rare opportunity to examine both costs and clinical outcomes in a careful and comprehensive evaluation of the implementation of an innovative system of care.

THE FORT BRAGG DEMONSTRATION PROJECT

On June 1, 1990, after a 10-month start-up period, mental health and substance abuse services were offered to more than 42,000 child and adolescent dependents of military personnel in the Fort Bragg catchment area. The initial subcontract established a four-year period for the Demonstration, but the services contract between the Army and the state of North Carolina was extended through September 1995. The current contract for services was competitively bid and is operated by a managed care company.

The Demonstration required that families seeking services for their children use the Demonstration's clinical services, which were free, or seek and pay for services on their own. The services included both community-based nonresidential and residential service components. The Rumbaugh Clinic, located off-post in Fayetteville, North Carolina, was the coordinator, fiscal intermediary, quality assurance monitor, and umbrella organization for all mental health and substance abuse services for CHAMPUS beneficiaries. As such, it was responsible for preauthorizing services and for utilization reviews through its individual treatment teams and the quality assurance process. The clinic provided mental health services by using its own in-house staff or by contracting with community providers already offering traditional mental health services (such as outpatient therapy and acute inpatient hospitalization) and provided intensive outpatient services itself. For the intermediate level of the continuum, the clinic developed services that included in-home therapy, after-school group services, day treatment services, therapeutic homes, specialized group homes, and 24-hour crisis management teams. All families who requested services received a comprehensive intake and assessment.

Children using intermediate- or more intensive-level services were assigned a case manager who coordinated services with the other child-serving agencies and practitioners in the community. Thus, services in the continuum and across other agencies were linked by case managers and interdisciplinary treatment teams led by a doctoral-level staff person. Additional services, such as transportation and other wraparound services, were also provided.

The American Psychological Association's (APA's) section on Child Clinical Psychology and the Division of Child, Youth, and Family Services joint task force considered the Demonstration a model

[2]CHAMPUS refers to insurer of the dependent, the Civilian Health and Medical Program of the Uniformed Services.
[3]From p. C-1, Amendment 0002 of Contract DADA 10-89-R-0018 between the Army Health Services Command and the North Carolina Department of Human Resources, Division of Mental Health, Developmental Disabilities, and Substance Abuse Services.

program because it was seen as "the most comprehensive program to date, integrating many of the approaches demonstrated by other service programs," and its approach was considered "integrated and flexibly constructed, yet comprehensive, [with] services ... available to be adapted to meet the needs of children and their families, rather than a simplistic application of a single approach to all presenting problems" (Roberts, 1994, p. 215). The Demonstration was recognized for its continuum of care in a single location and its close ties to other services and agencies.

The Demonstration was to provide the best possible services for children without the typical limitations placed on providers by insurance companies or public agencies. A cost-reimbursement contract allowed the Demonstration autonomy in initiating a continuum of care. This contract theoretically placed no limits on the types or costs of services to be offered if they were judged to be therapeutically appropriate by the Demonstration's staff. This was to be a test of the continuum of care model without the usual financial restraints and the typical implementation problems found when multiple agencies need to collaborate and pool funds.

The philosophy of the Demonstration called for controlling costs not by the conventional method of limiting services or cost per child but by providing a continuum of services designed to be more "appropriate" for each child. The wide ranges of services were designed to permit placement in less restrictive and hypothetically less expensive services. It was assumed that this rational–clinical approach to managing benefits would be a more effective means of controlling costs than placing fixed, and often arbitrary, limits on care. The Demonstration, however, did operate under the scrutiny of the state, the Army, and Congress and was under pressure to provide the most cost-effective services possible. The Demonstration was monitored by an on-site Army representative and a contracting officer. In addition, there were monthly advisory meetings led by an Army medical officer. At these meetings, the Demonstration staff presented utilization and expense data and reviewed any problems. The Demonstration submitted monthly utilization and cost reports to the Army. Consultants to the Army reviewed level of care placements on a regular basis. Each year, the contract had to be reviewed and funds allocated. The next section describes the standard care children received outside the Fort Bragg catchment area in the control site.

TRADITIONAL CHAMPUS SERVICES

In fiscal year 1991, CHAMPUS allowed 45 days of inpatient or hospital care, 150 days of Residential Treatment Center (RTC) care, and 23 outpatient visits per year. Unlike many other insurers, CHAMPUS imposes no lifetime benefit or dollar limit (Baine, 1992). Health Management Systems, Inc. (HMS) was responsible for providing utilization management for all inpatient and RTC stays and for outpatient visits exceeding 23 visits per year. CHAMPUS coverage is generous. Nevertheless, it does not contain any of the key features of a continuum of care, in other words, no systematic centralized intake, case management and treatment teams, or intermediate-level services.

PROGRAM THEORY: WHY THE CONTINUUM SHOULD BE MORE COST-EFFECTIVE

Program theory has been defined as "a plausible and sensible model of how a program is supposed to work" (Bickman, 1987, p. 5). Describing the program theory was an important first step in planning the evaluation. The theory provided the hypothesized links between program features and planned outcomes to be tested. Program evaluation theorists (Bickman, 1987, 1990; Chen & Rossi, 1992; Lipsey, 1990) differentiate between program theory failure and program implementation failure. In this evaluation, the theory tested is that a comprehensive, integrated, and coordinated continuum of

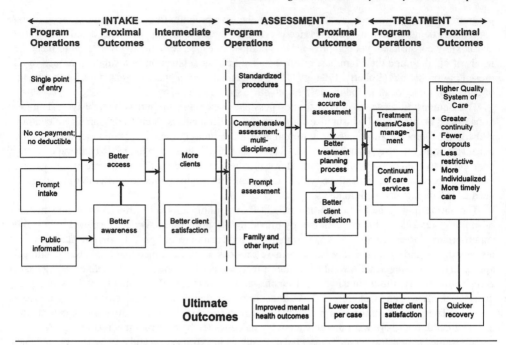

Figure 1. Fort Bragg child and adolescent demonstration: Program theory. (*Note:* From Evaluating Managed Mental Health Services: The Fort Bragg Experiment (p. 68), by L. Bickman, P. R. Guthrie, E. M. Foster, E. W. Lambert, W. T. Summerfelt, C. S. Breda, and C. A. Heflinger, 1995, New York: Plenum. Copyright 1995 by Plenum. Adapted with permission.)

care is more cost-effective than a fragmented service system with a limited variety of services. The theory could be tested only if the Demonstration implemented this theory sufficiently well and if the evaluation methods were valid. Because a continuum of care had never been implemented on this scale, the evaluation did not assume that such an undertaking necessarily would be successful. Thus, it was important to conceptualize and describe the Demonstration theory and its actual implementation.

Figure 1 shows the logic model or program theory of the Demonstration developed by the evaluators. This theory served as the organizing principle of the evaluation and identified key assumptions underlying the program. The intake characteristics of this system are on the left side of Fig. 1. Unlike many nonsystems or more complex systems, the eligible population can receive mental health services only through a single point of entry, the Demonstration. This feature allows the Demonstration to control access to services. Moreover, this feature should make it easy for potential clients to know where mental health services can be obtained. Strict standards of time-liness are not part of "services as usual" provided under CHAMPUS. However, for nonemergency cases, the Demonstration had to ensure that clients would receive intake and subsequent services within three weeks of a request for services.

As indicated in the lower left-hand column of Fig. 1, at the beginning of the Demonstration, providers and potential clients were informed about the new system of care. These activities were hypothesized to produce a proximal outcome of increased access to services. This increased access should have resulted in two intermediate outcomes: (a) an increase in the number of clients served by reducing barriers to obtaining services, and (b) an increase in client satisfaction with the intake process through a reduced financial burden and increased ease of access.

The second major section of Fig. 1 illustrates program operations during the assessment process. All families were to participate in a standard intake process, including a comprehensive evaluation and a review by an interdisciplinary treatment team. The Demonstration contract set standards for prompt assessment (within three weeks), including obtaining input from family and other relevant professionals. These program activities were hypothesized to lead to three proximal outcomes: (a) a more accurate assessment of the problem, which led to (b) a better treatment plan, and (c) an increase in client satisfaction with the assessment process. A more accurate assessment of the problem was predicted because of the comprehensive intake and assessment process, family participation, involvement of the multidisciplinary team, and the fact that reimbursement was not tied to diagnosis. Treatment planning should have been improved because of the increased accuracy in judgments of the child's problems and the input from a multidisciplinary team. The involvement of the family and the perceived accuracy of the assessment process should have improved consumer satisfaction as well.

The actual services (characterized on the far right-hand side of Fig. 1) provided by the Demonstration included access to the wide variety of services available in the continuum of care and the management of more complex cases by a treatment team and a clinical case manager. As noted earlier, the Demonstration offered inpatient and residential treatment, in-home therapy, after-school services, day treatment services, therapeutic homes, specialized group homes, 24-hour crisis management teams, wraparound services, and intensive outpatient services. These program activities should have led to the proximal outcome of a higher quality system of care that provided a better match between the services and the needs of the child and family. Operationally defined here, a *quality system of care* has (a) individualized treatment, (b) timely transitions between levels of care, (c) continuity of services, (d) services provided at the most appropriate and least restrictive level of services, and (e) few dropouts from treatment.

The Demonstration should have led to the following ultimate outcomes as compared with mental health services under CHAMPUS: improved mental health, lower costs per case, quicker recovery, and more client satisfaction. The higher quality service system should have increased the probability that services would be more effective. Although the total costs of the Demonstration should have been higher (because of a predicted increase in the number of clients treated), it was expected that similar cases would cost less to treat at the Demonstration (i.e., for similar cases, the Demonstration should have been more cost-effective than traditional care). The evaluation methodology was designed to test this program theory.

I should point out that this program model describes the logic underlying the Demonstration but is not empirical support for this model. The model attempts to explicate key linkages and assumptions made by the Demonstration's developers. However, the driving force behind the Demonstration was the beliefs and values that the continuum of care was the proper way to care for children. This Demonstration represented the type of system reform that advocates for children's services thought was critical.

METHODS AND RESULTS

Quality and Implementation

The Evaluation consisted of four substudies: (a) the Implementation Study, (b) the Quality Study, (c) the Mental Health Outcome Study, and (d) the Cost–Utilization Study. The Implementation and Quality Studies focused on documenting the Demonstration's activities. The primary purpose of the two substudies was to assess the degree to which the Demonstration implemented a high-quality system of care that was faithful to the program model. The Evaluation needed to be confident that the success or failure of the Demonstration could be attributed to the theory and not to a faulty implementation of the theory. The program implementation methodology was based on the theory-driven and component approaches to program evaluation (Bickman, 1985, 1987; Chen, 1990; Chen & Rossi, 1987) and followed a case study approach (Yin, 1986, 1993) to describe the structure and processes of the Demonstration. The case study used multiple methods and multiple sources of information and included a network analysis.

The Quality Study assessed the quality of two critical service components, intake assessment and case management, and one key administrative function, the Demonstration's Quality Improvement (QI) program. In the planning phase of the Evaluation, the developers acknowledged that the Quality Study was an indirect way to gauge the effectiveness of the individual components of care such as psychotherapy and hospitalization. These studies are described in Bickman, Bryant, and Summerfelt (1993); Bickman, Summerfelt, and Bryant (1996); and Heflinger (1993, 1996).

The Implementation Study concluded that the service delivery model specified by the Demonstration theory was well implemented. The Demonstration successfully executed a coordinated, individualized, community-based, and family-focused continuum of care. As indicated by measures of system coordination and fragmentation, on the basis of a network analysis, services were better coordinated at Fort Bragg than at the comparison site. Moreover, the Quality Study showed that the services provided at the Demonstration were of sufficient quality. The Demonstration maintained a QI program that supported quality clinical activities.[4] The two most significant nontherapeutic activities, case management and intake-assessment central to a continuum of care, also were judged to be of high quality.

Mental Health Outcomes

The Mental Health Outcome Study collected data from a sample of 984 children (574 at the Demonstration; 410 at the Comparison), between the ages of 5 and 17, and their families to determine the effect of the Demonstration on child and adolescent psychopathology and psychosocial functioning and family functioning. To serve as the Comparison group, children receiving traditional CHAMPUS services were recruited at two comparable army posts. Families were interviewed at the intake to services and 6 and 12 months later. Parents and children provided clinical information through in-person structured clinical interviews and self-report questionnaires. Areas of inquiry included level of functioning, competencies, pathologies, family environment, and client satisfaction with services. Multiple informants included children in treatment, their primary caretaker, the mental health provider, teachers, and trained interviewers. The specific instrumentation, fully described in Bickman, Guthrie et al. (1995), covered several domains and approaches that are listed in Table 1.

Because the study was a quasi-experiment, sample comparability was addressed after recruitment and at each wave of data collection. Analyses of demographic and outcome data showed that the samples were comparable at each wave of data collection. Of the 103 measures of mental health status of the children at intake, 14 suggested that the two sites differed significantly: Nine indicated that children at the Comparison site exhibited greater symptomatology than those at the Demonstration site, and 5 suggested the children at the Demonstration were more severely impaired. None of the effect sizes associated with the mental health status of children were greater than .25. The Evaluation

---

[4]The QI program should not be confused with the utilization review process. The former is concerned with enhancing the quality of services, whereas the latter is more concerned with cost control. Although the QI program functioned very well, the utilization review system had several problems that were documented by Heflinger (1993). Although there was constant pressure by the Army to control costs, the issue was not brought to a head until late in the project when the utilization review system was made fully operational.

TABLE 1
Eleven Key Measures of Outcome

Measure	Description
Standardized measures of child mental health	
Overall outcome Psychopathology + Functioning+ Family burden	Z-weighted average of P-CAS psychopathology, CAFAS functioning impairment, and BCQ family burden. A single overall measure of outcome as reported by parent and scored by a trained rater. Psychopathology high.
Child Behavior Check List (CBCL) psychopathology total	Total psychopathology score from Achenbach's CBCL. Data reported directly by parent, scored with Achenbach's methods and norms. Widely used measure of child psychopathology. Psychopathology high.
Parent–Child Assessment Schedule (P-CAS) psychopathology total	Total psychopathology score from Hodges's P-CAS. Parent reports observations that are scored by a trained rater with ongoing reliability checks. Regorous measure of child psychopathology in *DSM–III–R* terms. Psychopathology high.
Burden of Care (BCQ) total	Total burden (objective and subjective; internal and external) experienced by family as a result of having a troubled child. Measure of child's impact on the family that could be changed by effective treatment of the child. Psychopathology high.
Youth Self-Report (YSR) total psychopathology	Total psychopathology score from Achenbach's YSR, a variant of the CBCL self-reported by the child. Data reported directly by child, scored by Achenbach's methods and norms. Child-reported measures have fewer cases because only children 12 years old or older complete the YSR. Widely used measure of self-reported child psychopathology. Psychopathology high.
Child Assessment Schedule (CAS) psychopathology total	Total psychopathology score from Hodges's CAS. Children report observations about themselves that are scored by a trained rater with ongoing reliability checks. Only children eight years old or older take the CAS. Rigorous measure of child-reported psychopathology in *DSM–III–R* terms. Psychopathology high.
Child and Adolescent Functional Assessment Scale (CAFAS)	Overall functioning impairment from Hodges's CAFAS. Standardized rating of child functioning competence. Scored by a trained rater with ongoing reliability checks based on parent reports, child self-reports, and all biographical data available to interviewer. Psychopathology high.
Parent-reported individualized measures	
Presenting problem: Associated parent-reported psychopathology score	Using the parent's report of the child's main presenting problem, the corresponding parent-reported psychopathology score from the P-CAS is chosen to represent the child's key problem. Scores are standardized to eliminate differences among means of psychopathology measures.
Parent-reported "most severe" psychopathology	After psychopathology scores from the P-CAS and CBCL are standardized to the same mean and standard deviation, each child's highest (worst) score is chosen to represent his or her most severe mental health problem area.

TABLE 1 (*Continued*)

Measure	Description
Child-reported individualized measures	
Presenting problem: Child-reported psychopathology score	Using the parent's report of the child's main presenting problem, the corresponding child-reported psychopathology score from the CAS is chosen to represent the child's key problem. Scores are standardized to eliminate difference among means of psychopathology measures.
Child-reported "most severe" psychopathology	After psychopathology scores from the CAS and YSR are standardized to the same mean and standard deviation, each child's highest (worst) score is chosen torepresent his or her most severe self-reported mental health problem area.

Note: From *Evaluating Managed Mental Health Services: The Fort Bragg Experiment* (pp. 146–147), by L. Bickman, P. R. Guthrie, E. M. Foster, E. W. Lambert, W. T. Summerfelt, C. S. Breda, and C. A. Heflinger, 1995, New York: Plenum, Copyright 1995 by Plenum. Adapted with permission. *DSM–III–R = Diagnostic and Statistical Manual of Mental Disorders* (3rd ed., revised; American Psychiatric Association, 1987).

sample, particularly regarding mental health status, was nearly identical at the two sites at the time participants entered the Project. It is unlikely, therefore, that any differences in outcome at later waves could have been a result of initial differences between sites.

Analysis of covariance with Wave 1 data serving as[5] the covariate was the primary analytic technique at Waves 2 and 3. In this simple endpoint analysis, the Wave 1 covariate controls for individual differences in pathology at intake. Most of the outcome measures showed a large drop in pathology from Wave 1 to Wave 2 (6 months) followed by a smaller drop from Wave 2 to Wave 3 for both sites. Overall, at Wave 2, there were three significant site differences, two favoring the Comparison and all three having small ($SDs < .25$) effect sizes. At Wave 3 (12 months), there were two significant results favoring the Demonstration. Only five small differences suggest that mental health outcomes were equivalent at the Demonstration and Comparison.

More focused analyses that were based on the program theory predicted better outcomes at the Demonstration for those who received intermediate care, children who received more than outpatient services, children with severe psychopathology and impairment, children from families with multiple problems, and children with more than one type of clinical diagnosis. In each analysis, outcomes were measured by the key outcome variables at Wave 2 and Wave 3. Although overall there were slightly more findings than were expected from chance alone, the results favored the Demonstration and Comparison sites equally.

Client Satisfaction

Both adolescents and parents were surveyed about their satisfaction with individual service elements (e.g., outpatient) and overall satisfaction with services. Both sites showed a great deal of satisfaction with services, but there was significantly more satisfaction expressed at the Demonstration, especially about services unique to the Demonstration.

Cost–Utilization Outcomes

The Cost–Utilization Study compared service use and the costs of those services for all children treated (including, but not limited to, those participating in the Outcome, Study) at both the

---

[5]Random coefficients longitudinal models were also used, instead of endpoint analyses, with the same results (Lambert & Guthrie, 1996).

Demonstration and Comparison sites. The program theory predicted that the continuum should have provided better access to services, a greater diversity in the types of services used, less care in the more restrictive settings, and better timing and continuity of services.

The Demonstration served 14% of children who lived in the catchment area[6] in contrast to 7% served at the Comparison site. Clients in the Demonstration were seen more quickly. It took an average of 17 days between an assessment and the first services at the Demonstration in contrast to 38 days at the Comparison site. Children also remained in services much longer in the Demonstration. Six months after starting treatment, 41% of the children at the Demonstration still were receiving services compared with 13% at the Comparison site. Another indicator of greater continuity is the finding that more than 93% of the Demonstration children received a follow-up service within 30 days after leaving the hospital compared with only 47% in the Comparison group. Finally, defining a *dropout* as someone who received only one visit, 7% of the clients at the Demonstration dropped out as compared with more than 18% at the Comparison.

Only 9% of the children at the Demonstration were hospitalized or placed in an RTC compared with 16% at the Comparison site. Children at the Demonstration received an average of two to three different types of services compared with the one to two at the Comparison site. Parents at the Demonstration also reported that they were more satisfied with the match between their children's and family's needs and the services received.

Figure 1 summarizes the indicators of service utilization related to quality in the box labeled *higher quality system of care*. The Demonstration had greater continuity in care and fewer dropouts, used less restrictive settings, provided more individualized care, and delivered services quicker. All of the differences in utilization were statistically significant. As described in the next section, this enhanced system performance had important cost implications.

The Demonstration costs were much higher than the Comparison for the three-year study period. The Demonstration spent an average of $7,777 per treated child compared with $4,904 at the Comparison site for the three years studied. The cost per eligible child, determined by dividing the total cost by the number of children who were eligible to receive services in the catchment area, averaged $1.056 at the Demonstration compared with $321 at the Comparison site.

The costs of treating the average child at the Demonstration were higher because of longer time spent in treatment, greater volume of traditional services, heavy use of intermediate services, and higher per-unit costs. When considering only those services available at both sites (outpatient therapy, hospitalization, and RTC), the average expenditure per treated child for these services at the Demonstration was $4,696, only 4% less than that for the same services at the Comparison site. Children at the Demonstration received new additional services, but their use of traditional services was reduced only slightly.

The outcome sample was used to determine if the cost differences were in fact due to different services and not differences in the types of children treated. Data from comparable children in the Outcome Study showed that the average cost of Demonstration children, depending on the severity of the child's condition, was from 1.5 to 2.5 times more than the Comparison children. The difference in average expenditures per child does not reflect differences in the mix of children treated.

---

[6]The 14% figure is not a true measure of prevalence, but the number of children served divided by the average number of eligible children in the catchment area. Dividing by the average size served is a means of standardizing the measure for differences in catchment area size. A measure of prevalence, however, would use as a denominator the number of children who lived in the catchment area at any point during the Demonstration period. Because families moved in and out of the catchment area during the Demonstration, this figure is no doubt larger than that of the children living in the catchment area on a day in a particular year. A measure of the prevalence of mental health services use, therefore, would be less than 14%.

DISCUSSION

The Fort Bragg Demonstration was designed to examine the impact of a continuum of mental health care on children's mental health on the basis of the program theory shown in Fig. 1. According to this model, the Demonstration had to support multiple assumptions to obtain the predicted outcomes. If these assumptions were not met, then the Demonstration could not produce the ultimate effects, namely, improved mental health outcome, quicker recovery, lower costs per client, and better client satisfaction. This discussion focuses on the failure to find better mental health outcomes and lower costs. However, several alternative explanations for the clinical outcomes need to be reviewed before it can be concluded that there was no support for the continuum of care theory.

There are three assumptions underlying the model: (a) the successful implementation of a system of care (e.g., case management) and the clinical services (e.g., psychotherapy), (b) a more basic assumption that these services are clinically effective even when well implemented, and (c) the successful implementation of the evaluation. Thus, evidence concerning the implementation of the Demonstration's system of care and the evaluation's methods and evidence underlying the clinical effectiveness of services provided in community settings should be closely examined.

Null Effects Were Not Likely Caused by Implementation Failure

The Demonstration had to implement appropriate components of service and ensure that these components were well integrated. The services had to be available to clients quickly to produce smooth transitions from one service level to another. The service needs of clients had to be carefully monitored and changes in those needs adapted to quickly. If the Demonstration did not implement these features of the theory, then this study would not have been a valid test of the theory. Moreover, both services and their management had to be available and of sufficient quality (i.e., excellent case management cannot affect clinical outcomes unless appropriate mental health services are available to manage). Demonstration management and staff were responsible for the appropriate implementation of the theory at the systems level.

Data from the Implementation (Heflinger, 1993, 1996) and Quality Studies (Bickman et al., 1993, 1996) showed that the model was implemented with great fidelity. Services utilization data revealed that access to care increased dramatically and that children at similar levels of impairment were more likely to be treated without an institutional stay at the Demonstration. These findings are evidence that an implementation failure at the Demonstration site was unlikely to have occurred.

Were the Clinical Services Effective?

The second way the continuum could have appeared ineffective was if the clinical services themselves were not effective. In other words, the Demonstration could have faithfully implemented all the aspects of the theory and still there might have been no enhanced clinical impact found if the mental health services (e.g., outpatient therapy, hospitalization) provided by the Demonstration were not effective in altering clients' mental health status. These components of services could have failed to be effective for two reasons: They were themselves ineffective or the Demonstration did not implement them with sufficient quality.

The Evaluation documented the Demonstration's implementation of key aspects of the continuum of care theory and its proximal effects on utilization but was unable to judge the effectiveness of individual service components because it was not designed to test individual components of the system. The pragmatic and economical substitute for studying each component of care was an assessment of the Demonstration's own QI activities (Bickman et al., 1993, 1996). However, this approach is clearly not as desirable as evidence of actual effectiveness. Yet no single study can evaluate every aspect of care in a rigorous experimental design. Nevertheless, this limitation does not allow an unequivocal interpretation of the results.

The inability of the Evaluation to show that the clinical services were effective would not be a major impediment if there were a substantial scientifically valid body of evidence that showed that psychotherapy with children and adolescents is effective in community settings (Weisz & Weiss, 1993). Furthermore, no clear scientific evidence exists that the other forms of intervention (e.g., in-home services, hospitalization) used in the Demonstration were effective (Rivera & Kutash, 1994). Thus, the Demonstration may have very effectively delivered seemingly more appropriate services in a higher quality system of care that were nonetheless ineffective. A very impressive structure was built on a very weak foundation.

Implementation of the Evaluation

A poorly designed and implemented evaluation may also mask a treatment effect. The quality of the evaluation can be assessed from a validity framework that focuses on four different types of validity: (a) statistical validity, (b) internal validity, (c) construct validity, and (d) external validity (Hedrick, Bickman, & Rog, 1993).

Statistical validity. The statistical power (i.e., the ability of an evaluation to detect an effect that is really there) of an evaluation is crucial, especially when trying to explain nonsignificant effects. An underpowered design would result in a finding of *no difference* when, in fact, there may be a difference between the treatment and control groups. Whereas several variables contribute to the power of the design, the clearest and most easily controlled variable is sample size. The initial planning of the evaluation included a sufficiently large sample to detect an effect size of clinical importance. An empirical estimate of power that was based on Monte Carlo modeling (Lambert, 1993) showed that the evaluation had sufficient power (.80) to detect effect sizes as small as .25 standard deviations. The Evaluation's inability to find statistically significant differences was not likely caused by insufficient statistical power. The critical lesson here is that in a field with uncertain measures and effects, large sample sizes are necessary if there is going to be confidence that the possible null effects are true. From a policy perspective, this means that studies of this nature are going to be expensive and time-consuming.

Internal validity. Internal validity refers to the ability to link causally the Demonstration to an outcome (i.e., to have confidence that the Demonstration, and not another variable, caused any observed differences between the Demonstration and Comparison sites). The most plausible threats to internal validity in this study were the initial and subsequent equivalency of the Demonstration and Comparison samples most often called "selection artifacts" and "differential attrition." Bickman, Guthrie, et al. (1995) and Breda (1996) provide detailed information showing the initial and subsequent equivalency of the Demonstration and Comparison Evaluation samples. Again, confidence in the results would have been improved if a randomized experiment could have been conducted. Randomized designs in children's services at the systems level are difficult to implement but are possible. A randomized study currently being conducted in Stark County, Ohio, should provide further clarification about the relationship between system-level reform and clinical outcomes (Bickman, Summerfelt, & Douglas, in press).

Construct validity. Two different aspects of construct validity are of concern here, the construct of cause and construct of effect (Cook & Shadish, 1994). The Demonstration could be seen as ineffective if measurement of the outcomes or effects was faulty, a distinct possibility given the infancy of measurement in this field. To guard against the danger of selecting inappropriate or insensitive measures, several steps were taken in planning the evaluation. First, most of the outcome measures were widely used. Second, for the most critical outcome (mental health status), multiple measures were obtained from several informants. Third, the evaluation had validated the instruments on the project data (Bickman, Guthrie, et al., 1995).

Another measurement variable to consider was the length of the follow-up period. It is not clear how long clients, especially children and adolescents, need to be followed before an effect is manifested. A competitive renewal grant from the National Institute of Mental Health (NIMH) will allow us to follow the families in this study for up to four years after entering treatment. However, because the scores of both Demonstration and Comparison children are close to what is considered normal for the population on the Child Behavior Check List (CBCL), it is unlikely that differences will emerge in the future unless the Comparison children start getting worse instead of better. Because we know so little about the natural course of disorders in such a heterogeneous population, it is possible that as the adolescents pass through the critical transition to young adulthood that regression might occur.

Finally, some aspects of the model presented in Fig. 1 were not adequately measured in the Evaluation. In particular, there is no established method for determining whether the clinical assessments in the Demonstration led to better treatment plans as hypothesized. Both assessment and treatment planning are thought to be important in affecting outcomes, but the necessary research to demonstrate this has yet to be accomplished.

Our concern about the ability of clinicians to perform key tasks required in a continuum of care was heightened by the results of a study conducted subsequent to the evaluation. This study found that clinicians were not able to reliably agree on the assignment of children to different levels of care (Bickman, Karver, & Schut, 1995).

The other facet of construct validity, the construct of cause, could have been compromised if the Comparison site system of care was equivalent to the Demonstration (i.e., the Comparison site also provided a continuum of care). However, the Comparison site provided (a) no single point of entry, (b) no comprehensive and standardized intake procedure, (c) no multidisciplinary treatment teams, (d) no case management, and (e) no intermediate services. It is not likely that the equivalent clinical outcomes found could be explained by pointing to equivalent systems of care.

External validity. Generalizability, or the external validity of the results, is concerned with whether the results generalize to other populations and to other operationalizations of the continuum of care (Costner, 1989; Sussman & Robertson, 1986). The external validity of this study was examined by (a) comparing it with other systems interventions, (b) examining the similarity of the client population to other populations, and (c) analyzing the degree to which client characteristics differentially influenced the success of a continuum of care.

Other system interventions. It is illuminating to compare the Fort Bragg Demonstration with other recent major system reform efforts, in particular two other demonstration projects and a new federal program. The two demonstration projects, sponsored by the Robert Wood Johnson Foundation (RWJF), were conducted contemporaneously with the Demonstration. These resembled the Demonstration in that they examined the implementation and effects of integrating mental health services through a centralized continuum of care. However, the RWJF projects were more ambitious and broader in scope in attempting to show that multiple public agencies could pool resources and develop and implement a system of care. The RWJF provided funds for project management, technical assistance, program evaluation, and case management, while the communities were to develop the financing required to support the full array of services. In contrast, in the Fort Bragg Demonstration, the development and management of the system and all services were fully funded from the start.

The program model of the RWJF Program on Chronic Mental Illness for Adults proposed that a centralized mental health authority would result in expanded services and resources and thus would improve client outcomes. The evaluation concluded that

> a mental health authority might be necessary, but not sufficient to create a comprehensive system of services. Most of the cities improved the availability of services, especially case management, but none had a truly comprehensive system of community support services by the end of the Demonstration. (Goldman, Morrissey, & Ridgely, 1994, p. 42)

Given the shortfall in services, it was not surprising that the evaluators found that this RWJF demonstration did not affect client outcomes, such as quality of life, when compared with other sites (Goldman et al., 1994; Lehman, Postrado, Roth, McNary, & Goldman, 1994; Shern, Wilson, & Coen, 1994). Similar in program design to the adult demonstration, the Mental Health Services Program for Youth (MHSPY) was conducted by Brandeis University (England & Cole, 1992; Saxe, Cross, Lovas, & Gardner, 1995). Unfortunately, the evaluation of the MHSPY did not include collection of comprehensive and systematic outcome data at the client level nor any comparison sites. Both demonstrations illustrate some difficulties in making systems of care changes in the community, as observed by the U.S. General Accounting Office (1992).

The passage of the Comprehensive Community Mental Health Services Program for Children and Adolescents with Severe Emotional Disturbances (SED), signed into law on July 10, 1992 (Part E of Title V, section 561 et seq. of the Public Health Service Act), provides funds for assessment, case management, outpatient services, day treatment, in-home services, respite care, therapeutic foster care, and group homes for children with SED. This $60-million program, now in more than 20 sites, is comparable in some ways to the Fort Bragg continuum of care. Because the Demonstration and this program share a common heritage and they are based on similar principles, the results of this evaluation are relevant to this major federal initiative.

The continuum was central to these three system reform efforts in that the system that was to be developed in each community was a continuum of care, but the continuum had to be preceded by interagency coordination and pooling of funds. These initial efforts can be described as developing a system of care in contrast to a continuum of care. For these programs to show positive clinical and cost outcomes, both a system of care and a continuum of care had to be successfully implemented. The Fort Bragg Demonstration, because of the single funding source, was required only to implement a continuum of care. The Fort Bragg Demonstration was a less complicated and more direct test of the continuum of care theory.

Systems of care cannot affect clinical outcomes unless children receive services that they would not have received had there not been a change at the system level. Graphically, this flow model is shown below:

$$\text{system change} \rightarrow \text{continuum of care} \rightarrow \text{clinical outcomes.}$$

The results of this study apply to these other interventions because they were based on a continuum of care similar to Fort Bragg's.

Other populations of children. A comparison of children in the Fort Bragg Demonstration and other populations (Breda, 1996) showed that the military dependent children who participated in the Evaluation were similar to middle- and lower-middle-class children and adolescents treated in the civilian sector. Thus, the population that was studied in this Demonstration is most similar to the estimated 68% of the children in the United States who are covered by private health insurance (Cutler & Gruber, 1995). However, the Demonstration differed in a major way from the RWJF youth project and the Comprehensive Community Mental Health Services Program. The clients in these programs were mainly poor, publicly funded children from multiproblem families. The Demonstration's children were primarily from two-parent families with good education and middle to lower incomes. Would the continuum of care operate the same why with children who were from poorer environments?

The complexity of the continuum and its demands on the primary caretaker's time and commitment also may make it more difficult for families with multiple problems to stay in treatment. For example, parents in the Demonstration reported expending significantly more resources on travel related to their child's treatment. However, a continuum may have been more effective with these families because it would have provided the support that they needed to receive and stay in services. The inability to specify how client characteristics would function in a continuum may reflect the immaturity of the continuum of care theory. However, the results of the Evaluation show that the impact of the continuum on mental health outcomes was not different for multiproblem families or for those clients of different socioeconomic status or demographic characteristics. The present study provided no indication that the continuum would be expected to work better with clients who were more impoverished.

The Demonstration provided the optimal conditions under which to test a continuum of care theory. As Palumbo and Olivrio (1989) recognized, "The concern of external validity is generalizing to future applications. In doing this, we should be concerned with whether a better program can be put into place in future locations" (p. 342). Future system reform efforts are not likely to have the extensive financial and personnel resources of the Demonstration. If the continuum was not effective under these advantageous conditions (i.e., abundant funds, small interagency problems, intact families), then it is unlikely it will be more successful in more difficult and complex contexts.

Relevance to managed care. The Demonstration was planned and implemented before most of the current managed care systems were begun. Clearly, the cost control assumptions made in the Demonstration are not followed in contemporary managed care operations. In fact, this study provided little support for placing so much control in the hands of clinicians and their managers. After the Evaluation results were reported, the Demonstration removed much of the direct control of placement and length-of-care determination from case managers and treatment teams to more distally located personnel. This move may have contributed to the cost reductions reported by the clinical director (Lane, 1996). However, the managed care (in contrast to managed costs) aspects of the Demonstrations have more relevance to current managed care efforts.

The Demonstration can be described as one variety of managed care. A leader in this field suggested the following:

> Managed care has taken on a number of different meanings. To some it means any form of peer review to limit utilization, while others interpret it to mean active case management of a patient's treatment to coordinate and assure continuity of care. (Broskowski, 1991, p. 8).

Goodman, Brown, and Deitz (1992) provided a simpler definition of *managed behavioral health care* as "any patient care that is not determined solely by the provider" (p. 5). Case managers and treatment teams assigned the Demonstration children to a level of care using written guidelines, as suggested by Olsen, Rickles, and Travlik (1995) in their definition of the managed care process. Reimbursement strategies are another aspect of managed care in some definitions. Landress and Bernstein (1993) stated, "Managed mental health care organizations provide comprehensive inpatient and outpatient services, including alcohol and drug abuse, using a variety of reimbursement techniques" (p. 36). The Demonstration management qualified all providers and negotiated payment rates. There was a utilization review function that was especially effective for restrictive forms of residential care. The Demonstration can be considered an example of managed care because it contained elements thought necessary for managing care, namely, case managers and treatment teams who assigned and reviewed provider care decisions as well as required treatment plans and their review by management; level-of-care criteria; a utilization review process; certification of and contracting with providers; and a quality improvement system. Financial risk is not necessary to describe the Demonstration as managed care.

Why Did the Continuum Cost More?

It was reported earlier that the Demonstration kept children in care longer, had higher per-unit costs, had a higher volume of traditional services, and extensively used intermediate services. It is not possible, in this study, to disaggregate the relative contributions of several causal variables that can be hypothesized to have affected the utilization and costs at the Demonstration. All of the following variables could have been related to higher Demonstration costs: no cost to clients, the cost-reimbursement contract for the Demonstration (but not to providers), the Demonstration's belief that primarily controlling hospitalization would reduce costs, the lack of a fully operational utilization review process, the strong belief that significant cost control would be achieved by the assumed ability to assign children to the "appropriate" level of care, the lack of a clear procedure for determining when treatment should be terminated, and so on. All these variables could have been responsible for the utilization pattern obtained and the subsequent higher costs at the Demonstration. Future research needs to focus on these variables. Approaches both to study and to train individuals to make judgments about level and length of care are needed, especially in a managed care environment where these decisions are often centralized. Again, there are major gaps in our knowledge about basic treatment decisions.

CONCLUSIONS

This study has shown that systems reforms can be successfully implemented with sufficient resources that can increase access, treat children in less restrictive environments, and significantly improve satisfaction. However, the notion that costs can be controlled by clinicians and their managers by placing children in what they believe to be the most "appropriate" level of care for the most "appropriate" length of time was not supported. This clinical judgment model was not cost-effective. These higher costs were primarily related to longer treatment and to the use of more expensive intermediate-level services, without a significant reduction in the use of the traditional services (i.e., outpatient, hospital, and RTC). However, this method of cost control is not an intrinsic aspect of a continuum of care. Although costs per treated child were much higher at the Demonstration, we should not conclude that a continuum of care is necessarily more expensive than other services systems. A continuum of care model may be less expensive under a capitated or fixed-price cost model.

The most unanticipated finding of the evaluation is the lack of differences in clinical outcomes between the Demonstration and Comparison sites. These results should raise serious doubts about some current clinical beliefs. For example, Whittington (1992), in a very informative chapter on clinical myths, asserted that "there can be no doubt of the clinical value of a system that promotes continuity within a managed care environment" (p. 235). There is widespread support for reforming systems of care, apparently on the basis of their presumed clinical effectiveness.

The Evaluation showed that the Demonstration had (a) a more systematic and comprehensive assessment and treatment planning approach, (b) more parent involvement, (c) case management, (d) more individualized services, (e) fewer treatment dropouts, (f) a greater range of services, (g) enhanced continuity of care, (h) more services in less restrictive environments, and (i) better match between services and needs as judged by parents. Still, better clinical outcomes were not found. Thus, conventional wisdom about what is a better quality system of care is called into question. A fragmented system of care, without these features, did as well clinically and was less expensive. Moreover, the ability of a system of care to influence clinical outcomes is limited by the logical difficulty in expecting that distal events such as systems changes affect clinical outcomes (Salzer & Bickman, in press). Apparently, similar counterintuitive findings have been reported for primary care settings. For example, a recent study reported that there was no relationship between cost of services and quality and outcomes for six selected medical procedures (Starfield et al., 1994).

An alternative to considering the continuum of care model unsuccessful is to question the assumption that clinical services provided in the community are effective. Whereas only a few scientifically credible studies have examined psychotherapy in community settings, a metanalysis showed that the average effect size was very close to zero (Weisz, Donenberg, Han, & Weiss, 1995). This result is in contrast to hundreds of studies of psychotherapy in research settings that showed significant and clinically meaningful effects (Weisz & Weiss, 1993). Therapeutic interventions can work. We have just not been able to establish their effectiveness in real-world conditions. There is just a handful of studies that have examined clinical effectiveness in realistic community settings in contrast to the laboratory-like university settings (Shadish et al., 1995). However, the present study was not designed to examine the effects of treatment because it did not contain a no-treatment control group. Thus, this alternative explanation for the null effects remains speculative.

This study raises significant questions about the validity of several widely held beliefs. The cost-effectiveness of the continuum of care has been challenged, as has, more generally, the effectiveness of services as delivered in community settings. Nevertheless, it is also recognized that this study is just a single study with accompanying limitations. The Demonstration was just one example of a continuum of care. Other variations of systems of care should be subject to rigorous evaluations. The Evaluation was also limited in the number of issues it could address. For example, we do not know the cost to society of leaving children untreated.

However, the patter of results found in the present study are consistent with the findings from similar child and adolescent mental health services research. Recent studies have found that changes in the service delivery system (e.g., case management) do result in different services being received, but no study has reported a significant consistent enhancement in clinical outcomes (Burns, Farmer, Angold, Costello, & Behar, in press; Catron & Weiss, 1994; Cauce et al., 1994; Cauce, Morgan, Wagner, & Moore, 1995; Clark et al., 1994; Evans et al., 1994; Harris, Jacobs, Weiss, & Catron, 1995; Huz, Evans, Morrissey, & Burns, 1995; Lee, Clark, Knapp-Inez, Factor, & Stewart, 1995). This and similar research suggest that the mental health field has skipped over a whole generation of research in moving directly from the laboratory-based treatment efficacy studies to system reform efforts without sufficiently studying the effectiveness of clinical services as delivered in community settings.

This study also implies that if managed care focuses only on system reform, it can be expected to influence access, cost, and satisfaction, but is unlikely to improve clinical outcomes unless it also reforms the actual services delivered. However, there is little research to provide guidance as to what changes in services are required. As managed behavioral health care matures as an industry, it is necessary that it invest in research and development to improve the quality of services and client outcomes. The private sector, besides government, needs to assume responsibility in this area.

Researchers need to move outside their comfortable laboratory settings to study services in community settings. Although this exhortation has been repeated in the past (e.g., Bickman & Henchy, 1969), the need is urgent now. The mental health community is in desperate need of methodological advances and data to support its efforts. The need to show impact on client outcomes has never been greater. Moreover, providers in the community should be more willing to work closely with researchers to help to discover which interventions are effective in the real world.

REFERENCES

American Psychiatric Association. (1987). *Diagnostic and statistical manual of mental disorders* (3rd ed., rev.). Washington, DC: Author.

Baine, D. P. (1992). Prepared statement to the select committee on children, youth and families of the United States House of Representatives. In *The profits of misery: How inpatient psychiatric treatment bilks the system and betrays our trust* (GPO Publication No. 1992-52-362, pp. 172–214). Washington, DC: U.S. Government Printing Office.

Behar, L. (1985). Changing patterns of state responsibility: A case study of North Carolina. In J. Knitzer (Ed.), Mental health services to children (Special issue). *Journal of Clinical Child Psychology, 14*, 188–195.

Bickman, L. (1985). Improving established statewide programs: A component theory of evaluation. *Evaluation Review, 9*, 189–208.

Bickman, L. (1987). The functions of program theory. In L. Bickman (Ed.), *Using program theory in evaluation.* San Francisco: Jossey-Bass.

Bickman, L. (Ed.). (1990). *Advances in program theory.* San Francisco: Jossey-Bass.

Bickman, L., Bryant, D., & Summerfelt, T. (1993). *Final report of the Quality Study of the Fort Bragg Evaluation Project.* Unpublished manuscript, Vanderbilt University Center for Mental Health Policy.

Bickman, L., Guthrie, P. R., Foster, E. M., Lambert, E. W., Summerfelt, W. T., Breda, C. S., & Heflinger, C. A. (1995). *Evaluating managed mental health services: The Fort Bragg experiment.* New York: Plenum.

Bickman, L., & Henchy, T. (1969). *Beyond the laboratory: Field research in social psychology.* New York: McGraw-Hill.

Bickman, L., Karver, M. S., & Schut, L. J. A. (1995). *Clinician accuracy and reliability in judging appropriate level of care.* Unpublished manuscript, Vanderbilt University Center for Mental Health Policy.

Bickman, L., Summerfelt, W. T., & Bryant, D. (1996). The quality of services in a children's mental health managed care demonstration. In L. Bickman (Ed.), The evaluation of the Fort Bragg Demonstration [Special issue]. *The Journal of Mental Health Administration, 23,* 30–39.

Bickman, L., Summerfelt, W. T., & Douglas, S. (in press). Evaluation of an innovative system of care: The Stark County Project. In D. Northrup & C. Nixon (Eds.), *Evaluating mental health services: How do programs for children "work" in the real world?* Newbury Park, CA: Sage.

Breda, C. S. (1996). Methodological issues in evaluating mental health outcomes of a children's mental health managed care demonstration. In L. Bickman (Ed.), The evaluation of the Fort Bragg Demonstration [Special issue]. *The Journal of Mental Health Administration, 23,* 40–50.

Broskowski, A. (1991). Current mental health care environments: Why managed care is necessary. *Professional Psychology: Research and Practice, 22,* 6–14.

Burns, B. J., Farmer, E. M. Z., Angold, A., Costello, E. J., & Behar, L. (in press). A randomized trial of case management for youths with serious emotional disturbance. *Journal of Clinical Child Psychology.*

Catron, T., & Weiss, B. (1994). The Vanderbilt school-based counseling program: An interagency, primary-care model of mental health services. *Journal of Emotional and Behavioral Disorders, 2,* 247–253.

Cauce, A. M., Morgan, C. J., Wagner, M. A., & Moore, E. (1995, February). *Effectiveness of intensive case management for homeless adolescents after nine months.* Paper presented at the Eighth Annual Research Conference: A System of Care for Children's Mental Health: Expanding the Research Base, Tampa, FL.

Cauce, A. M., Morgan, C. J., Wagner, V., Moore, E., Sy, J., Wurbacher, K., Weeden, K., Tomlin, S., & Blanchard, T. (1994). Effectiveness of intensive case management for homeless adolescents: Results of a 3-month follow-up. *Journal of Emotional and Behavioral Disorders, 2,* 219–227.

Chen, H. (1990). *Theory-driven evaluations.* Newbury Park, CA: Sage.

Chen, H., & Rossi, P. H. (1987). The theory-driven approach to validity. *Evaluation and Program Planning, 10,* 95–103.

Chen, H., & Rossi, P. H. (1992). *Using theory to improve program and policy evaluation.* New York: Greenwood Press.

Clark, H. B., Prange, M. E., Lee, B., Boyd, L. A., McDonald, B. A., & Stewart, E. S. (1994). Improving adjustment outcomes for foster children with emotional and behavioral disorders: Early findings from a controlled study on individualized services. *Journal of Emotional and Behavioral Disorders, 2,* 207–218.

Cook, T., & Shadish, W. (1994). Social experiments: Some developments over the past fifteen years. *Annual Review of Psychology, 45,* 545–580.

Costner, H. (1989). The validity of conclusions in evaluation research: A further development of Chen & Rossi's theory-driven approach. *Evaluation and Program Planning, 12,* 345–353.

Cutler, D. M., & Gruber, J. (1995). *Does public insurance crowd out private insurance?* (Working Paper No. 5082). Cambridge, MA: National Bureau of Economic Research, Inc.

England, M. J., & Cole, R. F. (1992). Building systems of care for youth with serious mental illness. *Hospital and Community Psychiatry, 43,* 630–633.

Evans, M. E., Armstrong, M. I., Dollard, N., Kuppinger, A. D., Huz, S., & Wood, V. M. (1994). Development and evaluation of treatment foster care and family-centered intensive case management in New York. *Journal of Emotional and Behavioral Disorders, 2*, 228–239.

Goldman, H. H., Morrissey, J. P., & Ridgely, S. M. (1994). Evaluating the Robert Wood Johnson Foundation program on chronic mental illness. *Milbank Quarterly, 72*, 37–48.

Goodman, M., Brown, J., & Deitz, P. (1992). *Managing managed care: A mental health practitioner's survival guide.* Washington, DC: American Psychiatric Press.

Harris, V. S., Jacobs, J., Weiss, B., & Catron, T. (1995, February). *One year findings for the Vanderbilt School-Based Counseling Evaluation Project.* Paper presented at the Eighth Annual Research Conference: A System of Care for Children's Mental Health: Expanding the Research Base, Tampa, FL.

Hedrick, T., Bickman, L., & Rog, D. (1993). *Planning applied social research.* Newbury Park, CA: Sage.

Heflinger, C. A. (1993). *Final report of Fort Bragg Evaluation: The Implementation Study.* Unpublished manuscript, Vanderbilt University Center for Mental Health Policy.

Heflinger, C. A. (1996). Implementing a system of care: Findings from the Fort Bragg Evaluation Project. In L. Bickman (Ed.), The evaluation of the Fort Bragg Demonstration [Special issue]. *The Journal of Mental Health Administration, 23*, 16–29.

Huz, S., Evans, M. E., Morrissey, J., & Burns, B. (1995, February). *Outcomes from research on case management with serious emotional disturbances.* Papers presented at the Eighth Annual Research Conference: A System of Care for Children's Mental Health: Expanding the Research Base, Tampa, FL.

Lambert, E. W. (1993). Monte Carlo modeling. In L. Bickman (Ed.), *Response to the directorate of health care studies and clinical investigations final report: Assessing power analysis approaches for the Fort Bragg Evaluation Project, Appendix G* (Rev.). Unpublished manuscript, Vanderbilt University Center for Mental Health Policy.

Lambert, E. W., & Guthrie, P. R. (1996). Clinical outcomes of a children's mental health managed care demonstration. In L. Bickman (Ed.), The evaluation of the Fort Bragg Demonstration [Special issue]. *The Journal of Mental Health Administration, 23*, 51–68.

Landress, H. J., & Bernstein, M. A. (1993). Managed care 101: An overview and implications for psychosocial rehabilitation services. *Innovations and Research, 3*, 33–38.

Lane, T. (1996). Comment on the final report of the Fort Bragg Project. In L. Bickman (Ed.), The evaluation of the Fort Bragg Demonstration [Special issue]. *The Journal of Mental Health Administration, 23*, 125–127.

Lee, B., Clark, H. B., Knapp-Inez, K., Factor, M., & Stewart, E. (1995, February). *Children lost in the foster care system: Analysis of placement changes, services, and outcomes.* Paper presented at the Eighth Annual Research Conference: A System of Care for Children's Mental Health: Expanding the Research Base, Tampa, FL.

Lehman, A. E., Postrado, L. T., Roth, D., McNary, S. W., & Goldman, H. H. (1994). Continuity of care and client outcomes in the Robert Wood Johnson Foundation program on chronic mental illness. *Milbank Quarterly, 72*, 105–122.

Lipsey, M. W. (1990). *Design sensitivity.* Newbury Park, CA: Sage.

Olsen, D. P., Rickles, J., & Travlik, K. (1995). A treatment-team model of managed mental health care. *Psychiatric Services, 46*, 252–256.

Palumbo, D. J., & Olivrio, A. (1989). Implementation theory and the theory-driven approach to validity. *Evaluation and Program Planning, 12*, 337–344.

Rivera, V. R., & Kutash, K. (1994). *Components of a system of care: What does the research say?* Tampa: Florida Mental Health Institute, Research and Training, Center for Children's Mental Health, University of South Florida.

Roberts, M. C. (1994). Models for service delivery in children's mental health: Common characteristics. *Journal of Clinical Child Psychology, 23*, 212–219.

Salzer, M., & Bickman, L. (in press). Delivering effective children's services in the community: Reconsidering the benefits of system interventions. *Applied and Preventive Psychology.*

Saxe, L., Cross, T. P., Lovas, G. S., & Gardner, J. K. (1995). Evaluation of the mental health services program for youth: Examining rhetoric in action. In L. Bickman & D. J. Rog (Eds.), *Creating a children's mental health service system: Policy, research and evaluation* (pp. 206–235). Newbury, CA: Sage.

Shadish, W. R., Navarro, A. M., Crits-Christoph, P., Jorn, A., Nietzel, M. T., Robinson, L., Svartberg, M., Matt, G. E., Siegle, G., Hazelrigg, M., Lyons, L. S., Prout, H. T., Smith, M. L., & Weiss, B. (1995). *Clinically representative psychotherapy.* Unpublished manuscript.

Shern, D. L., Wilson, N. R., & Coen, A. S. (1994). Client outcomes II: Longitudinal client data from the Colorado treatment outcome study. *Milbank Quarterly, 72,* 123–148.

Starfield, S., Powe, N. R., Weiner, J. R., Stuart, M., Steinwachs, D., Scholle, S. H., & Gerstenberger, A. (1994). Costs vs. quality in different types of primary care settings. *Journal of the American Medical Association, 272,* 1903–1908.

Stroul, B. A., & Friedman, R. (1986). *A system of care for children and youth with severe emotional disturbances* (Rev. ed.). Washington, DC: Georgetown University Child Development Center, CASSP Technical Assistance Center.

Sussman, M., & Robertson, D. U. (1986). The validity of validity: An analysis of validation study design. *Journal of Applied Psychology, 71,* 461–468.

U.S. General Accounting Office. (1992). *Integrating human services: Linking at-risk families with services more successful than system reform efforts.* Washington, DC: Author.

Weisz, J. R., Donenberg, G. R., Han, S. S., & Weiss, B. (1995). Bridging the gap between lab and clinic in child and adolescent psychotherapy. *Journal of Consulting and Clinical Psychology, 63,* 688–701.

Weisz, J. R., & Weiss, B. (1993). *Effects of psychotherapy with children and adolescents.* Newbury Park, CA: Sage.

Whittington, H. G. (1992). Managed mental health care: Clinical myths and imperatives. In S. Feldman (Ed.), *Managed mental health services* (pp. 223–244). Springfield, IL: Charles C Thomas.

Yin, R. K. (1986). *Case study research.* Newbury Park, CA: Sage.

Yin, R. K. (1993). *Applications of case study research.* Newbury Park, CA: Sage.

Part VI

SOCIOCULTURAL ISSUES

The three papers in this section are on children at risk. To determine the influence of role models and living conditions on boys' occupational aspirations, Cook and his colleagues posed the following question to inner-city boys: "What do you want to be when you grow up?" The unemployment rates among inner-city males are high, and legitimate jobs with reasonable pay are often scarce. Thus, inner-city children do not grow up with images of men going to a variety of occupations. Children in the second, fourth, sixth, and eighth grades were asked what type of job they would like to have and what type of job they thought they might have when they grew up. After the open-ended questions, children were presented with closed-ended measures of occupational aspirations and expectations. They were also asked questions about educational aspirations and expected educational obstacles. The total sample of 220 consisted of inner-city minority boys living in poor neighborhoods and White boys living in more economically advantaged circumstances. Results indicate that as early as Grade 2, inner-city boys experience a larger gap between job aspirations and expectations than economically advantaged youth. This gap remains fairly steady as the youth age. Thus, well before high-school age, minority youth anticipate limited occupational opportunities. This study is intriguing because it takes a topic of normal development and places it in the context of sociocultural influences.

The next paper elaborates more on ways to study normal development within minority populations. Garcia Coll and colleagues present a model for conducting research with minority children. They delineate important issues that need to be considered when studying children who are growing up out of the mainstream. Omissions in previous research are detailed, including the absence of longitudinal investigations of normal development in minorities and a disregard for intragroup variability with an emphasis on between-group comparisons. Coll et al. describe social stratification variables, including racism, prejudice, discrimination, and segregation. The integrative model that they present includes eight factors: (a) social position variables (e.g., race, gender), (b) racism, (c) segregation (e.g., residential, economic, and psychological), (d) promoting/inhibiting environments (schools, neighborhoods), (e) adaptive culture (e.g., traditions and legacies), (f) child characteristics (temperament, health status), (g) family (structure, beliefs, SES), and (h) developmental competencies (e.g., cognitive, social and linguistic, and coping with racism). Although race is often included in studies, its dimensions, such as skin color, are rarely considered.

This is an interesting paper because of its rich discussion of social stratification variables and their effect on development. The paper also leaves one with many questions unanswered. Are there aspects of development that are "culture free," or is development so embedded in the social/cultural environment that it can only be understood within that context? If competence is only defined within the subculture, how do we evaluate children who must succeed not only within subculture, but also within society at large?

The final paper in this section deals with an ethical dilemma often faced by researchers studying urban, low-income youth. What does one do if he or she finds that a participant is in trouble? The research subject has been assured confidentiality; in return, the researcher hopes for honest reporting. In this simple but intriguing study, Fisher and colleagues asked urban youth what they thought researchers should do with different types of information. The children were 7th, 9th, and 11th graders. They were asked to pretend that they were in a research study in which they had consented to participate because the researcher promised not to tell anybody what they said. The child was then presented with three options for what the researcher could do when he finds out the child has a problem: Should the researcher not tell anyone, talk to the child, and suggest the child get help, or should the researcher tell a parent? There were 12 different developmental risks ranging in severity from cutting classes, drinking or drug problem, being physically or sexually abused, having a sexually transmitted disease, or thinking about suicide. The risks were rated for perceived severity by younger and older children and by boys and girls. Youth were more likely to favor telling an adult when the risks were maltreatment or suicide. Facilitating a self-referral was the most preferred option for almost all risks.

It is important to note that current ethical guidelines are unclear as to how researchers should behave when they discover participants are in jeopardy. Asking potential participants what they think should be done, albeit in a hypothetical situation, provides important information for researchers to consider in making their decisions.

22

The Development of Occupational Aspirations and Expectations Among Inner-City Boys

Thomas D. Cook
Northwestern University

Mary B. Church, Subira Ajanaku, and William R. Shadish, Jr.
University of Memphis

Jeong-Ran Kim
Northwestern University

Robert Cohen
University of Memphis

The occupational aspirations and expectations of two populations of boys in grades 2, 4, 6, and 8 were examined in order (1) to describe what is unique about the development of job preferences among urban ghetto children who live in settings where many adult males are not well attached to the labor force and (2) to examine 6 reasons for any age- and population-dependent patterns there might be in job aspirations and job expectations. Findings show that boys tend to be more realistic about occupational aspirations and expectations the older they are; that from second grade on the occupational expectations of inner-city boys mirror existing race and class differences in adult job holdings; that the gap between occupational aspirations and expectations is greater for the ghetto boys and remains roughly constant in size across the grades examined; and that the lower occupational expectations of the inner-city boys are strongly related to their lower educational expectations, with these educational expectations being associated with fewer poor boys having a biological father at home and with more of these boys seeing obstacles to success in the local social setting. But, the lower occupational expectations of the ghetto boys are not due to having fewer positive role models or believing that schooling will not pay off for them in the future as it does for others.

Income inequality is still growing in the United States (Danziger & Gottschalk, 1991), and a group especially suffering from this change are those adult males of color who live in the inner core of

Reprinted with permission from *Child Development*, 1996, Vol. 67, 3368–3385. Copyright © 1996 by the Society for Research in Child Development, Inc.

This article has benefited from discussions in the MacArthur Foundation's Network on Successful Adolescent Development in High-Risk Settings and from comments by Jacquelynne Eccles and Meredith Phillips.

large cities (Bound & Freeman, 1992). The unemployment rate of such ghetto males—predominantly African-American—is much higher than that of their female counterparts and, between the ages of 18 and 25, routinely exceeds 30%. Even this is probably an underestimate, for many local men are prematurely deceased, are incarcerated, or have ceased looking for work. Moreover, the legitimate jobs available to them offer low wages, few benefits, inconvenient work hours, and sometimes less peer prestige than work in the illegitimate labor market (Bound & Freeman, 1992).

This article is about one aspect of what it means to grow up male in settings where work is scarce but is nonetheless still the preferred path to economic independence (Sullivan, 1989; Williams & Kornblum, 1985). Given the contradiction between inner-city work norms that are quite conventional and the reality that local work opportunities are limited, we will explore the nature and prestige of the jobs inner-city boys in grades 2–8 *want* to hold and the nature and prestige of the jobs they *expect* to hold. We will also explore what accounts for any discrepancies we might observe between such occupational aspirations and expectations.

To address these issues requires a sample of inner-city boys and a description of how their occupational aspirations and expectations vary with age. But these age trends alone would tell us nothing about what is *unique* about the development of job preferences in the inner city. This is because we would not know whether any age trends observed there are identical to the trends that would be found with boys from other social backgrounds. Comparison data are needed. Many comparisons are possible and desirable, with each being desirable for a different purpose. For instance, if we were to contrast the age trends for minority boys from the inner city with the trends for both inner-city white and middle class minority boys, we would come closer to understanding how race and class separately contribute to the development of job preferences. But as useful as these comparisons are, we would still not know whether the relevant inner-city age trends differ from those we would find with most American boys. This is because the national "mode" (or "mainstream") does not depend on middle class blacks or poor whites living in ghetto-like surroundings, since each makes up such a small share of the overall American population. Much more numerous are middle class white boys, and they therefore provide a better comparison for assessing how age trends in occupational preferences differ for inner-city minority boys when compared to most other boys. If we were to find that inner-city trends are indeed unique by this criterion, then an obvious next step would be to assess how race and class contribute to this uniqueness.

Most past research on job preferences has involved high school students, rather than the elementary and middle school students who were sampled in the research to be reported here. The assumption underlying the use of high schoolers is that they are more realistic about their job choices, presumably because most of them have already worked and are close to making career choices that have serious personal consequences (Gottfredson, 1981). But it does not follow from this that younger children are totally fantasy-based when they consider jobs. Indeed, existing research on the occupational preferences of elementary and middle school children already indicates that (a) "understandings of occupational roles are relatively well developed by the fourth grade" (McGee & Stockard, 1991); (b) "at least by the fourth grade, children understand status or prestige differences between occupations" (McGee & Stockard, 1991); (c) by grade 4, children can also distinguish between occupational aspirations and expectations (Gottfredson, 1981); (d) elementary school children can rank the status of occupations in much the same ways as adults (Lauer, 1974); (e) they can also accurately attribute various job characteristics to a wide range of occupations (McGee & Stockard, 1991); and (f) their preferences for jobs for themselves reflect their own social class standing (Henderson, Hesketh, & Tuffin, 1988; Simmons & Rosenberg, 1971; Tudor, 1971). It seems, then, that pre-high school students have some concrete knowledge about jobs and the social contexts in which these jobs are embedded and that they use this information to make judgments about the world of work.

Even so, we know very little about the specific occupational choices of boys of different ages. Casual observation suggests that boys prefer jobs like professional athlete, fireman, policeman, lawyer, or doctor at a much higher rate than these jobs are represented in the current American occupational structure. But we do not know at what age preferences for these jobs peak and whether older boys make choices that are more realistic in that they more closely mirror the distribution of jobs found in today's occupational structure (Gottfredson, 1981). Nor do we know how boys from different social backgrounds vary in their job preferences at different ages. Some media accounts portray inner-city children as especially susceptible to the influence of high profile professional athletes whom they try to imitate, often to the detriment of schoolwork. But given the low odds of attaining such jobs, we need to ask: Do inner-city boys really differ from others in their expectations about becoming professional athletes? And if they do, how are their higher expectations related to age? Do they increase or diminish relative to the case with other boys?

Research with high school and college students has consistently shown a gap between the prestige of desired and expected jobs, with the gap being larger for African-Americans and the poor (Bogie, 1976; Cosby & Picou, 1971; Curry & Picou, 1971; Dillard & Perrin, 1980; Kuvlesky & Bealer, 1966; Kuvlesky & Ohlendorf, 1968). But we still do not know how the size of this gap changes with age or for different population groups. Inner-city children see many more men around them who are unemployed, hold dead-end jobs, or are active in the illegitimate labor market (MacLeod, 1987; Sullivan, 1989; Williams & Kornblum, 1985). And at some age they will presumably come to realize that their own job choices are particularly constrained because of past school performance, the quality of their family networks, the paucity of local jobs, and the prejudices of potential employers (Gottfredson, 1981). Thus, at some time during childhood we expect that occupational expectations will be lower for inner-city boys, perhaps creating an especially wide gap between their occupational aspirations and expectations.

Although we cannot predict the age at which young boys' occupational expectations decrease, some interesting hypotheses about timing are still possible. For one, if nearly all inner-city children come to understand the job realities facing them *within a fairly narrow age range*, then we should expect to find an age-specific drop in the prestige of expected jobs that is larger among inner-city boys than others of the same age. For another, if knowledge of poor job prospects is pervasive within the inner city, then even very young children could come to acquire such diminished expectations that then remain lower across all the elementary and middle-school years. And finally, if understanding the personal implications of inner-city job realities depends on higher-order cognitive skills, then it should be the older boys who are better able to do the cognitive work, resulting in a steeper decrease in job expectations at older ages. We will examine these possibilities.

We assume that occupational expectations are more dependent on the surrounding contexts of a child's life than are occupational aspirations. Inner-city children learn from their schools, the media, and their parents about the need to set their sights high in order to take advantage of a supposedly open social mobility system that has recently created new job openings for minorities. They are also enjoined to emulate conspicuously successful individuals of their own race and to disregard low expectations that teachers and others might hold for them and others like themselves. All these factors might help set and maintain high aspirations.

But even so, in their daily life inner-city children are also exposed to many forces that signal how difficult it will be for them to get ahead, perhaps depressing their expectations. These forces include the following: (a) The inner-city boys may anticipate more local obstacles to occupational attainment, whether because of poor schools, fewer (or prejudiced) employers, or poor transportation to jobs (MacLeod, 1987; Sullivan, 1989; Wilson, 1987); (b) They see fewer local men working in steady jobs that pay a family wage and so they may calibrate their own expectancies accordingly (Anderson, 1990; Brooks-Gunn, Duncan, Kato, & Sealand, 1993; Jencks & Mayer, 1990; Williams

& Kornblum, 1985); (c) They have fewer mentors, especially fathers who can advocate for them and teach them about the job market and what it takes to be well positioned in it (Hamilton & Darling, 1989; Werner, 1987); (d) On the average, their grades and test scores are lower than for other children, and as early as fourth grade children know that their school performance will influence later job quality (Gottfredson, 1981); (e) They are more likely to believe that hard work there will not pay off for them in school as it does for children from more advantaged backgrounds (Ogbu, 1989); and (f) They live in environments they see as unsafe for themselves and for potential employers (Bound & Freeman, 1992; Wilson, 1987), and so it is possible that they equate a lack of physical safety with fewer opportunities for good jobs. Any of these factors could explain population differences in occupational aspirations or—more likely—occupational expectations.

To summarize, we want to sample two contrasting populations of boys in order to study how job preferences vary by population across the grades 2, 4, 6, and 8. We will describe how some especially popular boyhood occupational preferences vary by grade and population group; for each group, we will also describe the form of the relation between grade level and occupational expectations; and finally, we will explore six possible explanations for why grades and population groups are related to occupational aspirations and expectations in whatever way we uncover.

METHOD

Sampling Design

The boys were recruited from four elementary schools (grades 1–6) and two junior high schools (grades 7 and 8) in Memphis, Tennessee. The schools differ radically in racial composition and income. The percentage of students receiving federally subsidized lunches averages 96% in the two low-income elementary schools and 74% in the low-income junior high. In the middle-income schools the corresponding percentages are 17% and 12%. The three low-income schools each average 99% African-American students, while the three middle-income schools average 70% European-Americans. In interviews, 22% of the boys from the poorest schools report living with both biological parents, whereas 65% of the other boys do. These are neighborhood schools, and Table 1 displays 1990 census data on some attributes of the tract in which each school is located and on the average of the tracts physically adjacent to the school tract. It can be seen that the two student populations differ radically in the material quality of social settings, especially as regards median household income and the percent poor in the tract. There can be little doubt that we sampled two populations: inner-city minority boys from densely poor neighborhoods that could legitimately be called ghettos, and white boys living in more advantaged material circumstances.

For grade 2, the mean student age was 8.30 years (range = 7.08–10.92); for grade 4 the mean was 10.41 (range = 9.58–11.92); for grade 6 the mean age was 12.53 years (range = 11.25–14.75); and for grade 8 the mean age was 14.51 (range = 13.33–16.92).

Interviewers

Two female interviewers, one African-American and one European-American, conducted all interviews. Children were randomly assigned to interviewers. Since analyses showed no statistically significant differences between interviewers, the results were pooled over interviewers for all the analyses presented here.

TABLE 1

Characteristics of Census Tracts Surrounding Study Schools

| | Schools in Poor Minority Neighborhoods | | | | | | Schools in Affluent White Neighborhoods | | | |
| | Elementary School 1 | | Elementary School 2 | | Junior High | | Elementary School 1 | | Elementary School 2, plus Junior High | |
Census Attribute	Tract of School	Adjacent Tracts	Tract of School	Adjacent Tracts	Tract of School	Adjacent Tracts	Tract of School	Adjacent Tracts	Tract of School	Adjacent Tracts
Median household income ($)	6,868	8,232	6,742	12,600	10,502	18,469	42,067	38,345	44,663	49,057
% poverty	56.8	42.9	69.7	46.6	39.5	30.4	2.2	4.8	1.7	2.0
% college graduate or higher	3.4	11.1	1.7	9.7	4.1	10.7	23.0	19.0	48.8	43.9
% white	1.6	19.9	.5	11.9	.0	.0	88.6	85.6	93.6	93.3

Procedure

Parental permission forms were distributed by teachers to each male child in all classes in the second, fourth, sixth, and eighth grades in each school; and a second form was sent to nonrespondents 1 week later. Students who returned forms indicating approval were selected for study. The school system allowed interviewing students only during their art, music, physical education, or health classes. If the number of available students exceeded the planned sample size of 25 for each combination of grade and population group, we then selected students whose schedule optimized our ability to maintain a full interview schedule during each day. The total sample included 255 students attending school in spring 1990.

This total includes one European-American child attending a school in a densely poor Black inner-city setting, and a total of two Hispanic and 32 African-American children attending the three schools in more affluent settings. Most of the latter children were bussed voluntarily and, as interesting as they are, there are too few of them to analyze by grade level. Hence, they were excluded from further analysis. This leaves 220 boys with usable data. The achieved sample sizes are 25, 25, 26, and 25 for each age group of inner-city boys, and 34, 27, 28, and 30 for the boys from more affluent areas.

Each child was interviewed individually in a room outside the class so that he could answer questions without direct influence from other students. Each child was reminded of the permission form that he returned and asked if he understood and was willing to be interviewed; all students agreed. Then each student was introduced to the study by being told that we were interested in what children wanted to do when they grow up. After about 5 min of interaction to establish rapport, the interview was conducted according to an interview script. Each interview lasted approximately 30 min. At the end of the interview, each student was given the opportunity to ask questions about the study, thanked for his participation, and escorted back to class.

Measures

It was not easy to construct items that would be easily understood by a second grader and that were not condescending to an eighth grader. Pilot studies were conducted on a sample of children from a local university school to develop items meeting this goal. Some questions called for an answer on an ordered polychotomy, and for this we devised a graphical response format that approximates the more commonly used Likert format. Boys were presented with four glasses, each filled with successively larger quantities of fluid from one-fifth to four-fifths of the glass's volume. Children were instructed to answer each question by pointing to the glass which best described their response. Generically, the four glasses represented "very . . ." (four-fifths full glass; score of 4), "pretty . . ." (glass three-fifths full; score of 3); "a little . . ." (glass two-fifths full; score of 2); and "not . . ." (glass one-fifth full; score of 1). A precise descriptor tailored to each question followed these generic descriptors. For example, if the question was about how sure the child was that he would attend college, response options included "very sure," "pretty sure, " "a little sure," and "not sure." Standardized practice trials were conducted until the child appeared to understand the use of this response format. Each time the precise descriptor changed over items (e.g., how *sure*, how *true*, how *much*) the use of the new descriptor was discussed. *Independent variables.* Grade level was recorded from school records. Population group was defined by the type of school attended. All minority boys attending the schools in poor African-American sections of the city were treated as inner city, and all the white boys attending more affluent schools were treated as the comparison group from which to infer the uniqueness of inner-city age trends in occupational preference.
Dependent variables. The research depends on children's ability to distinguish between occupational aspirations and expectations, and so we prepared a script for rehearsing this distinction with each child.

The script dealt with whether the child *would like* to do something (e.g., Would you like to go to Walt Disney World tomorrow?) versus whether the child thought he *would* do the same thing within the same time frame (e.g., How sure are you that you *will* be going to Walt Disney World tomorrow?). A list of such examples was prepared (win $1,000,000, eat ice cream now); and rehearsal continued until the interviewer judged that the child understood the distinction. The interviewers reported that the children seemed to grasp the distinction after only a few rehearsals, and the analyses we report later are generally consistent with that contention.

Two different assessment methods were used—one open-ended and the other closed-ended. To assess *open-ended occupational aspirations* we asked each child, "If you could have any job you wanted when you grow up, what job would you really like to have?" To assess *open-ended occupational expectations* we asked, "Of all the jobs there are, what job do you think you'll probably get when you grow up?" These assessments tap into a child's set of unconstrained occupational possibilities.

To assess close-ended occupational aspirations and expectations, we also presented each child with 4-inch × 5-inch photographs of nine occupations, selected from each decile of Duncan's occupational prestige scale. These were: physician, reporter, teacher, insurance agent, mail carrier, policeman, plumber, auto mechanic, and taxicab driver. Persons actually holding these jobs served as models for the photographs, and each child got to see photographs in which the depicted person's race corresponded with his own. However, for each job the composition of the picture was held as constant as possible over the race of the person depicted. Children's attention was focused on each individual picture by the interviewer who pointed to each occupation while also giving its name. (A label on each picture also included this name.) For the aspirations measure, children were asked, "If these were the only jobs that people could do and you could have any of them when you grow up, which one would you really like to have?" For the occupational expectations measure, children were asked, "Pretending these are the only jobs that people can do when they grow up, which one do you think you would probably get when you grow up?" The *closed-ended measures of occupational aspirations and expectations* constrain a child to select from nine named occupations whose understanding may vary by age and population group.

Irrespective of the method of measurement, all occupational choices were converted to occupational prestige scores using the Nakao and Treas (1990) conversion table. Since only boys were tested, there is no gender bias in the transformation of occupational choices into rankings, as Maxwell and Cummings (1988) claim is often the case.

Explanatory variables. We also gathered data on constructs to explain how occupational choices vary by grade and population group. Four items assessed *the child's educational expectations* (alpha = .75) by asking how sure the child was that he would (a) go to high school, (b) finish high school, (c) go to college, and (d) finish college. Six items assessed *the child's perceptions of parental educational expectations* (alpha = .86), with each child reporting how sure he was that each parent thought he would (a) finish high school, (b) go to college, and (c) finish college. These two scales correlated .47 to give an overall educational expectations construct.

Each child also answered a nine-item cartoon-based pictorial assessment of his *expected educational obstacles* (alpha = .69), with each child seeing cartoons depicting characters of his own race. The obstacles were (a) not knowing what to do to get a good education; (b) having no good schools nearby, (c) not having enough money, (d) parental disinterest, (e) lack of ability, (f) not wanting to move to an area with better schools, (g) friends not going to the school, (h) not trying hard enough, and (i) having no quiet place to study at home. After the child examined each cartoon and was told the problem it represented, he was asked whether the problem would keep from going to school, with response options being yes, maybe, or no (scored 2, 1, 0). Six cartoons assessed *expected occupational obstacles* in a similar manner (alpha = .69), with the obstacles being (a) lack of ability, (b) not enough jobs, (c) don't want to move, (d) parental disinterest, (e) not knowing what to do, and (f) not trying hard enough. These two scales correlated .61, to give a composite obstacles score.

Three items assessed the *benefits the child attributed to finishing high school* (alpha = .85). The items used the four-point water glass response format to ask how true the child thought it was that if they graduate from high school they will (a) get a good job, (b) live in a nice home, and (c) have money to buy nice clothes. Three additional items assessed the same *benefits attributed to finishing college* (alpha = .79). These two scales correlated .48 to give a composite benefits score.

One item used the four-point water glass format to assess *how safe the child believed his neighborhood to be.*

Each child was also asked *"Who lives in your house with you?"* Responses received a score of 2 for both biological mother and father; 1 if either biological parent was present but not both—the father was nearly always the missing parent; and 0 if neither biological parent lived in the child's home.

Finally, we questioned each child about role models in the family, neighborhood, school, church, and television. Specifically, in each domain we asked the child whom he would most like to be like when he grows up. We then summed the number of spontaneous nominations to create *the total number of role models score.*

RESULTS

The Development of Some Popular Occupational Choices

Many young boys in the USA want to be professional athletes, though the chances of achieving this are minuscule. Using data from the open-ended measure, the first two rows of Table 2 show the percentage of children who aspired and expected to be professional athletes. Among the poorer African-American children, the percentage peaks in the fourth grade at 36% for aspirations but at a much lower 12% rate for expectations. The peak is less noticeable for the other boys, coming at the sixth grade (19% for aspirations and 15% for expectations). But by the eighth grade, fewer than 10% of all the boys aspire to be professional athletes and fewer than 5% expect to be one, with the percentages not differing by population group. Indeed, only 4% of the poor African-American boys expect to work as professional athletes. It seems, then, that boys from each group "grow" into *and out* of wanting to be sports stars.

TABLE 2
Percentage of Boys Selecting Some Visible Occupations: By Population Group, School Grade, and Occupational Aspirations versus Expectations

	Aspirations				Expectations			
	Second	Fourth	Sixth	Eighth	Second	Fourth	Sixth	Eighth
Professional athlete:								
Inner-city boys	8	36	19	8	0	12	15	4
Other boys	9	7	18	3	9	0	4	3
Policeman/fireman:								
Inner-city boys	48	16	12	4	36	0	4	8
Other boys	15	4	0	0	12	4	0	0
Doctor/lawyer:								
Inner-city boys	16	4	23	12	4	8	15	4
Other boys	9	19	25	27	15	26	18	27

Very young boys also often talk of being policemen and firemen, visible uniformed (and stable working-class) roles in our society. The next two rows of the table give the percentages of children selecting these jobs. As early as grade 2, aspirations for these jobs are frequent but differ by population group. However, the frequency declines precipitously by grade for each group, reaching zero for the more advantaged children by grade 8. Since expectations follow the same down-ward trend, it seems that both types of boys outgrow whatever masculine image or glamour is associated with the policeman and fireman roles, just as they outgrow expecting to work as athletes. However, at the eighth grade the less advantaged boys are still more likely to expect to work as policemen or firemen—jobs that are presumably more desirable for them than the others. The same relations are observable for becoming a doctor or lawyer. Preference for each decreases with age, and there is a population difference such that, by eighth grade, 27% of the more advantaged boys expect to be a doctor or lawyer whereas only 4% of the inner-city boys do. These last percentages are higher than we would expect to find in adult life; but they may still approximate the relative advantage the more affluent children have over others with respect to becoming a doctor or lawyer.

These findings indicate that, from second grade on, the jobs boys expect to hold recreate the system of class- and race-based occupational differentiation found in the United States today. That is, economically advantaged boys disproportionately expect to be doctors or lawyers, the ghetto boys disproportionately expect to be policemen or firemen. This differentiation is even more apparent when *all* the jobs children spontaneously mentioned are coded as either blue- or white-collar jobs. As can be seen in Fig. 1, at all grades, the inner-city African-American boys are less likely to want and expect white-collar jobs.

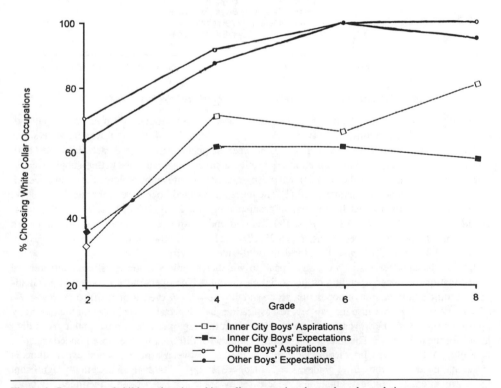

Figure 1. Percentage of children choosing white-collar occupations by grade and population group.

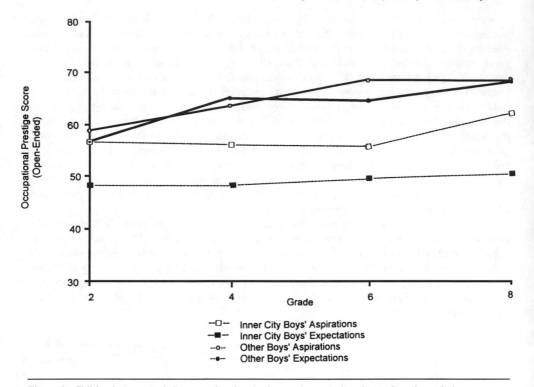

Figure 2. Childern's (open-ended) occupational aspirations and expectations by grade and population group.

How Are Grade and Population Group Related to Occupational Preferences?

Figures 2 and 3 present the data for the open-ended and closed-ended measures of occupational expectations and aspirations. The data were analyzed using a $2 \times 4 \times 2$ multivariate analysis of variance with population groups and grades as between-subjects factors. Since each child rated both aspirations and expectations, the aspiration/expectation distinction served as the within-subjects factor. The dependent variable was the occupational prestige score of whatever occupation the child selected.

The analyses show two main effects: (1) The more advantaged boys have higher aspirations and expectations, the main effect for population groups being $F = 21.10$, $df = 1,212$, $p < .001$, open-ended; and $F = 10.57$, $df = 1,212$, $p < .001$, closed-ended; and (2) occupational aspirations are consistently higher than expectations, $F = 8.28$, $df = 1,212$, $p < .004$, for the open-ended measure; and $F = 19.41$, $df = 1,212$, $p < .001$, for the closed-ended measure.

The statistical interactions we tested speak to whether a child's grade is differentially related to occupational choice depending on his social background. The open-ended data reveal a statistically significant interaction of population group and the aspiration/expectation distinction, $F = 4.94$, $df = 1,212$, $p < .05$, because the gap between aspirations and expectations is larger for the inner-city boys than for others. However, there is no evidence that the gap opens up at a particular grade or is larger for the older boys. The interaction pattern is somewhat different for the closed-ended measure (see Fig. 3). A two-way interaction suggests that the gap between aspirations and expectations is larger at the later than the earlier grades, $F = 5.28$, $df = 3,212$, $p < .002$; and a marginally significant three-way interaction indicates that the gap increases by grade at a faster rate for the inner-city boys,

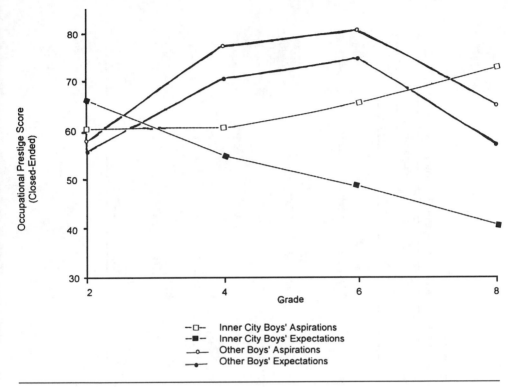

Figure 3. Children's (closed-ended) occupational aspirations and expectations by grade and population group.

overall three-way interaction, $F = 2.36$, $df = 3,212$, $p < .08$, and for linear trend within it, $F = 6.94$, $df = 1,212$, $p < .01$. Thus, the closed-ended measure shows an age-dependent group difference in the size of the gap between aspirations and expectations, while the open-ended measure suggests an invariant age relation However, the measures converge for other findings. First, the gap between aspirations and expectations is almost always larger for the inner-city boys. Second, the two groups of boys differ more in occupational expectations than aspirations, suggesting that expectations are more sensitive to whatever contextual factors are responsible for the different occupational choices boys make. And third, neither measure provides evidence of a sudden discontinuity in gap size at any grade level.

Explaining Occupational Preferences

To explore why the two population groups differ, mediational analyses were computed in the structural equations modeling program EQS (Bentler, 1992)—separately for occupational aspirations and expectations. We report robust test statistics, though the variable distributions approximated multivariate normality fairly well. Our plan is to develop a model on the data using the open-ended method of assessing outcomes and then to cross-validate this model on the closed-ended picture method.

The means for the explanatory variables are presented in Table 3, as are the results of MANOVA tests designed to estimate the effects of group, grade, and their interaction. The grade main effect

TABLE 3
Mediational Variables by Population Group and School Grade Means (and Standard Deviations)

	Grade 2	Grade 4	Grade 6	Grade 8	Group	Grade	Group*Grade
						Magnitude of F Value	
Number of role models:							
Inner-city boys	3.14 (1.06)	3.05 (1.00)	3.18 (.80)	2.55 (.89)	5.68*	6.53***	.40
Other boys	2.89 (.99)	2.60 (1.10)	3.15 (.83)	2.30 (1.02)			
Benefits from graduating high school/college:							
Inner-city boys	22.84 (1.62)	21.64 (2.58)	19.85 (2.96)	18.28 (2.98)	10.73**	23.88***	.24
Other boys	21.09 (2.82)	20.85 (3.30)	18.46 (3.98)	16.80 (3.58)			
Educational/occupational obstacles:							
Inner-city boys	9.04 (6.43)	6.38 (6.65)	6.09 (5.35)	5.56 (5.26)	3.23	9.23***	.88
Other boys	9.42 (7.62)	4.88 (4.16)	4.70 (3.99)	2.42 (2.25)			
Educational expectations:							
Inner-city boys	36.71 (5.19)	36.21 (4.56)	33.28 (5.42)	32.13 (5.43)	4.44*	.92	5.38**
Other boys	35.34 (4.38)	35.15 (5.20)	37.07 (3.25)	36.44 (4.35)			
Lives with both parents:							
Inner-city boys	1.24 (.44)	1.30 (.47)	1.05 (.49)	1.10 (.72)	56.83***	3.28*	1.36
Other boys	1.73 (.45)	1.80 (.41)	1.73 (.45)	1.48 (.51)			
Safety of neighborhood:							
Inner-city boys	2.95 (1.20)	2.50 (1.15)	2.41 (.91)	2.75 (.85)	34.85***	.84	.93
Other boys	3.39 (.85)	3.50 (.61)	3.31 (.74)	3.35 (.83)			

* $p < .05$.
** $p < .01$.
*** $p < .001$.

results show that younger boys from both groups are more likely (a) to live with both biological parents, (b) to list multiple role models, (c) to believe that significant rewards accrue to those who finish high school or college, and (d) to perceive more obstacles to success. The population group main effects reveal that the inner-city boys are less likely to live with both biological parents and to see their neighborhood as safe. However, they report having more role models and being more prone to believing that significant rewards accure to finishing high school or college. These last two findings are opposite to our initial expectations. There was only one statistically significant interaction of group and grades. This indicates that the inner-city boys tend to have slightly higher expectations of educational attainment in the two earliest grades but lower expectations thereafter, entailing a steeper rate of age decline for them than for the others.

Modeling occupational aspirations. Table 4 presents the correlation matrix (with standard deviations on the diagonal) on which all the model analyses that follow are based. Figure 4 presents a mediational model that fits the data for predicting children's occupational aspirations *using the open-ended method*, $\chi^2 = 23.93$, $df = 18$, $p = .19$, $CFI = .98$. Both grade and group membership affect most of the potential mediators, but their interaction does not affect any mediators. All coefficients in Fig. 4 are significantly different from zero.

Figure 4 shows three pathways to higher occupational aspirations. Only one is a direct path—from being in a higher grade to higher aspirations. The first indirect path suggests that boys in the higher grades are less likely to live with both biological parents; the latter factor raises occupational aspirations, so boys in higher grades have lower aspirations. The other indirect path suggests that more advantaged boys are more likely to live with both parents, and inner-city boys are also less likely to do so, thereby again lowering aspirations for the inner-city boys. Taken together, these results indicate that the advantage age confers on occupational aspirations is attenuated among the inner-city boys because they are the least likely group to live with a biological father. The same model also fits the closed-ended aspirations data, $\chi^2 = 18.97$, $df = 18$, $p = .39$, $CFI = .995$, and the coefficients in the two models are nearly identical and all still significant (see the coefficients in parentheses in Fig. 4). None of the other mediators is related to occupational aspirations.

Modeling occupational expectations. We next predict children's occupational expectations using the open-ended data. We initially tested the model in Fig. 4, but it did not fit well. So, we added the composite measure of educational expectations which had not fit well when modeling aspirations. Various fit statistics and model modification indices—especially the residual errors of prediction—suggested that a better model was achieved with this addition. Figure 5 presents the new model, and it fits well, $\chi^2 = 27.84$, $df = 31$, $p = .63$, $CFI = 1.00$.

The relations between the independent variables and the first column of mediators in Fig. 5 remain identical to those in Fig. 4. But there are now several causal paths from grade level to occupational expectations—one via family composition and a second via the number of role models. Each of these paths then influences occupational expectations *through modifying educational expectations*. There are also several paths from the population group to occupational expectations—one via family composition and a second via the number of role models. Once again, each influences occupational expectations *by modifying educational expectations*. Figure 5 also shows that the statistical interaction of group and grade predicts occupational expectations and that the mediating pathway is, once again, *through educational expectations*. (The latter tend to be slightly higher for the inner-city boys to the earlier grades but lower thereafter.) This model also shows a direct effect of group on occupational expectations, with more advantaged boys having higher expectations. Finally, an indirect path exists from group to occupational expectations through the number of obstacles to success: the effect of this indirect path is to raise expectations of the inner-city boys. We cross-validated the model

TABLE 4
Correlations (Standard Deviations on Diagonal) of Variables in Mediational Models

	1	2	3	4	5	6	7	8	9	10	11	12	13
1. Grade	1.14												
2. Group	-.02	.50											
3. Interaction	.03	.00	.56										
4. Living with both parents	-.17*	.45**	-.00	.56									
5. Safety of neighborhood	-.06	.38**	.03	.23**	1.00								
6. Number of role models	-.17**	-.16*	.01	.05	-.07	1.04							
7. Benefits of school	-.48**	-.18**	-.01	.06	-.01	.06	.36						
8. Obstacles to success	.10	.15*	.06	.02	.01	-.11	-.03	.62					
9. Educational expectations	-.15*	.08	.15*	.22**	.09	.27**	.11	-.14*	.79				
10. Open-ended aspirations	.14*	.18**	.06	.17**	.13	.06	-.18**	-.04	.05	.23			
11. Pictured aspirations	.09	.30**	.06	.14*	.12	-.06	-.16*	-.13	.19**	.41**	.27		
12. Open-ended expectations	.14*	.11	.01	.20**	.19**	.01	-.06	-.02	.07	.25**	.25**	.28	
13. Pictured expectations	-.14*	.21**	.20**	.18**	.22**	.05	-.09	-.07	.17*	.25**	.41**	.36**	.28

* $p < .05$.
** $p < .01$.

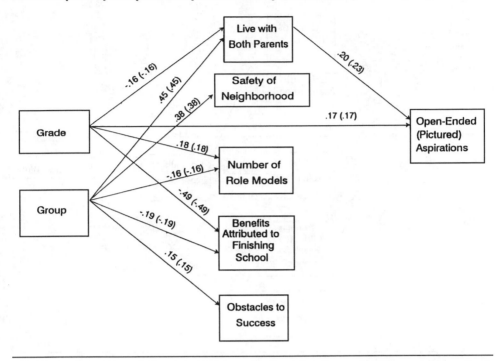

Figure 4. Mediators of children's occupational aspirations. Open-ended measures without parentheses; closed-ended measures within parentheses. All coefficients are significantly different from zero. Error variances are omitted.

in Fig. 5 using the closed-ended picture measures of occupational expectations. The resulting model fit adequately, $\chi^2 = 41.66$, $df = 31$, $p = .10$, $CFI = .95$, and the coefficients in parentheses in Fig. 5 indicate a similar interpretation to that offered for the open-ended measure, except that the indirect path to expectations through obstacles is no longer significant.

It seems, then, that a number of ecological factors are important for understanding how boys' occupational expectations are related to grade level, population group, and the statistical interaction of the two. Foremost among these are living with both biological parents, having more role models, seeing fewer obstacles to advancement and—especially—having higher expectations for educational attainment. In contrast, occupational aspirations are not as complexly mediated, probably because they depend less on the actual social context in which a child lives.

DISCUSSION

Table 2 and Figs. 1 and 2 show that as early as grade 2 a boy's social background is reflected in the prestige and blue-collar status of his occupational aspirations and expectations, with the inner-city boys experiencing the larger gap between the jobs they would like and the jobs they expect. Since the two populations are closer in aspirations than expectations, this suggests that group differences in expectation are mostly responsible for the larger inner-city gap, though the inner-city boys still aspire to less prestigious and more blue-collar jobs than their counterparts.

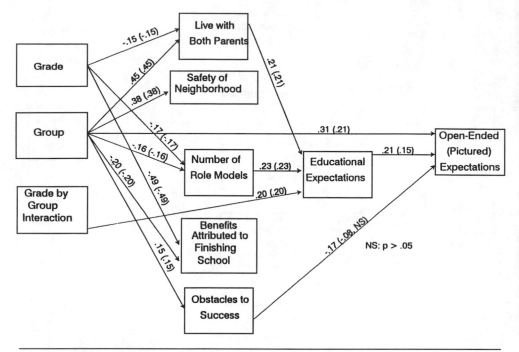

Figure 5. Mediators of children's occupational expectations. Open-ended measures without parentheses; closed-ended measures within parentheses. All coefficients are significantly different from zero except where indicated as nonsignificant (NS). Error variances are omitted.

These findings conflict with the normative system of occupational stratification in the United States where all jobs are supposed to be open to everyone, irrespective of color, class, or residence. Talent, interests, and industry should alone decide who gets which job. To buttress this ideological belief system, schools and the media present all children of color with same-race models of high achievement; they teach that preferential treatment is sometimes given to minorities for college admissions and entry into some jobs; and minority children are frequently exhorted not to aspire too low and so sell themselves short. But despite the ideology and its exemplification in schools, the media, and some families (Clark, 1983), as early as second grade the poorer African-American boys' expectations and aspirations reflect the realities in the world the boys see around them. They do not see an unconstrained world of occupational choices and, in selecting jobs based on the world they know, they inadvertently recreate in the next generation the very social divisions found in the present (Bourdieu & Passeron, 1977). What is surprising is how early this process of social reproduction begins. It is observable in the open-ended data as early as second grade!

Our results offer little support to those persons who contend that many inner-city boys persist in wanting to become professional athletes and work so hard at this that they downplay school work. By the eighth grade fewer than 5% of the boys from either population expect to be professional athletes, perhaps because they understand the low odds of achieving such a career. Boys from both settings also grow out of an earlier fascination with popular uniformed jobs like policeman and fireman; and almost all the poorer boys also abandon earlier hopes to become doctors or lawyers. We interpret this as evidence of a developing realism about the occupational structure that is underway well before high school. An exclusive concern with high school and college students misses some of the earlier developmental action that probably influences late adolescent and early adult job preferences and choices, though realism undoubtedly continues to increase during this later period (Gottfredson, 1981).

The present findings produced no support for the hypothesis that most inner-city boys come to realize *at a specific age* that the odds of social mobility are stacked against them. We found no evidence that the prestige of the jobs boys expect to hold dropped precipitously at any grade. Indeed, Figs. 1 and 2 show that the gap between expectations and aspirations remains roughly constant after grade 2. There is some visual evidence that the differential might increase with age, but this is only statistically significant with the less valid closed-ended measure (see Fig. 3).[1] Thus, the safest generalization is that the group difference in the size of the gap between occupational expectations and aspirations starts very early and remains constant thereafter. This is a surprising result. We had originally surmised that occupational expectations depend on observing and processing details about the contextual factors in urban ghettos that negatively influence employment possibilities—details that the youngest boys would be less capable of processing. But the evidence for such a cognitive processing interpretation is weak compared to the evidence for the simple social modeling hypothesis that can be inferred from the age-invariant group difference in the size of the gap between aspirations and expectations.

Willis's (1977) work suggests a disclaimer to the preceding discussion. He argues that working-class British boys do not value professional and other white-collar jobs like middle-class children do. They assign greater utility to any work that requires physical force and projects a stereotypical view of masculinity. Does the larger gap between the prestige of job aspirations and expectations obtained for inner-city boys simply reflect middle-class values being inadvertently embedded in the procedures used to scale specific occupational choices as "prestigious"? We doubt whether such a bias can account for all the results presented, primarily because the two populations of boys are more similar to each other in occupational aspirations than expectations. This suggests that when the two sets of boys make their least constrained job choices their judgments reflect a more similar set of values than when expectations (and the constraints associated with them) come into play.

We discovered that occupational aspirations depend on age and on whether both biological parents live at home, but not on any of the other factors in the model. Expectations, on the other hand, depend on grade level, population group and the interaction of the two in a complex way that involves mediational influences from family structure, the number of role models a boy reports, the number of obstacles to success he perceives, and the educational expectations he holds for himself and that he believes his parents hold for him. Occupational expectations are embedded in the proximal world of family and neighborhood, while aspirations probably depend on such distal cultural influences as the media, school policies, and general norms about how open the American social mobility system is.

Occupational expectations are mediated by a complex multifactor causal chain. It is initiated by such sociologically and developmentally relevant variables as grade level and social group. These demographic factors then affect how boys perceive their family and neighborhood contexts. Such perceived contexts then influence a boy's self-cognitions, particularly regarding how much he will progress educationally. These self-cognitions then affect his occupational expectations and the size

---

[1] The open- and closed-ended methods of rating occupational preferences usually produced the same results. In the few cases where they did not, we believe that the closed-ended measure is probably less valid because it requires boys to have some understanding of the content of the nine occupations presented to them. But what do boys of various ages make of, say, a journalist's job—one of the depicted roles? and how can a boy evaluate the relative desirability of one job from the others? The problems with the open-ended measure are less severe. A boy has only to nominate a job whose title he knows and that he currently finds attractive.

of the gap between what he wants and expects from a job. In this explanatory system that Fig. 5 exemplifies, demography influences perceived context; perceived context influences cognitions about self; and such cognitions then influence job choices. Involved here are the context, the person, and some of the processes linking context and person, creating the type of theory Bronfenbrenner (1986) has made popular. But in postulating such a *chain* of influence we are subject to all the limitations associated with a single wave of data and the use of multivariate modeling procedures that do not probe whether other models fit the data better than the one we have advanced. However, it is at least possible to claim that the data are not inconsistent with Fig. 5.

The contextual variables seem to influence occupational expectations through their covariation with educational expectations. A practical implication of this is that interventions to raise the occupational sights of inner-city boys should concentrate on how far they expect to go in school and on how well their parents think they will do there. There are obvious limitations to such an approach because educational expectations presumably depend on how well boys are actually performing in school. If the lower educational expectations of older boys are due to schoolwork becoming more difficult or to grading becoming tougher, then it will not be easy to modify educational expectations without actually improving school performance. A theoretical implication of the crucial mediating role played by educational expectations is that we can now see how relevant they are, not only for sustaining motivation in school and for contributing to improved school performance (Eccles & Midgley, 1989) but also for sustaining boys' hopes about the kinds of jobs they will eventually get.

In this study, beliefs about the positive payoff from additional schooling are higher among the boys living in the inner city and are not related to occupational expectations. This seems to contradict that part of Ogbu's (1989) theory which postulates that ghetto boys believe that improved school performance will not pay off for them. In Ogbu's work, the respondents are typically high school students, and it may well be that older students believe as his theory claims. But elementary and middle-school children from the poorest sections of Memphis are not dispirited about the returns they anticipate from doing well in school.

These same children also report having more—and not fewer—local role models, suggesting that their lower occupational expectations are not due to a paucity of role models (contrast this with Wilson, 1987). Moreover, analysis of the roles the persons the poorer boys nominated as models (e.g., preacher) indicated that none was unconventional in the sense of living from the underground economy or otherwise diverting children from mainstream norms. Even so, the number of positive models may not be as important as who they are and how they function to guide individual behavior. We do not mean to suggest that the types of role models are similar across contexts. Indeed, biological fathers are likely to be particularly conscientious mentors and models, and this study showed that having a biological father at home is less prevalent in the inner city but, when present, is associated with a preference for higher-quality jobs. Having a biological father around may be particularly important, then, in protecting inner-city boys from the consequences of their surroundings.

We have only just begun the process of explaining occupational preferences among children and early adolescents. Future research should involve better measurement plans and sampling plans than we achieved. It will also have to struggle with the best method to assess occupational preferences, since one of our present findings depended on a single method. It will have to be longitudinal rather than cross-sectional. It would also be highly desirable if girls and high school students were sampled. Future research should also try to unconfound race and class. We deliberately confounded the two since we did not have the resources for many comparison groups and, to assess the uniqueness of inner-city age trends, we thought it advisable to contrast such trends with those from the majority of American boys of the same age. The latter happen to be white and middle class. However, it would definitely be desirable to examine race and class variation separately.

REFERENCES

Anderson, E. (1990). *Streetwise: Race, class and change in an urban community*. Chicago: University of Chicago Press.

Bentler, P. M. (1992). *EQS: Structural Equations Program Manual*. Los Angeles, CA: BMDP Statistical Software.

Bogie, D. W. (1976, March). Occupational aspiration-expectation discrepancies among high school seniors. *Vocational Guidance Quarterly*, 50–58.

Bound, J., & Freeman, R. (1992, February). What went wrong? The 1980's erosion of the economic well-being of black men. *Quarterly Journal of Economics, 107*, 201–232.

Bourdieu, P., & Passeron, J. (1977). *Reproduction in education, society and culture*. London: Sage.

Bronfenbrenner, U. (1986). Ecology of the family as a context for human development: Research perspectives. *Developmental Psychology, 22*, 723–742.

Brooks-Gunn, J., Duncan, G. J., Kato, P., & Sealand, N. (1993). Do neighborhoods influence child and adolescent behavior? *American Journal of Sociology, 99*, 353–395.

Clark, R. (1983). *Family life and school achievement: Why poor black children succeed or fail*. Chicago: University of Chicago Press.

Cosby, A. G., & Picou, J. S. (1971). Agricultural students and anticipatory occupational deflection. *Rural Sociology, 37*, 211–214.

Curry, E. W., & Picou, J. S. (1971). Rural youth and anticipatory occupational goal deflection. *Journal of Vocational Behavior, 1*, 317–330.

Danzinger, S., & Gottschalk (Eds.), (1991). *Uneven tides*. New York: Russell Sage.

Dillard, J. M., & Perrin, D. W. (1980). Puerto Rican, black and anglo adolescents' career aspirations, expectations, and maturity. *Vocational Guidance Quarterly, 24*, 43–49.

Eccles, J. S., & Midgley, C. (1989). Stage-environment fit: Developmentally appropriate classrooms for young adolescents. In R. E. Ames & C. Ames (Eds.), *Research on motivation in education* (Vol. 3, pp. 139–179). New York: Academic Press.

Gottfredson, L. S. (1981). Circumscription and compromise: A developmental theory of occupational aspirations (Monograph). *Journal of Counseling Psychology, 28*, 545–579.

Hamilton, S. F., & Darling, N. (1989). Mentors in adolescents' lives. In K. Hurrelmann & V. Engel (Eds.), *The social world of adolescents: International perspectives*. Berlin: de-Gruyter.

Henderson, S., Hesketh, B., & Tuffin, K. (1988). A test of Gottfredson's theory of circumscription. *Journal of Vocational Behavior, 33*, 37–48.

Jencks, C., & Mayer, S. (1990). The social consequences of growing up in a poor neighborhood. In L. Lynn & M. McGeary (Eds.), *Inner-city poverty in the U.S.* Washington, DC: National Academy Press.

Kuvlesky, W. P., & Bealer, R. C. (1966). A clarification of the concept "occupational choice." *Rural Sociology, 31*, 265–276.

Kuvlesky, W. P., & Ohlendorf, G. W. (1968). A rural-urban comparison of the occupational status orientations of Negro boys. *Rural Sociology, 33*, 141–152.

Lauer, R. H. (1974). Socialization into inequality: Children's perception of occupational status. *Sociology and Social Research, 50*, 176–183.

MacLeod, J. (1987). *Ain't no makin' it*. Boulder, CO: Westview Press.

Maxwell, G. S., & Cummings, J. J. (1988). Measuring occupation aspiration in research on sex differences—an overview and analysis of issues. *Journal of Vocational Behavior, 32*, 60–73.

McGee, J., & Stockard, J. (1991). From a child's view: Children's occupational knowledge and perceptions of occupational characteristics. In N. Mandell (Ed.), *Sociological studies of child development: Vol. 4. Perspectives on and of children* (pp. 113–136). Greenwich, CT: JAI Press.

Nakao, K., & Treas, J. (1990). *Computing 1989 occupational prestige scores*. General Social Survey Methodological Report Number 70.

Ogbu, J. U. (1989). Cultural boundaries and minority youth orientation toward work preparation. In D. Stern & D. Eichorn (Eds.), *Adolescence and work: Influences of social structure, labor markets, and culture*. Mahway, NJ: Erlbaum.

Simmons, R. G., & Rosenberg, M. (1971). Functions of children's perceptions of the stratification system. *American Sociological Review, 36*, 235–249.

Sullivan, M. L. (1989). *Getting paid: Youth, crime and work in the inner city*. Ithaca, NY: Cornell University Press.

Tudor, J. F. (1971). The development of class awareness in children. *Social Forces, 49*, 470–476.

Werner, E. B. (1987). Vulnerability and resiliency in children at risk for delinquency: A longitudinal study from birth to young adulthood. In J. D. Burchard & S. N. Burchard (Eds.), *The prevention of delinquent behavior*. Beverly Hills, CA: Sage.

Williams, T., & Kornblum, W. (1985). *Growing up poor*. Lexington, MA: Lexington Books.

Willis, P. E. (1977). *Learning to labor*. Aldershot: Gower.

Wilson, W. J. (1987). *The truly disadvantaged: The inner city, the underclass and public policy*. Chicago: University of Chicago Press.

23

An Integrative Model for the Study of Developmental Competencies in Minority Children

Cynthia García Coll
Brown University

Gontran Lamberty
Maternal and Child Health Bureau

Renee Jenkins
Howard University

Harriet Pipes McAdoo
Michigan State University

Keith Crnic
Pennsylvania State University

Barbara Hanna Wasik
University of North Carolina

Heidie Vázquez García
Brown University

In this article, a conceptual model for the study of child development in minority populations in the United States is proposed. In support of the proposed model, this article includes (a) a delineation and critical analysis of mainstream theoretical frameworks in relation to their attention and applicability to the understanding of developmental processes in children of color and of issues at the intersection of social class, culture,

Reprinted with permission from *Child Development*, 1996, Vol. 67, 1891–1914. Copyright © 1996 by the Society for Research in Child Development, Inc.

Preparation of this article was supported by cooperative agreement MCU-117007 between the Maternal and Child Health Bureau (Title V, Social Security Act) and the National Center for Education in Maternal and Child Health of Georgetown University. Portions of this paper were presented at the Second National Head Start Research Conference, November 4–7, 1993, in Washington, DC. We gratefully acknowledge the more than 75 scholars who contributed ideas to this paper as part of study groups held in Boston, Washington, DC, and San Juan, Puerto Rico. Special contributions were also made by Margaret B. Spencer, Mary Melo, Shelley Spisak, Wendy K. K. Lam, and Katherine Magnuson.

ethnicity, and race, and (b) a description and evaluation of the conceptual frameworks that have guided the extant literature on minority children and families. Based on the above considerations, an integrative conceptual model of child development is presented, anchored within social stratification theory, emphaszing the importance of racism, prejudice, discrimination, oppression, and segregation on the development of minority children and families.

This article proposes a conceptual model for the study of child development in minority populations in the United States. This work is the product of a multidisciplinary collaboration among the authors who share a strong collective concern with the absence of appropriate conceptual models or frameworks for conducting research that addresses the diversity and strengths of minority populations. A conceptual framework that incorporates and emphasizes essential factors for understanding the growth and development of minority children and their families is critical to address omissions in existing theoretical formulations and research. The proposed integrative model differs from previous sociodevelopmental frameworks and models in that it introduces considerations of both social position and social stratification constructs at the *core* rather than at the periphery of a theoretical formulation of children's development.

A new model is needed because, traditionally, the interaction of social class, culture, ethnicity, and race has not been included at the core of mainstream theoretical formulations in the discipline of child development. For example, most of the prevalent conceptual frameworks do not emphasize the social stratification system, or the social positions that comprise the scaffolding or structure of the system (i.e., social class, ethnicity, and race) and the processes and consequences that these relative positions engender for a child's development. This shortcoming is found even in most of the contextually based theoretical frameworks identified in the developmental literature as organizational, transactional, and ecological.

Accordingly, reviews of published research suggest a pattern of omission and neglect (García Coll, 1990; McLoyd, 1990a; McLoyd & Randolph, 1984, 1985). They indicate (1) the conspicuous absence of longitudinal investigations on the normative development of minority children; (2) an emphasis on outcomes rather than on process in what little research is being done on children of color; (3) a lack of attention to intragroup variability and an emphasis on between-group comparisons; (4) a disregard for the diversity inherent in some of the minority group categories in use; and (5) a minimization of the effects of such social stratification derivatives as racism, prejudice, discrimination, and segregation on the development of minority children. These exclusions and lack of attention to crucial aspects of the context in which children's development takes place undermine a more comprehensive scientific understanding of the minority child and raise questions about the validity of empirical knowledge about children in general (McKinney, Abrams, Terry, & Lerner, 1994). Moreover, they hamper our ability to intervene efficaciously and to lessen the deleterious effects of the less-than-optimal conditions experienced by most minority and other low-income children.

This article includes (a) a critical analysis of mainstream theoretical frameworks in relation to the understanding of developmental processes in children of color and of issues at the intersection of social class, culture, ethnicity, and race, and (b) a description and evaluation of the dominant conceptual frameworks that have guided the extant literature on minority children and families and that exemplify the need for mainstream models to incorporate and delineate other important sources of influence. Based on the above considerations, an integrative conceptual model of child development is presented. The model is anchored within social stratification theory (Attewell & Fitzgerald, 1980; Barber, 1957; Bendix & Lipset, 1966; Laumann, 1970; Tumin, 1967) and emphasizes the importance of racism, prejudice, discrimination, oppression, and segregation to the development of minority children and families.

African-Americans and mainland Puerto Ricans will be used as examples throughout this article, although most of the issues raised are generalizable to other ethnic and minority groups (Ogbu, 1981, 1987). Aside from space considerations that preclude the inclusion of all minority groups, there are two main reasons for using these two groups as examples. First, for most indicators of development and social well-being (e.g., infant mortality, low birthweight, teenage pregnancy, and school drop-out), these two groups occupy the most unfavorable positions in comparison to other minority groups (Arcia, Keyes, & Gallagher, 1994; Becerra, Hogue, Atrash, & Peréz, 1991; Collins & Shay, 1994; Mendoza, Glenn, Takata, & Martorell, 1994; Rodriguez, 1994; Ventura, 1994; Wise, Kotelchuck, Wilson, & Mills, 1985). Second, these two groups are examples of involuntary minorities (Ogbu, 1987) who were originally brought into the United States through slavery, conquest, or colonization. Although both groups have often been relegated to menial positions and denied integration into the mainstream, their contrasting social histories, languages, and cultures provide two distinct reference groups.

This article has several recurrent themes. One is that neither early theorists nor researchers have proposed a realistic understanding of racial and ethnic groups in the United States and their experiences within a white, mainstream society. Certain beliefs and practices such as ignoring minorities, maintaining false stereotypes, and/or distorting their life styles have hindered the understanding of different groups (Sue & Sue, 1990). Second, the expanded role that family and kin networks play in developmental processes for minority children may serve to protect them from economic hardships and social and psychological sources of oppression derived from their relative position in society (Harrison, Wilson, Pine, Chan, & Buriel, 1990; McAdoo, 1982). Third, there is the need to more fully include contexts other than the family because of their particular saliency in the development of minority children. Consequently, health and education should be viewed not only as important contributors to children's development, but also as outcomes in themselves that share with other more traditionally considered developmental outcomes many of the same determinants and causal sequencing.

MAINSTREAM THEORETICAL MODELS: CONSIDERATIONS OF RACE, CULTURE, AND ETHNICITY IN CHILD DEVELOPMENT

Throughout Western history, developmental theories have evolved toward a greater understanding of the child, progressing from a lack of acknowledgment of developmental differences between children and adults (see Locke, 1690/1913; Rousseau, 1762/1938) toward recognition of the unique characteristics of childhood and also of its complexity and diversity (see Darwin, 1859; Erickson, 1950; Sears, Maccoby, & Levin, 1957; Vygotsky, 1978). These theories have not only influenced social values, but have also been shaped by society's views. These bidirectional influences are discernible in the treatment of race, ethnic status, and gender, as well as other issues in child development (Young, 1974).

There is no theoretical or empirical reason to assume that individual primary developmental processes operate differently for children of color than for Caucasian children in Western society. Developmental processes (e.g., cognitive, affective, and social) probably emerge in similar fashion across racially and ethnically diverse populations. However, developmental differentiation, beyond that related to constitutionally based individual differences, is largely a function of the dynamic interaction between the child and both proximal and distal ecologies. As such, understanding the normal developmental process of children of color requires more explicit attention to the unique ecological circumstances (e.g., the pervasive influence of racism) these children face. Defining and integrating these unique ecological circumstances that are not shared by Caucasian children becomes the basis for the formulation of theories of normal development in children of color because their influences often inhibit rather than facilitate development. Indeed, as Spencer (1990) suggests, developmental adaptations of children of color require insights not readily available from traditional paradigms.

Early theoretical foundations of child development generally failed to address issues related to life-course processes for children of color within a larger sociocultural context (Sue & Sue, 1990). Though differences in gender were frequently recognized as important by early researchers, race was rarely considered (e.g., Goodenough & Anderson, 1931; Parten, 1932; Thomas, 1929). When ethnic and racial factors were taken into account, they were typically incorporated within an evolutionary framework that described differences between racial/ethnic groups rather than within groups and conceptualized these differences as evidence for either the genetic or the cultural inferiority of ethnic/racial groups relative to the white mainstream standard (see Darwin, 1859; de Gobineau, 1915; Galton, 1869; Jensen, 1969; Reissman, 1962; Terman, 1916). Moreover, the focus on environmental influences on human learning and development was limited primarily to immediate situational events, and therefore sociocultural factors were largely excluded from research efforts (e.g., Sears et al., 1957).

Mainstream developmental theories may nevertheless have an heuristic value in guiding the study of the normative developmental process in children of color. Global developmental theories can provide a general framework for the development of more specific predictive models. In particular, the interplay of organizational (Cicchetti & Schneider-Rosen, 1986; Sroufe, 1979; Werner, 1948), transactional (Sameroff & Chandler, 1975; Sameroff & Fiese, 1990), life span (Lerner, 1989), and ecological theories (inclusive of person-process-context concepts) (Bronfenbrenner, 1977, 1979; Bronfenbrenner & Crouter, 1983) has the capability of addressing particular issues critical to developmental process in diverse populations of color, although both expansion and greater specification are needed to realize this potential.

Although mainstream developmental models could contribute to the conceptualization of developmental processes in children of color (Slaughter-Defore, Nakagawa, Takanishi, & Johnson, 1990), they have not met this promise. To date, these models have been too narrowly defined and applied, without elaborating those considerations unique to populations of children of color (e.g., the culturally diverse physical and psychological attributes of individual children of color, the contexts specific to their daily experience, the racial and ethnic values that influence their competencies, and the societal structures that limit them). Further, the literature has proven to be more exclusive than inclusive. However, a call to become more inclusive does not represent a call to approach all populations from a similar view, nor does it imply that all populations can be understood from a single explanatory model. Indeed, a "one model fits all"approach exposes the well-documented dangers of race-comparative research (McLoyd & Randolph, 1985). Further, it detracts from efforts to describe models that account for intragroup variability in diverse populations of color (McLoyd, 1990a). Given the variability within populations of children of color (e.g., differing ethnicities, socioeconomic classes, or skin colors), these populations provide ideal samples with which to test our theories and the specific models to be developed.

Developing more inclusive models requires the rigorous specification and integration of contextual influences far beyond what has been done to date in either ecological theory or transactional theory. For example, although cultural influence may well be subsumed under the broad notion of macrosystem influence, specific notions of culture have been only marginally integrated into ecological theory. Sameroff and Fiese (1990) have incorporated culture more specifically within transactional theory by discussing the importance of the cultural code as the primary regulator of family processes that directly influence children's development; however, these authors failed to specify the mechanisms by which these distal considerations shape development.

In addition, social mechanisms such as racism, discrimination, and prejudice have not been routinely specified in analyses of macrosystem influences, even though these may well be the critical factors that underlie the more commonly studied sociopsychological aspects of developmental processes in children of color. McAdoo (1992) has suggested that ecological models may be appropriate in describing environments of diverse families and children, but only when they are extended to include societal racism, classism, and sexism. These mainstream theories have not yet provided a specific framework with which development of children of color can be best studied and understood.

DEVELOPMENT IN CHILDREN OF COLOR: DOMINANT CONCEPTUAL FRAMEWORKS

The lack of attention to issues of race, ethnicity, and culture in developmental science has resulted in a literature on minority children and their families that concentrates on explaining developmental deviations in comparison to white middle class populations rather than examining normative developmental processes and outcomes. This comparative paradigm has been exacerbated by a heavy reliance on two theoretical models that have been used over the past 150 years to explain or describe differences among ethnic/racial groups. The genetically deficient model (see Dunn, 1987; Herrnstein, 1971; Jensen, 1969; Shuey, 1966) posits that differences in physical, intellectual, and psychological capacities between races are innate. The culturally deficient model (see Sears, 1975; Senn, 1975) conceives of the "culturally deprived" as those who lack the benefits and advantages of white middle-class America and thus end up with developmental deficiencies and deviancies.

The conceptual and empirical literatures on Puerto Rican and African-American children and their families have been guided primarily by these deficiency models (Anastasi & Cordova, 1953; Anastasi & de Jesús, 1953; Armstrong, Achilles, & Sacks, 1935; Dunn, 1987; Glazer & Moynihan, 1963; Herrnstein, 1971; Jensen, 1969; Lewis, 1965; Miller, 1952; the Puerto Rican Forum, 1964; the Puerto Rican Study, 1953–1957, 1958; Sears, 1975; Senn, 1975). Genetic and environmental deficiencies are still considered to be the primary explanations for the poor school performance of African-American and Puerto Rican children (Dunn, 1987; Ogbu, 1985). In addition, African-American and Puerto Rican parents are blamed for not transmitting the right educational values (i.e., white, middle-class competencies) to their children (see Bloom, Davis, & Hess, 1965; Dunn, 1987; Passow, 1963).

Moreover, current research on African-American and Puerto Rican children and their families continues to concentrate on standard definitions of high risk and competency. Although studies are addressing the contributions of stress, poverty, and lack of social support (rather than assuming genetic or cultural deficits), the emphasis still remains on negative developmental outcomes. McLoyd (1990b) argues that the racecomparative research model encourages researchers to document how minority children compare unfavorably with white children, and therefore concentrate on how they are abnormal or incompetent. Similarly, Barbarin (1993) notes that most research on Africa-American and Latino school-age children has focused on aggression, delinquency, attention deficits, and hyperactivity, but it has not informed areas such as emotional development or resiliency.

In contrast to these deficiency models, there is a growing theoretical and empirical literature using culturally diverse/difference models to guide the conceptualization and investigation of minority children. The culturally different model (see Boykin, 1978; Gibson, 1976; Ogbu, 1981; Ramirez & Castaneda, 1974) proposes that cultures and lifestyles different from the white middle-class mainstream are not pathological, deviant, or deficient relative to the mainstream but rather legitimate and valuable in their own right. This literature adapts existing concepts, measures, and diagnostic instruments to the specific sociocultural contexts and creates new measures of competencies for these populations. This body of work argues, for example, that by assuming that African-Americans and Puerto Ricans should have the same cultural imperatives (Cohen, 1971) as middle-class whites, research is decontextualizing these competencies from their cultural, economic, and social realities

(Ogbu, 1985). In other words, the establishment and maintenance of white middle-class childrearing patterns as the standard for normal development of intellectual, cognitive, and social competencies not only obscures cultural differences in child rearing, but assumes that anything other than mainstream competencies are inferior.

Although culturally diverse/different models can capture the strengths within these populations, they have not yet addressed in depth some of the critical factors in the analyses of developmental competencies in children of color. These models include contextual variables but have yet to fully articulate how variables but have yet to fully articulate how variables such as racism, prejudice, discrimination, and other sources of oppression operate and influence developmental outcomes. In addition, studies of children of color need to move from conceptualizing developmental outcome as either negative or positive to a more balanced conceptualization that reflects both the strengths and weaknesses in developmental processes and competencies of these children.

AN INTEGRATIVE MODEL

We propose an integrative theoretical model that both incorporates and expands current formulations of mainstream developmental theoretical frameworks as well as culturally different/diverse models. This model addresses two major considerations: (1) constructs salient only to populations of color that contribute unique variance to their developmental processes, and (2) constructs that are also relevant to the developmental processes in other populations, but are differentiated on the basis of individual factors that affect developmental processes. Figure 1 presents the model in schematic form, showing eight major constructs hypothesized eight major constructs hypothesized to influence developmental processes for children of color.

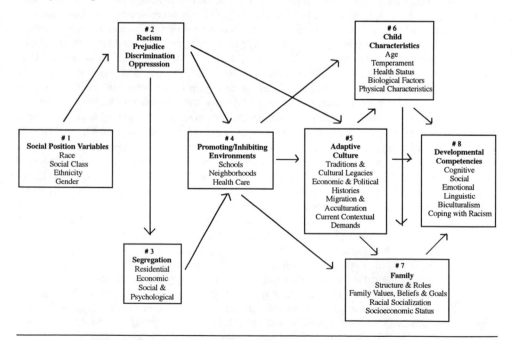

Figure 1. Integrative model for the study of developmental competencies in minority children.

We first provide a brief overview of the model as a framework for understanding the relations among the eight constituent constructs. Of primary concern in this framework is the preeminence of social position factors. These are attributes of individuals that societies use to stratify or place individuals in the social hierarchy and that pertain to children of color. These factors include (but are not limited to) race, social class, ethnicity, and gender. For example, included within considerations of race are factors such as skin color and racial features. These position factors represent social addresses that influence or create alterantive developmental pathways to competence in these children. Further, these social position factors are not simply additive in their contributions; rather, they have the potential to interact in ways that magnify or diminish the importance of the factors that follow (Bronfenbrenner & Crouter, 1983).

Although considered a primary construct, social position does not directly affect developmental outcomes and the immediate environments in which children of color grow. Rather, the effect of social position is mediated through the pervasive social mechanisms of racism, prejudice, discrimination, and oppression. These factors, in turn, create the segregated environments to which children of color and their families are subjected. We hypothesize that the effects of racism on children of color operate through the creation of segregated contexts, as opposed to a simple direct pathway of influence. Segregation must be considered as multifaceted, combining residential, economic, and social and psychological dimensions. These elements create unique conditions that more directly influence individual developmental processes of children of color. The interplay of these three major derivatives of social stratification (social position, racism, and segregation) creates the unique conditions faced by children of color and affects the nature of the developmental processes that operate and the eventual competencies that result. These are "nonshared" experiences with mainstream populations and define the unique pathways of development for children of color.

Moreover, we propose that segregation (residential, economic, and social and psychological) directly influences the various inhibiting and promoting environments that children of color experience. Within these multiple environments (e.g., the school, the neighborhood, and other institutions such as health care) children are directly affected by the macrosystem factors. Although previously we have posited that racism and its concomitant processes provide a macrosystem context that *indirectly* influences the nature of the opportunities available to children of color, processes such as racism, discrimination, and prejudice *directly* affect children's experience through social interactions in specific inhibiting and promoting environments. Through these social interactions the influence of the macrosystem factors (derived from the social stratification system in place) directly affects developmental processes in children of color.

Inhibiting and promoting environments in turn directly influence the adaptive cultures that are created in response to children's and families' experience within these environments. An adaptive culture involves a social system defined by sets of goals, values, and attitudes that differs from the dominant culture. The adaptive culture evolves from a combination of both historical forces and current demands. As Boykin and Toms explain, "though a Black cultural orientation might be present, Blacks must still possess distinctly pragmatic and expedient ways of responding to racially and economically problematic life circumstances" (Boykin & Toms, 1985, p. 44).

Both inhibiting/promoting environments and the adaptive culture directly influence the nature of specific individual family processes (the day-to-day interactions and experiences) and interact with the children's biological, constitutional, and psychological characteristics. Children are not simply passive recipients of their experience; rather, they influence their family processes and contribute to their own socialization. Finally, children's developmental competencies emerge as a direct function of individual contributions of adaptive culture, family processes, and the child's own characteristics opeating through the interactions among these systems of influence. Each of the models' constructs are discussed in more detail in the following sections.

Social Position Variables

A fundamental assumption of this model is that developmental outcome is profoundly affected by the individual's social position derived from the social stratification system of any given society. Although no standard definition of social stratification exists, most definitions denote a process that sorts individuals into a hierarchy of groups based on their imputed relative worth, utility, or importance to the society in which they live (Tumin, 1967).

Three assumptions are embedded in the concept of social stratification: (a) a social position such as social class, ethnicity, or race carries with it varying degrees of segregation in the spatial, physical, social, and psychological environments; (b) the degree of social mobility is a consequence of one's relative social position; and (c) individuals develop a hierarchical attribution system that consists of attitudes and beliefs about the self, as well as the persons both above and below on the social ladder.

Theoretically, the bases for imputing relative worth, utility, or importance can be any personal or group attribute. The critical prerequisite is that the characteristics or attribute is defined by the society as desirable/undesirable and consequently merits differential rewards, such as access to scarce resources (Tumin, 1967). In the United States, race, social class, and ethnicity are the most important attributes on which our society is startified. These categories are overlapping, with resultant additive and multiplicative effects, depending on the degree to which an individual child occupies specific combinations of these social positions (e.g., a child who is poor, dark skinned, and Puerto Rican). Gender further compounds the adversities faced (Krieger, Rowley, Herman, Avery, & Phillips, 1993).

A recent article by Entwisle and Astone (1994) emphasizes the defficulty that researchers have had incorporating these social constructs in developmental research. Although the need to include and appropriately measure these demographic characteristics in studies is being addressed, their article highlights the difficulties that researchers have had defining and measuring these constructs.

Race. There are two definitions of the concept of race: the biological and the social. UNESCO's Statement on Race summarizes the biological definition as "... a group or population characterized by some concentration, relative as to frequency and distribution, of hereditary particles (genes) or physical characters, which appear, fluctuate, and often disappear in the course of time by reason of geographic and/or cultural isolation" (Montague, 1972). Even at the biological level, there is great controversy about the validity and origin of the concept of race (Yee, Fairchild, Weizmann, & Wyatt, 1993).

As socially defined, the construct of race constitues a way of classifying individuals and groups in the context of daily living, usually on the basis of externally visible physical characteristics (Simpson & Yinger, 1953). The classification that ensues implicitly or explicitly attributes an inferior/superior social position to the group or individual in question. This attribution of social position is often institutionalized, either formally or informally, and guides to varying degrees public as well as private behavior. The social valuation of race and ethnicity evolves in response to changes in historical and economic circumstances.

Skin color, hair texture, and facial characteristics are often used as indicators of race. This has been true especially when considering the racial identity and social position of individuals with multiracial or biracial backgrounds. Historically in U.S. culture, there has been a conceptual racial dichotomy. Children of mixed ancestry are categorized as either white or black, depending on their features, and those who are considered black are relegated to an inferior social status (Hirschfeld, 1995; Massey, 1993). Hirschfeld (1995) has demonstrated that by the end of their grade school years children expect that a child with one black parent will have a black external anatomy. Moreover, these children's thinking was specific to racial categorization and asymmetrical, in that they did not believe a child would have brown hair if they had one parent with brown hair and one with blond hair, nor did they predict that dark hair or skin dominated in animals. Therefore, racial categorization is a cultural construct sustained by beliefs about the inheritability of identity which are passed on from generation to generation.

Moreover, the darker the skin color the more social penalties accrue (West, 1993). This situation exists across all race and ethnic groupings within the United States, and derives from ". . . the salience of race in the United States . . . and . . . the unique status of African ancestry" (Massey & Denton, 1988). Differences in innate abilities, poverty, and culture are frequently imputed to be the causes of racial and ethnic differentials in health and develoment to avoid acknowledging that racism may be the culprit (Ogbu, 1991a).

Social class. As used most often today, the term social class refers to a unit of social stratification in which individuals are classified on the basis of economic considerations (Gordon, 1963). Such classification implicitly or explicitly posits commonalities in psychosocial and cultural characteristic among the classified individuals arising from their unit's economic rank in the overall social structure (Tumin, 1967).

More recent conceptualizations of social class include multiple levels, which are individual, household, and neighborhood, both independently and in their interactions (Krieger et al., 1993). Research also suggests that age plays a significant role in how social class affects the self-esteem of individuals. For example, Rosenberg and Pearlin (1978) suggest that social class is achieved by adults and assigned to children. Consequently, they argue that the principles of self-esteem formation in children, adolescents, and adults are affected by social class differently as each age group organizes their "social class" experiences differently. Similarly, Wiltfang and Scarbecz (1990) found that adolescents' self-esteem was significantly related to their own achievement rather than their parents' social class. Yet, they also found that some dimensions of parental social class, such as measures of neighborhood unemployment, had a negative effect on adolescents' self-esteem.

Social class has also been examined as it relates to values and orientation. For example, Kohn (1977) suggests that social class variables influence parental values and child-rearing practices, thereby influencing how children develop and acquire the knowledge and skills to cope with change and the conditions of life. Furthermore, Kohn posits that systematic differences in conditions of life (e.g., occupation, education) have an important influence on people's behavior, social class position, and value orientation and therefore in the transmission of these values to their children.

Ethnicity. The term ethnicity is used principally to convey cultural distinctness deriving mostly from national origin, language, religion, or a combination thereof (Broom & Selznick, 1970; Harrison, Serafica, & McAdoo, 1984; Morris, 1968). Because it is socially acquired, this cultural distinctness is subject to change over time through the process of acculturation and assimilation, unless other social barriers such as race prevent full participation in the society.

As in the concepts of social class and race, ethnie identification for the most part includes valuation and attribution of inferior/superior social status, and it changes as a function of historical processes. For example, Masson and Verkuyten (1993) found that ethnic identity was highly correlated with in-group formation and preference. In addition, they found that more frequent crossethnic contact was associated with a decrease in in-group preference and formation, suggesting that in-group preferences and orientations may shift as a function of exposure and contact with out-groups. However, while it has been widely noted that intergroup contact lessens discrimination and hostility, negative intergroup contact can also reinforce hostility and prejudice (Masson & Verkuyten, 1993).

Gender. As with race, there are both biological and social aspects of the definition of gender. One refers to the biological primary and secondary characteristics pertaining to the ability to reproduce. Socially defined gender involves the culture-bound conventions about the appropriate roles and behaviors for, as well as relations between, women and men (Krieger et al., 1993). Gender relations, as part of society's social stratification system, are supported by assumptions of the innate superiority of men over women and the subsequent subordination of women by men. For minority children, their expected role in society as a function of their gender also influences access to resources, social interactions, and expectations, and will consequently influence their developmental outcomes. For example, Stevenson, Chen, and Uttal (1990) found that African-American girls received significantly higher scores for comprehension at first grade and computation at third grade when compared to boys. In addition, Spencer, Dobbs, and Swanson (1988) reported that poverty has more detrimental effects for black boys that it does for black girls. These findings may help explain why black boys and girls differ academically. The social valuation of gender, therefore, also evolves with changes in economic and historical circumstances and can lead to differential developmental outcomes within particular groups.

Social Stratification Mechanisms

Classification in terms of social position does not itself explain how these variables eventually influence developmental outcome. Four macrosystem-level mechanisms mediate between an individual's social position and various other contexts that may more directly affect developmental outcome: (a) racism, (b) prejudice, (c) discrimination, and (d) oppression.

Racism. Racism refers to the pervasive and systematic assumptions of the inherent superiority of certain races, and consequent discrimination against other races. Racism occurs when the ideology and concepts of social stratification are actualized and persons are deemed to be more or less inferior solely on the basis of their membership in a racial group (Essed, 1991; Montague, 1942). In Western societies, the preferred group is Caucasoid. Persons who are descendants of all other racial groups are placed into an inferior class status. Whereas an individual's position can be modified or buffered through the acquisition of wealth or higher social status, it can never be completely changed. Racism is considered to be the primary mechanism of influence within this categorization system, as it refers to different social attitudes and treatment based solely on race. In contrast, prejudice, discrimination, and oppression may be experienced not only as a function of race, but also on the basis of social class, ethnicity, and gender.

Racism also can vary in its expression from institutionalized racism to symbolic racism (McConahay & Hough, 1976). Research on symbolic racism demonstrates that racism in the United States has not actually declined but is now expressed in a more subtle and complex manner (Duckitt, 1992; Frey & Gaertner, 1986). While majority individuals may increasingly support the principle of racial or ethnic equality, they still maintain a set of moral abstractions and attitudinal predispositions concerning how minorities ought to act, whether or not they are treated equitably, and what they deserve. Behaviorally this is manifested in a set of acts (such as voting against minority candidates or opposing affirmative action) that are rationalized on a nonracial basis but that operate to maintain the racial status quo. Thus, while in the past racism was rooted in legal barriers that prevented minority children from having access to the same educational institutions as white children, today minority children are faced with more subtle forms of educational racism such as "low teacher expectations and attitudes, clinical definitions of black academic problems, testing and tracking, biased curriculum and textbooks, and socializing into lower expectations and inferior jobs" (Ogbu, 1991a, p. 269).

Prejudice. Prejudice refers to the preconceived judgment or opinion made about a person or a group based on social position variables, and it is usually accompanied by an unreasonable predilection or objection. Prejudice is operationalized by the automatic attribution of certain (often pejorative) characteristics to a person regardless of whether that person indeed has these particular characteristics (Feagin, 1992). Even when evidence is presented that a specific attribute may not be applicable, a prejudiced person does not incorporate this new information into the perception of the other individual or into their conceptual framework (Duckitt, 1992). Under such informational conditions, the person is seen as an exception to the ongoing prejudicial rule of status. Prejudice is likely based on a complex interaction of the attributes of race, social class, ethnicity, and gender.

Children, even at the preschool level, make judgments about people based on ethnic, racial, and social categories and also identify themselves as members of particular groups, compete for resources, and segregate themselves based on social and physical characteristics (see García Coll & Vázquez García, 1995a). While these are normative processes, it is not necessary that they result in prejudicial attitudes against children of color. García Coll and Vázquez García (1995a) argue that certain environmental conditions and socialization patterns, such as de-emphasizing in-group/out-group distinctions, providing positive models, and reducing social distance, can contribute to reducing the development of prejudicial attitudes in children.

Discrimination. Discrimination has been defined as "any behavior which denies individuals or groups of people equality of treatment which they may wish" (Stroebe & Insko, 1989, elaborated from Allport, 1954, p. 50). As a manifestation of prejudice, individuals are discriminated against on the basis of preconceived notions or stereotypes. The systematic inclusion or exclusion of members of a specific group can also stem from social distance or social desirability. Discrimination may be subtle as well as overt. Discrimination not only limits the quantity of resources available to a particular group but also places limits on their access to those resources.

One of the most detrimetal forms of discrimination today is employment discrimination. Although this form of discrimination was made unlawful by the Civil Rights Act of 1964, there are still occupational fields in which women and minorities are paid less than their white male counter-parts (Haberfeld & Shenav, 1990). In addition, several studies have shown that discrimination persists in hiring practices, and therefore minorities have a harder time than whites securing employment (Coontz, 1992; Shulman, 1990; Turner, Fix, & Struyk, 1991). Bowman's (1990) national survey of young black adults portrays a group of individuals whose hope and expectations have been eroded by their own experiences in and observations of the job market. As Bowman explained, "chronic job search strain and related psychosocial problems among black youth do not occur at one point in time; they evolve from past student-role expectations and adaptations to pressing labor market barriers" (Bowman, 1990, p. 99).

Oppression. Oppression is the systematic use of power or authority to treat others unjustly. Oppression is an omnipresent atmosphere that exists when a group of persons find that they are in a devalued position, a position from which they can not escape (Turner & Singleton, 1978). There is a pervasive element of oppression that comes from the acting out of a racial or ethnic classification. Research has shown that the psychological internalization of the devalued status and feelings of oppression can tend to limit the mobility of families and individuals and lead to the adoption of denigrating views and judgments both about themselves and others in their racial and ethnic group (Essed, 1991; Feagin, 1989).

Segregation

Aside from the ideological social stratification mechanisms described above, another salient mediator between social position variables and developmental outcome is segregation. Segregation refers to the systematic separation of groups and individuals based on attributions made in regard to their social position (Taeuber & Taeuber, 1965). Separation and segregation are ongoing facts of life in the United States. No longer by law or de jure, but de facto, segregation continues to be pervasive in today's society (Feagin, 1992). The proposed model denotes three types of segregation that can affect the family's and the child's ongoing transactions with the environment: (a) residential, (b) economic, (c) social and psychological.

Residential. The most pervasive form of segregation in the United States is residential. Where a family lives determines many of the elements of the environment that will either promote or inhibit the child's development (Blau, 1981). Barriers in the housing market, which create residential segregation, have been perceived to have a direct and constraining effect on the resources available to a population within a segregated area (Massey & Bitterman, 1985; Santiago, 1992). Despite the mitigation of legal barriers, members of the same ethnic and racial groups still tend to cluster in specific residential areas because of social position variables and stratification mechanisms (e.g., ethnic and racial discrimination that does not allow families to freely live in any area that they can afford) (Massey & Bitterman, 1985). The higher concentration of poor blacks than poor whites in impoverished neighborhoods suggests that black children are more likely to live in dangerous neighborhoods and thus more likely to be exposed to violence, inadequate housing, and other environmental health risks (Krieger et al., 1993).

Economic. Socioeconomic status of the family is another major determinant of segregation. The persistence of employment discrimination in both salary levels and hiring practices has contributed to economic segregation of miniroity populations. Economic segregation is critical to children's development because families with higher economic status have greater access to the resources that enhance the development of their children's competencies than families of lower economic status. However, even an upwardly mobile minority family with an increased income will not have accumulated available resources from previous generations that often are necessary for a family to meet emergency needs (Landry, 1980). In addition, families are also forced into forming protective groups because of differential education and occupational opportunities that are available under segregation (McAdoo, 1995; McAdoo & Villarruel, in preparation).

Employment discrimination and subsequent economic segregation are particularly troublesome given the detrimental effects of poverty on children's development (see Huston, McLoyd, & García Coll, 1994b). For example, Duncan, Brooks-Gunn, and Klebanov (1994) found that children who lived in poverty, even only occasionally, demonstrated lower IQ scores and more internalizing behavior than children who had never experienced poverty. Furthermore, economic hardship heightens a parent's psychological strain, which in turn creates a tendency for parents to be erratic, punitive, and nonsupportive of their children (McLoyd, 1990a). This type of parenting has been found to be a critical contributor to the socioemotional problems of children.

Social and psychological. Residential and economic segregation provides the background for social and psychological segregation. Social and psychological segregation occurs when families and children of color are not permitted access to important social and emotional resources as a result of social stratification mechanisms. Social and emotional isolation among groups only serves to widen the gap between them. As the emotional intensity of discord between these groups escalates, their separation increases, fostering feelings of fear and distrust (Harry, 1992). Social and psychological disconnection is compounded by the cultural, racial, and ethnic characteristics of the groups that initially separated them from one another (Harry, 1992). For the most part, minority families of diverse heritages find themselves living in different worlds from each other, as well as from mainstream society. By remaining separate, groups are unable to find commonalities between their cultures and their experiences. This situation enhances the power positions of those who control environmental resources (Harry, 1992).

Social and psychological segregation also can occur within environments that are residentially and economically integrated. The experience of middle-class African-Americans in predominantly white communities clearly exemplifies these mechanisms (Tatum, 1987). The distinction made between old-fashioned racism and modern or symbolic racism captures these different types of segregation (McConahay & Hough, 1976). Although negative attitudes about the desirability of segregation, miscegenation laws, or the innate intelligence of people of color are less prevalent in modern society than they were earlier, negative attitudes and beliefs continue to affect the non-white population. For example, the notions that blacks are getting more money or attention than they deserve and that blacks do not have the right to push themselves into situations where they are not wanted are currently prevalent (McConahay, Hardee, & Batts, 1981). These attitudes can provide the foundation for subtle forms of racism, prejudice, and discrimination that promote social and psychological segregation.

Promoting/Inhibiting Environments

Children are exposed to similar settings across cultures, ethnic groups, and socioeconomic backgrounds (i.e., schools, neighborhoods, and health care settings). Yet the structure, function, and relative importance of these systems for the development of competence vary according to cultural influences, values, and goals (Sameroff & Fiese, 1990). Within these settings, macrosystem variables such as poverty and segregation become operationalized in these children's lives (Bronfenbrenner & Crouter, 1983). It is necessary both to specify how these environmental factors affect children of color and to consider the relevance of these "mainstream" environments to the realities, experiences, and necessities of these particular populations. In the case of minority families and children, there is the need to evaluate how the environments of these children can either promote, inhibit, or simultaneously inhibit and promote their developmental competencies.

Inhibiting environments can result from a limitation in resources (e.g., inadequate health care). These resource deficits create conditions that do not facilitate and might actually undermine the development of competencies in children. In addition, inhibiting environments can result from an incongruence between the expectations, goals, and values of the child and the family and those held in a particular environment. For example, familial and cultural values can conflict with school ideologies, thereby influencing the child's school performance (Harry, 1992).

Promoting environments, on the other hand, can result not only from an appropriate number and quality of resources (e.g., neighborhoods that can adequately respond to social, emotional, and economic needs) but also from the compatibility between the two sets of systemic variables. In other words, an environment that would be considered inhibiting (e.g., such as school segregation) can become a promoting environment for a child when that setting is supportive of the developmental outcome of children and prepares them to deal with the societal demands imposed by prejudice or discrimination. Rosenberg (1979) asserts that a child's self-esteem is affected by whether he or she operates in a dissonant or consonant environment. In a consonant environment, which can be segregated but supportive, not only is a minority child protected from the prejudice of the majority world, but the environment and norms are more comprehensible and congenial and the social reference group is appropriate. In a dissonant context, the minority child faces greater discrimination, an unfamiliar environment and norms, and a less appropriate reference group, and consequently is more apt to suffer from a lower sense of self-esteem.

Among the multiple environments that can be both promoting and inhibiting to children of color, we will highlight three: the school, the neighborhood, and the health care system.

Schools. Children enter school with a rich background that includes the child's unique characteristics, family characteristics, and community characteristics. This background influences the child's ability to learn and develop within the context of the school setting. School variables that can influence child behavior can be viewed as a set of nested environments: (a) the school district or system (including organizational and instructional philosophies, policies, and procedures); (b) the individual schools (which includes school personnel and resources); (c) and the individual classrooms (which includes child, teacher, and peer characteristics and classroom structure, curriculum, and instructional strategies) (Wasik, 1992). Each of these nested environments can be inhibiting, promoting, or both. Very little systematic research has been done to address how these different school variables influence the social and academic competence of children of color. Most literature discussing issues of multicultural education focuses on the individual classroom teachers (Sleeter & Grant, 1987). However, an analysis of multicultural education should include other important variables such as the role of administrators and school boards, the school's policies on staffing and tracking, and the extent to which the school promotes parental involvement (Harry, 1992; Sleeter & Grant, 1987).

There is some evidence that compatibilities between school and culture have fortuitous effects on student achievement and school satisfaction (Tharp, 1989). Tharp's (1989) review of studies revealed that the sociocultural compatibility of classroom instruction and children's natal-culture patterns could lead to an improvement in learning. The studies surveyed included factors such as social organization, participation structures, speech patterns, and the contextualization of instruction. For example, a study by Mohatt and Erickson (cited in Tharp, 1989) found that when Anglo teachers did not employ a Native American's rhythm and patterns of speech during their instruction with Native American children, "a more disorganized and less efficient pattern of interaction as well as a lower level or rapport between teacher and students resulted" (Tharp, 1989, p. 352).

Delgado-Gaitan's work (1994) also illustrates how the cultural gap between schools and homes can be bridged for more effective schooling experiences. She examined how Mexican-American immigrant parents in Carpenteria, California, changed their child-rearing practices after participating in a Latino parent/community program to help families address school-related issues. She found that the parent support group was effective in two ways. First, the group enabled Mexican-American parents to learn how to convey to the schools their interest in bilingual programs and other curriculums. Second, it helped them socialize their children to meet the expectations of the school. Although both first-generation and immigrant families verbally communicated to their children, parents who participated in the program spoke to their children with the intent of encouraging specific verbal skills, expressive language, and critical thinking, which would help them academically.

Neighborhoods. Neighborhoods also are a crucial component of children's development. Barbarin and Soler (1993) suggest that the persistent prevalence of anxiety-based behaviors (problems with concentration, restlessness, and noncompliance) in African-American adolescents is based in an anxiety response to environmental stresses, particularly the concern for personal safety.

However, while the tendency for many is to label poor and ghetto neighborhoods as inhibiting environments and categorize middle-class communities as promoting environments for the development of children of color, these environments can be both inhibiting and promoting. Children develop subsistence tasks and acquire instrumental competencies according to their surroundings (Ogbu, 1981). Although a child who grows up in a poor, all Puerto Rican neighborhood might not have the availability or access to adequate resources (i.e., health care or good schools), the community can still encourage and provide the child with the instrumental competencies needed to be successful outside of that community. Conversely, while a middle-class environment can provide a minority child with some sort of economic stability, better schools, and access to adequate health services, it might not buffer the effects of prejudice, racism, and discrimination to which the child might be exposed within as well as outside of the community (Rodriguez, 1975; Tatum, 1987). Barnes (1991) argues that a sense of belonging in an ethnic or racial community can filter out the harmful effects of mainstream society, either by rejecting harmful messages or transforming them so they are harmless. Initial data analysis of a study conducted by Barnes in four schools in Dayton, Ohio, showed that parental involvement in the black community and black consciousness were associated positively with a more positive self-concept in their children. Neighborhoods need to be examined not only on the basis of the external resources available (i.e., better housing, better schools, good health care), but also on the internal resources of the community that may support or interfere with a child's social, academic, and psychological competencies.

The ability of predominantly African-American neighborhoods to provide economic and social support for residents is a strong theme in Tatum's (1987) qualitative study of African-American families living in a predominantly white community. Eight of the 10 sets of parents interviewed lamented that their children were not a part of a black peer group, and four of the families actively sought to create a black peer group for their children. Tatum's work suggests that black families see a link between having black friends and the establishment of a positive racial identity, an important source of protection from white racism.

Health care environments. The development of competencies also is affected by the individual's health status, which is partly a reflection of adequate health care resources. By this we mean a system with reasonable accessibility that can screen for diseases or conditions that would impede normal development and that can respond appropriately to injury, infection, or health problems to avoid further complication or disability.

Research has shown that underutilization of health services among minority families, especially preventive care, is due to socioeconomic, linguistic, and cultural barriers (Anderson, Giachello, & Aday, 1986; Boyce et al., 1986; Chavez, Cornelius, & Jones, 1986). Guendelman & Schwalbe (1986) compared rates of Hispanic, black, and non-Hispanic whites' contact with physicians during a 1 year period and found that the rates of health care utilization were significantly different. They found that Hispanic children were least likely to have had contact with a doctor, followed by black children and then non-Hispanic white children (68.3%, 72.2%, and 78.5%, respectively). This occurred despite the fact that Hispanic families were more likely to report that their children had only fair or poor health.

In addition, the presence or absence of family stressors and social networks operates to enhance or diminish the likelihood that a child can take advantage of available health resources. Traditional sociocultural practices can operate as buffering mechanisms against negative health conditions (Dowling & Fisher, 1987; Swenson, Erickson, Ehlinger, Swaney, & Carlson, 1986). A child's environment can also operate to inhibit or promote better health status. Health risk conditions (i.e., an area of high crime or violence, unsafe playgrounds, older housing with lead-based paints or hazardous waste) can expose children of color to environmental influences that can have negative consequences for developmental outcomes (Krieger et al., 1993).

The most frequently noted health risk for children is lead poisoning. Between 1988 and 1991, one in four black children younger than age 6 were affected by elevated levels of lead in their bloodstream, which can result from inhaling lead dust or from paint chips (Sherman, 1994). Children in poverty are at particular risk for lead exposure. High levels of lead in childhood have caused hearing loss, stunted growth, damage to blood production and kidney development, and poor vitamin D metabolism (Sherman, 1994). Health care environments can be important influences in the development of competencies in children of color, affecting use of health care services, adoption of health-promoting life-styles, exposure to environmental risk conditions, and ultimately health status.

Adaptive Culture

Social stratification deriving from prejudice, discrimination, racism, or segregation and the differential access to critical resources such as good schools, employment, and health care influence families and children of color to develop goals, values, attitudes, and behaviors that set them apart from the dominant culture. This adaptive culture is the product of the group's collective history (cultural, political, and economic) and current contextual demands posed by the promoting and inhibiting environments.

Work by Ogbu (1981, 1985) and Boykin (Boykin, 1983; Boykin & Toms, 1985), among others, contributes to the conceptualization of adaptive culture. Ogbu (1981) describes a series of subsistence tasks and survival strategies that are developed in response to the environmental demands of the inner city, such as scarcity of jobs, deadend peripheral and unstable jobs, and low wages and little social credit as measured by the values of the larger society. Boykin and Toms (1985) postulate that African-American families must negotiate three different realms of experience: the mainstream, the minority, and the black cultural experience. These different survival strategies and realms of experience are integrated into the development of an adaptive African-American culture.

These responses largely reflect culturally defined coping mechanisms to the demands placed by the promoting and inhibiting environments. A good example is the development of kinships or extended social networks to cope with the demands of childcare and employment. At the collective level, three sources of historical processes are operating to influence the development of these responses: traditions and other cultural legacies, economic and political events, and migration and acculturation patterns.

Traditions and cultural legacies. This first source of adaptation refers to traditions and other cultural legacies that have been part of the group's collective history for generations (i.e., for Puerto Ricans, internalized and externalized expressions of a mixed cultural heritage that incorporates Taino, colonial Spanish, and African influences, as well as influences from the United States). Boykin (1983) has specified nine interrelated but distinct dimensions of black culture that are incorporated into the socialization processes of African-American families, including an emphasis toward the affective-feeling domain and an enhanced responsiveness to variability. These dimensions, according to Boykin, are an integral part of black culture and permeate the child-rearing processes of African-American families.

Economic and political history. Adaptation is also rooted in the economic and political events that have shaped the group's collective history. For African-Americans, the system of enslavement and its subsequent economic and political ramifications have had tremendous consequences for adaptation (Herskovits, 1930; McAdoo, 1993). For Puerto Ricans, the history of colonization from Spain and the United States has been postulated as a major contributor to psychosocial development (e.g., García Coll & Vázquez García, 1995b).

Migration and acculturation patterns. A third influence is the migration and acculturation patterns of a group. These patterns include the initial reasons for migration (i.e., slavery and seasonal employment), length of the settlement of the particular community, and the ease of back and forth, or circular, migration. Patterns of acculturation are also important, including the ease of acculturation and the community's ideal of biculturalism versus assimilation to the mainstream culture. Minority parents residing in the United States must decide what aspects of ethnic parenting they wish to retain and those they wish to relinquish in favor of the dominant culture's parental values, attitudes, and practices. Subsequently, parental acculturation levels might have an impact on parenting styles by influencing developmental expectations, mother infant interactions, feeding and caregiving practices, and the role of the extended family (García Coll, Meyer, & Brillon, 1995). For example, Gutierrez and Sameroff (1990) found that bicultural Mexican-American mothers' levels of acculturation were associated with their perceptions of child development. Mothers who were more acculturated had more complex conceptualizations of their child's development and therefore could better understand their children's behavior than mothers who were less acculturated or monocultural. They suggest that a bicultural living circumstance may enable a mother to more easily understand and differentiate multiple influences on a child's development and thus enhance her parenting skills. Similarly, Rueschenberg and Buriel (1989) found that Mexican-American families became more acculturated they became increasingly involved with formal social support services outside the family.

These collective forces of migration and acculturation provide the background from which adaptive responses are generated at both the family and the community level. Cohort effects need to be considered when assessing the impact of migration and acculturation, as each are ongoing processes and can be experienced as much by recent immigrants as by those living in the United States who move from an ethnic neighborhood to one that is predominantly white (García Coll, Meyer, & Brillon, 1995). In addition, the distinction made by Ogbu (1991b) between voluntary and involuntary minorities might be important in that involuntary minorities might be less likely to embrace the dominant culture than voluntary minorities. Finally, the consequences of these historical processes should be recognized as relevant for both dominant and minority groups.

Current contextual demands. More contemporary and immediate sources of influence also contribute to the development of an adaptive culture. Rates of unemployment, neighborhood safety, and other aspects of the promoting/inhibiting environments are current influences on children and families (Krieger et al., 1993). Also operating at this level are racism, prejudice, and other ideological stratification mechanisms that are transmitted through systems of formal education, the media, and interpersonal interactions.

Thus, the adaptive culture is the product of the group's prior collective history (cultural, political, and economic) and the contextual demands placed by the promoting and inhibiting environments.

Child Characteristics

The developmental principle that children are not passive recipients of environmental influences is no less the case for children of color, such as African-Americans and Puerto Ricans, than for any other groups. In the proposed model, child characteristics play a key role, both in how they are influenced by promoting and inhibiting environments and adaptive cultures and in how they influence family functioning and the emergence of developmental competencies. While the range of potential characteristics to consider is wide and shares some similarities with those of majority culture children, a number of others might be considered particularly relevant for children of color.

Age and temperamental characteristics are obvious considerations. Few studies explicitly assess temperamental characteristics of children of color; however, previous findings suggest that African-American and Puerto Rican children differ from Caucasian infants on Brazelton indices assessed neonatally (García Coll, Sepkoski, & Lester, 1981). Temperament also has been incorporated into previous models of the connections between poverty and African-American children's socioemotional functioning (McLoyd, 1990a). Although important, such considerations are less unique to children of color than other potential factors such as health, maturational timing, and racial features.

There are clear indications that the health status of children of color is less satisfactory than is the health status of majority culture children (see García Coll, 1990). Rates of prematurity in both African-American and Puerto Rican populations are higher than in Caucasian populations, thereby creating greater developmental risk (see Vohr & García Coll, 1988). Further, African-American infants have been found to have a greater incidence of iron deficiency, which has been associated with decreased attention, greater fatigue, and impaired performance on measures of cognitive ability (Carter, 1983; Webb & Oski, 1974).

Biological factors may have specific significance for children of color. García Coll (1990) reviewed a number of studies that demonstrate differences in neonatal behavior in various populations of infants of color. Lester and Brazelton (1982) suggested that neonatal behavior may be a phenotype that expresses the complex relations among genetic endowment, intrauterine environment, and mothers' obstetrical history, and these characteristics can elicit specific adaptive behaviors from the caregiving environment and contribute to the practices and expectations of the culture. In a different developmental period, biology, as manifested in maturational timing during adolescence, may be important. Spencer, Dobbs, and Swanson (1988) note that African-American adolescent boys tend to be taller and heavier that their Caucasian counterparts and may mature earlier as well. These authors suggest that early maturation and increased size are risk factors for social and academic competence. They posit that larger, early maturing African-American boys may be perceived as a threat in their environment and therefore receive less positive support from the contexts in which they interact, which in turn affects the development of competencies.

Physical characteristics, such as racial features and skin color, also may affect minority children's development, although the impact of such characteristics has not been fully studied. Spencer and Markstrom-Adams (1990) have suggested that skin color may affect development of identity and social relationships in African-American children, although they note that this possibility is seldom addressed either empirically or conceptually. Lightness of skin color is perceived as more desirable, even within groups of African-American and Puerto Rican children, and is associated with greater opportunity (Russell, Wilson, & Hall, 1992).

Gender has been discussed in previous sections of this model, but also has relevance as an individual characteristic. Spencer et al. (1988) showed that poverty appears to have more detrimental effects on black boys than black girls, although the extent to which this finding is culturally unique is unclear. Nevertheless, documented gender differences in various competencies (Patterson, Kupersmidt, & Vaden, 1990) suggest that the impact of gender must be taken into account in multivariate models of developmental competence.

Family

Minority families tend to have certain characteristics that differentiate them from mainstream families and that affect family processes in very profound ways. Among these characteristics we will highlight the following: the structure and roles of the family; family beliefs, values, and goals; racial socialization; and socioeconomic status and resources.

Structure and roles of the family. The presence in the family of at least one or more persons who unconditionally love a child (Bronfenbrenner, 1979) is considered a minimum requirement for the development of competencies in children. In families of color, there is a tendency for a more integral use of persons other than the birth parents to perform some of the tasks of parenting, through the support of extended family members, familism, and fictive kin (friends who become as close as kin) (García Coll, 1990; Harrison et al., 1990; McAdoo, 1982). African-American, Puerto Rican, and other minority populations have a high percentage of single heads of households (Center for the Study of Social Policy, 1986; Vázquez Nuttall, 1979), but the reliance on extended kin by some of these family systems might provide enough resources to meet the child's needs.

Reliance on the social support of extended kin is maintained as part of the adaptive culture because of cultural patterns that have been brought from other lands (Harrison et al., 1990). These patterns have been maintained because of the economic and discriminatory environments of the societies in which these groups live (McAdoo, 1982). These families are not able to rely on mainstream institutions to provide assistance and help to meet the differential developmental needs of family members.

The roles that individuals play in the family are based on culturally defined gender, parental, and age-appropriate expectations as well as the family structure (i.e., the persons living in the home). In families of color, there can be flexibility of roles as an adaptive response to cultural and societal pressures, as well as adherence to traditional culturally defined roles (McAdoo, 1993). Interactions between family members, therefore, will be reflective of the adaptive culture and the stressors and pressures that the family must cope with.

Family values, beliefs, and goals. Family values, beliefs, and goals embody the elements that are held dear and important to family members. A growing literature documents the differences between ethnic and minority groups in child-rearing values, beliefs, and goals (McAdoo, 1993). These beliefs are rooted in cultural and religious traditions that can be traced to the countries of origin (Boykin & Toms, 1985; Fitzpatrick, 1988; García Coll, 1990; García Coll, Meyer, & Brillon, 1995; Harrison et al., 1990; Ogbu, 1981) and the adaptive culture, as well as the unique experiences of parents. These factors will not only determine the basis of the behavior displayed during family interactions, but will also influence family structure and roles and therefore interactions with other members of the extended family.

Racial socialization. Positioning families and children of color within their environment requires incorporating the ways in which minority families cope with racism and discrimination in the confines of family life (Cross, 1992; McAdoo, 1993). Families of color face chronic stressors when they attempt to socialize their children and simultaneously protect them from the negative effects of racism, segregation, and the resulting inhibiting environments (Peters, 1985).

Racial socialization has been postulated as an important aspect of family processes within minority populations from diverse socioeconomic backgrounds (Branch & Newcombe, 1986; García Coll, Meyer, & Brillon, 1995; Hale-Benson, 1982; Renne, 1970; Tatum, 1987; Thornton, Chatters, Taylor, & Allen, 1990). Children of color must learn to function in both white and black realms (Boykin & Toms, 1985; Cross, 1991; Thornton et al., 1990). Parents teach their children how to cope with the demands of a society that devalues their heritage, race, and culture (McAdoo, 1992). While children of color may demonstrate preferences for being members of the dominant culture, parents have the task of ensuring that their children maintain a positive view of their ethnic and racial group. In fact, Brigham (1974) found that African-American children were more likely than white children to attribute positive traits to their own group. The importance of racial socialization is emphasized by findings that relate these practices to the child's motivation, achievement, prospects for upward mobility, and racial attitudes (Bowman & Howard, 1985; Branch & Newcombe, 1980, 1986).

Socioeconomic status/resources. The socioeconomic resources available to families of color and how they are used also are important influences on the developmental competencies of minority children (see Huston et al., 1994b). While measures of socioeconomic status can be good indicators of social class variables, they fail to pick up within-group nuances. For example, a first-generation middle-class family of color may react differently to a financial crisis than a fourth-generation middle-class family, with greater uncertainty about socioeconomic status. Given the fact that most minority families experience higher, more extreme, and more long-lasting poverty (U.S. Bureau of the Census, 1991), the consequences of differences in socioeconomic status on the development of competencies in children of color need further attention (Huston, McLoyd, & García Coll, 1994a).

Developmental Competencies

Developmental competencies represent the "outcome" portion of the model and reflect both the functional competencies of a child at any one point in time and the developing/emerging skills that children bring to the multiple ecologies in which they exist. Nevertheless, it is critical to determine and appropriately measure the emergence and salience of specific skills that define the functional or adaptive competence of children of color in specific developmental periods. According to organizational models, development in children of color cannot be judged solely in relation to a specific "standard norm" applied to all children, but must be considered within the context of specific ecological circumstances. Further, within-group variability in ecological niches and developmental outcome in children of color is as great as is the between-group variability that necessitates the development of this model.

The evaluation of meaningful developmental competencies will continue to involve important traditional skill areas such as cognitive, social, emotional, and linguistic skills. However, functional outcome measures must also recognize manifestations of these skills that reflect competent adaptation to circumstances created by social stratification, the effects of racism and its concomitant processes, and the influence of segregation on the nature of the environments faced by children of color. For example, assertive behavior with members of the peer group may be more appropriate in some contexts for African-American children (Heath, 1989; Rotheram-Borus & Phinney, 1990), and the lack of eye contact with authority figures is an appropriate social response by Puerto Rican children (Fitzpatrick & Travieso, 1980).

Notions of competence also must be expanded to include a broader range of adaptive responses beyond the traditional areas of concern and to incorporate additional and alternative abilities, such as the child's ability to function in two or more different cultures, to cope with racism, subtle and overt discrimination, and social and psychological segregation. Both culture-specific and bicultural competencies are needed to promote these children's development. Children must learn the codes that are appropriate to both cultures if they are to master the activities that are called upon in each (LaFromboise, Coleman, & Gerton, 1993). Szapocznik and colleagues (Szapocznik, Kurtines, & Fernandez, 1980; Szapocznik, Santisteban, Kurtines, Perez-Vidal, & Hervis, 1984) found that Hispanic children with bicultural skills were less likely to experience school and family conflicts or to become involved in illegal drug use. Children of color also must effectively cope with racism and its derivatives and maintain a strong sense of self despite multiple threats. Parents who are successful in preparing their children for these tasks thus can be considered to be effective teachers of a culture who foster the adaptive racial socialization of their children (see García Coll et al., 1995).

Competency for children of color involves a wide range and multiple levels of abilities that are intertwined and cannot be defined by any one single index, indicator, or measure. The adaptive competency of children of color at any one point in time is, in turn, an important influence on the subsequent ecological processes that will continue to affect the developmental course of these children. The process is recursive and operates at multiple levels, but is most represented in reciprocal influences on the child's psychological and social segregation, promoting/inhibiting environments, and family processes.

CONCLUSIONS

Both historically and in the present, mainstream developmental sciences have not emphasized the unique normative processes among minority children and their families or the development of competencies within these populations. This omission reflects, in part, the inability of existing theoretical models to address critical aspects of the environment that have profound influences in the developmental processes in these populations. By placing these influences (social position, racism and its derivatives, and segregation) at the core rather than at the periphery of a causal framework and by specifying how they influence more immediate settings, the proposed model is a heuristic guide to research in the development of competencies in children of color. Patterns of family interaction can then be conceptualized as a reflection of an adaptive culture—a mix of history, traditions, and adaptive responses to present contextual demands—and not solely as individual patterns of interactions.

Several challenges are posed by this model. The first is to identify the alternative competencies in children of color that are not measured by traditional assessment tools, not only in the realms of established developmental competencies but in areas of bicultural adaptation and coping with racism. The second is to analyze the implications for social policy and interventions. For example, the present analysis implies that bilingual education should foster the development of balanced bilingualism so that the children develop mastery in two languages and the family is not negatively affected by the creation of a linguistic gap between family members. Alternatively, bilingual education for children can be paired with English as a Second Language instruction for family members so that, as the child's communicative skills evolve toward greater mastery in a second language, so do other family members'.

The third challenge is to recognize that we cannot continue to waste human talent because of outdated racial/ethnic conceptualizations. The competence and productivity of minority populations are crucial to our collective well-being (McLoyd, 1990a). Indeed, people of color from various national origins will be close to a majority in the United States (Exter, 1992) early in the next century. The proposed model and the consequent research and social policies can contribute to a necessary change in societal views of children's development and the characteristics of racial and ethnic groups.

REFERENCES

Allport, G. W. (1954). *The nature of prejudice.* Reading, MA: Addison-Wesley.

Anastasi, A., & Cordova, F. (1953). Some effects of bilingualism upon the intelligence test performance of Puerto Rican children in New York City. *Journal of Education Psychology, 44*(1), 1–19.

Anastasi, A., & de Jesús, C. (1953). Language development and nonverbal IQ of Puerto Rican preschool children in New York City. *Journal of Abnormal and Social Psychology, 48*(3), 357–366.

Anderson, R. M., Giachello, A. L., & Aday, L. A. (1986). Access of Hispanics to health care and cuts in services: A state-of-the-art overview. *Public Health Reports, 101,* 238–252.

Arcia, E., Keyes, L., & Gallagher, J. J. (1994). Indicators of developmental and functional status of Mexican-American and Puerto Rican children. *Developmental and Behavioral Pediatrics, 15*(1), 27–33.

Armstrong, C. P., Achilles, E. M., & Sacks, M. J. (1935). *Reactions of Puerto Rican children in New York City to psychological tests.* Report of the Special Commission on Immigration and Naturalization, New York State Chamber of Commerce.

Attewell, P., & Fitzgerald, R. (1980). Comparing stratification theories. *American Sociological Review, 45,* 325–328.

Barbarin, O. A. (1993). Coping and resilience: Exploring the inner lives of African-American children. *Journal of Black Psychology, 19*(4), 478–492.

Barbarin, O. A., & Soler, R. E. (1993). Behavioral, emotional, and academic adjustment in national probability sample of African-American children: Effects of age, gender, and family structure. *Journal of Black Psychology, 19*(4), 423–446.

Barber, B. (1957). *Social stratification: A comparative analysis of structure and process.* New York: Harcourt.

Barnes, E. J. (1991). The black community as the source of positive self concept for black children: A theoretical perspective. In R. L. Jones (Ed.), *Black psychology* (3d ed., pp. 667–692). Berkeley, CA: Cobb & Henry.

Becerra, J. E., Hogue, C. J. R., Atrash, H. K., & Pérez, N. (1991). Infant mortality among Hispanics: A portrait of heterogeneity. *JAMA, 265(2),* 217–221.

Bendix, R., & Lipset, S. M. (Eds.). (1966). *Class, status and power: A reader in social stratification in comparative perspective.* New York: Free Press.

Blau, Z. S. (1981). *Black children/white children: Competence, socialization, and social structure.* New York: Free Press.

Bloom, B. S., Davis, A., & Hess, R. (1965). *Compensatory education for cultural deprivation.* New York: Holt Rinehart & Winston.

Bowman, P. J. (1990). The adolescent-to-adult transition: Discouragement among jobless black youth. In V. C. McLoyd & C. A. Flannagan (Eds.), Economic stress: Effects on family life and child development. *New Directions for Child Development, 46,* 87–105.

Bowman, P. J., & Howard, C. (1985). Race related socialization, motivation and academic achievement: A study of black youth in three generation families. *Journal of the American Academy of Child Psychiatry, 24,* 1134–1141.

Boyce, W. T., Schaefer, C., Harrison, H. R., Haffner, W. H. J., Lewis, M., & Wright, A. L. (1986). Social and cultural factors in pregnancy complications in Navajo women. *American Journal of Epidemiology, 124,* 242–253.

Boykin, A. W. (1978). Psychological/behavioral verve in academic/task performance: A pretheoretical consideration. *Journal of Negro Education, 47,* 343–354.

Boykin, A. W. (1983). The academic performance of Afro-American children. In J. Spence (Ed.), *Achievement and achievement motives* (pp. 321–371). San Francisco: Freeman.

Boykin, A. W., & Toms, F. (1985). Black child socialization: A conceptual framework. In H. McAdoo & J. McAdoo (Eds.), *Black children: Social, educational, and parental environments* (pp. 33–52). Newbury Park, CA: Sage.

Branch, C. W., & Newcombe, N. (1980). Racial attitudes of black preschoolers as related to parental civil rights activism. *Merrill–Palmer Quarterly, 26,* 425–428.

Branch, C. W., & Newcombe, N. (1986). Racial attitude development among young black children as a function of parental attitudes: A longitudinal and cross-sectional study. *Child Development, 57*, 712–721.

Brigham, J. C. (1974). Views of black and white children concerning the distribution of personality characteristics. *Journal of Personality, 42*, 144–158.

Bronfenbrenner, U. (1977). Toward an experimentaly ecology of human development. *American Psychologist, 32*, 513–531.

Bronfenbrenner, U. (1979). *The ecology of human development.* Cambridge, MA: Harvard University Press.

Bronfenbrenner, U., & Crouter, A. C. (1983). The evolution of environmental models in developmental research. In W. Kessen (Ed.), P. H. Mussen (Series Ed.), *Handbook of child psychology: Vol. 1. History, theory, and methods* (4th ed., pp. 357–414). New York: Wiley.

Broom, L., & Selznick, P. (1970). *Principles of sociology.* New York: Harper & Row.

Carter, J. H. (1983). Vision or sight: Health concerns for Afro-American children. In G. Johnson-Powell (Ed.), *The psychosocial development of minority group children* (pp. 13–25). New York: Brunner/Mazel.

Center for the Study of Social Policy. (1986). The "flip-side" of black families headed by women: The economic status of black men. In R. Staples (Ed.), *The black family: Essays and studies* (pp. 232–238). Belmont, CA: Wadsworth.

Chavez, L. R., Cornelius, W. A., & Jones, O. W. (1986). Utilization of health services by Mexican immigrant women in San Diego. *Women and Health, 11*, 3–20.

Cicchetti, D., & Schneider-Rosen, K. (1986). An organizational approach to childhood depresion. In M. Rutter, C. E. Izard, & P. B. Read (Eds.), *Depression in young people: Developmental and clinical perspectives* (pp. 71–134). New York: Guilford.

Cohen, Y. A. (1971). The shaping of men's minds: Adaptation to the imperatives of culture. In M. L. Wax, S. Diamond, & F. O. Gearing (Eds.), *Anthropological perspectives on education* (pp. 19–50). New York: Basic.

Collins, J. W., & Shay, D. K. (1994). Prevalence of low birth weight among Hispanic infants with United States born and foreign-born mothers: The effect of urban poverty. *American Journal of Epidemiology, 139*(2), 184–192.

Coontz, S. (1992). *The way we never were.* New York: Basic.

Cross, W. (1991). *Shades of black: Diversity in African-American identity.* Philadelphia: Temple University Press.

Cross, W. (1992). *Shades of blackness.* Philadelphia: Temple University Press.

Darwin, C. R. (1859). *On the origin of species by natural selection.* London: J. Murray.

de Gobineau, A. (1915). *The inequality of human races.* New York: Putman.

Delgado-Gaitan, C. (1994). Socializing young children in Mexican-American families: An intergenerational perspective. In P. M. Greenfield & R. R. Cocking (Eds.), *Cross cultural roots of minority child development* (pp. 55–86). Hillsdale, NJ: Erlbaum.

Dowling, P. T., & Fisher, M. (1987). Maternal factors and low birth weight infants: A comparison of Blacks with Mexican-Americans. *Journal of Family Practice, 25*, 153–158.

Duckitt, J. (1992). Psychology and prejudice. *American Psychologist, 47*(10), 1182–1193.

Duncan, J. D., Brooks-Gunn, J., & Klebanov, P. D. (1994). Economic deprivation and early childhood development. *Child Development, 65*, 296–318.

Dunn, L. M. (1987). *Bilingual Hispanic children on the U.S. mainland: A review of research on their cognitive, linguistic and scholastic development.* Circle Pines, MN: American Guidance Service.

Entwisle, D. R., & Astone, N. M. (1994). Some practical guidelines for measuring youth's race/ethnicity and socioeconomic status. *Child Development, 65*, 1521–1540.

Erickson, E. H. (1950). *Childhood and society.* New York: Norton.

Essed, P. (1991). *Understanding everyday racism.* Newbury Park, CA: Sage.

Exter, T. G. (1992). Demographic forecasts: Blacks to 2010. *American Demographics, 14*(12), 63.

Feagin, J. R. (1989). *Racial and ethnic relations* (3d ed.). Englewood Cliffs, NJ: Prentice-Hall.

Feagin, J. R. (1992). *Racial and ethnic relations.* Englewood Cliffs, NJ: Prentice-Hall.

Fitzpatrick, J. P. (1988). The Puerto Rican family. In C. H. Mindel & R. W. Habenstein (Eds.), *Ethnic families in America: Patterns and variations* (pp. 192–217). New York: Elsevier.

Fitzpatrick, J. P., & Travieso, L. (1980). The Puerto Rican family: Its role in cultural transition. In M. D. Fatini & R. Cárdenas (Eds.), *Parenting in a multicultural society* (pp. 103–113). New York: Longman.

Frey, D., & Gaertner, S. (1986). Helping and the avoidance of inappropriate interracial behavior: A strategy that perpetuates a nonprejudiced self-image. *Journal of Personality and Social Psychology, 50,* 1083–1090.

Galton, F. (1869). *Hereditary genius: An inquiry into its laws and consequences.* London: Macmillan.

García Coll, C. (1990). Developmental outcome of minority infants: A process-oriented look into our beginnings. *Child Development, 61,* 270–289.

García Coll, C. T., Meyer, E. C., & Brillon, L. (1995). Ethnic and minority parenting. In M. Bornstein (Ed.), *Handbook of parenting: Vol. 2. Biology and ecology of parenting* (pp. 189–209). Hillsdale, NJ: Erlbaum.

García Coll, C. T., Sepkoski, C., & Lester, B. M. (1981). Cultural and biomedical correlates of neonatal behavior. *Developmental Psychobiology, 14,* 147–154.

García Coll, C. T., & Vázquez García, H. A. (1995a). Developmental processes and their influence on interethnic and interracial relations. In W. D. Hawley & A. W. Jackson (Eds.), *Toward a common destiny* (pp. 103–130). San Francisco: Jossey-Bass.

García Coll, C. T., & Vázquez García, H. A. (1995b). Hispanic children and their families: On a different track from the very beginning. In H. E. Fitzgerald, B. M. Lester, & B. Zuckerman (Eds.), *Children of poverty: Research, health care, and policy issues* (pp. 57–83). New York: Garland.

Gibson, M. A. (1976). Approaches to multicultural education in the United States: Some concepts and assumptions. *Anthropology and Education Quarterly, 7,* 7–18.

Glazer, N., & Moynihan, D. P. (1963). *Beyond the melting pot.* Cambridge, MA: MIT Press and Harvard University Press.

Goodenough, F. L., & Anderson, J. E. (1931). *Experimental child study.* New York: Century.

Gordon, M. M. (1963). *Social class in American sociology.* New York: McGraw-Hill.

Guendelman, S., & Schwalbe, J. (1986). Medical utilization by Hispanic children. *Medical Care, 26*(10), 925–940.

Gutierrez, J., & Sameroff, A. (1990). Determinants of complexity in Mexican-American mothers' conceptions of child development. *Child Development, 61,* 384–394.

Haberfeld, Y., & Shenav, Y. (1990). Are women and blacks closing the gap? Salary discrimination in American science during the 1970s and 1980s. *Industrial and Labor Relations Review, 44*(1), 68–82.

Hale-Benson, J. E. (1982). *Black children: Their roots, culture and learning styles.* Baltimore: Johns Hopkins Press.

Harrison, A. O., Serafica, F., & McAdoo, H. (1984). Ethnic families of color. In R. D. Parke (Ed.), *The family: Review of child development research* (Vol. 7, pp. 329–371). Chicago: University of Chicago Press.

Harrison, A. O., Wilson, M. N., Pine, C. J., Chan, S. Q., & Buriel, R. (1990). Family ecologies of ethnic minority children. *Child Development, 61,* 347–362.

Harry, B. (1992). Restructuring the participation of African-American parents in special education. *Exceptional Children, 59*(2), 123–131.

Heath, S. B. (1989). Oral and literate traditions among black Americans living in poverty. *American Psychologist, 44*(2), 367–373.

Herrnstein, R. (1971, September). IQ. *Atlantic Monthly,* 43–64.

Herskovits, M. (1930). The Negro in the New World. *American Anthropologist, 32,* 145–155.

Hirschfeld, L. A. (1995). The inheritability of identity: Children's understanding of the cultural biology of race. *Child Development, 66,* 1418–1437.

Huston, A. C., McLoyd, V. C., & García Coll, C. (1994a). Children and poverty: Issues in contemporary research. *Child Development, 65,* 275–282.

Huston, A. C., McLoyd, V. C., & García Coll, C. (Guest Eds.). (1994b). Children and poverty [Special issue]. *Child Development, 65*(2).

Jensen, A. (1969). How much can we boost IQ and school achievement? *Harvard Educational Review, 39*, 1–123.

Kohn, M. L. (1977). *Class and conformity.* Chicago: University of Chicago Press.

Krieger, N., Rowley, D. L., Herman, A. A., Avery, B., & Phillips, M. T. (1993). Racial differences in preterm delivery—Developing a new research paradigm. *American Journal of Preventive Medicine, 9*(Suppl. 6), 82–122.

LaFromboise, T., Coleman, H. L. K., & Gerton, J. (1993). Psychological impact of biculturalism: Evidence and theory. *Psychological Bulletin, 114*(3), 395–412.

Landry, L. B. (1980). The social and economic adequacy of the black middle class. In J. R. Washington, Jr. (Ed.), *Dilemmas of the new black middle class.* University of Pennsylvania Afro-American Studies Symposium Proceedings.

Laumann, E. O. (Ed.). (1970). *Social stratification research and theory for the 1970's.* New York: Bobs-Merrill.

Lerner, R. M. (1989). Individual development and the family system: A life-span perspective. In K. Kreppner & R. M. Lerner (Eds.), *Family systems and life-span development* (pp. 15–31). Hillsdale, NJ: Erlbaum.

Lester, B. M., & Brazelton, T. B. (1982). Cross-cultural assessment of neonatal behavior. In H. Stevenson & D. Wagner (Eds.), *Cultural perspectives on child development* (pp. 20–53). San Francisco: W. H. Freeman.

Lewis, O. (1965). *La vida.* New York: Vintage.

Locke, J. (1913). *Some thoughts concerning education: Sections 38 and 40.* London: Cambridge University Press. (Original work published 1690).

Massey, D. S. (1993). Latinos, poverty, and the underclass: A new agenda for research. *Hispanic Journal of Behavioral Sciences, 15*(4), 449–475.

Massey, D. S., & Bitterman, B. (1985). Explaining the paradox of Puerto Rican segregation. *Social Forces, 64*(2), 306–331.

Massey, D. S., & Denton, N. A. (1988). Suburbanization and segregation in U.S. metropolitan areas. *American Journal of Sociology, 94*, 592–626.

Masson, C. N., & Verkuyten, M. (1993). Prejudice, ethnic identity, contact and ethnic group preferences among Dutch young adolescents. *Journal of Applied Social Psychology, 23*(2), 156–168.

McAdoo, H. P. (1982). Stress absorbing systems in black families. *Family Relations, 31*, 379–488.

McAdoo, H. (1992). Reaffirming African-American families and our identities. *Psychology Discourse, 23*(3). (Excerpted from the Distinguished Psychologist Address, Aug. 17, 1991, New Orleans).

McAdoo, H. (1993). The social cultural contexts of ecological developmental family models. In P. G. Boss, W. J. Doherty, R. LaRossa, W. R. Shumm, & S. K. Steinmetz (Eds.), *Sourcebook of family theories and methods: A contextual approach* (pp. 298–301). New York: Plenum.

McAdoo, H. P. (1995). African-American families: Strength and realities. In H. I. McCubbin, E. A. Thompson, A. I. Thompson, & J. A. Futrell (Eds.), *Resiliency and ethnic minority families: African American families* (Vol. 2, pp. 17–30). Madison: University of Wisconsin.

McConahay, J. B., Hardee, B. B., & Batts, V. (1981). Has racism declined in America? *Journal of Conflict Resolution, 25*(4), 563–579.

McConahay, J. B., & Hough, J. C. (1976). Symbolic racism. *Journal of Social Issues, 32*(2), 23–45.

McKinney, M., Abrams, L. A., Terry, P. A., & Lerner, R. M. (1994). Child development research and the poor children of America: A call for a developmental contextual approach to research and outreach. *Family & Consumer Sciencs Research Journal, 23*, 26–42.

McLoyd, V. C. (1990a). The impact of economic hardship on Black families and children: Psychological distress, parenting, and socioemotional development. *Child Development, 61*, 311–346.

McLoyd, V. C. (1990b). Minority children: Introduction to the special issue. *Child Development, 61*, 263–266.

McLoyd, V. C., & Randolph, S. (1984). The conduct and publication of research on Afro-American children: A content analysis. *Human Development, 27*, 65–75.

McLoyd, V. C., & Randolph, S. (1985). Secular trends in the study of Afro-American children: A review of *Child Development*. In A. B. Smuts & J. W. Hagen (Eds.), History and research in child development. *Monographs of the Society for Research in Child Development, 50*(4–5, Serial No. 211).

Mendoza, F., Glenn, S., Takata, S., & Martorell, R. (1994). In G. Lamberty & C. García Coll (Eds.), *Puerto Rican women and children: Issues in health, growth, and development*. New York: Plenum.

Miller, H. (1952). New York City's Puerto Rican pupils: A problem of acculturation. *School and Society, 76*(1967), 129–132.

Montague, A. (1942). *Man's most dangerous myth: The fallacy of race*. New York: Columbia University Press.

Montague, A. (1972). *Statement of race* (3rd ed.). New York: Oxford University Press.

Morris, H. S. (1968). Ethnic groups. In D. Sill (Ed.), *International encyclopedia of the social sciences* (Vol. 15, p. 167). New York: Conwell, Collier & MacMillian.

Ogbu, J. U. (1981). Origins of human competence: A cultural-ecological perspective. *Child Development, 52*, 413–429.

Ogbu, J. U. (1985). A cultural ecology of competence among inner-city blacks. In M. B. Spencer, G. K. Brookins, & W. R. Allen (Eds.), *Beginnings: The social and affective development of black children*. Hillsdale, NJ: Erlbaum.

Ogbu, J. U. (1987). Variability in minority school performance: A problem in search of and explanation. *Anthropology and Education Quarterly, 18*, 312–334.

Ogbu, J. U. (1991a). Low school performance as an adaptation: The case of blacks in Stockton, California. In M. A. Gibson & J. U. Ogbu (Eds.), *Minority schooling and status* (pp. 249–285). New York: Garland.

Ogbu, J. U. (1991b). Minority coping responses and school experience. *Journal of Psychohistory, 18*(4), 433–456.

Parten, M. B. (1932). Social participation among pre-school children. *Journal of Abnormal and Social Psychology, 27*, 243–269.

Passow, H. A. (Ed.). (1963). *Education in depressed areas*. New York: Teachers College, Columbia University.

Patterson, C. J., Kupersmidt, J. B., & Vaden, N. A. (1990). Income level, gender, ethnicity, and household composition as predictors of children's school-based competence. *Child Development, 61*, 485–494.

Peters, M. F. (1985). Racial socialization of young Black children. In H. McAdoo & J. McAdoo (Eds.), *Black children: Social, educational, and parental environments* (pp. 159–173). Newbury Park, CA: Sage.

Puerto Rican Forum. (1964). *A study of poverty conditions in the New York Puerto Rican community*. New York: Puerto Rican Forum, Inc.

Puerto Rican Study 1953–1957. (1958). New York: New York City Board of Education.

Ramirez, M., & Castaneda, A. (1974). *Cultural democracy, bicognitive development, and education*. New York: Academic Press.

Reissman, F. (1962). *The culturally deprived child*. New York: Harper & Row.

Renne, K. (1970). Correlates of dissatisfaction in marriage. *Journal of Marriage and the Family, 32*, 54–67.

Rodriguez, C. (1975). A cost benefit analysis of subjective factors affecting assimilation: Puerto Ricans. *Ethnicity, 2*, 66–80.

Rodriguez, C. (1994). A summary of Puerto Rican migration to the United States. In G. Lamberty & C. García Coll (Eds.), *Puerto Rican women and children: Issues in health, growth, and development* (pp. 11–28). New York: Plenum.

Rosenberg, M. (1979). *Conceiving the self*. Malabar, FL: Krieger.

Rosenberg, M., & Pearlin, L. (1978). Social class and self esteem among children and adults. *American Journal of Sociology, 84*(1), 53–77.

Rotheram-Borus, M. J., & Phinney, J. S. (1990). Patterns of social expectation among black and Mexican-American children. *Child Development, 61*, 542–556.

Rousseau, J. J. (1938). Emile: Or concerning education: Book 2. New York: Dutton, 1938. Cited in P. H. Mussen, J. J. Conger, & J. Kagan (Eds.), *Child development and personality* (2d ed., p. 9). New York: Harper & Row. (Original work published 1762).

Rueschenberg, E., & Buriel, R. (1989). Mexican family functioning and acculturation: A family system perspective. *Hispanic Journal of Behavioral Sciences, 11*(3), 232–244.

Russell, K., Wilson, M., & Hall, R. (1992). *The color complex: The politics of skin color among African-Americans.* New York: Harcourt Brace Jovanovich.

Sameroff, A. J., & Chandler, M. (1975). Reproductive risk and the continuum of caretaking casualty. In F. D. Horowitz, E. M. Hetherington, & S. Scarr-Salapatek (Eds.), *Review of child development research* (Vol. 4, pp. 187–244). Chicago: University of Chicago Press.

Sameroff, A. J., & Fiese, B. H. (1990). Transactional regulation and early intervention. In S. J. Meisels & J. P. Shonkoff (Eds.), *Handbook of early childhood intervention* (pp. 119–191). New York: Cambridge University Press.

Santiago, A. (1992). Patterns of Puerto Rican segregation and mobility. *Hispanic Journal of Behavioral Sciences, 14*(1), 107–133.

Sears, R. R. (1975). Ancients revisited: A history of child development. *Review of Child Development Research* (Vol. 5, pp. 1–73). Chicago: University of Chicago Press.

Sears, R. R., Maccoby, E. E., & Levin, H. (1957). *Patterns of child rearing.* Evanston, IL: Row & Peterson.

Senn, M. (1975). Insights on the child development movement. *Monographs of the Society for Research in Child Development, 40*(3–4, Serial No. 161).

Sherman, A. (1994). *Wasting America's future: The Children's Defense Fund report on the costs of child poverty.* Boston: Beacon.

Shuey, A. (1966). *The testing of Negro intelligence.* New York: Social Science Press.

Shulman, S. (1990). The causes of black poverty: Evidence and interpretation. *Journal of Economic Issues, 24*(4), 995–1016.

Simpson, G. E., & Yinger, M. J. (1953). *Racial and cultural minorities.* New York: Harper & Brothers.

Slaughter-Defoe, D. T., Nakagawa, K., Takanishi, R., & Johnson, D. J. (1990). Toward cultural/ecological perspectives on schooling and achievement in African- and Asian-American children. *Child Development, 61,* 363–383.

Sleeter, C. E., & Grant, C. A. (1987). An analysis of multicultural education in the United States. *Harvard Educational Review, 57,* 421–444.

Spencer, M. B. (1990). Development of minority children: An introduction. *Child Development, 61,* 267–269.

Spencer, M. B., Dobbs, B., & Swanson, D. P. (1988). Afro-American adolescents: Adaptational processes and socioeconomic diversity in behavioral outcomes. *Journal of Adolescence, 11,* 117–137.

Spencer, M. B., & Markstrom-Adams, C. (1990). Identity processes among racial and ethnic minority children in America. *Child Development, 61,* 290–310.

Sroufe, L. (1979). The coherence of individual development: Early care, attachment and subsequent developmental issues. *American Psychologist, 34*(10), 834–841.

Stevenson, H. W., Chen, C., & Uttal, D. H. (1990). Beliefs and achievement: A study of black, white, and Hispanic children. *Child Development, 61,* 508–523.

Stroebe, W., & Insko, C. A. (1989). Stereotype, prejudice and discrimination: Changing conceptions in theory and research. In D. BarTal, C. F. Graumann, A. W. Kruglanski, & W. Stroebe (Eds.), *Stereotyping and prejudice: Changing conceptions* (pp. 3–34). New York: Springer-Verlag.

Sue, D. W., & Sue, D. (1990). *Counseling the culturally different.* New York: Wiley.

Swenson, I., Erickson, D., Ehlinger, E., Swaney, S., & Carlson, G. (1986). Birthweight, apgarscores, labor and delivery complications and prenatal characteristics of Southeast Asian adolescents and older mothers. *Adolescence, 21,* 711–722.

Szapocznik, J., Kurtines, W., & Fernandez, T. (1980). Bicultural involvement and adjustment in Hispanic-American youths. *International Journal of Intercultural Relations, 4,* 353–365.

Szapocznik, J., Santisteban, D., Kurtines, W., Perez-Vidal, A., & Hervis, O. (1984). Bicultural effectiveness training: A treatment intervention for enhancing intercultural adjustment in Cuban American families. *Hispanic Journal of Behavioral Sciences, 6,* 317–344.

Taeuber, K. E., & Taeuber, A. F. (1965). *Negroes in cities: Residential segregation and neighborhood change.* Chicago: Aldine.

Tatum, B. (1987). *Assimilation blues.* Westport, CT: Greenwood.

Terman, L. M. (1916). *The measurement of intelligence: An explanation of and a complete guide for the use of the Stanford revision and extension of the Binet-Simon Intelligence Scale.* Boston: Houghton Mifflin.

Tharp, R. G. (1989). Psychocultural variables and constants: Effects on teaching and learning in schools. *American Psychologist, 44*, 349–359.

Thomas, D. S. (1929). Some new techniques for studying social behavior. *Child development monographs* (No. 1). New York: Teachers College, Columbia University.

Thornton, M. C., Chatters, L. M., Taylor, R. J., & Allen, W. R. (1990). Sociodemographic and environmental correlates of racial socialization by black parents. *Child Development, 61*, 401–409.

Tumin, M. M. (1967). *Social stratification.* Englewood Cliffs, NJ: Prentice-Hall.

Turner, J. H., & Singleton, R. (1978). A theory of ethnic oppression: Toward a reintegration of cultural and structural concepts in ethnic relations theory. *Social Forces, 56*(4), 1001–1018.

Turner, M., Fix, M., & Struyk, R. J. (1991) *Opportunities denied, opportunities diminished: Discrimination in hiring.* Washington, DC: Urban Institute Press.

U.S. Bureau of the Census. (1991). *Poverty in the United States.* (Current Population Reports: Consumer Income, Series P-60, No. 175). Washington, DC: Government Printing Office.

Vázquez Nuttall, E. (1979). The support system and coping patterns of the female Puerto Rican single parent. *Journal of Non-White Concerns, 7*(3), 128–137.

Ventura, S. J. (1994). Demographic and health characteristics of Puerto Rican mothers and their babies. In G. Lamberty & C. García Coll (Eds.), *Puerto Rican women and children: Issues in health, growth, and development* (pp. 71–84). New York: Plenum.

Vohr, B. R., & García Coll, C. T. (1988). Follow-up studies of high-risk low-birthweight infants. In H. E. Fitzgerald, B. M. Lester, & M. W. Yogman (Eds.), *Theory and research in behavioral pediatrics* (Vol. 4, pp. 1–65). New York: Plenum.

Vygotsky, L. S. (1978). *Mind in society.* Cambridge, MA: Harvard University Press.

Wasik, B. H. (1992, January). The context of the classroom and children's learning. In J. Belsky (Chair), *The context of schooling.* Symposium conducted at the School Readiness: Scientific Perspectives National Conference, Columbia, MD.

Webb, T. E., & Oski, F. A. (1974). Behavioral status of young adolescents with iron deficiency anemia. *Journal of Special Education, 8*, 153.

Werner, H. (1948). *The comparative psychology of mental development.* New York: Harper & Row.

West, C. (1993). *Race matters.* Boston: Beacon.

Wiltfang, G. L., & Scarbecz, M. (1990). Social class and adolescents' self-esteem: Another look. *Social Psychology Quarterly, 53*(2), 174–183.

Wise, P. H., Kotelchuck, M., Wilson, M. L., & Mills, M. (1985, August), Racial and socioeconomic disparities in childhood mortality in Boston. *New England Journal of Medicine, 313*(6), 360–366.

Yee, A. H., Fairchild, H. H., Weizmann, F., & Wyatt, G. E. (1993). Addressing psychology's problem with race. *American Psychologist, 48*(11), 1132–1140.

Young, V. H. (1974). A black American socialization pattern. *American Ethnologist, 1*(2), 405–413.

24

Referring and Reporting Research Participants at Risk: Views from Urban Adolescents

Celia B. Fisher, Ann Higgins-D'Alessandro, Jean-Marie B. Rau,
Tara L. Kuther, and Susan Belanger
Fordham University

Researching developmental risks of urban youth raises ethical concerns when an investigator discovers a participant is in jeopardy. This study collected data on 147 seventh, ninth, and eleventh graders' views of 3 investigator options: (1) taking no action and maintaining confidentiality, (2) reporting the problem to a concerned parent or adult, and (3) facilitating adolescent self-referrals. Participants judged these options within the context of 5 risk domains: substance abuse, child maltreatment, life-threatening behaviors, delinquency, and shyness. Judgments of reporting options were related to grade and ratings of risk severity, but not to moral reasoning. Confidentiality was viewed favorably for risk behaviors of low perceived severity or for which the consequences of adult discovery might introduce greater risk. Confidentiality was viewed unfavorably and reporting to adults favorably for child maltreatment and threats of suicide. Self-referral was viewed favorably across all grades and risk behaviors. Implications of adolescent perspectives for research ethics are discussed.

The past 15 years have witnessed a significant shift in the way developmental scientists view their roles and responsibilities. Economic, social, political, and disciplinary factors have converged to foster increased attention to the social and applied relevance of the developmental data base (Fisher & Lerner, 1994; Fisher et al., 1993; Horowitz & O'Brien, 1989). In particular, developmental scientists are being called upon to generate knowledge about many of the societal problems jeopardizing the development of adaptive and productive life skills during the critical years of adolescence (Dougherty, 1993; Jessor, 1993; Lerner, 1993; Zaslow & Takanishi, 1993). Scholars engaged in research on developmental processes in adolescence have begun to shift the focus of their work from the laboratory to the streets in response to societal demands for knowledge and techniques that can help stem the tide of psychological risk associated with urban poverty, violence, and despair. Concern about the current risk-opportunity imbalance (Takanishi, 1993) in the lives of urban adolescents has risen with increases in the number of teenagers: living in poverty, abusing drugs and alcohol, becoming victimized by or engaged in violence, manifesting depressive symptomology, and engaging in high-risk sexual activities and other health compromising behaviors (Chase-Lansdale & Brooks-Gunn, 1994; Children's Safety

Reprinted with permission from *Child Development*, 1996, Vol. 67, 2086–2100. Copyright © 1996 by the Society for Research in Child Development, Inc.

Network, 1991; Cicchetti & Toth, 1993; Gans & Blyth, 1990; Jessor, 1992; Petersen et al., 1993; Richters & Martinez, 1993; Sum & Fogg, 1991; Takanishi, 1993).

Referring and Reporting Adolescent Research Participants: An Ethical Challenge

As developmental scientists move out of the laboratory to examine developmental correlates of adolescent risk and to design and evaluate interventions that may alter such risk, participant welfare evolves from an abstract ethical issue to a concrete daily concern (Fisher & Tryon, 1990). For example, investigation of the developmental correlates of adaptive and maladaptive behaviors in hitherto underresearched urban adolescent populations has the potential to tap previously undetected problems facing individual research participants (Fisher, 1993; Fisher & Rosendahl, 1990). During the course of such data collection, adolescent participants may reveal information suggesting that they may be thinking about suicide, have been or are being abused by an adult, are engaging in health-compromising behaviors, or are planning to engage in activities that might be illegal or harmful to others. This raises ethical questions concerning whether an investigator should take steps to help the participant address these problems.

Current Ethical Guidelines on Referring and Reporting Issues

Current federal and professional guidelines offer incomplete answers about what investigators should do if during the course of experimentation they discover that an adolescent's well-being or the well-being of others may be in jeopardy. For example, Federal Regulations Part 46 Subpart D on Protections for Children Involved as Subjects in Research (Department of Health and Human Services [DHHS], 1991) does not address whether an investigator has a responsibility to report or refer adolescent research participants to parents or appropriate authorities when a problem has been discovered during the course of research. Similarly, while the American Psychological Association's (APA) *Ethical Principles of Psychologists and Code of Conduct* allows a psychologist to disclose confidential information without the consent of the individual when it is mandated by law or to protect an individual or others from harm (APA, 1992, Standard 5.05), the current terminology of the code (e.g., references to "patients" and "clients") leaves uncertain the extent to which this standard refers to research participants.

More specific guidelines appear in the Society for Research in Child Development's (SRCD) *Ethical Standards for Research with Children* (SRCD, 1993). Principle 9 of the *Ethical Standards* states that when research-derived information suggests that a child's well-being may be in jeopardy, an investigator has a responsibility to inform guardians or those expert in the field in order to arrange necessary assistance for the child (SRCD, 1993, Principle 9, p. 338). While the SRCD *Ethical Standards* raises expectations regarding investigator responsibility, it does not resolve the complex issue of deciding when it is appropriate or how to report or provide referrals for adolescent participants whose well-being is judged to be in jeopardy (Fisher, 1994).

Referring and Reporting Options
Taking no action. In the course of conducting studies with adolescent populations, researchers may utilize assessment instruments or interviewing techniques that yield previously undetected information about conditions that place an adolescent participant at developmental risk. When such facts have been uncovered, the scientific community has traditionally been reluctant to act upon such information, whether out of concern for participant confidentiality, a healthy skepticism that behaviors measured may not have "diagnostic" validity, or a commitment to scientific controls that may be jeopardized

by humanitarian actions (Fisher, 1993, 1994; Fisher & Brennan, 1992; Fisher, Hoagwood, & Jensen, 1996).

The decision to take no action when such information is revealed during the course of research is supported by the importance federal and professional guidelines have placed upon the maintenance of confidentiality for research-derived information (e.g., APA, 1992, Standard 5.02; Office for Protection of Research Risks [OPRR], 1993, pp. 3–27; SRCD 1993, Principle 11). Implicit in these guidelines is the assumption that protection of privacy is a fundamental right of those who have agreed to participate in research. Moreover, developmental scientists are aware that sharing with parents or other concerned adults research-derived information about the behaviors of individual adolescents can sometimes create stressful or harmful consequences for teenage participants, especially if adults react to such revelations with punitive measures.

The decision to take no action when confronted with information suggesting developmental risk is also supported in research situations in which assessment instruments valid for identifying group differences in the experimental setting may not have the psychometric properties sufficient to draw meaningful conclusions about individual risk (Fisher, 1993, 1994; Fisher & Brennan, 1992). For example, while adolescent alcohol use has been associated with a number of risk factors, including delinquency and unprotected sex (Kandel, Davies, Karus, & Yamaguchi, 1986), empirical information does not yet exist regarding the degree of alcohol consumption, personal characteristics, or social factors that can identify which individual adolescent might progress to alcohol abuse (Pentz, 1994). Under such circumstances, discussing the implications of specific drinking patterns with adolescents or their parents might be misleading and outside the boundaries of good ethical practice (Fisher, 1993).

A third factor influencing the decision to take no action when research-derived information indicates potential participant risk concerns the ways in which many investigators perceive their responsibilities and obligations to the community. Such research-derived information places investigators in what Veatch (1987) has coined the scientist-citizen dilemma: the need to reconcile the scientist's professional commitment to the implementation of well-controlled research designs with his or her humanitarian commitment to protect participant welfare (Fisher, 1993, 1994; Fisher & Rosendahl, 1990; Scarr, 1994). In such situations, investigators may be concerned that acting to assist an adolescent research participant may threaten the internal validity of an experiment (especially in longitudinal designs) or jeopardize the trust and participation of other adolescents involved in the research. This act utilitarian position (an act is morally justified if it promotes the greatest good for the greatest number of persons) has traditionally been adopted in human subjects research (e.g., Beauchamp, Faden, Wallace, & Walters, 1982). Consequently, when a conflict arises between scientific rigor and the immediate welfare of a research participant, investigators often see the production of well-controlled data that can benefit society as superseding their obligation to facilitate or procure services for individual participants (Fisher, 1994).

Reporting risk-related information. In some research contexts, investigators may become aware of information suggesting delinquent behavior, the use of addictive products, or threats of harm or violence to the adolescent participant or others that appear to require immediate attention. As indicated previously, under such conditions, professional guidelines could be interpreted as encouraging an investigator to report the problem to adults who could arrange necessary assistance for the participant (e.g., APA, 1992, Standard 5.05; SRCD, 1993, Principle 9). Moreover, some investigators may take the position that under certain circumstances the immediate welfare of research participants outweighs the distal contributions to society that may be jeopardized by potential threats to the integrity of the research design created by reporting.

Investigators studying adolescent development need to also be aware that certain reporting decisions, such as the decision to report to authorities suspected child abuse, threats of violence, or certain illegal conduct, may not only be an ethical decision, but a legal requirement (Fisher, 1993, 1994;

Fisher et al., 1996). Since the 1976 Child Abuse Prevention and Treatment Act, all 50 states have enacted statutes to mandate the reporting of suspected child abuse or neglect. Since states vary as to whether researchers are included in the list of individuals mandated to report child abuse (see Liss, 1994), investigators must review their own state laws to determine their personal responsibility to report child abuse and neglect as well as the responsibility of other professionals (e.g., pediatricians, school psychologists) who may be part of their research team (Fisher, 1991, 1993).

Recently, Appelbaum and Rosenbaum (1989) have raised concerns about the possibility that social science researchers may, under certain conditions, share with their practitioner colleagues the responsibility to warn third parties about suspected dangers posed by research participants (see *Tarasoff v. Regents of the University of California*, 1976). The possibility that some researchers working with violence-prone adolescents may have a duty to protect potential victims underscores the importance of considering ethical issues associated with reporting high-risk participant behaviors to adults when appropriate (Fisher, 1993; Fisher et al., 1996). There are also situations in which confidential records regarding illegal behaviors of adolescent research participants may be subject to subpoena (Melton, 1990). While researchers may obtain a Certificate of Confidentiality from the Department of Health and Human Services to protect the privacy of research participants against legally compelled disclosure of identifying information, the certificate's protection has yet to be tested in the courts (Hoagwood, 1994). Thus, investigators studying adolescent delinquency or use of illegal drugs may need to consider the extent to which reporting such behaviors to adults who can assist a participant may, in the long run, be a better form of participant protection than taking no action.

Assisting adolescent participants to self-refer. There may be situations in which research-derived information suggests that an adolescent research participant would benefit from medical, social, or psychological services, but would not benefit from reporting the adolescent's risk status to concerned adults. For example, a researcher may learn that an adolescent participant has not sought medical consultation for a suspected sexually transmitted disease. While failure to receive medical attention in the era of AIDS may in fact be a life-threatening risk for the participant, informing the parent about risks associated with sexual activity may violate a teenager's privacy or even jeopardize his or her welfare. In such situations, investigators may look to the legal-medical model defining the rights of adolescents to consent to medical intervention as a guide for determining whether they should report the risk to a parent or discuss with the adolescent ways in which he or she can independently obtain services (Fisher, 1993, 1994; Fisher et al., 1996; Holder, 1981). Asher (1993) has developed and tested an innovative procedure of self-referral following research on peer rejection and loneliness in a normative sample. In his model, after completing the study, participants indicate on a form whether they would like to speak to a school social worker about "things that bother you." The adaptation of such a procedure for normative middle and high school samples may be an appropriate reporting option in studies examining individual behaviors observed to predict poor social adaptation (e.g., shyness) or delinquent behaviors judged inappropriate for formal reporting.

Adolescents as Partners in Ethical Decision Making

When considering the implications of taking no action, reporting a suspected risk to an appropriate and concerned adult, or helping an adolescent self-refer, investigators must be wary of the potential to either overestimate or underestimate the impact of their decision on the research participant. A relatively untapped resource for assisting in such ethical decision making is the perspective of members of the population who will serve as research participants (Bok, 1978; Fisher & Fyrberg, 1994; Gergen, 1973; Levine, 1986; Melton, Levine, Koocher, Rosenthal, & Thompson, 1988; Wilson & Donnerstein, 1976). Data on adolescent perceptions of referring and reporting alternatives can help developmental scientists judge the impact that a decision to maintain confidentiality, report at-risk conditions to an appropriate adult, or assist in self-referrals may have on the research participants themselves.

Eliciting the opinions of adolescents from communities representative of prospective samples supports the moral principle of *respect for personhood* by recognizing that prospective participants are themselves moral agents, with the right to apply a moral judgment to the ethical procedures that will be used in research in which they or members of their cohort will be asked to participate (Fisher & Fyrberg, 1994). Surveying the opinions of adolescents on reporting and referring decisions can also guard against researchers either erroneously assuming that such procedures will have a devastating impact on urban youth or underestimating the potential distress associated with a particular procedure (Farr & Seaver, 1975; Fisher & Fyrberg, 1994; Veatch, 1987). Moreover, such surveys may have generalizability to the ethical decision making of investigators studying common developmental risks across a variety of settings. Finally, including members of a participant community in decision making about ethical procedures has the potential to reduce participant anxiety and increase the perceived justice of reporting decisions made during the course of research (Melton et al., 1988).

In summary, teenagers participating in research, as well as developmental scientists, stand to benefit from research investigating participant perspectives on reporting options available to investigators who discover that a research participant is in developmental jeopardy. Our goal for the present study was to provide empirical information that could assist the ethical decision making of investigators studying adolescent risk behaviors. We sought the opinions of teenagers living in a low-income urban environment since lower socioeconomic and ethnic minority youth have been the focus of recent research on adolescent risk behavior and are disproportionately vulnerable to the social problems currently facing American children and youth (Fisher, Jackson, & Villarruel, in press; Hammond & Yung, 1993; Jessor, 1992). In this investigation, we defined participant jeopardy in terms of 12 risks that have generated a significant amount of attention in the developmental literature and that might vary in perceived severity: alcohol consumption, illicit drug use, cigarette smoking, physical abuse, sexual abuse, suicide, sexually transmitted diseases (STD), truancy, vandalism, theft, violence, and shyness (Berman & Jobbs, 1991; Chase-Lansdale & Brooks-Gunn, 1994; Cicchetti & Toth, 1993; DiLalla & Gottesman, 1989; Duckworth & Dejung, 1989; Gans & Blyth, 1990; Hauck, Martens, & Wetzel, 1986; Kandel et al., 1986; Lester & Anderson, 1992; Petersen et al., 1993; Quadrel, Fischhoff, & Davis, 1993; Richters & Martinez, 1993; Stiffman & Davis, 1990; Windle, 1990). To further broaden our understanding of adolescent perspectives on these options, we sought to examine participant responses within the context of their judgments regarding the perceived severity of the risks under consideration as well as their level of moral reasoning.

METHOD

Participants

The sample consisted of 44 seventh graders (mean age = 12.7 years), 42 ninth graders (mean age = 15.1 years), and 61 eleventh graders (mean age = 17.1 years) attending a New York City Public middle and high school. These two neighborhood schools served adolescents from lower- to lower-middle-class families, as indicated by an average Hollingshead (1957) score of 4 (range = 2–7) based on student reports of parents' occupations. Eighty-three percent of fathers and 62% of mothers were reported to have employment outside the home. Females comprised 66%, 43%, and 52% of seventh-, ninth-, and eleventh-grade respondents, respectively. The seventh graders primarily identified themselves as Hispanic/Latino (85.4%). In ninth and eleventh grades, self-identification was predominantly Hispanic/Latino (26.8% and 32.8%, respectively) and non-Hispanic white (29.3% and

36.2%, respectively). Students in seventh, ninth, and eleventh grades also described themselves as Asian American (2.4%, 26.8%, 19%), black (4.9%, 2.4%, 1.7%), or other (7.3%, 34.1%, 10.3%), respectively.

Approximately one-third of the students in each grade returned both parental permission and student assent forms. While this response rate can be considered moderate to low with respect to those obtained in contemporary studies on adolescent risk, our use of both active parental and child assent is a more ethically stringent participation criteria than is typically reported in the child and adolescent research literature (Fisher & Brennan, 1992).

Procedure

Guardian permission and participant assent forms written in both English and Spanish were distributed in class for the students to take home. Students also were given the opportunity to ask for consent forms in other languages; this option was never requested, however. To encourage a joint-decision-making approach for informed consent, the guardian forms encouraged parents to discuss the study with their child prior to granting permission for the student to participate (Fisher & Rosendahl, 1990; Weithorn, 1983). The parental permission and participant assent forms informed parents and adolescents about the study's purpose and procedures, the voluntary nature of participation, and the confidential nature of the data. Information was collected anonymously: Students did not write their names on any of the response forms. After completing the questionnaires, one child approached one of the investigators and spontaneously revealed several personal problems. The investigator suggested the child see the school counselor, and, with the child's agreement, an appointment with the counselor was arranged.

Instruments

Reporting options rating scale. Following a description of the purpose of the study and a brief presentation on what research psychologists do, participants were instructed as follows:

> Pretend there is a research study going on in your school and the researcher finds out that you have a problem. The researcher can help you by talking to you or by telling somebody about your problem. But, you agreed to be in the study because the researcher promised not to tell anybody what you said. We want to know if you were in this pretend situation, what you think the researcher should do. Do you think the researcher should keep the promise to you and not tell anyone what you said? Do you think the researcher should talk to you first and let you get help? Or do you think the researcher should tell a parent or another concerned adult?

Participants were then asked to judge the acceptability of each of the three reporting options for each of 12 developmental risks. On the response sheets, the three reporting options (maintain confidentiality, help the adolescent self-refer, and report the problem to an adult) were listed as "Keep the promise; do not tell anyone"; "Talk to me first and let me get help"; and "Tell a parent or another concerned adult," respectively. For each reporting option, students were asked to rate what they thought a researcher should do *if you told the researcher*: "you had a drinking problem," "you had a drug problem," "you were smoking cigarettes," "you were being physically abused (hit or beaten) by an adult," "you were being sexually abused by an adult," "you were thinking about suicide," "you had a sexually transmitted disease like herpes, gonorrhea, or HIV," "you were into doing graffiti (tagging or writing on walls)," "you were cutting classes," "you were stealing," "you were planning to hurt someone else," "you were shy." Students were asked to indicate what they "would want the researcher to do" by rating the reporting options on 4-point Likert-type scales in which 1 = "definitely yes," 2 = "probably yes," 3 = "probably no," and 4 = "definitely no."

Risk rating scale. While many studies attempt to quantify the extent to which adolescents are exposed to developmental risks (Farrell, Danish, & Howard, 1992; Jessor, 1993; Windle, 1990), little is known of adolescents' perceptions of these problems (Dubow, Lovko, & Kausch, 1990). Immediately following completion of the Reporting Options Rating Scale, students rated the seriousness of each of the 12 risks. They were asked to "Please tell us how serious or how big of a problem the issues below are to teenagers you may know." Each risk was rated on a 4-point Likert-type scale in which 1 = "not a problem," 2 = "a small problem," 3 = "a problem," and 4 = "a big problem."

The sociomoral reflection measure—short form (SRM-SF). Since decisions concerning whether to refer or report adolescent research participants raise ethical and moral conflicts for developmental scientists, we were interested in whether adolescents would also construe the situations as calling for ethical reasoning. We hypothesized that adolescents who used higher-stage moral reasoning would be less likely to value conventional promise keeping (maintaining confidentiality) when it conflicted with participant welfare. To test this hypothesis, we used the SRM-SF (Gibbs, Basinger, & Fuller, 1992), an 11-item, group-administered, short answer questionnaire designed to assess students' sociomoral values within the context of Kohlberg's theory of moral development. Items focus on the values of contract and truth, affiliation, life, property and law, and legal justice. Respondents are asked to rate how important the value is and to give an explanation for their answer. The SRM-SF scoring manual (Gibbs et al., 1992) is organized into the Immature Level, which includes Stage 1 (unilateral and physicalistic reasoning) and Stage 2 (exchange and instrumental reasoning), and the Mature Level, which includes Stage 3 (mutual and prosocial reasoning) and Stage 4 (systematic reasoning). The total stage score is the mean of the 11 scores registered on a 10-point scale. A continuous score, the SRMS, can also be calculated. The minimally acceptable interrater reliability is 80% agreement within one interval on the 10-point scale for the total global stage score and a difference of 0.2 on the continuous SRMS total score.

RESULTS

The primary purpose of this study was to gather information on how urban youth evaluate three reporting options available to investigators when a research participant tells them he or she is involved in or the victim of behaviors that present different developmental risks. To provide a context in which to interpret adolescent evaluations of reporting options, we first briefly present data on the extent to which seventh, ninth, and eleventh graders view the risks under question as serious problems for teenagers they know. Analyses of student responses to each reporting option across the various risk categories are then described. We conclude this section with a description of the relation between student levels of moral reasoning, perceived risk severity, and evaluations of different reporting options.

Perceived Severity of Each Risk Category

Table 1 provides the mean ratings on the extent to which adolescents viewed each risk category as a serious problem. A 3 (grade) × 2 (sex) × 12 (risk) mixed ANOVA on perceived problem severity yielded main effects of grade, $F(2, 125) = 5.05$, $p = .008$, and problem, $F(11, 115) = 21.39$, $p < .001$, and the grade × problem interaction, $F(22, 230) = 1.75$, $p = .022$. As indicated in Table 1, univariate F tests yielded significant grade differences for drugs, alcohol use, child maltreatment, sexually transmitted diseases, and theft. Scheffé tests (alpha = .05) indicated that these differences reflected the fact that seventh graders perceived the problems as significantly more serious when

TABLE 1

Means, Standard Deviations, Percentage of Ratings Indicating Serious Risk, and Univariate F Tests on Adolescent Evaluations of the Severity of Each Risk Category

Risk Category	Grade 7 ($n = 44$)			Grade 9 ($n = 42$)			Grade 11 ($n = 61$)			
	M	SD	%	M	SD	%	M	SD	%	F
Substance abuse:										
Drugs	3.80	.69	95	3.03	1.30	70	3.23	1.14	72	4.72*
Alcohol	3.48	.72	93	2.83	1.18	61	3.04	1.10	72	3.48*
Cigarettes	2.95	.88	71	2.78	1.07	65	2.50	1.16	46	2.88
Child maltreatment:										
Sexual abuse	3.63	.89	90	2.94	1.37	65	2.84	1.39	60	4.05*
Physical abuse	3.65	.66	95	2.94	1.29	67	2.84	1.32	63	4.84**
Life threatening:										
Suicide	3.55	.90	88	3.00	1.39	58	2.96	1.29	66	2.55
STD	3.70	.79	90	2.78	1.38	62	2.93	1.35	68	5.00**
Delinquency:										
Cutting	2.93	.94	68	2.67	.89	56	2.73	.88	58	.45
Graffiti	2.55	1.01	46	2.53	1.03	45	2.29	.85	34	1.23
Theft	3.10	.71	80	2.53	1.06	52	2.59	1.06	63	4.76**
Violence	2.85	1.05	68	2.83	1.08	59	2.75	1.10	61	.20
Shyness	1.43	.68	5	1.53	.81	8	1.57	.78	14	.47

Note: Risk categories were scored on 4-point Likert-type scales, with 1 and 2 indicating the category was not perceived as a serious problem and 3 and 4 indicating it was a serious problem. Percentages indicate the proportion of adolescents rating the risk as serious with scores of 3 or 4.
* $p < .05$.
** $p < .01$.

compared to ninth and eleventh graders, with the exception of drinking, which seventh graders rated as significantly more serious than did ninth graders, but not eleventh graders.

Table 1 also illustrates the percentage of students who rated each risk problem as serious (ratings of 3 or 4). Binomial tests indicated that a significant majority of students from all grades rated shyness as either "not a problem" or a "small problem" ($ps = .000$). All other risks, with the exception of graffiti, were rated as serious problems by a majority of seventh graders ($ps = .029 - .0000$). By contrast, ninth graders were more ambivalent about the extent to which the 12 developmental risks were problems among teenagers they knew. Only drugs and physical abuse were rated as serious by a significant majority of ninth graders, $ps = .02$ and .04, respectively. And, with the exception of shyness, none of the other risks yielded significant ninth grader majority opinions. Eleventh graders were somewhat more differentiating than younger students. A significant majority agreed that graffiti was not a problem ($p = .02$) and rated substance abusing behaviors (using drugs and drinking alcohol) and life-threatening behaviors (sexually transmitted diseases and suicide) as serious problems ($ps = .0001$, .001, .007, and .02, respectively).

Student Evaluations of Reporting Options

Take no action. Mean ratings for an investigator's decision to take no action when informed about a participant risk and the percentage of students who gave favorable responses (ratings of 1 and 2) for this option are illustrated in Table 2. A 3 (grade) × 2 (sex) × 12 (risk) mixed ANOVA on the extent to which students agreed that an investigator should maintain confidentiality and take no action when

TABLE 2
Means, Standard Deviations, and Percentage of Favorable Ratings for Adolescent Evaluations
of the Three Reporting Options

Reporting Option and Risk Category	Grade 7 (n = 44)			Grade 9 (n = 42)			Grade 11 (n = 61)		
	M	SD	%	M	SD	%	M	SD	%
Take no action:									
Substance abuse:									
Drugs	2.54	1.35	49	2.54	1.27	51	2.33	1.33	54
Alcohol	2.07	1.08	66	2.21	1.15	59	2.26	1.17	62
Cigarettes	2.10	1.06	69	2.15	1.10	67	1.79	.81	79
Child maltreatment:									
Sexual abuse	2.98	1.28	35	2.78	1.33	40	2.41	1.39	52
Physical abuse	2.91	1.25	40	2.83	1.20	35	2.54	1.25	48
Life threatening:									
Suicide	2.52	1.40	73	2.38	1.30	57	2.81	1.20	39
STD	2.48	1.42	52	2.03	1.27	71	1.85	1.20	74
Delinquency:									
Cutting	1.91	1.01	73	1.80	1.03	83	1.77	1.05	79
Graffiti	2.30	1.15	58	1.98	1.10	73	1.76	.90	83
Theft	2.33	1.19	60	2.21	1.22	62	1.84	1.10	75
Violence	2.50	1.35	50	2.55	1.24	49	2.53	1.23	45
Shyness	2.19	1.31	62	2.18	1.14	62	1.73	.91	78
Tell a parent or concerned adult:									
Substance abuse:									
Drugs	2.49	1.24	49	2.28	1.28	58	2.49	1.30	54
Alcohol	2.70	1.23	42	2.48	1.13	53	2.62	1.17	45
Cigarettes	2.74	1.19	43	2.85	1.03	40	3.21	.89	24
Child maltreatment:									
Sexual abuse	1.72	1.03	81	1.78	1.06	78	2.12	1.26	66
Physical abuse	1.91	1.13	74	1.66	.91	81	2.12	1.15	66
Life threatening:									
Suicide	2.02	1.33	69	2.10	1.09	66	1.84	1.07	79
STD	2.12	1.21	64	2.05	1.18	75	2.47	1.25	55
Delinquency:									
Cutting	3.02	1.17	58	3.15	1.04	72	3.31	.90	57
Graffiti	2.58	1.18	47	3.10	1.03	28	3.29	.88	14
Theft	2.63	1.25	47	3.00	1.12	26	3.18	1.04	28
Violence	2.29	1.15	60	2.43	1.13	53	2.33	1.07	57
Shyness	2.17	1.25	62	2.74	1.04	39	2.91	.96	39
Facilitate self-referrals:									
Substance abuse:									
Drugs	1.51	.84	88	1.53	.89	85	1.36	.75	90
Alcohol	1.66	1.06	86	1.61	.82	85	1.35	.62	97
Cigarettes	1.66	.79	83	1.74	.83	88	1.87	.86	82
Child maltreatment:									
Sexual abuse	1.71	1.08	84	1.50	.95	90	1.60	.85	85
Physical abuse	1.93	1.23	67	1.53	.89	85	1.46	.72	92
Life threatening:									
Suicide	1.76	1.16	76	1.47	.83	90	1.40	.71	91
STD	1.61	1.07	83	1.40	.76	95	1.38	.65	95

TABLE 2 (Continued)

Reporting Option and Risk Category	Grade 7 (n = 44)			Grade 9 (n = 42)			Grade 11 (n = 61)		
	M	SD	%	M	SD	%	M	SD	%
Delinquency:									
Cutting	2.02	1.01	70	1.84	1.05	74	1.66	.75	88
Graffiti	2.17	1.18	65	2.11	1.06	70	1.76	.74	88
Theft	1.83	1.05	84	1.79	.94	82	1.49	.74	93
Violence	1.90	1.16	78	1.87	1.07	75	1.64	.87	86
Shyness	2.15	1.28	64	1.90	.92	77	1.93	.94	71

Note: Risk categories were scored on 4-point Likert-type scales, with 1 and 2 indicating favorable ratings for the reporting option and 3 and 4 indicating unfavorable ratings. Percentages indicate the proportion of adolescents giving favorable ratings of 1 or 2.

confronted with a participant at risk yielded a significant main effect of problem, $F(11, 119) = 8.74$, $p < .000$, and a sex × problem interaction, $F(11, 119) = 2.76$, $p = .004$.

Adolescent males and females differed in their views with respect to only a few areas of risk. For example, a Tukey Multiple Comparison Test (alpha = .05) indicated that males were more likely than females to favor taking no action (indicated by lower mean scores) when risks involved the use of illegal drugs (males = 2.15, females = 2.60), alcohol use (males = 1.83, females = 2.41), delinquent violence (males = 2.24, females = 2.68), and shyness (males = 1.73, females = 2.07). While the mean ratings on suicide indicated that females were significantly more likely than males to favor no action (females = 2.53, males = 2.90), it should be noted that approximately half (52%) of both females and males disagreed with the statement that no action should be taken when suicide was a risk. Binomial tests of significance further indicated that a significant majority of males and females favored an investigator taking no action when informed about a sexually transmitted disease, cutting, graffiti, or shyness ($ps = .001 - .0001$). However, a significant majority of males (73%, $p = .0004$), but not females (54%), believed investigators should take no action when risk involved drinking alcohol, and only females formed a majority opinion against acting upon information that a participant smoked (females = 81%, $p = .0000$; males = 63%) or was involved in theft (females = 71%, $p = .0005$; males = 63%).

A Newman-Keuls Multiple-Range Test (alpha = .05) on the mean scores collapsed across grades indicated that adolescent opinions formed two significantly different clusters: Students more strongly agreed with the decision to take no action when the risks involved cigarette smoking, sexually trans-mitted diseases, nonviolent delinquent acts, and shyness (risks that the majority of urban youth did not view as serious problems) than when the risks involved drugs, child maltreatment, suicide, and violent delinquency. Drinking fell in between these two clusters, with a mean significantly different from all risks in both categories except for drug use. Binomial tests indicated a significant majority ($ps = 0001 - .0000$) of students believed that no action should be taken when research participants revealed they were smoking cigarettes, had a sexually transmitted disease, were engaged in nonviolent delinquency (cutting, graffiti, theft), or were shy.

Telling a parent or concerned adult. Mean ratings for this reporting option and the percentage of adolescent participants viewing this option favorably (ratings of 1 and 2) are provided in Table 2. A 3 (grade) × 2 (sex) × 12 (risk) mixed ANOVA on the extent to which students agreed that an investigator should inform a parent or adult when confronted with a participant at risk yielded significant main effects of grade, $F(2, 128) = 3.57$, $p = .031$, and problem, $F(11, 118) = 18.35$, $p = .000$.

On average, seventh graders' ratings were more in agreement with telling a parent or adult ($M = 2.31$) than were ninth graders' ($M = 2.48$) or eleventh graders' ($M = 2.74$). However, individual univariate tests for grade effects for each of the 12 risk categories yielded significance only for graffiti,

$F(2, 144) = 6.16$, $p = .003$, and shyness, $F(2, 144) = 5.99$, $p = .003$. Scheffé tests (alpha $= .05$) further indicated that for these two categories seventh graders were significantly more in favor of reporting these behaviors to adults than were the older students, although binomial tests did not yield significant seventh-grade majority opinions for these two risks. Binomial tests of significance did demonstrate that a significant majority of ninth and eleventh graders strongly disagreed with the decision to report graffiti to a parent or adult ($ps = .007$ and $.001$, respectively).

A Newman-Keuls Multiple-Range Test (alpha $= .05$) on the mean scores collapsed across grade indicated that ratings for child maltreatment (physical and sexual abuse) and suicide were significantly more favorable toward telling a concerned adult than ratings for other risks. By contrast, mean ratings for cigarette smoking and nonviolent delinquency were significantly more unfavorable toward the decision to tell another concerned adult than mean ratings for other risks. Newman-Keuls Multiple-Range Tests did indicate that, as a group, the urban youth surveyed in this study rated telling a concerned adult about participant risks related to child maltreatment (sexual abuse and physical abuse) and suicide significantly more favorably than telling an adult about cigarette smoking and nonviolent delinquency. Binomial tests further confirmed this pattern, demonstrating that a significant majority of students were in favor of reporting information about child maltreatment (physical and sexual abuse) and life-threatening risks (suicide and STD) and were not in favor of reporting cigarette smoking, graffiti, or theft ($ps < .0003$).

When responses were evaluated by grade, a majority of seventh, ninth, and eleventh graders thought an investigator should tell a parent or adult if he or she was told by a participant that they had been physically or sexually abused ($ps = .02-.0001$). A significant majority of ninth graders thought an adult should be informed if students told an investigator they had a sexually transmitted disease ($p = .0027$), while a significant majority of eleventh graders thought threats of suicide should be reported ($p = .0000$). In contrast, the majority of ninth and eleventh graders strongly believed that adults should not be told if an investigator discovered that a research participant was stealing or writing graffiti (ps ranged $.004-.0000$). In addition, most ninth graders disagreed with the decision to tell an adult if cutting was involved ($p = .03$), and most eleventh graders disagreed with reporting to an adult if cigarette smoking was involved ($p = .0001$). An overview of the means in Table 2 indicates that the urban youth surveyed clearly differentiated among risk categories when judging the appropriateness of an investigator's decision to either take no action or tell an adult when the investigator learned a participant was at risk. For example, for each of the 12 risk categories, judgments favoring reporting the information to an adult were negatively correlated with judgments favoring keeping the information confidential ($rs = .27-.66$, $p < .01-.001$).

Facilitating self-referrals. As indicated by the mean ratings and percentage of adolescents viewing this option favorably (see Table 2), across all grades and risk categories, the majority of students thought favorably about an investigator's decision to talk about a problem with the research participant and let the participant seek help. A 3 (grade) $\times$ 2 (sex) $\times$ 12 (risk) mixed ANOVA on student responses to this reporting option yielded a main effect for problem, $F(11, 118) = 4.90$, $p = .000$. No other significant main or interaction effects emerged.

A Newman-Keuls analysis (alpha $= .05$) indicated few significant differences across risk categories. With grade collapsed, responses regarding self-referrals for graffiti and shyness were significantly higher than responses to speaking to the participant about drugs, drinking, child maltreatment, and life-threatening risks. Additionally, ratings for cutting were significantly higher than for drugs and sexually transmitted diseases. No meaningful significant patterns emerged when risk ratings were analyzed by grade. This is not surprising since binomial tests of probability indicated that this rating option was viewed favorably by a significant majority of the urban youth surveyed for all 12 risk categories ($ps = .0000$). Similar patterns emerged when binomials were conducted by grade, with two exceptions: (1) a significant ninth-grade majority favoring self-referrals did not emerge for graffiti, signaling more ambivalence, and (2) a significant seventh-grade majority did not emerge for physical abuse, cutting, graffiti, or shyness, perhaps reflecting the seventh graders' preference for the more definitive solutions of either taking no action or reporting to an adult.

Levels of Moral Reasoning

Interrater reliability for scoring student responses to the Sociomoral Reflection Measure—Short Form (SRM-SF) was calculated as percent agreement within one interval and as the difference between raters on the continuous SRMS total score for three pairs of raters. Percent agreement for the three rater pairs on half the sample protocols was 90%, 86%, and 100%. The difference on the SRMS continuous scores between pairs ranged from .07 to .18; all were below the allowed scoring difference of .20.

Moral reasoning as a developmental variable. The range of global stage scores for this sample was from Stage 1(2) to Stage 3(4). One protocol was scored as Stage 1(2), identified as an outlier, and dropped from all analyses. In addition, 14 seventh-grade, 4 ninth-grade, and 5 eleventh-grade protocols were unscorable, leaving 123 cases for analyses. The global stage scores for these cases ranged across 9 points on Gibbs et al.'s (1992) 10-point interval scale; they were thus grouped into three levels corresponding to preconventional reasoning (Stages 2(1) and 2), transition to conventional reasoning (Stages 2(3) and 3(2)), and solid conventional reasoning (Stages 3 and 3(4)).

A 3 (grade) × 2 (sex) ANOVA yielded a main effect for grade only, $F(2, 117) = 16.21, p < .0001$. A Scheffé contrast showed that eleventh graders reasoned significantly higher than both seventh and ninth graders, and that seventh and ninth graders were not different from each other. As expected, the majority (70%) of seventh graders reasoned at Level 1, the majority (73%) of ninth graders reasoned at Level 2, and 57% and 37% of eleventh graders reasoned at Level 2 and Level 3, respectively. The urban youth sampled in this study demonstrated developmental trends in moral reasoning consistent with those reported in previous studies of similar populations (Black, Paz, & DeBlassie, 1991; Gregg, Gibbs, & Basinger, in press). Neither sex nor the sex × grade interaction were significant.

Moral level, perceived severity of risks, and student evaluation of reporting options. A 3 (grade) × 3 (moral level) × 12 (risk) mixed ANOVA revealed no significant main effects or interactions on level of perceived risk. Contingency coefficients calculated between moral level and perceived severity for each of the 12 risks also failed to yield significant alpha levels. A 3 (moral level) × 2 (sex) × 12 (risk) mixed MANOVA with each of the three reporting options as a dependent variable also failed to reveal any significant main or interaction effects. The lack of relationship between level of moral reasoning and perceived risk severity is congruent with previous findings suggesting that, when faced with situations that could affect their peers or themselves, adolescents who score at the preconventional (Stage 2) or beginning conventional level (Stages 2/3, 3/2, and 3) on hypothetical tests of moral reasoning do not consistently apply these reasoning strategies to real-life situations (Kohlberg, 1984; Power, Higgins, & Kohlberg, 1989).

DISCUSSION

Research methodologies aimed at describing and understanding the developmental strengths and vulnerabilities of adolescence have the potential to tap previously undetected problems facing individual participants. Investigators who learn of potential participant risks need to consider whether they should take no action, alert an adult who can help the adolescent, or assist participants in making self-referrals. Current ethical guidelines offer incomplete answers as to what investigators should do if during the course of experimentation they discover that an adolescent's well-being may be in jeopardy.

As a consequence, developmental scientists have relied on their individual ethical perspectives, advice from colleagues, and evaluations from institutional review boards and funding agencies. An equally important but untapped resource for ethical decision making is empirical data on how adolescents prospectively evaluate the reporting options available to investigators.

1In the past, developmental scientists have shown a healthy skepticism toward the ethical benefits of facilitating services for research participants perceived to be at risk out of concern for the validity of such risk estimates, participant autonomy, and the maintenance of essential experimental controls. In recent years, researchers working with vulnerable and disenfranchised populations of urban youth have struggled with decisions that can allow them to meet dual obligations of scientific responsibility and participant care (Fisher, 1993, 1994; Fisher et al., 1996). Until now, these struggles have gone on in the absence of data on how adolescents themselves view investigator responsibilities. Perhaps the most important contribution of the present study to research ethics is the finding that urban youth do not view the maintenance of confidentiality favorably in situations in which an investigator learns that a research participant is a victim of or engaged in behaviors adolescents perceive to be serious problems.

The extent to which reporting a problem to a concerned adult was viewed favorably by the urban youth in our sample was influenced by both perceived risk severity and developmental level. Across grade, the majority of adolescents favored reporting child maltreatment and threats of suicide to a concerned adult. Younger adolescents were more likely to see other risks as serious and were also more in favor of reporting these risks to adults. Ninth graders were more ambivalent in their perceptions of risk severity and reporting, while eleventh graders were more likely to differentiate among severity of risks and all reporting options. Favorable responses for reporting certain risk behaviors were paralleled by unfavorable responses to taking no action, even when the investigator had promised confidentiality. These findings raise the disconcerting possibility that even under traditional informed consent procedures, in which participant confidentiality is assured, adolescents, especially middle schoolers, may expect to be helped when they tell an adult investigator that they are a victim of abuse or involved in high-risk behaviors. An investigator's failure to help a teenager who has disclosed such problems may unintentionally send messages that the problem is unimportant, that no services are available, or that knowledgeable adults can not be depended upon to help children in need.

Perhaps not surprisingly, facilitating self-referrals (Asher, 1993) was viewed favorably by a majority of seventh, ninth, and eleventh graders across risk contexts that drew mixed or strongly negative views for no action or reporting to an adult. While allowing for self-referral protects adolescent autonomy, it runs the risk of compromising participant welfare and parental responsibility (Fisher, 1993; Scarr, 1994). The increasing rise in health-endangering behaviors and life-threatening experiences of urban youth have raised ethical questions regarding the conditions under which adolescents can participate in research without guardian consent (Fisher, 1993; Fisher et al., 1996; Holder, 1981). Researchers and ethicists have raised concerns about situations in which guardian consent is in the best interests of the child or may violate an adolescent's privacy or jeopardize his or her welfare (Brooks-Gunn & Rotheram-Borus, 1994; Gaylin & Macklin, 1982). Facilitating self-referrals for adolescents at risk raises similar issues. For example, across grades, students favored no action concerning sexually transmitted diseases, and female students strongly believed that a researcher should keep information regarding cigarette smoking and theft confidential, while males favored no action if drinking behaviors were revealed. While these risks were more likely to have been judged as serious problems in some grades, students may have thought that the consequences of others finding out about these activities (e.g., law enforcement officials finding out about theft or parents learning of sexual activity, smoking, or drinking behaviors) outweigh any gain that might occur if the investigator sought intervention.

One way to address this problem is to determine the adequacy of school and community services for urban youth as well as whether or not adolescent participants have the maturity to utilize and benefit from these services independent of parental guidance. That adolescents in our sample appeared to view reporting options within the practical context of problem severity rather than the hypothetical context of moral reasoning underscores the need for researchers to familiarize themselves with the practical aspects of providing self-referrals or reporting behaviors to parents or adults in the community. This would include becoming familiar with local mental health and social service resources for urban adolescents and their families as well as the personal and legal consequences of reporting abusive or life-threatening behaviors. Once an investigator has determined these issues to her or his satisfaction, information clarifying how risks will be identified, and if and to whom (parents or adolescents) referrals will be made, should be included in both parental consent and participant assent forms (Fisher, 1993, 1994; Fisher et al., 1996). Along similar lines, both parents and adolescents need to be informed of the limitations of confidentiality, including statutory obligations to report suspicions of child abuse, at the outset of a research project.

Investigators considering reporting options for urban adolescent research participants must also be sensitive to the possibility of overreporting or overreferring minority or low-income youth. At present there is a paucity of information on developmental patterns in various urban cultural groups, a lack of culturally appropriate assessment instruments and services, and among urban youth a disproportionate amount of exposure to and participation in abusive or delinquent behaviors (Edelbrock, 1994; Richters & Martinez, 1993). Accordingly, investigators may find that service options for self-referrals are inadequate or that reports to concerned adults create an unjust burden on poor and minority youth (Fisher, 1993; Jackson, 1993; Scarr, 1994; Scott-Jones, 1994).

In conclusion, empirical investigation of adolescent expectations regarding the reporting responsibilities of developmental scientists can inform ethical decisions and enhance the investigator-participant relationship through mutual respect (Fisher & Fyrberg, 1994; Melton et al., 1988). This research is the first of which we are aware that explicitly assessed both adolescents' views of risk-taking behaviors and what they would want investigators to do if they were to reveal those behaviors during the course of a research study. Since this study was a fact-finding mission to begin to determine whether there is a context of legitimation for breaking confidentiality within the culture of urban adolescents, we chose to recruit a normative sample and use hypothetical situations, rather than target adolescents whom we could identify as specifically engaged in the risk behaviors. Conclusions drawn from these findings are by their very nature limited to students' responses to hypothetical problems as well as to the specific community surveyed. We hope that our efforts will encourage other investigators to empirically examine the implications of their ethical practices for participant development and well-being and to consider designing methodological and statistical procedures that include reporting and referring actions as factors in research designed for adolescents with identified risks.

Maintaining a balance between scientific responsibility and participant welfare will continue to be a difficult ethical challenge for scientists engaged in expanding our knowledge of the developmental strengths and vulnerabilities of urban youth. Incorporating participant perspectives into our ethical decision making has the potential to contribute to both the continued development of our science and the individuals whose participation make this science possible.

REFERENCES

American Psychological Association. (1992). Ethical principles of psychologists and code of conduct. *American Psychologist, 47*, 1597–1611.

Appelbaum, P. D., & Rosenbaum, A. (1989). Tarasoff and the researcher: Does the duty to protect apply in the research setting? *American Psychologist, 44*, 885–894.

Asher, S. R. (1993, March). *Inviting children to self-refer.* Paper presented as part of the invited symposium on "Ethical issues in the reporting and referring of research participants" at the biennial meeting of the Society for Research in Child Development, New Orleans.

Beauchamp, T. L., Faden, R. R., Wallace, R. J. Jr., & Walters, L. (1982). *Ethical issues in social science research.* Baltimore, MD: Johns Hopkins University Press.

Berman, A. L., & Jobbs, D. A. (1991). *Adolescent suicide assessment and intervention.* Washington, DC: American Psychological Association.

Black, C., Paz, H., & DeBlassie, R. R. (1991). Counseling the Hispanic male adolescent. *Adolescence, 26,* 223–232.

Bok. S. (1978). *Secrets: On the ethics of concealment and revelation.* New York: Pantheon.

Brooks-Gunn, J., & Rotheram-Borus, M. J. (1994). Rights to privacy in research: Adolescents versus parents. *Ethics and Behavior, 4,* 109–123.

Chase-Lansdale, P. L., & Brooks-Gunn, J. (1994). Correlates of adolescent pregnancy and parenthood. In C. B. Fisher & R. M. Lerner (Eds.), *Applied developmental psychology* (pp. 207–236). New York: McGraw-Hill.

Children's Safety Network. (1991). *A data book of child and adolescent injury.* Washington, DC: National Center for Education in Maternal and Child Health.

Cicchetti, D., & Toth, S. L. (1993). *Child abuse, child development, and social policy.* Norwood, NJ: Ablex.

Department of Health and Human Services. (1991, August). *Code of federal regulations, protection of human subjects* (DHHS Title 45 Public Welfare, Part 46). Washington, DC: Government Printing Office.

DiLalla, L. F., & Gottesman, I. I. (1989). Heterogeneity of causes for delinquency and criminality: Lifespan perspectives. *Development and Psychopathology, 1,* 339–349.

Dougherty, D. M. (1993). Adolescent health: Reflections on a report to the U.S. Congress. *American Psychologist, 48,* 193–201.

Dubow, E. F., Lovko, K. R., & Kausch, D. F. (1990). Demographic differences in adolescents' health concerns and perceptions of helping agents. *Journal of Clinical Child Psychology, 19,* 44–54.

Duckworth, K., & Dejung, J. (1989). Inhibiting class cutting among high school students. *High School Journal, 72.*

Edelbrock, C. (1994). Assessment of child psychopathology. In C. B. Fisher & R. M. Lerner (Eds.), *Applied developmental psychology* (pp. 294–315). New York: McGraw-Hill.

Farr, J. L., & Seaver, W. B. (1975). Stress and discomfort in psychological research: Subject perceptions of experimental procedures. *American Psychologist, 30,* 770–773.

Farrell, A. D., Danish, S. J., & Howard, C. W. (1992). Relationship between drug use and other problem behaviors in urban adolescents. *Journal of Consulting and Clinical Psychology, 60,* 705–712.

Fisher, C. B. (1991). Ethical considerations for research on psychosocial interventions for highrisk infants and children. *Register Report, 17,* 9–12.

Fisher, C. B. (1993). Integrating science and ethics in research with high-risk children and youth. *SRCD Social Policy Report, 7*(4), 1–27.

Fisher, C. B. (1994). Reporting and referring research participants: Ethical challenges for investigators studying children and youth. *Ethics and Behavior, 4,* 87–95.

Fisher, C. B., & Brennan, M. (1992). Application and ethics in developmental psychology. In D. L. Featherman, R. M. Lerner, & M. Perlmutter (Eds.), *Life-span development and behavior* (pp. 189–219). Hillsdale, NJ: Erlbaum.

Fisher, C. B., & Fyrberg, D. (1994). Participant partners: College students weigh the costs and benefits of deceptive research. *American Psychologist, 49,* 417–427.

Fisher, C. B., Hoagwood, K., & Jensen, P. (1996). Casebook on ethical issues in research with children and adolescents with mental disorders. In K. Hoagwood, P. Jensen, & C. B. Fisher (Eds.), *Ethical issues in research with children and adolescents with mental disorders* (pp. 135–238). Hillsdale, NJ: Erlbaum.

Fisher, C. B., Jackson, J. F., & Villarruel, F. (in press). The study of ethnic minority children and youth in the United States. In R. M. Lerner (Ed.), W. Damon (Series Ed.), *Handbook of child psychology: Vol. 1. Theoretical models of human development* (5th ed.). New York: Wiley.

Fisher, C. B., & Lerner, R. M. (1994). Foundations of applied developmental psychology. In C. B. Fisher & R. M. Lerner (Eds.), *Applied developmental psychology* (pp. 3–20). New York: McGraw-Hill.

Fisher, C. B., Murray, J. P., Dill, J. R., Hagen, J. W., Hogan, M. J., Lerner, R. M., Rebok, G. W., Sigel, I. E., Sostek, A. M., Smyer, M. A., Spencer, M. B., & Wilcox, B. (1993). The national conference on graduate education in the applications of developmental science across the lifespan. *Journal of Applied Developmental Psychology, 14*, 1–10.

Fisher, C. B., & Rosendahl, S. A. (1990). Risks and remedies of research participation. In C. B. Fisher & W. W. Tryon (Eds.), *Ethics in applied developmental psychology: Emerging issues in an emerging field* (pp. 43–60). Norwood, NJ: Ablex.

Fisher, C. B., & Tryon. W. W. (1990). Emerging ethical issues in an emerging field. In C. B. Fisher & W. W. Tryon (Eds.), *Ethics in applied developmental psychology: Emerging Issues in an emerging field* (pp. 1–14). Norwood, NJ: Ablex.

Gans, J. E., & Blyth, D. A. (1990). *America's adolescents: How healthy are they?* (AMA Profiles of Adolescent Health series). Chicago: American Medical Association.

Gaylin, W., & Macklin, R. (1982). *Who speaks for the child: The problems of proxy consent.* New York: Plenum.

Gergen, K. J. (1973). The codification of research ethics: Views of a doubting Thomas. *American Psychologist, 8*, 907–912.

Gibbs, J. C., Basinger, K. S., & Fuller, D. (1992). *Moral maturity, Measuring the development of sociomoral reflection.* Hillsdale, NJ: Erlbaum.

Gregg, V., Gibbs, J. C., & Basinger, K. S. (in press). Patterns of delay in male and female delinquents' moral judgment. *Merrill-Palmer Quarterly.*

Hammond, W. R., & Young, B. (1993). Psychology's role in the public health response to assaultive violence among young African-American men. *American Psychologist, 48*, 142–154.

Hauck, W. E., Martens, M., & Wetzel, M. (1986). Shyness, group dependence, and self-concept: Attributes of the imaginary audience. *Adolescence, 21* (83), 529–534.

Hoagwood, K. (1994). The Certificate of Confidentiality at the National Institute of Mental Health: Discretionary considerations in its applicability in research on child and adolescent mental disorders. *Ethics and Behavior, 4*, 123–131.

Holder, A. R. (1981). Can teenagers participate in research without parental consent? *IRB: Review of Human Subjects Research, 3*, 5–7.

Hollingshead, A. B. (1957). *Two-Factor Index of Social Position.* Unpublished manuscript, Yale University.

Horowitz, F. D., & O'Brien, M. (1989). In the interest of the nation: A reflective essay on the state of our knowledge and challenges before us. *American Psychologist, 44*, 441–445.

Jackson, J. F. (1993). Multiple caregiving among African Americans and infant attachment: The need for an emic approach. *Human Development, 36*, 87–102.

Jessor, R. (1992). Risk behavior in adolescence: A psychosocial framework for understanding and action. In D. E. Rogers & E. Ginzburg (Eds.), *Adolescents at risk: Medical and social perspectives* (pp. 19–34). Boulder, CO: Westview.

Jessor, R. (1993). Successful adolescent development among youth in high-risk settings. *American Psychologist, 48*, 117–116.

Kandel, D., Davies, M., Karus, D., & Yamaguchi, K. (1986). The consequences in young adulthood of adolescent drug involvement. *Archives of General Psychiatry, 43*, 746–754.

Kohlberg, L. (1984). *Essays on moral development: Vol. 2. The psychology of moral development.* San Francisco: Harper & Row.

Lerner, R. M. (1993). Early adolescence: Toward an agenda for the integration of research, policy, and intervention. In R. M. Lerner (Ed.), *Early adolescence: Perspectives on research, policy, and intervention* (pp. 1–16). Hillsdale, NJ: Erlbaum.

Lester, D., & Anderson, D. (1992). Depression and suicidal ideation in African American and Hispanic American high school students. *Psychological Reports, 71*, 618.

Levine, R. J. (1986). *Ethics and regulation of clinical research.* Baltimore and Munich: Urban & Schwarzenberg.

Liss, M. B. (1994). Child abuse: Is there a mandate for researchers to report? *Ethics and Behavior, 4*, 133–146.

Melton, G. B. (1990). Certificates of confidentiality under the public health service act: Strong protection but not enough. *Violence and Victims, 5*, 67–71.

Melton, G. B., Levine, R. J., Koocher, G. P., Rosenthal, R., & Thompson, W. C. (1988). Community consultation in socially sensitive research: Lessons from clinical trials of treatments for AIDS. *American Psychologist, 43*, 573–581.

Office for Protection of Research Risks (OPRR), Department of Health and Human Services, National Institutes of Health, (1993). *Protecting human research subjects: Institutional review board guidebook.* Washington, DC: Government Printing Office.

Pentz, M. A. (1994). Primary prevention of adolescent drug abuse. In C. B. Fisher & R. M. Lerner (Eds.), *Applied developmental psychology* (pp. 435–474). New York: McGraw-Hill.

Petersen, A. C., Compas, B. E., Brooks-Gunn, J., Stemmler, M., Ey, S., & Grant, K. E. (1993). Depression in adolescence. *American Psychologist, 48*, 155–168.

Power, F. C., Higgins, A., & Kohlberg, L. (1989). *Lawrence Kohlberg's approach to moral education.* New York: Columbia University.

Quadrel, M. J., Fischhoff, B., & Davis, W. (1993). Adolescent (in)vulnerability. *American Psychologist, 48*, 102–116.

Richters, J. E., & Martinez, P. (1993). Children as victims of and witnesses to violence in a Washington, D.C. neighborhood. In L. A. Leavitt & N. A. Fox (Eds.), *The psychological effects of war and violence on children* (pp. 243–280). Hillsdale, NJ: Erlbaum.

Scarr, S. (1994). Ethical problems in research on risky behaviors and risky populations. *Ethics and Behavior, 4*, 147–156.

Scott-Jones, D. (1994). Ethical issues in reporting and referring in research with low-income minority children. *Ethics and Behavior, 4*, 97–198.

Society for Research in Child Development. (1993). Ethical standards for research with children. In *Directory of members* (pp. 337–339). Ann Arbor, MI: SRCD.

Sum, A. M., & Fogg, W. N. (1991). The adolescent poor and the transition to early adulthood. In P. B. Edelman & J. Ladner (Eds.), *Adolescence and poverty: Challenge for the 1990s* (pp. 37–109). Washington, DC: Center for National Policy Press.

Takanishi, R. (1993). The opportunities of adolescence—research, interventions, and policy: Introduction to the special issue. *American Psychologist, 48*, 85–86.

Tarasoff vs. Regents of the University of California (CA 1976). 131 Cal. Rptr. 14, 551 P.2d 334.

Veatch, R. M. (1987). *The patient as partner.* Bloomington: Indiana University Press.

Weithorn, L. A. (1983). Children's capacities to decide about participation in research. *IRB: A Review of Human Subjects Research, 5*, 1–5.

Wilson, D. W., & Donnerstein, W. (1976). Legal and ethical aspects of nonreactive social psychological research: An excursion into the public mind. *American Psychologist, 31*, 765–773.

Windle, M. (1990). A longitudinal study of antisocial behaviors in early adolescence as predictors of late adolescent substance use: Gender and ethnic group differences. *Journal of Abnormal Psychology, 99*, 86–91.

Zaslow, M. J., & Takanishi, R. (1993). Priorities for research in adolescent development. *American Psychologist, 48*, 185–192.